A Clinician's Guide to Sperm DNA and Chromatin Damage

Armand Zini • Ashok Agarwal
Editors

A Clinician's Guide to Sperm DNA and Chromatin Damage

Springer

Editors
Armand Zini, MD, FRCSC
Professor
Department of Surgery
Division of Urology
McGill University
Montreal, QC, Canada

Ashok Agarwal, PhD
American Center for Reproductive Medicine
Glickman Urological and Kidney Institute
Cleveland Clinic
Cleveland, OH, USA

ISBN 978-3-030-10116-9 ISBN 978-3-319-71815-6 (eBook)
https://doi.org/10.1007/978-3-319-71815-6

Printed on acid-free paper

This Springer imprint is published by Springer Nature
The registered company is Springer International Publishing AG
The registered company address is: Gewerbestrasse 11, 6330 Cham, Switzerland

Foreword

One of the great challenges for assessing male fertility is that with the microscope we can see the outside of a sperm and generally how it swims but that arguably the most important aspects of how it works to fertilize the egg and ultimately make a baby are hidden from view inside its head. One of the earliest ways of trying to crack that puzzle was to assess how deoxyribonucleic acid is packaged within the sperm and whether alterations in that packaging cause problems with male reproduction. Scientific and clinical studies abound, but the conclusions are varied and challenging to interpret. The editors and authors of this book have done a masterful job in assembling the most complete compendium to date on the subject of sperm DNA packaging and most importantly its clinical relevance. It's a reference work that will mark the era of sperm DNA assessment in the evaluation of male fertility and guide the clinician in what to order and how to interpret the results.

Craig Niederberger, MD, FACS
Department of Urology, UIC College of Medicine
Department of Bioengineering, UIC College of Engineering
Fertility and Sterility
Chicago, IL, USA

Preface

The essential role and pathophysiology of sperm DNA integrity in human reproduction has been increasingly recognized and extensively studied in the last few decades. Sperm DNA fragmentation (SDF) has emerged as a valuable tool for male infertility evaluation. Defects in sperm DNA integrity are associated with modifications during spermatogenesis, inflammatory processes, varicocele, and elevated post-testicular oxidative stress. Consequently, it has great potential as a functional diagnostic test that could complement the conventional sperm analysis. Clinical evidence is accumulating to show that the integrity of sperm DNA may also be linked with suboptimal embryo development, implantation failure, and recurrent miscarriage.

The focus on sperm DNA damage continues to generate enormous interest among reproductive health specialists and basic medical scientists, and this in part is fueled by the growing awareness that ICSI is not a panacea for all couples diagnosed with male infertility. Moreover, with the success rates of ICSI capping at 50–60%, the pursuit for a reliable test of sperm function which can accurately predict fertility in assisted reproduction has taken on a renewed sense of urgency.

Our book *A Clinician's Guide to Sperm DNA and Chromatin Damage* summarizes the role of SDF in male infertility. Firstly, the normal sperm chromatin structure and causative mechanisms of SDF are briefly introduced. Currently available SDF assays are also described. Secondly, the etiology of SDF and its implications on natural pregnancy and ART outcomes are presented. Finally, treatment options for high SDF and the clinical application of SDF tests are proposed.

The book is written by internationally recognized experts from 15 countries and is organized into five sections and 32 chapters. Part I contains three chapters on the basic aspects of sperm chromatin structure, whereas the various tests used to evaluate sperm DNA fragmentation are discussed in seven chapters under Part II. In Part III, the etiology of this enigmatic test is described within eight chapters, while the clinical usage of SDF tests, a must read, is well-elaborated in six chapters within the penultimate Part IV. The treatment options for men with clinically significant SDF are the subject of Part V which is highlighted in eight impressive chapters.

We are deeply grateful to our distinguished group of contributors for sharing their research and clinical knowledge and experience. Our book is an excellent and timely product of effective collaboration with members of the Springer Publishing House. The outstanding support of developmental editors Barbara Lopez-Lucio and Sarah Simeziane and editor Kristopher Spring was highly commendable. The editors are tremendously grateful to their families for their unwavering love and support.

Montreal, QC, Canada
Cleveland, OH, USA

Armand Zini, MD, FRCSC
Ashok Agarwal, PhD

Contents

Editors

Ashok Agarwal, PhD American Center for Reproductive Medicine, Glickman Urological and Kidney Institute, Cleveland Clinic, Cleveland, OH, USA

Armand Zini, MD, FRCSC Department of Surgery, Division of Urology, McGill University, Montreal, QC, Canada

Contributors

Ahmad H. Al-Malki, MB, BCh Department of Surgery, Division of Urology, McGill University, Montreal, QC, Canada

Elisabetta Baldi, BSc, PhD Center of Excellence DeNothe, University of Florence, Florence, Italy

Experimental and Clinical Biomedical Sciences, University of Florence, Florence, Italy

Rod Balhorn, BSc, PhD SHAL Technologies, Inc., Livermore, CA, USA

Noelia Fonseca Balvís, BSc, MS Department of Animal Reproduction, Spanish National Institute for Agricultural and Food Research and Technology (INIA), Madrid, Spain

Ferran Barrachina, MSc Molecular Biology of Reproduction and Development Research Group, Department of Biomedicine, Faculty of Medicine, and Biochemistry and Molecular Genetics Service, Institut d'Investigacions Biomèdiques August Pi i Sunyer (IDIBAPS), University of Barcelona, and Hospital Clínic, Barcelona, Spain

Guylain Boissonneault, PhD Department of Biochemistry, Université de Sherbrooke, Sherbrooke, QC, Canada

Mona Bungum, MedDr, MSc, PhD Reproductive Medicine Centre, Malmö University Hospital, Malmö, Sweden

Zeynep Cakar, BSc American Center for Reproductive Medicine, Cleveland Clinic, Cleveland, OH, USA

Eva Pericuesta Camacho, PhD Department of Animal Reproduction, Instituto Nacional de Investigación y Tecnología Agraria y Alimentaria (INIA), Madrid, Spain

Douglas T. Carrell, PhD Department of Surgery (Urology), Department of Human Genetics, Department of Obstetrics and Gynecology, University of Utah School of Medicine, Salt Lake City, UT, USA

Tiphanie Cavé, MSc Department of Biochemistry, Université de Sherbrooke, Sherbrooke, QC, Canada

Peter T.K. Chan, MD Department of Surgery (Urology), McGill University and the McGill Univeristy Health Centre, Montreal, QC, Canada

Elva I. Cortés-Gutiérrez, PhD Department of Genetics, Centro de Investigación Biomédica del Noreste, Instituto Mexicano del Seguro Social, IMSS, Monterrey, Mexico

Unit of Genetics, Department of Biology, Universidad Autónoma de Madrid, Madrid, Spain

Martha I. Dávila-Rodríguez, PhD Department of Genetics, Centro de Investigación Biomédica del Noreste, Instituto Mexicano del Seguro Social, IMSS, Monterrey, Mexico

Unit of Genetics, Department of Biology, Universidad Autónoma de Madrid, Madrid, Spain

Alejandro Chacón de Castro, MSc Reproduction Department, Instituto Nacional de Investigación y Tecnología Agraria y Alimentaria (INIA), Madrid, Spain

Hasan M. El-Fakahany, MD, PhD Department of Dermatology, STDs and Andrology, Al-Minya University, Al-Minya, Egypt

Juris Erenpreiss, MD, PhD Riga Stradins University, Riga, Latvia

Sandro C. Esteves, MD, MSc, PhD Andrology and Human Reproduction Clinic, ANDROFERT, Campinas, Brazil

Donald P. Evenson, PhD, HCLD SCSA Diagnostics, Inc., Brookings, SD, USA

Sarah K. Fatool, BS Medical School for International Health, Ben-Gurion University of the Negev, Be'er Sheva, Israel

Soroka University Medical Center, Ben-Gurion University of the Negev, Be'er Sheva, Israel

José Luis Fernández, MD, PhD Unidad de Genética, Complejo Hospitalario Universitario A Coruña (CHUAC), Instituto de Investigación Biomédica de A Coruña (INIBIC), A Coruña, Spain

Laboratorio de Genética Molecular y Radiobiología, Centro Oncológico de Galicia, A Coruña, Spain

Raul Fernández-González Department of Animal Reproduction, Instituto Nacional de Investigación y Tecnología Agraria y Alimentaria (INIA), Madrid, Spain

Shaghayegh Foroozan-Boroojeni, BSc Department of Reproductive Biotechnology, Reproductive Biomedicine Research Center, Royan Institute for Biotechnology, ACECR, Isfahan, Iran

Aleksander Giwercman, PhD Lund University, Malmö, Sweden

Jaime Gosálvez, BSc, Hons PhD Unidad de Genética, Facultad de Biología, Universidad Autónoma de Madrid, Spain

Marie-Chantal Grégoire, PhD Department of Biochemistry, Université de Sherbrooke, Sherbrooke, QC, Canada

Sezgin Gunes, PhD Ondokuz Mayis University, Samsun, Turkey

Alfonso Gutiérrez-Adan, PhD Department of Animal Reproduction, Instituto Nacional de Investigación y Tecnología Agraria y Alimentaria (INIA), Madrid, Spain

Avi Harlev, MD Soroka University Medical Center, Ben-Gurion University of the Negev, Be'er Sheva, Israel

Ralf Henkel, PhD Department of Medical Bioscience, University of the Western Cape, Bellville, South Africa

Meritxell Jodar, PhD Molecular Biology of Reproduction and Development Research Group, Department of Biomedicine, Faculty of Medicine, and Biochemistry and Molecular Genetics Service, Institut d'Investigacions Biomèdiques August Pi i Sunyer (IDIBAPS), University of Barcelona, and Hospital Clínic, Barcelona, Spain

Stephen Johnston, BSc, Hons PhD School of Agriculture and Food Sciences, The University of Queensland, Gatton, Australia

Michelle M. Kim, MD, PhD Urology Resident, Department of Urology, Massachusetts General Hospital, Harvard Medical School, Boston, MA, USA

Ricardo Laguna-Barraza, PhD Veterinarian Science, Department of Animal Reproduction, Instituto Nacional de Investigación y Tecnología Agraria y Alimentaria (INIA), Madrid, Spain

Angela Patricia López-Cardona, DZoot, MSc, PhD Department of Animal Reproduction, Instituto Nacional de Investigación y Tecnología Agraria y Alimentaria (INIA), Madrid, Spain

Carmen López-Fernández, PhD Unit of Genetics, Department of Biology, Universidad Autónoma de Madrid, Madrid, Spain

Ahmad Majzoub, MD Department of Urology, Hamad Medical Corporation, Doha, Qatar

Gayatri Mohanty, PhD Redox Biology Laboratory, Department of Zoology, School of Life Sciences, Ravenshaw University, Cuttack, India

Monica Muratori, BSc, PhD Center of Excellence DeNothe, University of Florence, Florence, Italy

Experimental and Clinical Biomedical Sciences, University of Florence, Florence, Italy

Mohammad Hossein Nasr-Esfahani, PhD Department of Reproductive Biotechnology, Reproductive Biomedicine Research Center, Royan Institute for Biotechnology, ACECR, Isfahan, Iran

Isfahan Fertility and Infertility Center, Isfahan, Iran

Krzysztof Oleszczuk, MD, PhD Reproductive Medicine Centre, Skåne University Hospital, Malmö, Sweden

Rafael Oliva, MD, PhD Molecular Biology of Reproduction and Development Research Group, Department of Biomedicine, Faculty of Medicine, and Biochemistry and Molecular Genetics Service, Institut d'Investigacions Biomèdiques August Pi i Sunyer (IDIBAPS), University of Barcelona, and Hospital Clínic, Barcelona, Spain

Serafín Perez-Cerezales, PhD Department of Animal Reproduction, Instituto Nacional de Investigación y Tecnología Agraria y Alimentaria (INIA), Madrid, Spain

Benjamin Planells, BSc, MSc Department of Animal Reproduction, Instituto Nacional de Investigación y Tecnología Agraria y Alimentaria (INIA), Madrid, Spain

Priscila Ramos-Ibeas, PhD, DVM, MsC Department of Animal Reproduction, Instituto Nacional de Investigación y Tecnología Agraria y Alimentaria (INIA), Madrid, Spain

Bernard Robaire, PhD Departments of Pharmacology & Therapeutics and of Obstetrics & Gynecology, McGill University, Montreal, QC, Canada

Matheus Roque, MD ORIGEN – Center for Reproductive Medicine, Rio de Janeiro, Brazil

Katherine Rotker, MD Department of Urology, UMASS Medical School & Memorial Healthcare System, Worcester, MA, USA

Denny Sakkas, PhD Boston IVF, Waltham, MA, USA

Luna Samanta, PhD Redox Biology Laboratory, Department of Zoology, School of Life Sciences, Ravenshaw University, Cuttack, India

Manesh Kumar Panner Selvam, PhD American Center for Reproductive Medicine, Glickman Urological and Kidney Institute, Cleveland Clinic, Cleveland, OH, USA

Semra Sertyel, MSc Embryology Laboratory, Centrum IVF Clinic, Ankara, Turkey

Rakesh Sharma, PhD American Center for Reproductive Medicine, Cleveland Clinic, Cleveland, OH, USA

Mark Sigman, MD Department of Surgery (Urology), Warren Alpert School of Medicine of Brown University, Rhode Island Hospital and The Miriam Hospital, Providence, RI, USA

Olivier Simard, BSc Department of Biochemistry, Université de Sherbrooke, Sherbrooke, QC, Canada

Luke Simon, PhD Department of Surgery (Urology), University of Utah, Salt Lake City, UT, USA

Ada Soler-Ventura, MSc Molecular Biology of Reproduction and Development Research Group, Department of Biomedicine, Faculty of Medicine, and Biochemistry and Molecular Genetics Service, Institut d'Investigacions Biomèdiques August Pi i Sunyer (IDIBAPS), University of Barcelona, and Hospital Clínic, Barcelona, Spain

Michael Solomon, PhD Department of Medical Bioscience, University of the Western Cape, Bellville, South Africa

Marcello Spanò, MD Laboratory of Biosafety and Risk Assessment, Division of Technologies and Methodologies for Health Protection, ENEA (Italian National Agency for New Technologies, Energy and Sustainable Economic Development), Rome, Italy

W. Steven Ward, PhD Institute for Biogenesis Research, John A. Burns School of Medicine, University of Hawaii at Manoa, Honolulu, HI, USA

Nirlipta Swain, MPhil School of Life Sciences, Redox Biology Laboratory, Department of Zoology, Ravenshaw University, Cuttack, India

Cigdem Tanrikut, MD MGH Fertility Center, Massachusetts General Hospital, Harvard Medical School, Boston, MA, USA

Marziyeh Tavalaee, PhD Department of Reproductive Biotechnology, Reproductive Biomedicine Research Center, Royan Institute for Biotechnology, ACECR, Isfahan, Iran

Ksenija Zubkova, MD Riga Stradins University, Riga, Latvia

Part I
Human Sperm Chromatin Structure

Chapter 1
Sperm Chromatin: An Overview

Rod Balhorn

1.1 Sperm Chromatin: The First 50 Years

Sperm chromatin research began with the discovery of the two primary molecular components that fill the head of mature sperm cells—DNA and protamine. Only a year after Gregor Mendel reported his work on the laws of heredity in 1865 [1], Ernst Haeckel suggested that the nuclei of cells must contain the material responsible for the transmission of genetic traits [2]. Friedrich Miescher, working in Felix Hoppe Seyler's laboratory in Germany, had become intrigued by cells and began conducting experiments to determine their chemical composition. Working initially with lymphocytes obtained from blood and later enriched populations of leukocytes he obtained from hospital bandages, Miescher noticed a precipitate that formed when he added acid to the cell extracts he was using to isolate proteins [3]. While he and the rest of the scientific community were unaware that this material, which he called nuclein, was the genetic material Mendel and Haeckel had referred to, he became fascinated by this acid-insoluble component of cells and continued to study its properties [4]. Walther Flemming's work over the next decade introduced the scientific community to the cellular substructures called chromosomes and the concept of mitosis, and Flemming was the first to introduce the term chromatin [5]. It took another 30 years, however, before cellular biologists began to realize the importance of individual chromosomes as the carriers of genetic information.

Miescher, who began his research career isolating and characterizing proteins, spent the majority of his later efforts investigating nuclein (DNA). When he discovered he could not obtain enough of the nuclein from human cells to properly examine its properties, he turned to working with fish sperm. Salmon provided an abundance of sperm, and the sperm cells were considered ideal because they had almost no cytoplasm to contaminate his nuclear preparations with other proteins.

R. Balhorn (✉)
SHAL Technologies, Inc., Livermore, CA, USA
e-mail: rod@shaltech.com; rodbalhorn@hughes.net

A. Zini, A. Agarwal (eds.), *A Clinician's Guide to Sperm DNA and Chromatin Damage*, https://doi.org/10.1007/978-3-319-71815-6_1

In addition to being the first to isolate DNA, Miescher was also the first to isolate protamine, which he called protamin, and to discover its highly basic nature [6]. He discovered that nuclein and protamin made up the majority of the mass of the sperm head, and he also provided the first insight into the fundamental interaction that bound these two components together inside the sperm nucleus—that nuclein was bound in a salt-like state to protamin. As the interest in DNA and protamine grew, other researchers began to examine the molecules present in sperm. The majority of the initial work characterizing the composition of protamine molecules was carried out by Kossel and his group, not Miescher, over several decades spanning from about 1890 to the 1920s [7–10]. The proteins bound to DNA in sperm were distinguished from those found in other cells very early on, but the real significance of this difference was not appreciated until almost half a century later when more detailed studies of spermatogenesis and spermiogenesis revealed significant differences in DNA packaging and sperm chromatin compaction. Up until this time, sperm chromatin was considered by many to be similar to the chromatin found in somatic cells.

1.2 Spermatogenesis: Terminal Differentiation and Reprogramming of the Testicular Cell Genome

The testicular cells of men and other mammals undergo a radical morphological transformation as they progress through a process of differentiation called spermatogenesis. Undifferentiated spermatogonia begin the process when they differentiate into primary spermatocytes. Diploid spermatocytes containing two complements of the genome divide in meiosis to produce haploid spermatids that retain only a single copy of each chromosome. In addition to dramatic changes that subsequently occur in the structure of the spermatid at the cellular level (the shape of its nucleus and the development of the flagellum), the chromatin inside these cells also undergoes a series of structural and functional changes. In humans and other mammals, specific genes within the male genome are imprinted to identify their "parent of origin" [11–15], epigenetic modifications in the DNA and proteins packaging the genome prepare the chromatin for early embryonic development [16], and the chromatin is transformed from a highly functional, genetically active state characteristic of somatic cells (spermatogonia and spermatocytes) to a quiescent or completely inactive state found in the fully mature sperm cell.

One might think of this transformation as the testicular cell embarking on a path of terminal differentiation similar to the process that occurs when a stem cell begins to differentiate into a liver, kidney, or brain cell. The final cell not only differs structurally from the stem cell, but it also performs very different functions. Unlike the genome in most stem cells, however, the genome of these spermatids undergoes an additional step in the process, a transient stage in which the entire genome is deprogrammed and shut down. This genome-wide inactivation bears some similarity to processes of heterochromatinization that have been observed to occur with one X chromosome in vertebrates [17, 18], the entire genome in avian erythrocytes [19], and one set of chromosomes in mealy bugs [20]. These changes, which are brought about by modifying or replacing the proteins that bind to and package DNA, enable the activity of the spermatid genome to be silenced, subsets of the genes to be marked for expression following fertilization, and the chromatin sequestered in a quiescent and protected state until the sperm enters the oocyte and its DNA is ready to be combined with the genome provided by the female to initiate embryogenesis. The process also provides a mechanism by which the genes contributed by the male can be reactivated in the proper temporal sequence and combinations to ensure the first cells function as embryonic stem cells, subpopulations of which later differentiate further into the other types of cells that are required for the development of a fully functional organism.

1.3 Chromatin Reorganization in Maturing Spermatids

Following the second meiotic division of mammalian spermatocytes, the chromatin of the haploid spermatids and their repertoire of functioning genes begin to change over a period of several days [21]. The entire genome of the early spermatid is initially packaged by histones in a manner that is identical to the structure of chromatin (Fig. 1.1) present in all other somatic cells [22]. Variants of histone H2B are

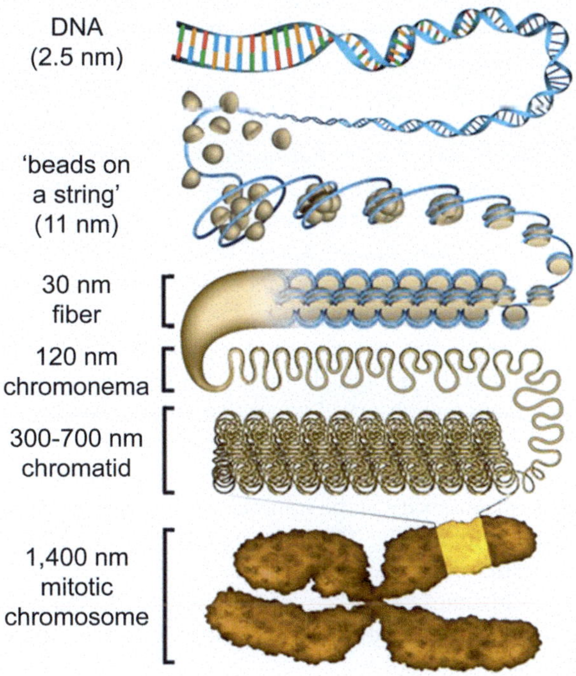

Fig. 1.1 The structure of chromatin (From Ou et al. [215]. Reprinted with permission from AAAS)

incorporated into the chromatin replacing a subset of their somatic counterparts prior to meiosis [23]. Other histones are posttranslationally modified by acetylation and methylation to modulate the interaction of the histone with DNA [24–29]. Acetylation of H3 has been observed to occur throughout spermatogenesis and is considered to relax the interaction of H3 with DNA. H4 acetylation appears to increase specifically during spermatid elongation [30, 31]. While the function of H4 acetylation has not been confirmed, it is thought to play a role in making it easier to displace the histone from DNA during spermiogenesis and also loosen the structure of the histone bound to regulatory regions of genes important for early embryonic development. H4 is increasingly methylated throughout spermatogenesis as spermatogonia differentiate into spermatids [24, 27, 32] and then this methylation is reduced during spermatid elongation [31]. H3 methylation, which occurs predominantly in round spermatids, has been reported to mark regulatory sites [26, 27, 33] on developmentally repressed genes [34] that play a role both in gamete differentiation and early embryonic development.

Only a small fraction of the chromatin in mature sperm retains its histone packaging [33–41]. This histone-containing subset of the genome appears to be present in the sperm of all mammals and is small, comprising not more than 1–2% of the sperm genome in mice and bulls. In human sperm, however, the fraction of DNA bound by histones is significantly larger, possibly as high as 10–15% [41–45]. The H2A, H2B, H3, and H4 histones and their variants that remain associated with DNA in the chromatin of fully mature sperm [43, 46], which will be described in more detail in Chap. 2, have been reported to be associated with centromeric and telomeric DNA [47, 48], matrix-associated regions [49], genes for epsilon and gamma globin [38], paternally imprinted genes [34, 50], retroposons [40], microRNA clusters [34], regulatory sequences [33, 51], genes that produce rRNA [52] and transcription factors such as those in the Hox family [34], genes known to be transcribed in the final stages of spermatogenesis [52], and the transcription initiation sites of a number of genes expressing signaling proteins important for early embryonic development [34, 35, 37, 38, 53]. Some studies suggest the retained histones may be associated with the transcription sites of all genes in sperm [54, 55], preserving the epigenetics of the paternal genome and providing markers to guide their expression in the early embryo [33, 34, 54, 56].

Although the incorporation of the histone variants and the acetylation and methylation of H3 and H4 do not visibly alter the structure of chromatin, a structural change is observed when two small basic transition proteins, TP1 and TP2, are expressed and incorporated into the spermatid chromatin (in human, step 1 for TP2 and step 3 for TP1) [57]. Coincident with the binding of TP1 and TP2 to DNA, the majority of the somatic histones are replaced, and the chromatin becomes more compact. The TP1 protein, which is half the size of a histone, appears to loosen the structure of the nucleosome and facilitate the displacement/replacement of the histones [58]. The larger protein TP2 has two bound zinc atoms and has been reported to stabilize and compact the DNA showing a preference for CG-rich sequences [59, 60].

During their short period of residence in spermatid chromatin, both TP1 and TP2 are posttranslationally modified at multiple sites by phosphorylation, acetylation, and methylation [61, 62]. In contrast to the methylation sites in histone, which occur on lysine residues, both lysine and arginine residues are methylated in the TPs. The presence of these modifications in the protein is likely to have a significant impact on the protein's ability to bind to DNA. Phosphorylation of the serine residues in the C-terminal domain of TP2, which has been shown to be the region of the protein that condenses DNA when it binds, reduces the ability of TP2 to condense DNA [63]. Since TP2 was found to be a poor substrate for phosphorylation when bound to DNA, it has been hypothesized that the phosphorylation of TP2 is more likely to occur prior to DNA binding. Lysine residues in this same region of TP2 have also been shown to be acetylated. In addition to reducing TP2 ability to condense DNA, the acetylation of TP2 has been shown to block the protein's ability to interact with NPM3, a histone chaperone similar to nucleoplasmin [64].

While the binding of TP1 and TP2 affect DNA differently and the two proteins appear to perform different functions, gene knockout studies have suggested the TP1 and TP2 proteins may work together with each being capable of compensating for the other in effecting the displacement of the majority of the somatic histones from the spermatid's DNA [65, 66]. As TP1 and TP2 displace the histones, both proteins also appear to facilitate the repair of DNA damage incurred as the genome is repackaged [67, 68]. Exactly how the TPs remove the histones and whether they work directly or indirectly to induce or initiate DNA repair are not yet known.

HMGB4 and the rat variant HMGB4L1 (previously identified as TP4 [69]), two members of the high mobility group box protein family, have also been observed to be synthesized and deposited in chromatin near the basal pole in elongating spermatids [70] around the same time as TP1 and TP2. Rat spermatids produce both proteins, while neither the HMGB4L1 gene nor the HMGB4L1 protein have been observed in the spermatids of mice or men. HMGB4 has also been detected in spermatocytes and in brain and neuronal cells [71]. RNA profiling and histological analyses in human and mouse testes suggest HMGB4 may play a role in the organization of chromatin in X and Y chromosomes [72]. Other studies have suggested it may also participate in regulating the transcription of genes through the posttranslational modification of histones [71].

The final proteins to be synthesized and deposited in late-stage spermatid chromatin are the protamines. In the mouse, synthesis of protamine P1 begins in step 12 spermatids approximately 24–30 h earlier than protamine P2 [73]. Unlike most mRNAs, those for protamines P1 and P2 are transcribed several days earlier [74–77], their translation is delayed, and protamine synthesis and its deposition into spermatid chromatin only begin after TP1 and TP2 have successfully replaced the majority of the histones. This delay has been shown to be essential for the proper completion of the histone-TP-protamine transition [78]. Without it, the synthesis of the protamines causes early condensation of the spermatid DNA, incomplete processing of the protamine P2 precursor, and induces the formation of abnormally shaped sperm heads. The binding of these protamines to DNA during the final steps of spermatid maturation completes the process of chromatin reorganization, packaging the male's haploid genome into a highly compact, genetically inactive state programmed for reactivation once the sperm head enters an oocyte.

1.4 Protamines P1 and P2

Two different types of protamines have been isolated from mammalian sperm. Protamine P1, the smaller of the two proteins, is found in the late-step spermatids and mature sperm of all mammals [79]. The P1 protamine of placental mammals is a small protein containing only 46–51 amino acids [80]. In marsupials and monotremes, the protamine P1s are slightly larger (typically 57–70 residues). Protamine P2, which is almost twice the size of P1 (typically 100–107 residues), is expressed at significant levels only in the spermatids and sperm of a subset of placental mammals. These include primates, most rodents, lagomorphs, and perissodactyls [79].

Protamine P1 and P2 are similar to the protamines isolated from the sperm of salmon, tuna, and many other fish in that they all contain a series of (Arg)n sequences that wrap around the phosphodiester backbone and bind the protein to duplex DNA. In protamine P1, these anchoring sequences, which are typically separated by one or two uncharged amino acids, make up a central DNA-binding domain that is very similar to the entire sequence of the fish protamines. In contrast to fish protamines, protamine P1 sequences from placental mammals also contain two N- and C-terminal peptide domains that do not bind to DNA [80, 81]. Both of these domains contain serine, threonine, or tyrosine residues that are phosphorylated shortly after the protein is synthesized [82–84]. These domains also contain multiple cysteine residues that form a series of inter- and intraprotamine disulfide bonds and link each protamine molecule to its neighbor as the spermatid matures and passes through the epididymis [81]. The formation of these disulfide cross-links occurs sequentially with the intraprotamine disulfides forming first, beginning in late-step spermatids and nearing completion by the time the sperm enter the caput epididymis [81, 85]. Once formed, the intraprotamine disulfides do not prevent the protein from being dissociated from DNA. As the sperm traverse the epididymis, a series of interprotamine disulfides are formed, cross-linking all the protamines to each other in such a manner that the protamines cannot be removed from the DNA. The resulting network of disulfide cross-links [81, 86] stabilize the structure of the completed sperm chromatin complex making it more difficult for other proteins (e.g., transcription factors and other enzymes) to gain access to the DNA until the protamines are removed following fertilization. With one exception, monotreme (platypus and echidna) [87] and marsupial [88–91] protamines differ from the P1 protamines of placental mammals in that they do not contain any cysteine residues. A shrewlike marsupial in the genus *Planigales* has been found to produce protamines that contain five to six cysteines [90, 92], a number similar to the number of cysteines that are typically found in the P1 protamines of placental mammals.

Unlike protamine P1, P2 is synthesized as a larger precursor protein (101 residues in human, 106 residues in mouse) that is deposited onto DNA and subsequently shortened over a several-day period [93]. Processing of the P2 precursor, which does not begin until several hours after its synthesis and deposition onto DNA, occurs by progressive and sequential cleavage (Fig. 1.2) and removal of a series of short peptide fragments from the amino-terminus of the precursor [93–97]. Each intermediate processed form of the protein persists for several hours before being

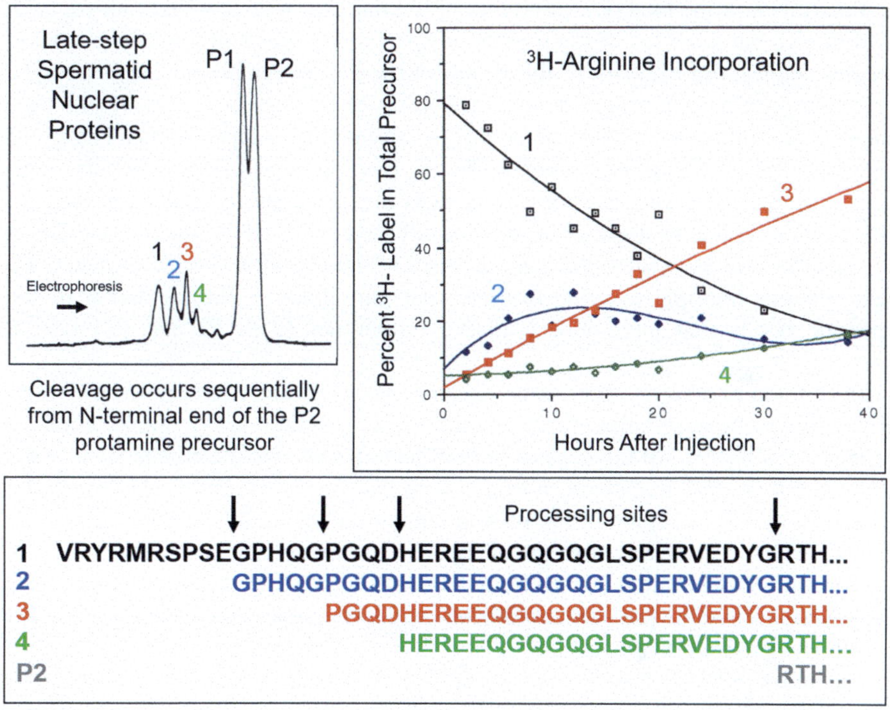

Fig. 1.2 Processing of the P2 precursor, which does not begin until several hours after its synthesis and deposition onto DNA, occurs by the sequential cleavage and removal of a series of short peptide fragments (black arrows) from the amino-terminal domain of the protamine P2 precursor. The intact P2 precursor (1, black) and partially processed forms of P2 (2, blue; 3, red; 4, green) migrate more slowly than P1 and P2 in acid urea gels. Changes in tritium labeling of the intact P2 precursor and its partially processed forms isolated from the spermatids of mice injected with 3H-arginine show the radiolabel appears first in the intact precursor (1, black; highest ^{3}H-arginine content at 2 h). As the labeling decreases in the intact precursor over time, the label moves next into processed form 2 (blue), followed by processed form 3 (red), and then processed form 4 (green)

processed further [81]. The final processing step occurs approximately 24–30 h after the intact precursor is synthesized and deposited onto DNA. While the function of this processing remains unknown, the sequential nature of segment removal and the observed delay in each step suggest the amino-terminal sequence being removed may have some time-dependent function that facilitates P2's integration into chromatin or modulates the protein's interaction with DNA or other protamines. P2 is also posttranslationally modified by phosphorylation [81, 98] on serine and threonine residues. Both the unprocessed precursor and the fully processed P2 are phosphorylated [98]. The P1 and P2 protamines appear to be phosphorylated prior to their binding to DNA and then repeatedly dephosphorylated and re-phosphorylated until they are properly bound to DNA. The level of phosphorylation progressively declines as the spermatids traverse the epididymis [98]. Once the sperm reach the vas deferens, the majority of the phosphorylation has been removed [83].

Precisely how the final processed form of P2 interacts with DNA has not yet been determined, but analyses of the protamines packaging sperm chromatin in several species suggest the majority of the length of the P2 molecule binds to DNA [42]. The "footprint" of P1 when bound to DNA has been estimated to be 10–11 base pairs, or one full turn of DNA, while the "footprint" of P2 appears to be larger (15 base pairs) [42]. Similar to protamine P1, the final processed form of P2 also contains a series of (Arg)n anchoring sequences that are used to bind the protein to DNA. These segments are shorter than those found in the DNA-binding domain of P1, and they are distributed throughout much of the length of the P2 sequence. P2 also contains multiple cysteine residues that participate in the formation of the disulfide bonds that interconnect all the protamines (both P1 and P2) late in spermiogenesis.

In addition to phosphorylation, mouse protamines P1 and P2 are posttranslationally modified by acetylation on lysine and serine residues and by methylation on lysine residues [99]. All three types of modifications change the charge state of the affected amino acid side chain in such a way that their presence could impact the conformation of the region of the protein containing the modification or disrupt its binding to DNA. In contrast to the acetylated and methylated sites, which can be found in the same protein molecule, phosphorylated and acetylated residues were not found in the same protamine molecule, suggesting they may have separate and possibly exclusive functions.

Protamine P2 also differs from protamine P1 in that it binds zinc [100–102]. Particle-induced X-ray emission (PIXE) analyses of individual mouse and hamster caudal sperm and ejaculated human and stallion sperm have shown the amount of zinc present in the sperm chromatin of each of these species is consistent with a single zinc atom being bound to each P2 molecule [101]. This zinc is already bound to hamster protamine P2 in late-step spermatids isolated from testes, and the stoichiometry (1 Zn/1 P2 protamine) remains constant as hamster sperm traverse the epididymis (Table 1.1). Nuclear zinc has been reported to increase once the sperm enters the zinc-rich seminal fluid [103, 104], but what role this zinc plays in sperm chromatin is currently unclear.

While analyses of zinc bound to protamine P2 in solution have suggested the coordination of zinc by histidine and cysteine residues may bear some similarity to zinc finger proteins [102, 105], other studies conducted with DNA-bound protamine P2 peptides and with intact hamster spermatid and sperm heads indicate zinc is

Table 1.1 Zinc is bound to hamster protamine P2 in late-step spermatids, and the stoichiometry (1 Zn/1 P2 protamine) remains constant as hamster sperm traverse the epididymis

Sperm source	DNA (pg)	P2 (10^{-15} mol)	Zn (10^{-15} mol)	Zn:P2
Cauda epididymis	3.3 ± 0.1	0.131 ± 0.007	0.16 ± 0.04	1.2 ± 0.3
Caput epididymis	3.4 ± 0.1	0.132 ± 0.008	0.15 ± 0.04	1.1 ± 0.3
Testis	3.4 ± 0.1	0.142 ± 0.008	0.15 ± 0.04	1.0 ± 0.3

DNA, protamine P2, and zinc contents were determined by PIXE analysis of individual spermatids and sperm using the nuclear microprobe at Lawrence Livermore National Laboratory as described previously [102]

Table 1.2 X-ray absorption fine structure (XAFS) analysis of zinc coordination by protamine P2 in sonication resistant Syrian hamster testicular sperm and caudal sperm

Chromatin source	Ligand	Coordination distance
Sperm (cauda)	1 S	At 2.33 Å
	3 N/O	At 2.04 Å
Testicular sperm	3 S	At 2.33 Å
	1 N/O	At 2.05 Å
MSH-treated sperm (cauda)	1 S	At 2.33 Å
	3 N/O	At 2.08 Å

coordinated differently when the protein is bound to DNA. Two potential zinc-binding sites were identified in the human protamine P2 peptide [100], one located near the amino-terminus of P2 and a second site near the carboxy-terminus. Only one zinc-binding site near the carboxy-terminus of hamster protamine P2 fits the hamster spermatid and sperm results [106]. What the analyses of P2-bound zinc in hamster sperm and spermatids also showed is that the amino acids in protamine P2 coordinating the zinc change during epididymal transit [106]. Extended X-ray absorption fine structure analyses of sonication-resistant (late-step) hamster spermatids have shown that, prior to the formation of the intraprotamine disulfides, the zinc is coordinated by three cysteines and one histidine or carboxyl group in protamine P2 (Table 1.2). Only one site located near the carboxy-terminal end of P2 (Fig. 1.3, structure A) has three cysteine residues and a histidine in close enough proximity to each other to coordinate zinc [106]. Once all the protamines have been deposited in sperm chromatin and the sperm pass through the epididymis, the coordination of zinc changes with two of the three cysteine residues coordinating zinc in late-step spermatids being replaced by two histidines or carboxyl groups (Fig. 1.3, structure B) in mature sperm. Following treatment of mature sperm chromatin with a reducing agent in vitro, the amino acids coordinating zinc change back to the arrangement observed in late step spermatids. This change in amino acids coordinating zinc, which occurs as the inter-protamine disulfide bonds are being formed, may reflect the initial protection and sequestration of specific cysteine residues until they are needed late in spermiogenesis for inter-protamine disulfide bond formation.

One interesting alternative theory proposed by Bjorndahl et al. [107] suggests that inter-protamine disulfides may not cross-link protamines together during the final stage of sperm chromatin maturation, but that the final step in the stabilization of the DNA-protamine complex is instead brought about by zinc forming inter-protamine zinc-dithiolate cross-links between neighboring protamine molecules [103, 107]. While this is unlikely to happen in the sperm of species whose DNA is packaged only by protamine P1 (all current studies indicate P1 does not bind zinc), zinc-mediated cross-linking of neighboring protamine P2 molecules (on same strand of DNA or neighboring strands in coiled toroid) could occur (Fig. 1.3, structures C and D) and might explain why the sperm chromatin containing protamine P2 is more easily decondensed in species that use protamine P2 to package their DNA [108]. Other cases have been reported in which tetrahedral zinc coordination by two different protein subunits or partners is used to stabilize an interaction [109, 110].

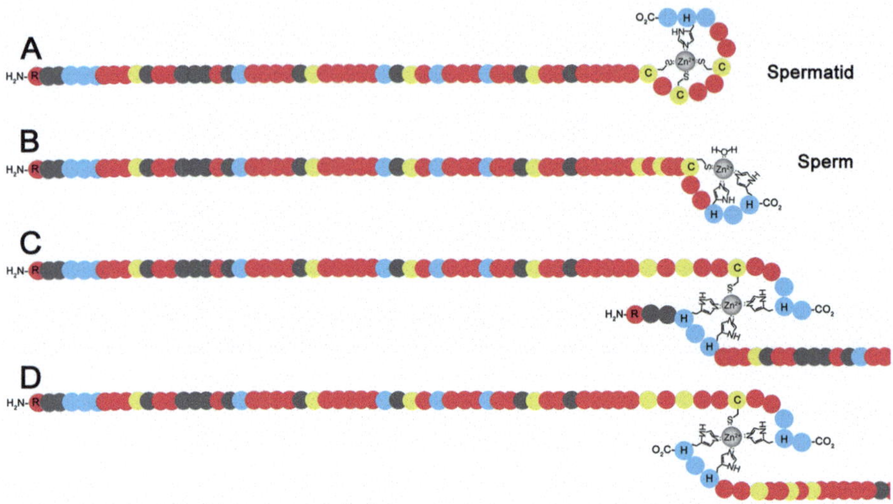

Fig. 1.3 Proposed mode of zinc coordination by protamine P2 in the Syrian hamster and changes that occur during the final stages of sperm chromatin maturation as the sperm traverse the epididymis. The site located near the carboxy-terminal end of Syrian hamster P2 has three cysteine and three histidine residues in close enough proximity to each other to coordinate zinc. The proposed zinc coordination shown in **A** is consistent with XAFS data obtained from analyses of Syrian hamster late-step spermatids (Table 1.2) which show the zinc bound to protamine P2 is coordinated by three cysteines and a histidine. By the time the sperm pass through the epididymis and reach the cauda, the amino acids coordinating the zinc in mature sperm have changed to a structure consistent with that shown in **B** where the zinc is coordinated by a single cysteine, two histidine residues, and a water molecule. Possible inter-protamine P2 zinc-mediated cross-links that could form between **C** the carboxy-terminal domain of one P2 and the amino-terminal domain of a different P2 or **D** the carboxy-terminal domain of one P2 and the carboxy-terminal domain of a different P2. Such zinc-coordinated cross-links could form between adjacent P2 molecules bound to the same DNA or between P2 molecules on different strands of DNA (such as those packed together during the coiling of the DNA-protamine complex into a toroid)

Artificial complexes with similar structures have also been generated to test the feasibility of using zinc coordination by a pair of partners to create novel peptide assemblies [111].

1.5 Protamine-DNA Interactions and Structure of the Complex

Differences in P1 and P2 protamine sequence, the synthesis of P2 as a precursor and its subsequent processing, the binding of zinc to P2 but not P1, the observation that sperm chromatins containing P2 are less stable than those containing only P1 [108], and the fact that no species has been identified that produces sperm with its DNA packaged only by protamine P2 suggest there are likely to be important differences in the way the P1 and P2 protamines bind to and "package" DNA. The observation that many species of mammals produce sperm with their DNA packaged only by protamine P1, while none are known to use only protamine P2, also suggests that P1 may be sufficient for the final packaging and that P2 contributes to the process but cannot be substituted entirely for P1. In those species whose sperm contain both protamines P1 and P2, the relative amounts of the P1 and P2 protamines found in the sperm chromatin of mammals varies widely between mammalian genera, but the relative proportion of the two proteins packaging the DNA appears to be conserved among the species within a genus [79].

Beyond the knowledge that both protamines P1 and P2 bind to DNA in some manner that allows the two proteins to be cross-linked together by disulfide bridges during the final stage of sperm maturation, we know very little about how protamines P1 and P2 are distributed along a segment of DNA. Experiments analyzing chemically cross-linked protamines and the disulfide bonds that are formed within and between protamine molecules in rodents, taken together with the variability in proportion of P2 present in the sperm of different mammalian species, have suggested protamine P2 molecules are likely to be clustered together along the DNA as dimers [112, 113]. This would be consistent with the observed conservation of cysteine residues (numbers and locations) in protamine sequences, and it could also explain how a similar pattern of disulfide bond formation could be used to interlink all the protamines together irrespective of the relative proportion of P1 and P2 [112, 113].

Protamines are unusual in that they are unstructured in solution [114] and only adopt a specific conformation when they bind to DNA. At the molecular level, protamines bind to duplex DNA in a manner that has been shown to be independent of base sequence [115, 116]. The primary interactions are electrostatic and involve the binding of the positively charged guanidinium groups in the arginine residues present in the DNA anchoring domains of protamine to the negatively charged phosphates that comprise phosphodiester backbone of DNA. The high affinity of binding is derived from two aspects of these interactions, the formation of a salt bridge and hydrogen bond between the guanidinium group and the phosphate and the multivalency achieved through the binding of multiple arginine residues in the DNA-binding domain of protamine to an equivalent number of phosphate groups in DNA. Computer modeling, X-ray scattering, and other experimental studies [114, 117–119] have provided evidence to suggest that the DNA-binding domain of protamine P1 wraps in an extended conformation around the DNA helix (Fig. 1.4), positioned above and stretching across the major groove. Adjacent arginine residues in the (Arg)n anchoring domains bind to phosphates on opposite strands of the duplex DNA molecule, interlocking the relative positions of the bases together and preventing strand separation or changes in DNA conformation throughout the period that the protamines remain bound to DNA. In order for alternating arginine residues in the (Arg)n anchoring sequences to bind to phosphates in opposing strands of the DNA helix, the amide backbone of the DNA-binding domain is forced into a unique conformation similar to a gamma-turn [114]. Following the binding of the protamines to DNA, a neutral, highly insoluble chromatin complex is produced that enables DNA strands to be packed tightly together without charge repulsion.

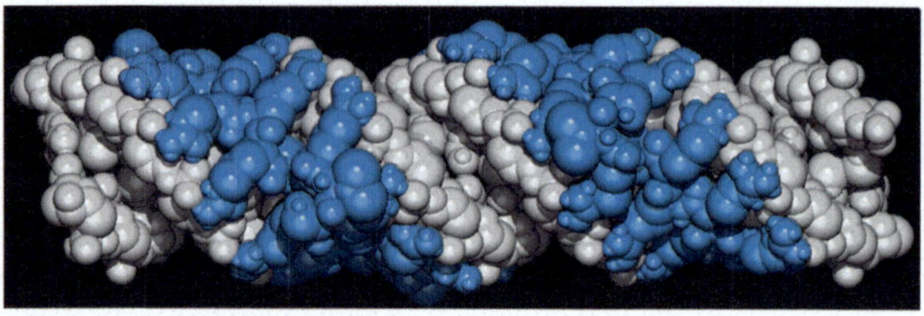

Fig. 1.4 A computer-generated molecular model of a DNA-protamine P1 complex shows how the DNA-binding domain of protamine P1 wraps in an extended conformation around the DNA helix, positioned above and stretching across the major groove. The structure contains four turns of DNA (white) and two bull protamine DNA-binding domains (blue)

Low-angle X-ray scattering experiments performed on intact sperm heads have confirmed the close packing of the DNA within sperm chromatin, showing the center-to-center distance between adjacent DNA molecules is approximately 2.7–3 nm [117, 120, 121]. To achieve this tight packing, the protamine-bound molecules must be organized in a hexagonal arrangement [86] with only 0.7 nm distance of separation between the surfaces of adjacent molecules. This is achieved by coiling the DNA into toroidal structures approximately 100 nm in diameter that contain ~50,000 bp of DNA. High-resolution EM studies of individual toroidal subunits [122] have confirmed the individual DNA molecules are tightly packed in a hexagonal arrangement, consistent with what has been observed by low-angle X-ray scattering.

1.6 Higher-Ordered Organization of Chromatin in Mature Sperm

Electron microscopy (EM) images of the chromatin in differentiating spermatids have shown that the DNA is initially organized similar to somatic chromatin (~11 nm nodules/nucleosomes and 30 nm fibers [22, 123]), which subsequently transforms into nodular structures or fibers in late-step spermatids with diameters (50–100 nm) much larger than individual nucleosomes. As the protamines are deposited in the chromatin, dephosphorylated and their disulfide bonds begin forming, these nodules coalesce into increasingly larger masses or fibers that eventually become so tightly packed and electron dense that the individual structures can no longer be resolved. Both the extreme degree of compaction of the DNA into the toroidal subunits and the insolubility of the DNA-protamine complex have made it difficult to obtain more detailed information about the higher-ordered arrangement of toroids and nucleosomes packed inside the nucleus by direct analyses of mature sperm.

Additional information has been obtained, however, by partially disrupting sperm chromatin using polyanions, reducing agents, high ionic strength, or following partial digestion by nucleases [112, 124–130]. EM and scanning probe microscopy

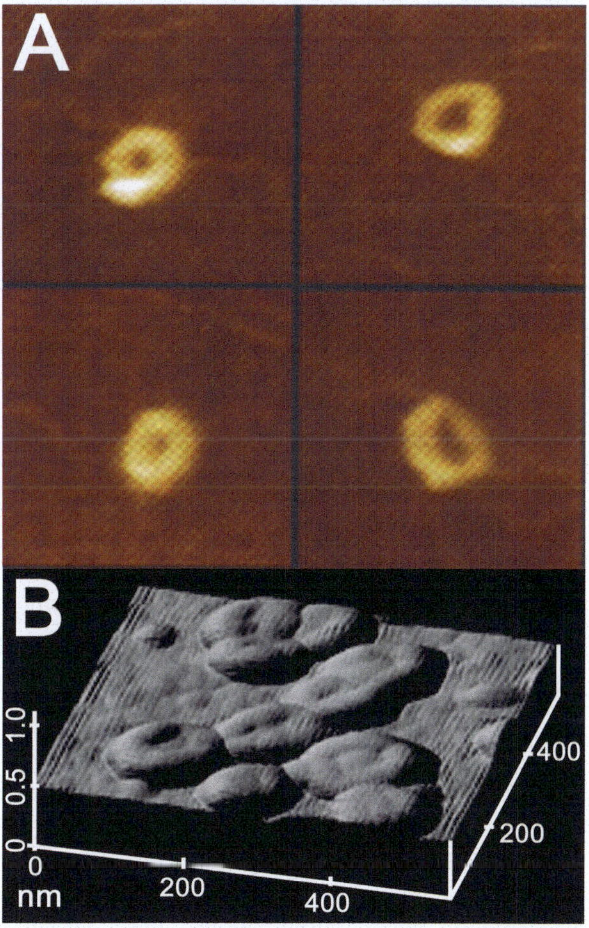

Fig. 1.5 Scanning probe microscopy images of **A** toroidal structures (100 nm) with lifesaver-like features generated in vitro when bull protamine P1 is added to dilute solutions of DNA (7.5 kb plasmid) loosely bound to a Mg+2 treated mica surface (dimensions of each toroid image is 325 × 325 nm) and **B** globular lifesaver-shaped toroid structures in dispersed human sperm chromatin. These native DNA-protamine toroids are approximately 100–150 nm in diameter and 20 nm thick with a hole or depression in the center

images of decondensed human sperm (Fig. 1.5) have revealed the presence of two types of structures, small subunits similar in diameter (~10 nm) and thickness (~5 nm) to somatic nucleosomes and larger globular lifesaver-shaped structures approximately 100 nm in diameter and 20 nm thick with a hole or depression in the center [112]. Toroidal structures with lifesaver-like features and similar dimensions (100 nm) are also spontaneously generated in vitro when protamine (Fig. 1.5) [112, 116], viral proteins involved in DNA encapsulation [131, 132], and other polycations are added to dilute solutions of DNA or to individual DNA molecules [133–135]. The size of the toroids, which have been generated using a wide variety of lengths of DNA and condensing agents, appears to represent a minimal energy state for DNA condensed by protamines and other polycations [122, 134, 136]. The toroids formed by protamine binding to DNA contain approximately 50,000 bp of DNA [112, 116]. Closely packed structures with diameters similar to these toroids were found by Koehler to comprise the lamellar sheets of chromatin packed inside rat, rabbit, bull, and human sperm [127, 128, 137]. Such a packing arrangement for

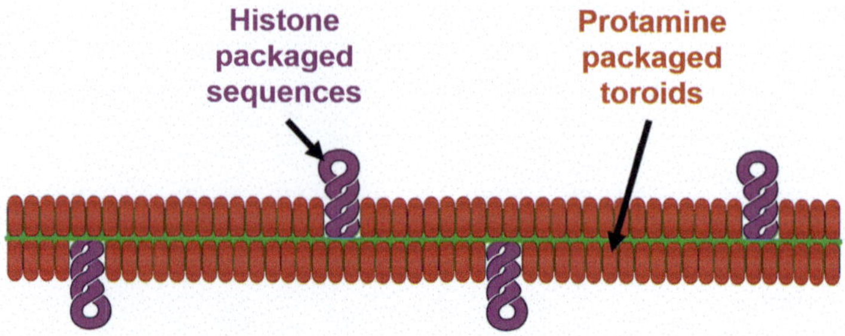

Fig. 1.6 Model showing arrangement of protamine-packaged DNA toroids (red) stacked side by side in sperm chromatin with interspersed regions of DNA packaged by histones (purple) as proposed by Ward et al. [49] (See Chap. 3, Fig. 3.2, for the complete model)

DNA would be consistent with the microscopy data obtained from stallion sperm heads [138] if the toroidal structures are stacked tightly together as lifesavers (Fig. 1.6 and see Chap. 3, Fig. 3.2) similar to the models presented by Ward [49] and Vilfan et al. [86]. While areas of less densely packed DNA similar to nucleosomal containing somatic chromatin were not observed by Koehler, images obtained from scanning probe microscopy studies of human and mouse sperm chromatin do show clusters of nucleosome-sized structures interspersed between much larger toroidal chromatin domains packaged by protamines [112].

1.7 Preservation of DNA Domains and Nuclear Matrix Associations

Following the multitude of nuclear protein transitions and the final compaction of the spermatid genome by protamines into a densely packed chromatin "particle," several aspects of somatic chromatin architecture still appear to be retained inside the sperm head. Confocal microscopy of somatic cells has shown in a number of cases that the DNA molecules that comprise individual chromosomes are not randomly distributed throughout the nucleus, but each appears to be confined to a specific domain or territory inside the interphase nucleus [139–143]. Similar observations have been made regarding the distribution of chromosomal DNA inside the heads of human, bull, mouse, echidna, and platypus sperm [47, 144–147]. While studies conducted with sperm from placental mammals have not provided strong evidence that the chromosomes are arranged in any particular order relative to each other, there is some evidence for a specific arrangement in echidna and platypus sperm.

Two other organizational features retained in sperm cell nuclei are the chromatin loop domains and the attachment of the chromatin to a nuclear protein scaffold or nuclear matrix [124, 148–151]. While protein content of the nuclear matrix changes as the spermatid differentiates [148], the DNA remains bound to the matrix at a very large number of sites (~50,000). This matrix appears in EM images as a network of dense protein filaments filling the interior of the head of the spermatid and sperm bounded by a peripheral structure, the lamina. The DNA in between the sites of attachment to the matrix retain the loop organization present in somatic cells [152, 153]. These loops, which contain ~40,000–50,000 bp of DNA in both the somatic and sperm nucleus, are anchored to the matrix through specific chromatin domains, called nuclear scaffold attachment regions/matrix attachment regions (SARs/MARs). The retention of the matrix and its associations with DNA in sperm are important to maintain because their presence would facilitate and speed up the process of genome reactivation following fertilization and the initiation of the first cycle of DNA replication in the male pronucleus [154, 155]. The loop domains play important roles in transcriptional regulation, DNA replication, and chromosome organization both prior to spermiogenesis and after fertilization. In sperm these loops may also aid in the packing of the DNA by protamines into toroids which also contain ~50,000 bp of DNA ([49, 112, 116] and (Fig. 1.6 and Chap. 3, Fig. 3.2).

1.8 Reactivation of Paternal Chromatin Following Sperm-Oocyte Fusion

Fertilization and the entrance of the haploid male genome into the oocyte trigger a cascade of events [156] that rapidly convert the genome back to nucleosome-organized chromatin and activate sets of genes within the male genome required for the first steps in embryonic development. Removal of the protamines and paternal histones and deposition of the histones provided by the oocyte onto DNA appears to be accomplished by a histone chaperone [157–165] similar to the nucleoplasmin first identified in frogs [162, 166, 167]. Sequence analyses of the frog and related mammalian nucleoplasmins have shown these proteins contain a series of polyglutamic acid sequences that may facilitate the removal of the protamines from the DNA prior to loading it with histones [168] by forming a series of salt bridges with the (Arg)n DNA-binding domains of the protamines [160, 164, 165]. The (Arg)n segments in the protamines, which have a higher affinity for polyglutamic acid than the phosphodiester backbone of DNA, would then release from the DNA and allow the chaperone to deposit the histones and regenerate the nucleosomal organization required to reactivate the new embryo's genome.

Another early event associated with the unpacking of the sperm chromatin that occurs almost immediately after removing the protamines is the initiation of a period of DNA synthesis associated with DNA damage repair [169–172]. This repair synthesis is required to repair DNA strand breaks and remove DNA adducts or other damage that is acquired during spermiogenesis and epididymal transit and storage when repair activities could not be performed due to the packaging of the genome by protamines. Studies have shown that the majority of the damage brought into the oocyte by the sperm is repaired during this period of DNA synthesis, and this process is considered to be critical for maintaining the integrity of the male genome and for ensuring normal embryonic development.

1.9 Consequences of Disrupting Sperm Chromatin Remodeling

A number of the chromatin protein-related changes associated with the repackaging of spermatid genome have been shown to be important for male fertility. These include the removal of the majority of the somatic histones by transition proteins TP1 and TP2, the deposition and posttranslational marking of a subset of paternal histones, and the replacement of the TP proteins by protamine. Numerous studies have suggested there is a positive correlation between male subfertility or infertility and elevated levels of histone in mature human sperm [95, 120, 173–178]. Alterations in the expression and/or translation of the protamine genes leading to a change in the proportion of the P1 or P2 proteins present in sperm chromatin have been shown to not only be linked to infertility [179–189] abnormal sperm head morphology and high levels of DNA fragmentation [186, 190] but to also adversely impact IVF (in vitro fertilization) outcome and early embryonic development [191–195]. The observed differences in protamine content of sperm obtained from infertile males ranged from sperm chromatin containing very little protamine to having too little protamine P1 or too little protamine P2. Defects in protamine P2 precursor processing, which have also been observed in infertile males [196, 197] and a male experiencing a high fever during an episode of influenza [198], may indirectly contribute to the reduction in the amount of P2 (the fully processed form of the P2 precursor).

Other studies have shown that the timely formation of the protamine disulfide cross-links that occur during the final stages of sperm maturation are also important for fertility. In mammals, both protamines P1 and P2 contain multiple cysteine residues. The thiol groups of these cysteines are in the reduced form (free thiols) when the protamines are synthesized and deposited onto DNA, and they remain reduced until the final stage of spermiogenesis when they participate in the formation of both intra-and intermolecular protamine disulfides as the spermatids elongate and the sperm pass through the epididymis [81, 199–202]. A number of cases of human, stallion, and bull infertility have been associated with what appear to be errors in disulfide cross-linking among the protamines. In the sperm of fertile males, the formation of the disulfide bonds is believed to stabilize the chromatin and protect it from physical damage. An equally feasible possibility is that these disulfide bonds not only stabilize the chromatin, but they also prevent the thiol groups from being oxidized or alkylated during the long period of time required for spermatid maturation and sperm storage prior to fertilization. This might be important if the cysteine residues in mammalian protamine also participate in the process of protamine removal from DNA after fertilization. Cysteine-free thiols are excellent free radical scavengers and are susceptible to oxidation to cysteic acid. If functional free thiols are required for efficient protamine removal, the oxidation or alkylation of even a few cysteines could potentially complicate or prevent the efficient removal of the modified protamine from the male genome, and its retention would block the gene it was bound to from being transcribed or replicated later in development.

Mice exposed to alkylating agents prior to protamine disulfide bond formation have been shown to produce sperm with alkylated protamine thiols [203–205]. Matings conducted with the treated males resulted in the production of embryos that died early in development from dominant lethal mutations [204]. The sperm containing the protamines with alkylated protamines succeeded in fertilizing oocytes and inducing embryonic development, but at some point the embryo died when a key gene could not be turned on.

Male infertility has also been linked to deficiencies in sperm chromatin-associated zinc. Zinc is known to be essential for several aspects of sperm development, ranging from contributions to structural elements in the tail to roles in chromatin organization and protamine structure and function [107]. A deficiency in zinc can affect the developing sperm directly, or it can impact the function of other testicular cells that contribute to or play a role in spermatid maturation, such as Sertoli cells. Because zinc plays multiple roles in spermatogenesis and testicular function, it has been difficult to decipher how sperm chromatin-bound zinc impacts the functionality of the sperm cell. Since sperm chromatin-associated zinc is almost exclusively bound to protamine P2 in mammals [101], it has been suggested that the coordination of the zinc by protamine P2 may influence the binding of the protamine to DNA [102, 105] or to other protamines [107].

An alternative possibility is that zinc coordination by cysteine residues in protamine might also protect the thiol groups and prevent their oxidation [206, 207] until it is time for the cysteines to form inter- and intramolecular disulfide bonds. Several studies have also suggested that exposures to other metals, such as copper and lead, may result in these metals binding to the cysteines in protamine in place of zinc (or prior to disulfide bond formation) and their being transported into the oocyte upon fertilization [201, 208–210]. In addition to potentially disrupting the function of sperm by altering chromatin decondensation or protamine P2 function, the delivery of these and other toxic metals into the oocyte would also be expected to have an adverse impact on early embryonic development.

DNA damage incurred during spermatid chromatin reorganization, deficiencies in transition protein synthesis and posttranslational modification, and defects in a number of epigenetic processes that contribute to imprinting [211, 212] and the reprogramming of the haploid genome during spermatogenesis have also been shown to adversely impact male fertility and the postfertilization function of the male genome [213]. Because sperm histones provide epigenetic information that regulates the transcription of genes in the two-cell embryo, environmental perturbations have the potential to change the pattern of gene expression in embryos via changes/differences in sperm chromatin composition during the reactivation of the male genome. Several of these processes will be described in the chapters that follow. A number of excellent reviews have been published describing others [14, 15, 30, 214].

Acknowledgments I would like to thank all the amazing students, postdocs, and collaborators whose curiosity and creativity have led to the discoveries described in this overview. I also thank Monique Cosman Balhorn for her invaluable contribution to, and constructive critique of, this chapter.

References

1. Mendel G, editor. Experiment in plant hybridization. Brunn: Brunn Natural History Society; 1865.
2. Haeckel E. Generelle morphologie der organismen. Berlin: Reimer; 1866.
3. Miescher F. Letter I to Wilhelm His; Tubingen, February 26th, 1869. In: His W, editor. Die Histochemischen und Physiologischen Arbeiten von Friedrich Miescher—Aus dem sissenschaft—lichen Briefwechsel von F. Miescher. Liepzig: F. C. W. Vogel; 1869. p. 33–8.
4. Miescher F. Uber die chemische Zusammensetzung der Eiter—zellen. Med-Chem Unters. 1871;4:441–60.
5. Flemming W. Uber das Verhalten des Kern bei der Zellltheilung und uber dei Bedeutung mekrkerniger Zellen. Arch Pathol Anat Physiol. 1879;77:1–29.
6. Miescher F. Das Protamin—Eine neue organishe Basis aus den Samenssden des Rheinlachses. Ber Dtesch Chem Ges. 1874;7:376.
7. Kossel A. Ueber die Constitution der einfachsten Eiweissstoffe. Z Pysiologische Chemie. 1898;25:165–89.
8. Kossel A, Dakin HD. Uber Salmin und Clupein. Z Pysiologische Chemie. 1904;41:407–15.
9. Kossel A, Dakin HD. Weitere Beitrage zum System der einfachsten Eiweisskorper. Z Pysiologische Chemie. 1905;44:342–6.
10. Kossel A, Edlbacher F. Uber einige Spaltungsprodukte des Thynnins und Pereins. Z Pysiologische Chemie. 1913;88:186–9.
11. Reik W, Walter J. Genomic imprinting: parental influence on the genome. Nat Rev Genet. 2001;2(1):21–32.
12. Solter D. Differential imprinting and expression of maternal and paternal genomes. Annu Rev Genet. 1988;22:127–46.
13. Ade H, Zhang X, Cameron S, Costello C, Kirz J, Williams S. Chemical contrast in X-ray microscopy and spatially resolved XANES spectroscopy of organic specimens. Science. 1992;258(5084):972–5.
14. Biermann K, Steger K. Epigenetics in male germ cells. J Androl. 2007;28(4):466–480. doi:jandr01.106.002048 [pii]. https://doi.org/10.2164/jandr01.106.002048.
15. Štiavnická M, García Álvarez O, Nevoral J, Králíčková M, Sutovsky P. Key features of genomic imprinting during mammalian spermatogenesis: perspectives for human assisted reproductive therapy: a review. Anat Physiol. 2016;6(5):236. https://doi.org/10.4172/2161-0940.1000236.
16. Canovas S, Ross PJ. Epigenetics in preimplantation mammalian development. Theriogenology. 2016;86(1):69–79. https://doi.org/10.1016/j.theriogenology.2016.04.020. S0093-691X(16)30051-6 [pii].
17. Pinheiro I, Heard E. X chromosome inactivation: new players in the initiation of gene silencing. F1000Research. 2017; 6(F1000 Faculty Rev):344 (doi: 10.12688/f1000research.10707.1)
18. Heard E, Clerc P, Avner P. X-chromosome inactivation in mammals. Annu Rev Genet. 1997;31:571–610.
19. Ney PA. Gene expression during terminal erythroid differentiation. Curr Opin Hematol. 2006;13(4):203–8.
20. Berlowitz L. Chromosomal inactivation and reactivation in mealy bugs. Genetics. 1974;78(1):311–22.
21. Montellier E, Boussouar F, Rousseaux S, Zhang K, Buchou T, Fenaille F, et al. Chromatin-to-nucleoprotamine transition is controlled by the histone H2B variant TH2B. Genes Dev. 2013;27(15):1680–92. https://doi.org/10.1101/gad.220095.113. gad.220095.113 [pii]
22. Annunziato A. DNA packaging: nucleosomes and chromatin. Nat Educ. 2008;1(1):26.
23. Hazzouri M, Pivot-Pajot C, Faure A-K, Usson Y, Pelletier R, Sèle B et al. Regulated hyperacetylation of core histones during mouse spermatogenesis: involvement of histone-deacetylases. Eur J Cell Biol 2000;79(12):950–960. doi: 10.1078/0171-9335-00123.

24. An J, Qin J, Wan Y, Zhang Y, Hu Y, Zhang C, et al. Histone lysine methylation exhibits a distinct distribution during spermatogenesis in pigs. Theriogenology. 2015;84(9):1455–62. https://doi.org/10.1016/j.theriogenology.2015.07.013. S0093–691X(15)00371–4 [pii].
25. Carrell DT. Epigenetics of the male gamete. Fertil Steril. 2012;97(2):267–74. https://doi.org/10.1016/j.fertnstert.2011.12.036. S0015–0282(11)02920–7 [pii]
26. Godmann M, Auger V, Ferraroni-Aguiar V, Sauro AD, Sette C, Behr R, et al. Dynamic regulation of histone H3 methylation at lysine 4 in mammalian spermatogenesis. Biol Reprod. 2007;77(5):754–64. https://doi.org/10.1095/biolreprod.107.062265.
27. Khalil AM, Boyar FZ, Driscoll DJ. Dynamic histone modifications mark sex chromosome inactivation and reactivation during mammalian spermatogenesis. Proc Natl Acad Sci U S A. 2004;101(47):16583–16587. doi:0406325101 [pii]. https://doi.org/10.1073/pnas.0406325101.
28. Song N, Liu J, An S, Nishino T, Hishikawa Y, Koji T. Immunohistochemical analysis of histone H3 modifications in germ cells during mouse spermatogenesis. Acta Histochem Cytochem. 2011;44(4):183–90. https://doi.org/10.1267/ahc.11027. AHC11027 [pii].
29. Luense LJ, Wang X, Schon SB, Weller AH, Lin Shiao E, Bryant JM, et al. Comprehensive analysis of histone post-translational modifications in mouse and human male germ cells. Epigenetics Chromatin. 2016;9:24. https://doi.org/10.1186/s13072–016–0072–6. 72 [pii].
30. Nair M, Nagamori I, Sun P, Mishra DP, Rheaume C, Li B, et al. Nuclear regulator Pyg02 controls spermiogenesis and histone H3 acetylation. Dev Biol. 2008;320(2):446–55. https://doi.org/10.1016/j.ydbi0.2008.05.553. S0012–1606(08)00920–2 [pii]
31. Sonnack V, Failing K, Bergmann M, Steger K. Expression of hyperacetylated histone H4 during normal and impaired human spermatogenesis. Andrologia. 2002;34(6):384–90. doi:524 [pii].
32. Shirakata Y, Hiradate Y, Inoue H, Sato E, Tanemura K. Histone h4 modification during mouse spermatogenesis. J Reprod Dev. 2014;60(5):383–7. doi:DN/JST.JSTAGE/jrd/2014–018 [pii].
33. Brykczynska U, Hisano M, Erkek S, Ramos L, Oakeley EJ, Roloff TC, et al. Repressive and active histone methylation mark distinct promoters in human and mouse spermatozoa. Nat Struct Mol Biol. 2010;17(6):679–87. https://doi.org/10.1038/nsmb.1821. nsmb.1821 [pii].
34. Hammoud SS, Nix DA, Zhang H, Purwar J, Carrell DT, Cairns BR. Distinctive chromatin in human sperm packages genes for embryo development. Nature. 2009;460(7254):473–8.
35. Arpanahi A, Brinkworth M, Iles D, Krawetz SA, Paradowska A, Platts AE, et al. Endonuclease-sensitive regions of human spermatozoal chromatin are highly enriched in promoter and CTCF binding sequences. Genome Res. 2009;19(8):1338–49. https://doi.org/10.1101/gr.094953.109. gr.094953.109 [pii].
36. Balhorn R, Gledhill BL, Wyrobek AJ. Mouse sperm chromatin proteins: quantitative isolation and partial characterization. Biochemistry. 1977;16(18):4074–80.
37. Erkek S, Hisano M, Liang CY, Gill M, Murr R, Dieker J, et al. Molecular determinants of nucleosome retention at CpG-rich sequences in mouse spermatozoa. Nat Struct Mol Biol. 2013;20(7):868–75. https://doi.org/10.1038/nsmb.2599. nsmb.2599 [pii].
38. Gardiner-Garden M, Ballesteros M, Gordon M, Tam PP. Histone- and protamine-DNA association: conservation of different patterns within the beta-globin domain in human sperm. Mol Cell Biol. 1998;18(6):3350–6.
39. Gatewood JM, Cook GR, Balhorn R, Bradbury EM, Schmid CW. Sequence-specific packaging of DNA in human sperm chromatin. Science. 1987;236(4804):962–4.
40. Pittoggi C, Renzi L, Zaccagnini G, Cimini D, Degrassi F, Giordano R, et al. A fraction of mouse sperm chromatin is organized in nucleosomal hypersensitive domains enriched in retroposon DNA. J Cell Sci. 1999;112(20):3537–48.
41. Wykes SM, Krawetz SA. The structural organization of sperm chromatin. J Biol Chem. 2003;278(32):29471–7.
42. Bench GS, Friz AM, Corzett MH, Morse DH, Balhorn R. DNA and total protamine masses in individual sperm from fertile mammalian subjects. Cytometry. 1996;23(4):263–71.

43. Gatewood JM, Cook GR, Balhorn R, Schmid CW, Bradbury EM. Isolation of four core histones from human sperm chromatin representing a minor subset of somatic histones. J Biol Chem. 1990;265(33):20662–6.
44. Gusse M, Sautière P, Bélaiche D, Martinage A, Roux C, Dadoune JP, et al. Purification and characterization of nuclear basic proteins of human sperm. Biochim Biophys Acta. 1986;884(1):124–34.
45. Tanphaichitr N, Sobhon P, Taluppeth N, Chalermisarachai P. Basic nuclear proteins in testicular cells and ejaculated spermatozoa in man. Exp Cell Res. 1978;117(2):347–56.
46. Kimmins S, Sassone-Corsi P. Chromatin remodelling and epigenetic features of germ cells. Nature. 2005;434(7033):583–9.
47. Zalenskaya IA, Zalensky AO. Non-random positioning of chromosomes in human sperm nuclei. Chromosom Res. 2004;12(2):163–73.
48. Zalenskaya IA, Bradbury EM, Zalensky AO. Chromatin structure of telomere domain in human sperm. Biochem Biophys Res Commun. 2000;279(1):213–8. https://doi.org/10.1006/bbrc.2000.3917. S0006–291X(00)93917–2 [pii]
49. Ward WS. Function of sperm chromatin structural elements in fertilization and development. Mol Hum Reprod. 2010;16(1):30–6. https://doi.org/10.1093/molehr/gap080. gap080 [pii].
50. Banerjee S, Smallwood A. Chromatin modification of imprinted H19 gene in mammalian spermatozoa. Mol Reprod Dev. 1998;50(4):474–84.
51. Castillo J, Amaral A, Azpiazu R, Vavouri T, Estanyol JM, Ballesca JL, et al. Genomic and proteomic dissection and characterization of the human sperm chromatin. Mol Hum Reprod. 2014;20(11):1041–53. https://doi.org/10.1093/molehr/gau079. gau079 [pii].
52. Sillaste G, Kaplinski L, Meier R, Jaakma U, Eriste E, Salumets A. A novel hypothesis for histone-to-protamine transition in Bos taurus spermatozoa. Reproduction. 2017;153(3):241–51. https://doi.org/10.1530/REP-16–0441. REP-16–0441 [pii].
53. Hammoud SS, Purwar J, Pflueger C, Cairns BR, Carrell DT. Alterations in sperm DNA methylation patterns at imprinted loci in two classes of infertility. Fertil Steril. 2010;94(5):1728–33. https://doi.org/10.1016/j.fertnstert.2009.09.010. S0015–0282(09)03689–9 [pii]
54. Ihara M, Meyer-Ficca ML, Leu NA, Rao S, Li F, Gregory BD, et al. Paternal poly (ADP-ribose) metabolism modulates retention of inheritable sperm histones and early embryonic gene expression. PLoS Genet. 2014;10(5):e1004317. https://doi.org/10.1371/journal.pgen.1004317. PGENETICS-D-13–01408 [pii]
55. Vavouri T, Lehner B. Chromatin organization in sperm may be the major functional consequence of base composition variation in the human genome. PLoS Genet. 2011;7(4):e1002036. https://doi.org/10.1371/journal.pgen.1002036.
56. Carrell DT, Hammoud SS. The human sperm epigenome and its potential role in embryonic development. Mol Hum Reprod. 2010;16(1):37–47. https://doi.org/10.1093/molehr/gap090. gap090 [pii].
57. Steger K, Klonisch T, Gavenis K, Drabent B, Doenecke D, Bergmann M. Expression of mRNA and protein of nucleoproteins during human spermiogenesis. Mol Hum Reprod. 1998;4(10):939–45.
58. Singh J, Rao MR. Interaction of rat testis protein, TP, with nucleic acids in vitro. Fluorescence quenching, UV absorption, and thermal denaturation studies. J Biol Chem. 1987;262(2):734–40.
59. Akama K, Sato H, Oguma K, Nakano M. Isolation of intact transition protein 2 with three zinc finger motifs from boar late spermatid nuclei. Biochem Mol Biol Int. 1997;42(5):865–72.
60. Kundu TK, Rao MR. DNA condensation by the rat spermatidal protein TP2 shows GC-rich sequence preference and is zinc dependent. Biochemistry. 1995;34(15):5143–50.
61. Gupta N, Madapura MP, Bhat UA, Rao MRS. Mapping of post-translational modifications of transition proteins, TP1 and TP2, and identification of protein arginine methyltransferase 4 and lysine methyltransferase 7 as methyltransferase for TP2. J Biol Chem. 2015;290(19):12101–22. https://doi.org/10.1074/jbc.M114.620443.
62. Ullas KS, Rao MR. Phosphorylation of rat spermatidal protein TP2 by sperm-specific protein kinase A and modulation of its transport into the haploid nucleus. J Biol Chem. 2003;278(52):52673–80. https://doi.org/10.1074/jbc.M308365200. M308365200 [pii]

63. Meetei AR, Ullas KS, Vasupradha V, Rao MR. Involvement of protein kinase A in the phosphorylation of spermatidal protein TP2 and its effect on DNA condensation. Biochemistry. 2002;41(1):185–95. doi:bi0117652 [pii].
64. Pradeepa MM, Nikhil G, Hari Kishore A, Bharath GN, Kundu TK, Rao MR. Acetylation of transition protein 2 (TP2) by KAT3B (p300) alters its DNA condensation property and interaction with putative histone chaperone NPM3. J Biol Chem. 2009;284(43):29956–67. https://doi.org/10.1074/jbc.M109.052043. M109.052043 [pii].
65. Yu YE, Zhang Y, Unni E, Shirley CR, Deng JM, Russell LD, et al. Abnormal spermatogenesis and reduced fertility in transition nuclear protein 1-deficient mice. Proc Natl Acad Sci U S A. 2000;97(9):4683–8. doi:97/9/4683 [pii].
66. Zhao M, Shirley CR, Yu YE, Mohapatra B, Zhang Y, Unni E, et al. Targeted disruption of the transition protein 2 gene affects sperm chromatin structure and reduces fertility in mice. Mol Cell Biol. 2001;21(21):7243–55. https://doi.org/10.1128/MCB.21.21.7243–7255.2001.
67. Caron N, Veilleux S, Boissonneault G. Stimulation of DNA repair by the spermatidal TP1 protein. Mol Reprod Dev. 2001;58(4):437–43.
68. Kierszenbaum AL. Transition nuclear proteins during spermiogenesis: unrepaired DNA breaks not allowed. Mol Reprod Dev. 2001;58(4):357–8. https://doi.org/10.1002/1098–2795(20010401)58:4<357::AID-MRD1>3.0.CO;2-T. [pii] 10.1002/1098–2795(20010401)58:4<357::AID-MRD1>3.0.CO;2-T.
69. Unni E, Meistrich ML. Purification and characterization of the rat spermatid basic nuclear protein TP4. J Biol Chem. 1992;267(35):25359–63.
70. Catena R, Escoffier E, Caron C, Khochbin S, Martianov I, Davidson I. HMGB4, a novel member of the HMGB family, is preferentially expressed in the mouse testis and localizes to the basal pole of elongating spermatids. Biol Reprod. 2009;80(2):358–66. https://doi.org/10.1095/biolreprod.108.070243. biolreprod.108.070243 [pii].
71. Rouhiainen A, Zhao X, Vanttola P, Qian K, Kulesskiy E, Kuja-Panula J, et al. HMGB4 is expressed by neuronal cells and affects the expression of genes involved in neural differentiation. Sci Rep. 2016;6:32960. https://doi.org/10.1038/srep32960.
72. Petit FG, Kervarrec C, Jamin SP, Smagulova F, Hao C, Becker E, et al. Combining RNA and protein profiling data with network interactions identifies genes associated with spermatogenesis in mouse and human. Biol Reprod. 2015;92(3):71. https://doi.org/10.1095/biolreprod.114.126250. biolreprod.114.126250 [pii].
73. Balhorn R, Weston S, Thomas C, Wyrobek AJ. DNA packaging in mouse spermatids. Synthesis of protamine variants and four transition proteins. Exp Cell Res. 1984;150(2):298–308.
74. Hecht NB. Mammalian protamines and their expression. In: Hnilica LS, Stein GS, Stein JL, editors. Histones and other basic nuclear proteins, CRC series in the biochemistry and molecular biology of the cell nucleus. Boca Raton: CRC Press; 1989. p. 347–73.
75. Kleene KC, Distel RJ, Hecht NB. Translational regulation and deadenylation of a protamine mRNA during spermiogenesis in the mouse. Dev Biol. 1984;105(1):71–9. doi:0012–1606(84)90262–8 [pii].
76. Yelick PC, Kwon YK, Flynn JF, Borzorgzadeh A, Kleene KC, Hecht NB. Mouse transition protein 1 is translationally regulated during the postmeiotic stages of spermatogenesis. Mol Reprod Dev. 1989;1(3):193–200.
77. Kleene KC, Flynn J. Translation of mouse testis poly (A)+ mRNAs for testis-specific protein, protamine 1, and the precursor for protamine 2. Dev Biol. 1987;123(1):125–35.
78. Lee K, Haugen HS, Clegg CH, Braun RE. Premature translation of protamine 1 mRNA causes precocious nuclear condensation and arrests spermatid differentiation in mice. Proc Natl Acad Sci U S A. 1995;92(26):12451–5.
79. Corzett M, Mazrimas J, Balhorn R. Protamine 1: protamine 2 stoichiometry in the sperm of eutherian mammals. Mol Reprod Dev. 2002;61(4):519–27.
80. Balhorn R. The protamine family of sperm nuclear proteins. Genome Biol. 2007;8(9):227.
81. Balhorn R. Mammalian protamines: structure and molecular interactions. In: Adolph KW, editor. Molecular biology of chromosome function. New York: Springer-Verlag; 1989. p. 366–95.

82. Dixon GH, Candido EPM, Honda BM, Louie AJ, Macleod AR, Sung MT. The biological roles of post-synthetic modifications of basic nuclear proteins. Ciba foundation symposium 28—The structure and function of chromatin. John Wiley & Sons, Ltd, Chichester, UK. doi:10.1002/9780470720103.ch2.
83. Ingles CJ, Dixon GH. Phosphorylation of protamine during spermatogenesis in trout testis. Proc Natl Acad Sci U S A. 1967;58(3):1011–8.
84. Oliva R, Dixon GH. Vertebrate protamine genes and the histone-to-protamine replacement reaction. Prog Nucleic Acid Res Mol Biol. 1991;40:25–94.
85. Balhorn R, Corzett M, Mazrimas J, Watkins B. Identification of bull protamine disulfides. Biochemistry. 1991;30(1):175–81.
86. Vilfan ID, Conwell CC, Hud NV. Formation of native-like mammalian sperm cell chromatin with folded bull protamine. J Biol Chem. 2004;279(19):20088–95. https://doi.org/10.1074/jbc.M312777200. M312777200 [pii].
87. Retief JD, Winkfein RJ, Dixon GH. Evolution of the monotremes. The sequences of the protamine P1 genes of platypus and echidna. Eur J Biochem. 1993;218(2):457–61.
88. Retief JD, Krajewski C, Westerman M, Winkfein RJ, Dixon GH. Molecular phylogeny and evolution of marsupial protamine P1 genes. Proc Biol Sci. 1995;259(1354):7–14.
89. Fifis T, Cooper DW, Hill RJ. Characterization of the protamines of the tammar wallaby (Macropus eugenii). Comp Biochem Physiol. 1990;95B:571–5.
90. Retief JD, Rees JS, Westerman M, Dixon GH. Convergent evolution of cysteine residues in sperm protamines of one genus of marsupials, the Planigales. Mol Biol Evol. 1995;12(4):708–12.
91. Winkfein RJ, Nishikawa S, Connor W, Dixon GH. Characterization of a marsupial sperm protamine gene and its transcripts from the North American opossum (Didelphis marsupialis). Eur J Biochem. 1993;215(1):63–72.
92. Retief JD, Krajewski C, Westerman M, Dixon GH. The evolution of protamine P1 genes in dasyurid marsupials. J Mol Evol. 1995;41(5):549–55.
93. Yelick PC, Balhorn R, Johnson PA, Corzett M, Mazrimas JA, Kleene KC, et al. Mouse protamine 2 is synthesized as a precursor whereas mouse protamine 1 is not. Mol Cell Biol. 1987;7(6):2173–9.
94. Carré-Eusèbe D, Lederer F, Lê KH, Elsevier SM. Processing of the precursor of protamine P2 in mouse. Peptide mapping and N-terminal sequence analysis of intermediates. Biochem J. 1991;277(Pt 1):39–45.
95. Chauviere M, Martinage A, Debarle M, Sautiere P, Chevaillier P. Molecular characterization of six intermediate proteins in the processing of mouse protamine P2 precursor. Eur J Biochem. 1992;204(2):759–65.
96. Elsevier SM, Noiran J, Carre-Eusebe D. Processing of the precursor of protamine P2 in mouse. Identification of intermediates by their insolubility in the presence of sodium dodecyl sulfate. Eur J Biochem. 1991;196(1):167–75.
97. Martinage A, Arkhis A, Alimi E, Sautiere P, Chevaillier P. Molecular characterization of nuclear basic protein HPI1, a putative precursor of human sperm protamines HP2 and HP3. Eur J Biochem. 1990;191(2):449–51.
98. Green GR, Balhorn R, Poccia DL, Hecht NB. Synthesis and processing of mammalian protamines and transition proteins. Mol Reprod Dev. 1994;37(3):255–63.
99. Brunner AM, Nanni P, Mansuy IM. Epigenetic marking of sperm by post-translational modification of histones and protamines. Epigenetics Chromatin. 2014;7(1):2. https://doi.org/10.1186/1756-8935-7-2. 1756-8935-7-2 [pii].
100. Bal W, Dyba M, Szewczuk Z, Jezowska-Bojczuk M, Lukszo J, Ramakrishna G, et al. Differential zinc and DNA binding by partial peptides of human protamine HP2. Mol Cell Biochem. 2001;222(1–2):97–106.
101. Bench G, Corzett MH, Kramer CE, Grant PG, Balhorn R. Zinc is sufficiently abundant within mammalian sperm nuclei to bind stoichiometrically with protamine 2. Mol Reprod Dev. 2000;56(4):512–9.

102. Bianchi F, Rousseaux-Prevost R, Sautiere P, Rousseaux J. P2 protamines from human sperm are zinc -finger proteins with one CYS2/HIS2 motif. Biochem Biophys Res Commun. 1992;182(2):540–7.
103. Kvist U, Björndahl L. Zinc preserves an inherent capacity for human sperm 104 decondensation. Acta Physiol Scand. 1985;124(2):195–200.
104. Kvist U, Björndahl L, Kjellberg S. Sperm nuclear zinc, chromatin stability, and male fertility. Scanning Microsc. 1987;1(3):1241–7.
105. Gatewood JM, Schroth GP, Schmid CW, Bradbury EM. Zinc-induced secondary structure transitions in human sperm protamines. J Biol Chem. 1990;265(33):20667–72.
106. Dolan CE. Structural and functional studies of the protamine 2-zinc complex from Syrian gold hamster (*Mesocricetus auratus*) spermatids and sperm. Davis: University of California; 2004.
107. Bjorndahl L, Kvist U. Human sperm chromatin stabilization: a proposed model including zinc bridges. Mol Hum Reprod. 2010;16(1):23–9.
108. Perreault SD, Barbee RR, Elstein KH, Zucker RM, Keefer CL. Interspecies differences in the stability of mammalian sperm nuclei assessed in vivo by sperm microinjection and in vitro by flow cytometry. Biol Reprod. 1988;39(1):157–67.
109. Auld DS. Zinc coordination sphere in biochemical zinc sites. Biometals. 2001;14(3–4):271–313.
110. Heinz U, Kiefer M, Tholey A, Adolph H-W. On the competition for available zinc. J Biol Chem. 2005;280(5):3197–207. https://doi.org/10.1074/jbc.M409425200.
111. Salgado EN, Lewis RA, Faraone-Mennella J, Tezcan FA. Metal-mediated self-assembly of protein superstructures: influence of secondary interactions on protein oligomerization and aggregation. J Am Chem Soc. 2008;130(19):6082–4. https://doi.org/10.1021/ja8012177.
112. Balhorn R, Cosman M, Thornton K, Krishnan VV, Corzett M, Bench G, et al. Protamine mediated condensation of DNA in mammalian sperm. In: Gagnon C, editor. The male gamete: from basic knowledge to clinical applications: proceedings of the 8th international symposium of spermatology. Vienna: Cache River Press; 1999. p. 55–70.
113. Corzett M, Kramer C, Blacher R, Mazrimas J, Balhorn R. Analysis of hamster protamines: primary sequence and species distribution. Mol Reprod Dev. 1999;54:273–82.
114. Hud NV, Milanovich FP, Balhorn R. Evidence of novel secondary structure in DNA-bound protamine is revealed by Raman spectroscopy. Biochemistry. 1994;33(24):7528–35.
115. Bianchi F, Rousseaux-Prevost R, Bailly C, Rousseaux J. Interaction of human P1 and P2 protamines with DNA. Biochem Biophys Res Commun. 1994;201(3):1197–204.
116. Brewer LR, Corzett M, Balhorn R. Protamine-induced condensation and decondensation of the same DNA molecule. Science. 1999;286(5437):120–3.
117. Feughelman M, Langridge R, Seeds WE, Stokes AR, Wilson HR, Hooper CW, et al. Molecular structure of deoxyribonucleic acid and nucleoprotein. Nature. 1955;175:834–8.
118. Prieto MC, Maki AH, Balhorn R. Analysis of DNA-protamine interactions by optical detection of magnetic resonance. Biochemistry. 1997;36(39):11944–51.
119. Wilkins MFH. Physical studies of the molecular structure of deoxyribonucleic acid and nucleoprotein. Cold Spring Harb Symp Quant Biol. 1956;21:75–90.
120. Foresta C, Zorzi M, Rossato M, Varotto A. Sperm nuclear instability and staining with aniline blue: abnormal persistence of histones in spermatozoa in infertile men. Int J Androl. 1992;15(4):330–7.
121. Sartori Blanc N, Senn A, Leforestier A, Livolant F, Dubochet J. DNA in human and stallion spermatozoa forms local hexagonal packing with twist and many defects. J Struct Biol. 2001;134(1):76–81. https://doi.org/10.1006/jsbi.2001.4365. S1047-8477(01)94365-5 [pii]
122. Hud NV, Vilfan ID. Toroidal DNA condensates: unraveling the fine structure and the role of nucleation in determining size. Annu Rev Biophys Biomol Struct. 2005;34:295–318.
123. Horowitz RA, Agard DA, Sedat JW, Woodcock CL. The three-dimensional architecture of chromatin in situ: electron tomography reveals fibers composed of a continuously variable zig-zag nucleosomal ribbon. J Cell Biol. 1994;125(1):1–10.

124. Allen MJ, Lee C, Lee JD 4th, Pogany GC, Balooch M, Siekhaus WJ, et al. Atomic force microscopy of mammalian sperm chromatin. Chromosoma. 1993;102(9):623–30.
125. Evenson DP, Witkin SS, de Harven E, Bendich A. Ultrastructure of partially decondensed human spermatozoal chromatin. J Ultrastruct Res. 1978;63(2):178–87.
126. Koehler JK. Fine structure observations in frozen-etched bovine spermatozoa. J Ultrastruct Res. 1966;16(3):359–75.
127. Koehler JK. A freeze-etching study of rabbit spermatozoa with particular reference to head structures. J Ultrastruct Res. 1970;33(5):598–614.
128. Koehler JK, Wurschmidt U, Larsen MP. Nuclear and chromatin structure in rat spermatozoa. Gamate Res. 1983;8:357–77.
129. Sobhon P, Chutatape C, Chalermisarachai P, Vongpayabal P, Tanphaichitr N. Transmission and scanning electron microscopic studies of the human sperm chromatin decondensed by micrococcal nuclease and salt. J Exp Zool. 1982;221(1):61–79.
130. Wagner TE, Yun JS. Fine structure of human sperm chromatin. Arch Androl. 1979;2(4):291–4.
131. Bera A, Perkins EM, Zhu J, Zhu H, Desai P. DNA binding and condensation properties of the herpes simplex virus type 1 triplex protein VP19C. PLoS One. 2014;9(8):e104640. https://doi.org/10.1371/journal.pone.0104640. PONE-D-14–16399 [pii].
132. Furlong D, Swift H, Roizman B. Arrangement of herpesvirus deoxyribonucleic acid in the core. J Virol. 1972;10(5):1071–4.
133. Allen MJ, Bradbury EM, Balhorn R. AFM analysis of DNA-protamine complexes bound to mica. Nucleic Acids Res. 1997;25(11):2221–6.
134. Bloomfield VA. Condensation of DNA by multivalent cations: considerations on mechanism. Biopolymers. 1991;31(13):1471–81.
135. Marquet R, Wyart A, Houssier C. Influence of DNA length on spermine-induced condensation. Importance of the bending and stiffening of DNA. Biochim Biophys Acta. 1987;909(3):165–72.
136. Hud NV, Downing KH. Cryoelectron microscopy of lambda phage DNA condensates in vitreous ice: the fine structure of DNA toroids. Proc Natl Acad Sci U S A. 2001;98(26):14925–30. https://doi.org/10.1073/pnas.261560398. 261560398 [pii].
137. Koehler JK. Human sperm head ultrastructure: a freeze-etching study. J Ultrastruct Res. 1972;39(5):520–39.
138. Livolant F. Cholesteric organization of DNA in the stallion sperm head. Tissue Cell. 1984;16(4):535–55.
139. Cremer T, Cremer C. Chromosome territories, nuclear architecture and gene regulation in mammalian cells. Nat Rev Genet. 2001;2(4):292–301.
140. Lichter P, Cremer T, Borden J, Manuelidis L, Ward DC. Delineation of individual human chromosomes in metaphase and interphase cells by in situ suppression hybridization using recombinant DNA libraries. Hum Genet. 1988;80(3):224–34.
141. Savage JR. Interchange and intra-nuclear architecture. Environ Mol Mutagen. 1993;22(4):234–44.
142. Schardin M, Cremer T, Hager HD, Lang M. Specific staining of human chromosomes in Chinese hamster x man hybrid cell lines demonstrates interphase chromosome territories. Hum Genet. 1985;71(4):281–7.
143. Weierich C, Brero A, Stein S, von Hase J, Cremer C, Cremer T, et al. Three-dimensional arrangements of centromeres and telomeres in nuclei of human and murine lymphocytes. Chromosom Res. 2003;11(5):485–502.
144. Manuelidis L. Individual interphase chromosome domains revealed by in situ hybridization. Hum Genet. 1985;71(4):288–93.
145. Manvelyan M, Hunstig F, Bhatt S, Mrasek K, Pellestor F, Weise A, et al. Chromosome distribution in human sperm—a 3D multicolor banding-study. Mol Cytogenet. 2008;1:25.
146. Mudrak O, Tomilin N, Zalensky A. Chromosome architecture in the decondensing human sperm nucleus. J Cell Sci. 2005;118(Pt 19):4541–50.
147. Zalensky A, Zalenskaya I. Organization of chromosomes in spermatozoa: an additional layer of epigenetic information? Biochem Soc Trans. 2007;35(Pt 3):609–11.

148. Chen JL, Guo SH, Gao FH. Nuclear matrix in developing rat spermatogenic cells. Mol Reprod Dev. 2001;59(3):314–21.
149. Santi S, Rubbini S, Cinti C, Squarzoni S, Matteucci A, Caramelli E, et al. Ultrastructural organization of the sperm nuclear matrix. Ital J Anat Embryol. 1995;100(Suppl 1):39–46.
150. Ward WS, Coffey DS. DNA packaging and organization in mammalian spermatozoa: comparison with somatic cells. Biol Reprod. 1991;44(4):569–74.
151. Yaron Y, Kramer JA, Gyi K, Ebrahim SA, Evans MI, Johnson MP, et al. Centromere sequences localize to the nuclear halo of human spermatozoa. Int J Androl. 1998;21(1):13–8.
152. Heng HH, Goetze S, Ye CJ, Liu G, Stevens JB, Bremer SW, et al. Chromatin loops are selectively anchored using scaffold/matrix-attachment regions. J Cell Sci. 2004;117(Pt 7):999–1008.
153. Heng HH, Krawetz SA, Lu W, Bremer S, Liu G, Ye CJ. Re-defining the chromatin loop domain. Cytogenet Cell Genet. 2001;93(3–4):155–61.
154. Shaman JA, Yamauchi Y, Ward WS. Function of the sperm nuclear matrix. Arch Androl. 2007;53(3):135–40.
155. Shaman JA, Yamauchi Y, Ward WS. The sperm nuclear matrix is required for paternal DNA replication. J Cell Biochem. 2007;102(3):680–8.
156. van der Heijden GW, Dieker JW, Derijck AA, Muller S, Berden JH, Braat DD, et al. Asymmetry in histone H3 variants and lysine methylation between paternal and maternal chromatin of the early mouse zygote. Mech Dev. 2005;122(9):1008–1022. doi:S0925–4773(05)00062–6 [pii]. https://doi.org/10.1016/j.mod.2005.04.009.
157. Burns KH, Viveiros MM, Ren Y, Wang P, DeMayo FJ, Frail DE, et al. Roles of NPM2 in chromatin and nucleolar organization in oocytes and embryos. Science. 2003;300(5619):633–6. https://doi.org/10.1126/science.1081813. 300/5619/633 [pii].
158. Dilworth SM, Black SJ, Laskey RA. Two complexes that contain histones are required for nucleosome assembly in vitro: role of nucleoplasmin and N1 in Xenopus egg extracts. Cell. 1987;51(6):1009–18. doi:0092–8674(87)90587–3 [pii].
159. Emelyanov AV, Rabbani J, Mehta M, Vershilova E, Keogh MC, Fyodorov DV. Drosophila TAP/p32 is a core histone chaperone that cooperates with NAP-1, NLP, and nucleophosmin in sperm chromatin remodeling during fertilization. Genes Dev. 2014;28(18):2027–40. https://doi.org/10.1101/gad.248583.114. 28/18/2027 [pii].
160. Iwata K, Hozumi K, Iihara A, Nomizu M, Sakairi N, Nishi N. Mechanism of salmon sperm decondensation by nucleoplasmin. Int J Biol Macromol. 1999;26(2–3):95–101. doi:S0141–8130(99)00071–9 [pii].
161. Laskey RA, Mills AD, Philpott A, Leno GH, Dilworth SM, Dingwall C. The role of nucleoplasmin in chromatin assembly and disassembly. Philos Trans R Soc Lond Ser B Biol Sci. 1993;339(1289):263–269.; discussion 8–9. https://doi.org/10.1098/rstb.1993.0024.
162. McLay DW, Clarke HJ. Remodelling the paternal chromatin at fertilization in mammals. Reproduction. 2003;125(5):625–33.
163. Okuwaki M, Sumi A, Hisaoka M, Saotome-Nakamura A, Akashi S, Nishimura Y, et al. Function of homo- and hetero-oligomers of human nucleoplasmin/nucleophosmin family proteins NPM1, NPM2 and NPM3 during sperm chromatin remodeling. Nucleic Acids Res. 2012;40(11):4861–78. https://doi.org/10.1093/nar/gks162. gks162 [pii].
164. Prieto C, Saperas N, Arnan C, Hills MH, Wang X, Chiva M, et al. Nucleoplasmin interaction with protamines. Involvement of the polyglutamic tract. Biochemistry. 2002;41(24):7802–10.
165. Ruiz-Lara SA, Cornudella L, Rodriguez-Campos A. Dissociation of protamine-DNA complexes by Xenopus nucleoplasmin and minichromosome assembly in vitro. Eur J Biochem. 1996;240(1):186–94.
166. Frehlick LJ, Eirin-Lopez JM, Jeffery ED, Hunt DF, Ausio J. The characterization of amphibian nucleoplasmins yields new insight into their role in sperm chromatin remodeling. BMC Genomics. 2006;7:99.
167. Philpott A, Leno GH. Nucleoplasmin remodels sperm chromatin in Xenopus egg extracts. Cell. 1992;69(5):759–67.

168. Katagiri C, Ohsumi K. Remodeling of sperm chromatin induced in egg extracts of amphibians. Int J Dev Biol. 1994;38(2):209–16.
169. Derijck A, van der Heijden G, Giele M, Philippens M, de Boer P. DNA double-strand break repair in parental chromatin of mouse zygotes, the first cell cycle as an origin of de novo mutation. Hum Mol Genet. 2008;17(13):1922–37.
170. Generoso WM, Cain KT, Krishna M, Huff SW. Genetic lesions induced by chemicals in spermatozoa and spermatids of mice are repaired in the egg. Proc Natl Acad Sci U S A. 1979;76(1):435–7.
171. Matsuda Y, Seki N, Utsugi-Takeuchi T, Tobari I. Changes in X-ray sensitivity of mouse eggs from fertilization to the early pronuclear stage, and their repair capacity. Int J Radiat Biol. 1989;55(2):233–56.
172. Matsuda Y, Yamada T, Tobari I. Studies on chromosome aberrations in the eggs of mice fertilized in vitro after irradiation. I. Chromosome aberrations induced in sperm after X-irradiation. Mutat Res. 1985;148(1–2):113–7.
173. Blanchard Y, Lescoat D, Le Lannou D. Anomalous distribution of nuclear basic proteins in round-headed human spermatozoa. Andrologia. 1990;22(6):549–55.
174. de Yebra L, Ballesca JL, Vanrell JA, Bassas L, Oliva R. Complete selective absence of protamine-P2 in humans. J Biol Chem. 1993;268(14):10553–7.
175. Hofmann N, Hilscher B. Use of aniline blue to assess chromatin condensation in morphologically normal spermatozoa in normal and infertile men. Hum Reprod. 1991;6(7):979–82.
176. Terquem A, Dadoune J. Aniline blue staining of human spermatozoa chromatin: evaluation of nuclear maturation. The sperm cell. The Hague: Martinus Nijhoff Publishers; 1983.
177. van Roijen HJ, Ooms MP, Spaargaren MC, Baarends WM, Weber RF, Grootegoed JA, et al. Immunoexpression of testis-specific histone 2B in human spermatozoa and testis tissue. Hum Reprod. 1998;13(6):1559–66.
178. Zhang X, San Gabriel M, Zini A. Sperm nuclear histone to protamine ratio in fertile and infertile men: evidence of heterogeneous subpopulations of spermatozoa in the ejaculate. J Androl. 2006;27(3):414–20.
179. Aoki VW, Liu L, Carrell DT. Identification and evaluation of a novel sperm protamine abnormality in a population of infertile males. Hum Reprod. 2005;20(5):1298–306.
180. Balhorn R, Reed S, Tanphaichitr N. Aberrant protamine 1/protamine 2 ratios in sperm of infertile human males. Experientia. 1988;44(1):52–5.
181. Belokopytova IA, Kostyleva EI, Tomilin AN, Vorobev VI. Human male infertility may be due to a decrease of the protamine-P2 content in sperm chromatin. Mol Reprod Dev. 1993;34(1):53–7.
182. Carrell DT, Emery BR, Hammoud S. Altered protamine expression and diminished spermatogenesis: what is the link? Hum Reprod Update. 2007;13(3):313–27.
183. Carrell DT, Liu L. Altered protamine 2 expression is uncommon in donors of known fertility, but common among men with poor fertilizing capacity, and may reflect other abnormalities of spermiogenesis. J Androl. 2001;22(4):604–10.
184. Chevaillier P, Mauro N, Feneux D, Jouannet P, David G. Anomalous protein complement of sperm nuclei in some infertile men. Lancet. 1987;2(8562):806–7.
185. Mengual L, Ballesca JL, Ascaso C, Oliva R. Marked differences in protamine content and P1/P2 ratios in sperm cells from percoll fractions between patients and controls. J Androl. 2003;24(3):438–47.
186. Oliva R. Protamines and male infertility. Hum Reprod Update. 2006;12(4):417–35.
187. Steger K. Haploid spermatids exhibit translationally repressed mRNAs. Anat Embryol (Berl). 2001;203(5):323–34.
188. Steger K, Fink L, Failing K, Bohle RM, Kliesch S, Weidner W, et al. Decreased protamine-1 transcript levels in testes from infertile men. Mol Hum Reprod. 2003;9(6):331–6.
189. Cho C, Willis WD, Goulding EH, Jung-Ha H, Choi YC, Hecht NB, et al. Haploinsufficiency of protamine-1 or -2 causes infertility in mice. Nat Genet. 2001;28(1):82–6. https://doi.org/10.1038/88313. 88313 [pii].

190. Torregrosa N, Dominguez-Fandos D, Camejo MI, Shirley CR, Meistrich ML, Ballesca JL, et al. Protamine 2 precursors, protamine 1/protamine 2 ratio, DNA integrity and other sperm parameters in infertile patients. Hum Reprod. 2006;21(8):2084–9.
191. Aoki VW, Christensen GL, Atkins JF, Carrell DT. Identification of novel polymorphisms in the nuclear protein genes and their relationship with human sperm protamine deficiency and severe male infertility. Fertil Steril. 2006;86(5):1416–22.
192. Aoki VW, Emery BR, Liu L, Carrell DT. Protamine levels vary between individual sperm cells of infertile human males and correlate with viability and DNA integrity. J Androl. 2006;27(6):890–8.
193. Aoki VW, Liu L, Jones KP, Hatasaka HH, Gibson M, Peterson CM, et al. Sperm protamine 1/protamine 2 ratios are related to in vitro fertilization pregnancy rates and predictive of fertilization ability. Fertil Steril. 2006;86(5):1408–15.
194. Cho C, Jung-Ha H, Willis WD, Goulding EH, Stein P, Xu Z, et al. Protamine 2 deficiency leads to sperm DNA damage and embryo death in mice. Biol Reprod. 2003;69(1):211–7.
195. Depa-Martynow M, Kempisty B, Lianeri M, Jagodzinski PP, Jedrzejczak P. Association between fertilin beta, protamines 1 and 2 and spermatid-specific linker histone H1-like protein mRNA levels, fertilization ability of human spermatozoa, and quality of preimplantation embryos. Folia Histochem Cytobiol. 2007;45(Suppl 1):S79–85.
196. de Mateo S, Ramos L, de Boer P, Meistrich M, Oliva R. Protamine 2 precursors and processing. Protein Pept Lett. 2011;18(8):778–85. doi:BSP/ PPL/ E pub/0319 [pii].
197. de Yebra L, Ballesca JL, Vanrell JA, Corzett M, Balhorn R, Oliva R. Detection of P2 precursors in the sperm cells of infertile patients who have reduced protamine P2 levels. Fertil Steril. 1998;69(4):755–9.
198. Evenson DP, Jost LK, Corzett M, Balhorn R. Characteristics of human sperm chromatin structure following an episode of influenza and high fever: a case study. J Androl. 2000;21(5):739–46.
199. Bedford JM, Calvin HI. The occurrence and possible functional significance of -S-S-crosslinks in sperm heads, with particular reference to eutherian mammals. J Exp Zool. 1974;188(2):137–55.
200. Calvin HI, Bedford JM. Formation of disulphide bonds in the nucleus and accessory structures of mammalian spermatozoa during maturation in the epididymis. J Reprod Fertil Suppl. 1971;13(Suppl 13):65–75.
201. Calvin HI, Yu CC, Bedford JM. Effects of epididymal maturation, zinc (II) and copper (II) on the reactive sulfhydryl content of structural elements in rat spermatozoa. Exp Cell Res. 1973;81(2):333–41.
202. Saowaros W, Panyim S. The formation of disulfide bonds in human protamines during sperm maturation. Experientia. 1979;35(2):191–2.
203. Sega GA, Generoso EE. Measurement of DNA breakage in spermiogenic germ-cell stages of mice exposed to ethylene oxide, using an alkaline elution procedure. Mutat Res. 1988;197(1):93–9.
204. Sega GA, Owens JG. Methylation of DNA and protamine by methyl methanesulfonate in the germ cells of male mice. Mutat Res. 1983;111(2):227–44.
205. Sega GA, Owens JG. Binding of ethylene oxide in spermiogenic germ cell stages of the mouse after low-level inhalation exposure. Environ Mol Mutagen. 1987;10(2):119–27.
206. Bray TM, Bettger WJ. The physiological role of zinc as an antioxidant. Free Radic Biol Med. 1990;8(3):281–91.
207. Maret W. Metallothionein/disulfide interactions, oxidative stress, and the mobilization of cellular zinc. Neurochem Int. 1995;27(1):111–7.
208. Hernandez-Ochoa I, Sanchez-Gutierrez M, Solis-Heredia MJ, Quintanilla-Vega B. Spermatozoa nucleus takes up lead during the epididymal maturation altering chromatin condensation. Reprod Toxicol. 2006;21(2):171–8.
209. Johansson L, Pellicciari CE. Lead-induced changes in the stabilization of the mouse sperm chromatin. Toxicology. 1988;51(1):11–24.

210. Quintanilla-Vega B, Hoover DJ, Bal W, Silbergeld EK, Waalkes MP, Anderson LD. Lead interaction with human protamine (HP2) as a mechanism of male reproductive toxicity. Chem Res Toxicol. 2000;13(7):594–600. doi:tx000017v [pii].
211. Laprise SL. Implications of epigenetics and genomic imprinting in assisted reproductive technologies. Mol Reprod Dev. 2009;76(11):1006–18. https://doi.org/10.1002/mrd.21058.
212. Marques PI, Fernandes S, Carvalho F, Barros A, Sousa M, Marques CJ. DNA methylation imprinting errors in spermatogenic cells from maturation arrest azoospermic patients. Andrology. 2017;5(3):451–9. https://doi.org/10.1111/andr.12329.
213. Miller D, Brinkworth M, Iles D. Paternal DNA packaging in spermatozoa: more than the sum of its parts? DNA, histones, protamines and epigenetics. Reproduction. 2010;139(2):287–301. https://doi.org/10.1530/REP-09–0281. REP-09–0281 [pii].
214. Jenkins TG, Aston KI, James ER, Carrell DT. Sperm epigenetics in the study of male fertility, offspring health, and potential clinical applications. Syst Biol Reprod Med. 2017;63(2):69–76. https://doi.org/10.1080/19396368.2016.1274791.
215. Ou HD, Phan S, Deerinck TJ, Thor A, Ellisman MH, O'Shea CC. ChromEMT: visualizing 3D chromatin structure and compaction in interphase and miotic cells.Science 2017; 357(6349): 370–383. pii: eaag0025. https://doi.org/10.1126/science.aag0025

Chapter 2
Sperm Nucleoproteins (Histones and Protamines)

Ferran Barrachina, Ada Soler-Ventura, Rafael Oliva, and Meritxell Jodar

2.1 Introduction

Diploid spermatogonial stem cells differentiate into haploid spermatozoa by an accurately controlled process termed spermatogenesis (Fig. 2.1). Spermatogenesis comprises three distinct phases: a mitotic proliferation phase, a meiotic phase, and the differentiation/maturation phase also known as spermiogenesis [1]. During this last phase, the round spermatids undergo significant nuclear, morphological, and cytoplasmic changes to end up becoming motile, haploid, and highly condensed spermatozoa.

One of the most remarkable features of spermatogenesis is the chromatin dynamics along the different phases (Fig. 2.1) [2–5]. Similarly to somatic cells, the DNA in differentiating spermatogonia is packaged by nucleosomes. Spermatogonia replicate by mitosis to ensure the maintenance of germinal stem cell population. However, certain spermatogonia will enter into meiosis to halve its chromosome content and give rise to haploid germ cells. In the prophase of the first meiotic division, the homologous chromosome recombination occurs. One prerequisite for the homologous recombination is the introduction of DNA double-strand breaks (DSB) and its subsequent repair. A high number of DSB are induced in meiotic cells, and only few of them will be resolved as chromosome crossovers, therefore

F. Barrachina • A. Soler-Ventura • R. Oliva (✉) • M. Jodar (✉)
Molecular Biology of Reproduction and Development Research Group, Department of Biomedicine, Faculty of Medicine, and Biochemistry and Molecular Genetics Service, Institut d'Investigacions Biomèdiques August Pi i Sunyer (IDIBAPS), University of Barcelona, and Hospital Clínic, Casanova 143, 08036 Barcelona, Spain
e-mail: roliva@ub.edu; m.jodar.bifet@gmail.com

A. Zini, A. Agarwal (eds.), *A Clinician's Guide to Sperm DNA and Chromatin Damage*, https://doi.org/10.1007/978-3-319-71815-6_2

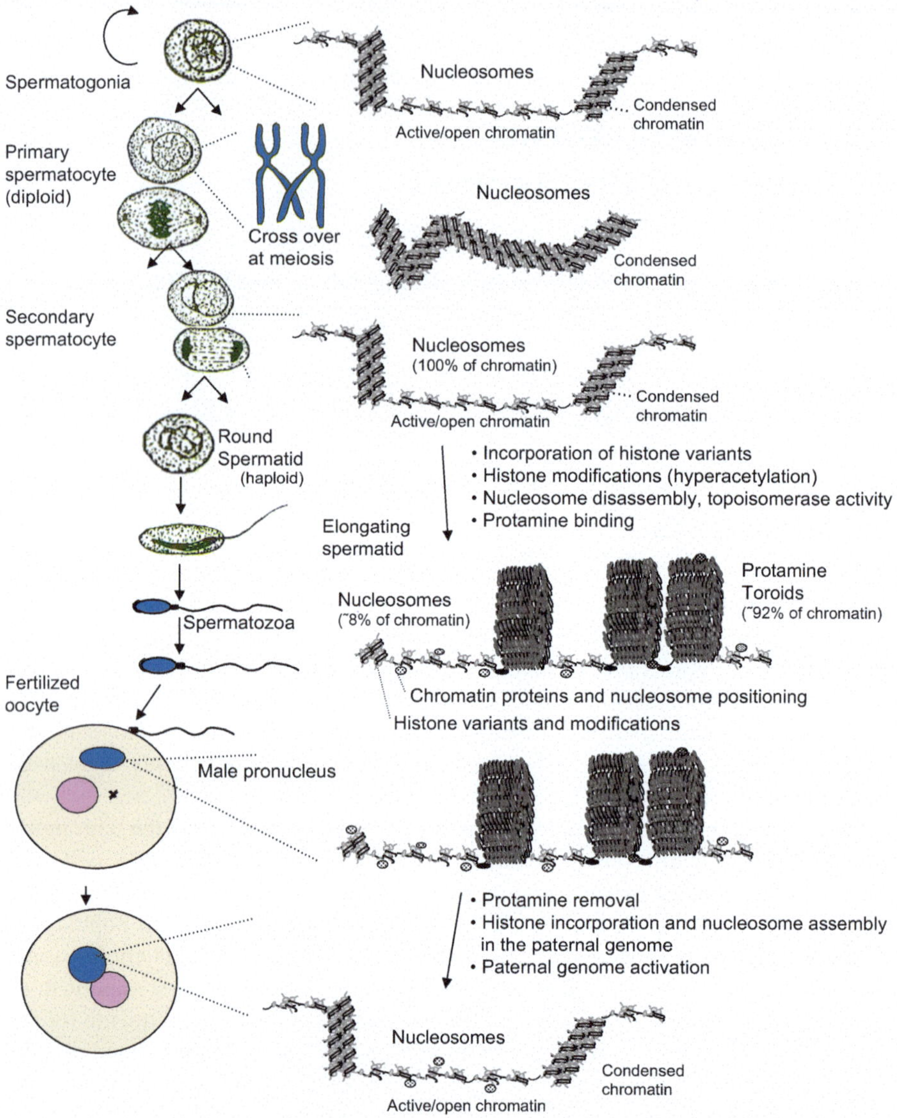

Fig. 2.1 Cellular and chromatin changes during spermatogenesis and fertilization. The main cellular changes (left) are represented together with the concomitant main chromatin changes (right). Spermatogonia replicate and differentiate into primary spermatocytes, which undergo crossing over at meiosis and genetic recombination, and give rise to the secondary spermatocytes after division. Secondary spermatocytes will then divide and give rise to the haploid round spermatids. The round spermatids possess a chromatin structure similar to that of the preceding cells and somatic cells formed by nucleosomes. However, a differentiation process called spermiogenesis is then initiated where the nucleosomal chromatin structure is disassembled and replaced by a highly compact nucleoprotamine complex. The disassembly of nucleosomes changes the superhelicity of the DNA and requires the action of topoisomerases. In the human sperm, about 92% of the chromatin DNA is condensed by protamines forming highly compact toroidal structures each packaging about 50 KB of DNA, and about 8% of the chromatin is formed by nucleosomes. The genes and repetitive sequences are specifically distributed in the nucleohistone and nucleoprotamine structure, and this peculiar chromatin structure is transferred to the oocyte at fertilization. After fertilization, the paternal chromatin must undergo the nucleoprotamine disassembly and the de novo assembly of nucleosomes before paternal gene expression starts

ensuring the genetic variability of the resulting germ cells [6]. In the meiotic and postmeiotic germ cells, the canonical histones are replaced sequentially, first by histone variants [7], subsequently, during spermiogenesis, by transition proteins (TNPs), and, finally, by protamines, following a precise and well-established timing (see Chap. 1) [2, 3, 5, 8]. This process results in a dramatic reorganization of the chromatin exchanging the nucleosomal histone-based structure in the diploid spermatogonia to a nuclear structure tightly packaged by protamines in the haploid spermatozoa, with a potential function in the sperm DNA protection [2, 3]. The multistep procedure of histone exchange requires the contribution of histone variants, as well as histone posttranslational modifications (PTMs); chromatin readers, for example, BRDT [9]; and the transient induction of DSB by topoisomerases to probably eliminate DNA supercoils formed during histone removal [10]. Of relevance, topoisomerases or topoisomerase activity also seems to be present in the final sperm chromatin and may be related to sperm DNA integrity (see Chap. 3) [11]. However, the underlying mechanisms of chromatin reorganization in developing spermatozoa are still poorly understood. Although most of the histones are replaced by protamines during spermatogenesis, the human sperm retains approximately 5–15% of its genome packaged by histones [12]. After fertilization, when the sperm nucleus enters into the oocyte cytoplasm, protamines are quickly replaced by maternal histones, although this process is also poorly understood [13]. However, it has been suggested that the sperm chromatin bound to histones could act as an epigenetic signature with a pivotal role during the activation of zygote genome in early embryogenesis, as well as on transgenerational epigenetic inheritance [14–16].

In this chapter, we highlight the most relevant proteins present in mature spermatozoa, the protamines, and histones, including their variants, their PTMs distribution in the sperm chromatin, and their potential correlation with male infertility.

2.2 Nucleoprotamine Complex in Sperm

Protamines are the most abundant sperm nuclear proteins in many species and in human are packing approximately the 85–95% of the paternal DNA [2, 3, 17–19]. Protamines are small basic proteins rich in positively charged arginine residues, allowing the formation of a highly condensed complex with the negatively charged paternal DNA. Additionally, protamines are rich in cysteine residues, which allow the formation of disulfide bonds and zinc bridges among intra- and inter-protamine molecules resulting in the compact toroidal nucleoprotamine complex [20, 21]. In mammals, two types of protamines have been described, the protamine 1 (P1) and the protamine 2 (P2) family. All mammal species harbor P1 in spermatozoa, but the P2 family, composed by the P2, P3, and P4 components, is solely expressed by some mammal species, such as humans and mice [18, 22]. Typically, the genes encoding protamines (*PRM1* and *PRM2*) are clustered together. In human, the protamine gene cluster is located in chromosome 16 together with the transition nuclear protein 2 (*TNP2*) gene [23]. Whereas P1 is synthesized as a mature form, P2 family is generated from the proteolysis of the protamine 2 precursor resulting in the different components of P2 family (P2, P3, P4), which differ among them only by one to four amino acid residues on the N-terminal extension, being the P2 the most abundant [17, 18].

Although several hypotheses of the P1 and P2 family functions have been proposed [2, 3, 18], the most accepted protamine functions are:

(i) To tightly package the paternal genome in a more compact and hydrodynamic nucleus required for a proper sperm motility
(ii) To protect the paternal genome from exogenous or endogenous mutagens or nucleases potentially present in the male and/or female tracts
(iii) To compete with and remove transcriptional factors and other nuclear proteins from the spermatid chromatin, leaving the paternal genome in a "blank state" so that the paternal genome could be reprogrammed by the oocyte
(iv) To be involved in the imprinting of the paternal genome during spermatogenesis and to confer new epigenetic marks in certain areas of the sperm genome, leading to gene reactivation or repression in the first steps of early embryo development [3, 18]

2.2.1 Protamine Post-translational Modifications

In contrast to the well-known roles of histone PTMs, such as acetylation, methylation, and phosphorylation (see Sect. 3.2), relatively little is known about protamine PTMs. The most well-studied protamine PTM has been phosphorylation (Fig. 2.1, Table 2.1) [2, 3]. Protamines are quickly phosphorylated after their synthesis in elongated spermatids, as a requisite for the proper protamine binding to sperm DNA [17]. However, after the protamine-DNA binding, protamines are extensively dephosphorylated except in some residues whose phosphorylation can still be observed in the mature sperm (Fig. 2.2, Table 2.1) [24, 27–29]. Another type of protamine PTM is the differential processing of protamine 2 precursors. In fact, protamine 2 is synthesized as a long precursor protein which is then proteolytically processed to give rise to the mature P2, P3, and P4 components [30]. More recently, the use of mass spectrometry has allowed to identify additional PTMs in both protamines, suggesting the existence of a protamine code similar to the histone code [31, 32] that could be relevant for zygote epigenetic reprogramming [26, 33, 34]. In mature human sperm, the analysis of the extracted intact protamines by mass spectrometry has enabled to identify mono-, di-, and tri-phosphorylations, di-acetylations, and a mono-methylation for P1 [25]. Using the same strategy, only the intact P3 component could be identified from the P2 family with two potential PTMs (one acetylation and one methylation) [25]. However, further studies are required in humans including the amino acid sequencing by mass spectrometry in order to identify new protamine PTMs and localize the modified residues, as has been recently described in mouse (Fig. 2.2, Table 2.1) [26].

Table 2.1 Posttranslational modifications (PTMs) detected in human and mouse protamine amino acid sequences

Specie	Protamine	Amino acid residue	Post-translational modification	Methodology	Reference
Human	Protamine 1	S8	Phosphorylation	Electrospray mass spectrometry	Chirat et al. [24]
				Phosphoserine conversion and protein sequencing	Pirhonen et al. [29]
		S10	Phosphorylation	Electrospray mass spectrometry	Chirat et al. [24]
				Phosphoserine conversion and protein sequencing	Pirhonen et al. [29]
		S28	Phosphorylation	Phosphoserine conversion and protein sequencing	Pirhonen et al. [29]
		ND	Phosphorylation	Mass spectrometry	Castillo et al. [25]
		ND	Acetylation	Mass spectrometry	Castillo et al. [25]
	Protamine 2	S50	Phosphorylation	Phosphoserine conversion and protein sequencing	Pirhonen et al. [29]
		S58	Phosphorylation	Electrospray mass spectrometry	Chirat et al. [24]
				Phosphoserine conversion and protein sequencing	Pirhonen et al. [29]
		S72	Phosphorylation	Phosphoserine conversion and protein sequencing	Pirhonen et al. [29]
Mouse	Protamine 1	S8	Phosphorylation	Mass spectrometry	Brunner et al. [26]
		S42	Phosphorylation	Mass spectrometry	Brunner et al. [26]
		S42	Acetylation	Mass spectrometry	Brunner et al. [26]
		T44	Phosphorylation	Mass spectrometry	Brunner et al. [26]
		K49	Methylation	Mass spectrometry	Brunner et al. [26]
		K49	Acetylation	Mass spectrometry	Brunner et al. [26]
		N-terminal	Acetylation	Mass spectrometry	Brunner et al. [26]
	Protamine 2	S55	Phosphorylation	Mass spectrometry	Brunner et al. [26]
		S55	Acetylation	Mass spectrometry	Brunner et al. [26]
		K57	Acetylation	Mass spectrometry	Brunner et al. [26]
		K64	Acetylation	Mass spectrometry	Brunner et al. [26]

The table shows the PTMs identified in human and mouse protamine 1 or protamine 2 amino acid residues and the methodology performed
ND Not determined

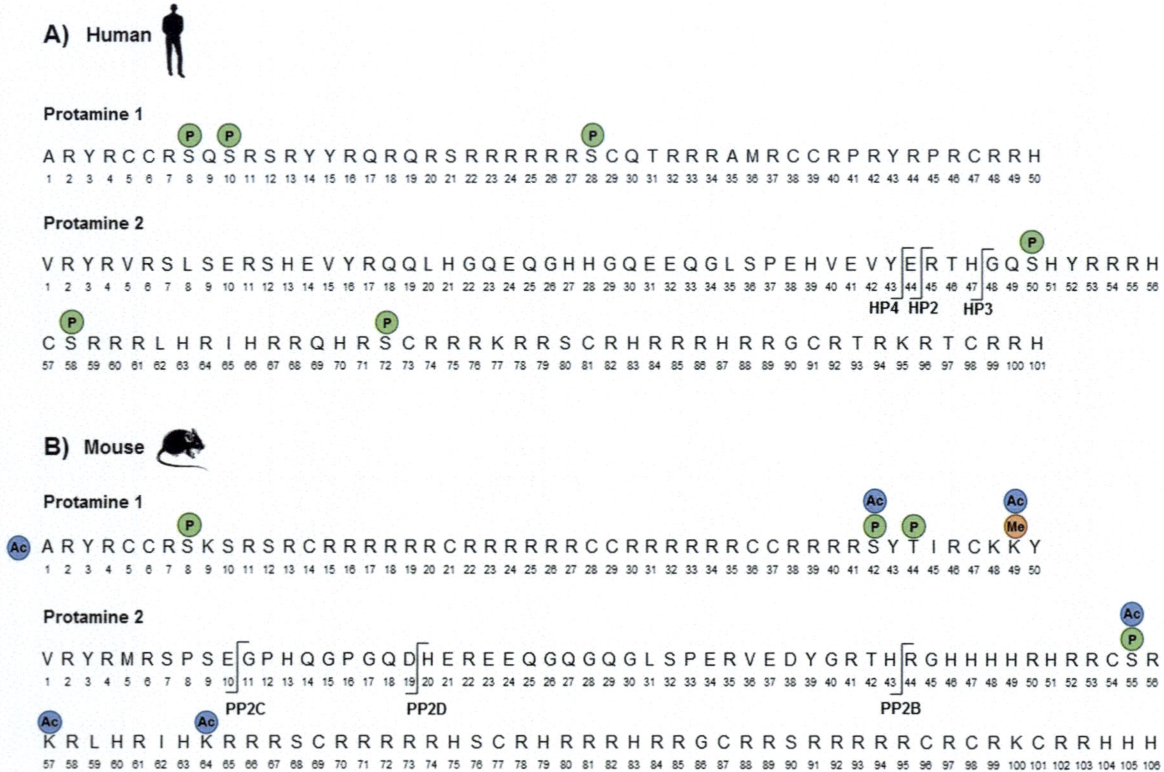

Fig. 2.2 Protamine amino acid sequences and posttranslational modifications (PTMs) detected in human and mouse spermatozoa. PTMs are indicated by Ac for acetylation, Me for methylation, and P for phosphorylation. Residues are numbered after the cleaved methionine. (**a**) Human protamine 1 and protamine 2 amino acid sequences with the described PTMs. The human HP2, HP3, and HP4 cleavage sites are indicated in the sequence. (**b**) Mouse protamine 1 and protamine 2 amino acid sequence with the described PTMs. The mouse PP2B, PP2C, and PP2D cleavage sites are indicated in the sequence

2.2.2 *Protamine Alterations in Infertile Patients*

The relative ratio of the abundance of the protamine 1 (P1) and the protamine 2 (P2) has been widely studied as a measure of sperm chromatin maturity and normality/abnormality [18]. A prospective study in the general population proposed the presence of a wide range for P1/P2 ratio that can oscillate between 0.5 and 1.5 [35]. However, from a reproductive view, several groups proposed a P1/P2 ratio around 1 (0.8–1.2) for fertile males [36, 37]. An altered P1/P2 ratio (below 0.8 or above 1.2) has been correlated among seminal parameter alterations, DNA damage, and low success rate of assisted reproduction techniques (Table 2.2). A recent meta-analysis comparing infertile and fertile patients, including data from nine different studies, has demonstrated a significantly increased P1/P2 ratio in subfertile patients [57].

P2 deregulation occurs more frequently than P1 deregulation, indicating that a P2 deregulation is normally responsible for the P1/P2 ratio alteration. Lower sperm count and sperm motility and/or abnormal sperm morphology have been correlated with abnormal P1/P2 ratio (Table 2.2) [38–45, 47, 48, 58, 59]. Furthermore, some studies have shown that the total absence of P2 or the incomplete processing of the P2 precursors reflected by a decreased pre-P2/P2 ratio is also linked to a lower sperm count, a lower sperm motility, and an abnormal sperm morphology (Table 2.2) [41, 44–46]. Additionally, an altered P1/P2 ratio or a decreased pre-P2/P2 ratio was also linked to an increased sperm DNA damage or to an augmented reactive oxygen species levels (Table 2.2) [41, 49–54, 58]. These studies suggest that an altered P1/P2 ratio results in a sperm DNA more accessible to nuclease activity and, therefore, DNA damage increases. A correct protamination, as a measure of a correct P1/P2 ratio, could be crucial for the DNA protection [49]. However, the meta-analysis performed by Ni et al. could not establish an association between an altered P1/P2 ratio and DNA damage [57]. Otherwise, several studies have also correlated an altered P1/P2 ratio with a low fertilization rate, a low implantation rate, a low embryo quality score, and a low pregnancy outcome using in vitro fertilization (IVF) with or without intracytoplasmic sperm injection (ICSI) treatments (Table 2.2) [40, 43, 45, 52, 55, 59]. Likewise, a decreased pre-P2/P2 ratio has been correlated to a low implantation rate and a poor pregnancy outcome [45], and the total absence of P2 has been correlated to a low sperm penetration ability in IVF [46]. Taken together, these results suggest that protamine deregulation could be involved in fertilization and early embryo development processes. Other parameters such as men's age and smoking have been proposed to alter the protamine P1/P2 ratio (Table 2.2) [38, 39, 54]. In addition, it has been reported that a mutation in the *PRM1* gene promoter (−191AA genotype) causes an increased P1/P2 ratio suggesting that genetic mutations could be the cause of a defective protamination [56]. All these studies suggest that a correct P1/P2 ratio is important for men's fertility and for proper embryo development.

Table 2.2 Altered P1/P2 ratio in infertile patients

Study	P1/P2 ratio	Outcome
Correlation with seminal parameters		
Simon et al. [38]	Altered P1/P2	Lower sperm count; lower semen volume
Hamad et al. [39]	Increased P1/P2	Lower sperm count; lower sperm vitality
Aoki et al. [40]	Altered P1/P2	Lower sperm count; lower sperm motility; abnormal sperm morphology
Torregrosa et al. [41]	Decreased pre-P2/P2	Lower sperm count; lower sperm motility; abnormal sperm morphology
Aoki et al. [58]	Altered P1/P2	Lower sperm count; lower sperm motility; abnormal sperm morphology
Mengual et al. [42]	Increased P1/P2	Lower sperm count
Khara et al. [43]	Altered P1/P2	Lower sperm count; lower sperm motility; abnormal sperm morphology
de Yebra et al. [44]	Altered P1/P2	Lower sperm count
	No P2	Lower sperm count; lower sperm motility; abnormal sperm morphology
De Mateo et al. [45]	Decreased P1/P2	Lower sperm motility
	Decreased pre-P2/P2	Lower sperm count; lower sperm motility
Aoki et al. [59]	Altered P1/P2	Lower sperm count; lower sperm motility; abnormal sperm morphology
	Decreased P1/P2	Abnormal sperm head morphology
Carrell and Liu [46]	No P2	Lower sperm motility; abnormal sperm morphology
Bach et al. [47]	Altered P1/P2	Altered seminal parameters
Lescoat et al. [48]	Altered P1/P2	Altered seminal parameters
Correlation with DNA damage		
Ribas-Maynou et al. [49]	Increased P1/P2	Increased DNA damage (SCD assay)
García-Peiró et al. [50]	Increased P1/P2	Increased DNA damage (SCD assay)
Castillo et al. [51]	Decreased P1/P2	Increased DNA damage (alkaline comet assay)
Simon et al. [52]	Increased P1/P2	Increased DNA damage (alkaline comet assay)
Aoki et al. [53]	Altered P1/P2	Increased DNA damage (TUNEL assay)
Torregrosa et al. [41]	Decreased pre-P2/P2	Increased DNA damage (TUNEL assay)
Aoki et al. [58]	Decreased P1/P2	Increased DNA damage (SCSA assay)
Hammadeh et al. [54]	Increased P1/P2	Increased reactive oxygen species (ELISA assay)
Correlation with assisted reproduction techniques		
Simon et al. [52]	Decreased P1/P2	Low fertilization rate (IVF)
De Mateo et al. [45]	Decreased P1/P2	Low fertilization rate (IVF); low implantation rate (IVF and/or ICSI); low pregnancy outcome (IVF and/or ICSI)
	Decreased pre-P2/P2	Low implantation rate (IVF and/or ICSI); low pregnancy outcome (IVF and/or ICSI)
Aoki et al. [40]	Altered P1/P2	Low fertilization rate (IVF)
	Decreased P1/P2	Low chemical-pregnancy and clinical-pregnancy rates (IVF and/or ICSI)

(continued)

Table 2.2 (continued)

Study	P1/P2 ratio	Outcome
Aoki et al. [59]	Decreased P1/P2	Low fertilization rate (IVF and ICSI)
Nasr-Esfahani et al. [55]	Increased P1/P2	Low fertilization rate (ICSI); low embryo quality score in day 3 (ICSI)
Khara et al. [43]	Altered P1/P2	Low fertilization rate (IVF)
Carrell and Liu [46]	No P2	Low sperm penetration ability (IVF)
Correlation with other parameters		
Simon et al. [38]	Altered P1/P2	Men's age
Hamad et al. [39]	Increased P1/P2	Smokers
Hammadeh et al. [54]	Increased P1/P2	Smokers
	Decreased P2	Smokers
Jodar et al. [56]	Increased P1/P2	Mutation in the PRM1 gene promoter (−191AA genotype)

Correlation of protamine P1/P2 ratio with seminal parameters, DNA damage, assisted reproduction techniques outcome, and other parameters
SCD sperm chromatin dispersion, *TUNEL* terminal deoxynucleotidyl transferase dUTP nick end labeling, *SCSA* sperm chromatin structure assay, *ELISA* enzyme-linked immunosorbent assay, *IVF* in vitro fertilization, *ICSI* intracytoplasmic sperm injection

2.3 Nucleohistone Complex in Sperm

As mentioned before, the human spermatozoon retains approximately a 5–15% of its chromatin packaged in nucleosomes [18]. The nucleosome structure in sperm seems to be similar to that from somatic cells and consists on 147 base pairs of DNA wrapped around an octameric histone core including two of each H2A, H2B, H3, and H4 histones [60, 61]. Adjacent nucleosomes are interconnected by a linker DNA that can be up to 80 bp long. Members of histone H1 family (linker histones) are situated at the site of DNA entry and exit from the core particle binding around 20 nt of linker DNA. Apart from acting as a linker, histone H1 plays an important role in the chromatin folding modulation. The final result is a constrained DNA that approximately achieves a fivefold compaction. Despite the high degree of compaction that nucleosomes confer, histone-packaged chromatin sperm is more open and dynamic than the protamine-packaged chromatin and could be modulated and regulated by the incorporation of histone variants [7, 62], histone PTMs [31], and nuclear factors that modulate the DNA and histone interactions [3, 63].

2.3.1 Histone Variants

During spermatogenesis, some canonical histones are replaced by histone variants, and a subset of those remains in the nucleus of mature spermatozoa. Several histone variants have been identified in mature sperm by mass spectrometry, including the histone H4, which is less diversified compared with the most diverse H2A and H2B histones (Table 2.3). Despite the fact that histone variants have only small changes

Table 2.3 Human sperm histone variants identified in mature sperm

Protein name	Gene name	Localization	♂KO effect on reproduction and embryogenesis	References
Histone H1 family				
Histone H1t	HIST1H1T	Testis	Normal phenotype	Lin et al. [64], Fantz et al. [65]
Testis-specific H1 histone (H1t2)	H1FNT	Testis	Oligozoospermia, asthenozoospermia, teratozoospermia, abnormal spermiogenesis, reduced male fertility, and impaired fertilization	Martianov et al. [66], Tanaka et al. [67]
Histone H1x	H1FX	All tissues	ND	–
Histone H1.2	HIST1H1C	All tissues	Normal phenotype	Fan et al. [68]
Histone H1.3	HIST1H1D	All tissues	Normal phenotype	
Histone H1.4	HIST1H1E	All tissues	Normal phenotype	
Histone H1.5	HIST1H1B	All tissues	ND	–
Histone H2 family				
Histone H2A type 1	HIST1H2AG	Testis	ND	–
Histone H2A type 1-A (TH2A)	HIST1H2AA	Testis	ND	–
Histone H2B type 1-A (TH2B)	HIST1H2BA	Testis	ND	–
Histone H2A-Bbd type 1	H2AFB1	Testis	ND	–
Histone H2A-Bbd type 2/3	H2AFB2	Testis	ND	–
Histone H2A type 1-B/E	HIST1H2AB	Enriched in testis	ND	–
Histone H2A type 1-H	HIST1H2AH	Enriched in testis	ND	–
Histone H2B type 1-B	HIST1H2BB	Enriched in testis	ND	–
Histone H2B type 1-J	HIST1H2BJ	Enriched in testis	ND	–
Core histone macro-H2A.1 (mH2A1)	H2AFY	All tissues	Normal phenotype	Changolkar et al. [69], Boulard et al. [70]
Histone H2A type 1-C	HIST1H2AC	All tissues	ND	–
Histone H2A type 2-A	HIST2H2AA3	All tissues	NP	–
Histone H2A type 2-C	HIST2H2AC	All tissues	ND	–
Histone H2A.V	H2AFV	All tissues	ND	–
Histone H2AX	H2AFX	All tissues	Seminiferous tubules reduced diameter, small testes, male meiosis arrest, and male infertility	Celeste et al. [71]

(continued)

Table 2.3 (continued)

Protein name	Gene name	Localization	♂KO effect on reproduction and embryogenesis	References
Histone H2A.Z	H2AFZ	All tissues	Not viable	Faast et al. [72]
Histone H2B type 1-C/E/F/G/I	HIST1H2BC	All tissues	ND	–
Histone H2B type 1-D	HIST1H2BD	All tissues	NP	–
Histone H2B type 1-H	HIST1H2BH	All tissues	ND	–
Histone H2B type 1-K	HIST1H2BK	All tissues	ND	–
Histone H2B type 1-L	HIST1H2BL	All tissues	ND	–
Histone H2B type 1-M	HIST1H2BM	All tissues	ND	–
Histone H2B type 1-N	HIST1H2BN	All tissues	ND	–
Histone H2B type 1-O	HIST1H2BO	All tissues	NP	–
Histone H2B type 2-E	HIST2H2BE	All tissues	KO not fertility related	Santoro et al. [73]
Histone H2B type 2-F	HIST2H2BF	All tissues	NP	–
Histone H2B type 3-B	HIST3H2BB	All tissues	ND	–
Histone H2B type F-S	H2BFS	All tissues	NP	–
Histone H2A type 1-D	HIST1H2AD	–	ND	–
Histone H2A type 2-B	HIST2H2AB	–	ND	–
Histone H3 family				
Histone H3.1	HIST1H3A	Testis	ND	–
Histone H3.1 t (H3t)	HIST3H3	Testis	NP	–
Histone H3.3C	H3F3C	Testis	NP	–
Histone H3.2	HIST2H3A	All tissues	ND	–
Histone H3.3	H3F3A	All tissues	Reduced male fertility	Tang et al. [74]
Histone H3-like centromeric protein A (CENP-A)	CENPA	All tissues	Not viable	Howman et al. [75], Kalitsis et al. [76]
Histone H4 family				
Histone H4	HIST1H4L	All tissues	ND	–
Histone H4	HIST1H4A	All tissues	ND	–
Histone H4-like protein type G	HIST1H4G	ND	NP	–

Integrative table of the human sperm histone families combining the protein/gene name, GTEx localization, and the knockout effect on reproduction/embryogenesis using Mouse Genome Informatics database

ND no data, *NP* not present in mouse

in their primary structure compared with the canonical histones, those little differences can lead to major changes in the nucleosome structure, stability, and function [62]. The destabilization of DNA-protein interaction by incorporation of histone variants during spermatogenesis allows the transition from the nucleohistone complex to the nucleoprotamine complex [7, 18, 62, 77].

Although there are histone variants widely expressed in all tissues, there are some testis-specific variants that are essentially expressed in spermatocytes [78]. Targeting the individual histone variants in mouse models (knockouts) has revealed which histone variants are crucial for male fertility and reproduction (Table 2.3). Unfortunately, there is a lack of information about a set of histone variants that are not present or have not been detected in mouse (NP) or the corresponding knockout model has not been generated yet (ND). In addition, it is not possible to assess the effect on male reproduction of some histone variants because the knockouts have resulted in embryonic lethality [72, 75, 76], pointing out the need to generate conditional knockout models to assess their importance in testes function (Table 2.3).

Knockouts of some histone variants display a normal phenotype without negative impact on fertility, for example, histone H1t, mH2A1, H2B type 2-E, H1.2, H1.3, and H1.4, suggesting that they are not essential for male fertility (Table 2.3) [64, 65, 68–70, 73]. However, it could be expected that different testis-specific histone variants should have a major importance for proper fertility. As observed in Table 2.3, the knockout models of some testis-specific histones or widely expressed histone variants seem to result in reproductive failure. This is the case of a testis-specific histone, the H1t2, and the widely expressed histones H2AX and H3.3. Each knockout of these three different histone variants displayed male infertility although due to different reasons. For example, H1t2 knockout displays an abnormal spermatogenesis, sperm defects, and impaired fertilization, because this histone is necessary for DNA condensation and nuclear modulation during the last steps of spermatogenesis [66, 67]. In contrast, the disruption of H2AX and H3.3 in mice results in male meiosis arrest, since H2AX is crucial for meiosis because it facilitates the repair of induced DSBs [62, 71] and H3.3 is essential for chromosome segregation that takes place during meiosis (Table 2.3) [74].

2.3.2 Histone Post-translational Modifications

The early events during the transition of histones to protamines throughout spermiogenesis involve the incorporation of histone variants and histone PTMs, which enable the chromatin remodeling and trigger the protamination. Both histones and histone variants are modified by different PTMs [79]. The most known histone PTMs are acetylation, methylation, phosphorylation, ubiquitination, sumoylation, and ribosylation, among other forms [79]. The different combinatorial patterns of the huge number of histone PTMs create a complex histone code that contributes to chromatin organization and dynamics, as well as to gene expression [7, 60]. For example, the massive increase of histone acetylation is one of the first signs that the protamine replacement during spermiogenesis will start [3, 18, 80–82]. Histone hyperacetylation relaxes the chromatin and decreases the affinity of the sperm histones to the DNA, allowing the removal and replacement of histones, firstly, by TNPs and, finally, by protamines [3, 18, 63, 83]. Actually, histone H4 hyperacetylation in elongating spermatids is a prerequisite for the histone-to-protamine replacement [84], and an aberrant H4 hyperacetylation pattern results in impaired spermatogenesis [3, 18, 81, 85]. Apart from histone acetylation, there are other histone modifications throughout spermatogenesis such as methylation, which could also be associated with nucleosome dismantlement and histone eviction. Histone methylation seems to modulate epigenetic signals necessary for spermatogenesis [14, 60]. This is the case of H3K4me, a methylation mark that is necessary to turn spermatogonia into spermatocytes [86, 87], and H3K9me and H3K27me, marks that regulate gene expression during spermatogenesis [88].

Although histone variants and histone PTMs allow chromatin remodeling and most of them are replaced by protamines during late spermatogenesis, some of the modified nucleosomes are not replaced and are retained in the mature sperm. More than 100 histone post-translational modifications have been identified in the remaining histones present in human sperm, including acetylation, methylation, phosphorylation, butyrylation, and crotonylation [31, 89, 90]. Surprisingly, some histone PTMs found in human mature sperm showed a high degree of conservation with mouse sperm, which further supports an evolutionary conserved role of histone PTMs [31]. Those modified paternal histones maintained in the sperm are inherited by the zygote, and they have been proposed to play a role in the epigenetic control of embryogenesis [34]. For example, alterations in the histone methylation (H3K4me2) pattern in mice sperm impair the development and survivability of the offspring, indicating the importance of the sperm epigenome in the health of the progeny [91].

2.3.3 Histone-Bound Sperm Chromatin

Many studies suggest that the 5–15% retained nucleosomes in mature sperm are not randomly distributed through the sperm genome but occupy specific loci [12, 14, 15, 19, 32, 89, 92, 93]. This is supported by recent sperm chromatin high-throughput genome-wide dissection studies indicating that there is a differential distribution of genes and repetitive sequences between nucleohistone and nucleoprotamine complexes.

The first studies using human sperm chromatin fractionation followed by microarrays or high-throughput sequencing concluded that mature sperm histones are associated with DNA enriched at gene regulatory regions and genes involved in developmental processes, including promoters of embryonic transcription factors and signaling pathway proteins, as well as miRNA clusters and imprinted genes (Table 2.4) [19, 89, 92]. In contrast, protamines seemed to be enriched at olfactory receptors genes and ZNF genes [92]. Interestingly, the use of sperm chromatin immunoprecipitation (ChIP) of specific histone PTMs followed either by microarray

Table 2.4 Sperm nucleosomal DNA distribution in healthy men

Study	Methodology	Main outcomes
Arpanahi et al. [92]	Sperm salt extraction and endonuclease digestion or micrococcal nuclease (MNase) digestion followed by a microarray-based genome-wide analysis. Additionally, after digestion, ChIP-chip for acH4 was also used	Endonuclease-sensitive DNA regions are enriched in gene regulatory regions including promoter sequences involved in the development and CTCF-recognized sequences
Hammoud et al. [89]	Sperm MNase digestion followed by either array analysis or high-throughput sequencing. Additionally, ChIP-chip and ChIP-seq for H3K9me3, H3K27me3, H3K4me2/me3, TH2B, and H2A.Z were performed	Sperm nucleosomes are enriched at loci of developmental importance including imprinted gene clusters, miRNA clusters, HOX gene clusters, and promoters of embryo developmental transcription and signaling factors. Histone modifications (H3K4me2/3 and H3K27me3) localize to particular developmental loci
Brykczynska et al. [32]	Sperm MNase digestion followed by mononucleosomal DNA isolation and ChIP for H3K4me2 and H3K27me3 combined with microarray analysis or high-throughput sequencing	Sperm nucleosomes are slightly enriched at TSS. H3K27me3 and H3K4me2 are retained at regulatory sequences in mature human spermatozoa and marks promoters of genes related with spermatogenesis and early embryonic development
Vavouri et al. [15]	Reanalysis of the data from Arpanahi et al. [92], Hammoud et al. [89], and Brykczynska et al. [32]	Nucleosome retention, which is determined by the base composition, occurs in both genic and nongenic regions of the genome. Nucleosomes at GC-rich sequences with high nucleosome affinity are retained at TSSs and at developmental regulatory genes, particularly TSSs of most housekeeping genes. Also, there is a link between nucleosome retention in sperm and DNA unmethylated regions in the early embryo
Samans et al. [93]	Sperm cell fractionation by micrococcal nuclease followed by DNA high-throughput sequencing of the nucleosomal fraction	Sperm chromatin nucleosomes are enriched in certain repetitive DNA elements, as centromere repeats and retrotransposons (LINE1 and SINEs), and the majority of nucleosomal binding sites are enriched in distal intergenic regions. Nucleosome depletion was observed within exons, the majority of promoters, 5′-UTRs, 3′-UTRs, TSS, and TTS. Function of paternally derived nucleosomes in postfertilization processes
Castillo et al. [19]	Sperm chromatin fractionation using salt extraction followed by restriction enzyme digestion or MNase digestion, followed by high-throughput sequencing and proteomic analyses (LC-MS/MS)	Nucleosomal and subnucleosomal DNA regions are highly enriched at gene promoters, CpG island promoters, and linked to genes involved in embryo development

TSS Transcription start site, *TTS* Transcription termination site

(ChIP-chip) or DNA sequencing (ChIP-seq) has revealed that H3K4me2 and H3K4me3 are enriched at developmental promoters expressed in the four- to eight-cell stage embryos, suggesting a potential epigenetic function of those modified sperm histones in early embryogenesis [89]. The specific study of sperm mononucleosomal DNA has shown slight differences, for example, H3K4me2 marks genes involved in spermatogenesis and cellular homeostasis, while H3K27me3 marks developmental regulators and HOX genes [32]. These differences could be attributed to different technical issues in the preparation of the human sperm mononucleosomal DNA in contrast to all nucleohistone complex [32]. In silico analysis from the studies mentioned above revealed that spermatozoal nucleosomes are retained at GC-rich loci and that nucleosome retention in the sperm cell is linked to demethylated DNA in the early embryo [15].

In contrast to the mentioned findings above, one study claimed that retained nucleosomes in sperm are enriched in certain repetitive DNA sequences, such as centromere repeats and retrotransposons (LINE1 and SINE), and the majority of nucleosomal binding sites were enriched at distal intergenic regions [93]. However, these contradictory observations are probably due to technical issues or differences in the computational methodology used [94].

As a summary, there is huge evidence suggesting the existence of a differential distribution between histone-packaged and protamine-packaged sperm chromatin, which is involved in a potential sperm epigenetic signature transferred into the oocyte. The sperm nucleosome enrichment at developmental regulatory genes and gene regulatory sequences suggest that it could regulate the gene expression in early embryogenesis when zygote genome activation occurs and indicate that sperm chromatin is much more complex than it was previously thought.

2.3.4 *Histone Alterations and Male Infertility*

In contrast to the vast number of studies assessing the potential correlation between protamines (P1/P2 ratio) and male infertility (see Sect. 2.2), very few studies have evaluated sperm histones in infertile patients. Early obervations already indicated that a large proportion of the sperm samples with an altered P1/P2 ratio also had increased levels of histones [3, 18, 44]. Focusing on specific histones, it has been described that γH2AX levels are higher in the sperm of infertile patients than in fertile men, and it has been correlated to an increased number of sperm DSBs [95]. It has also been reported that semen samples from infertile men have a significant higher H2B/(P1+P2) ratio than do fertile men, suggesting that an alteration of H2B/(P1+P2) ratio could reflect an abnormal chromatin structure that results in male infertility [96–98]. Moreover, it has also been found an increased H2B/(P1+P2) ratio in smokers [39], implying a negative effect between smoking cigarettes and male fertility. Finally, a correlation has been found between alterations of a testis-specific histone variant (TH2B) and male fertility, which indicates that TH2B is involved in sperm chromatin compaction and male pronucleus development [99].

Apart from the abovementioned alterations in histone content, the sperm of infertile men has also shown an altered histone localization pattern [100]. The study of these infertile men revealed a randomly distributed pattern of nucleosome retention in the sperm chromatin [100]. This alteration in nucleohistone-bound genome could be attributed to a disrupted chromatin remodeling machinery or due to an improper histone hyperacetylation signaling during the histone exchange by protamines [100]. On a different line of experiments, evidence for a substantial deregulation of histones has been detected in normozoospermic sperm cells from male infertile patients with failed assisted reproduction outcomes after ICSI [101]. Overall, these studies demonstrate the importance of an appropriate distribution of genes in the sperm chromatin structure. Therefore, the potential side effects in the embryo associated to an improper histone retention in the sperm are an aspect that deserves further investigation in the future.

2.4 Concluding Remarks

Protamines have been largely studied and correlated with male infertility, specifically by P1/P2 ratio measurement. Similarly, alterations of specific histones have also been associated with sperm defects. Recent studies support the idea that the distribution of the nucleohistone and nucleoprotamine complexes in the sperm chromatin is not random. The intracytoplasmic sperm injection (ICSI) of mouse round spermatids, that did not complete the histone replacement yet, into mature oocytes, derived in embryos with aberrant patterns of gene expression, thereby suggesting that the paternal chromatin structure is important for the first steps of early embryo development [5]. The complexity of sperm chromatin highlights the need to perform further studies in sperm nucleoproteins content and distribution, including the assessment of their variants and PTMs, in order to clarify the significance of the sperm chromatin in male infertility and early embryo development as well as to shed light into the possible effects across generations. Furthermore, it will be particularly interesting to determine the specific role of the hundreds of chromatin-associated proteins present in the normal sperm chromatin, in addition to histones and protamines, as derived from recent high-throughput proteomic studies [102–104].

Acknowledgments Supported by grants to RO from the Spanish Ministry of Economy and Competitiveness (Ministerio de Economía y Competividad; Instituto de Salut Carlos III, Fondos FEDER, "una manera de hacer Europa," PI13/00699, P16/00346, CP11/00312, BFU2011–29739), EUGIN-UB Research Excellence Program (EU-REP 2014), Fundación Salud 2000 (SERONO 13–015), and EU-FP7-PEOPLE-2011-ITN289880. FB is granted by the Spanish Ministry of Education, Culture and Sports (Ministerio de Educación, Cultura y Deporte para la Formación de Profesorado Universitario, FPU15). MJ is granted by the Government of Catalonia (Generalitat de Catalunya, pla estratègic de recerca i innovació en salut, PERIS 2016–2020).

References

1. Neto FTL, Bach PV, Najari BB, Li PS, Goldstein M. Spermatogenesis in humans and its affecting factors. Semin Cell Dev Biol. 2016;59:10–26.
2. Balhorn R. The protamine family of sperm nuclear proteins. Genome Biol. 2007;8:227.
3. Oliva R, Dixon GH. Vertebrate protamine genes and the histone-to-protamine replacement reaction. Prog Nucleic Acid Res Mol Biol. 1991;40:25–94.
4. Carrell DT, Aston KI, Oliva R, Emery BR, De Jonge CJ. The "omics" of human male infertility: integrating big data in a systems biology approach. Cell Tissue Res. 2016;363(1):295–312.
5. Rathke C, Baarends WM, Awe S, Renkawitz-Pohl R. Chromatin dynamics during spermiogenesis. Biochim Biophys Acta – Gene Regul Mech. 2014;1839(3):155–68.
6. Youds JL, Boulton SJ. The choice in meiosis – defining the factors that influence crossover or non-crossover formation. J Cell Sci. 2011;124:501–13.
7. Kimmins S, Sassone-Corsi P. Chromatin remodelling and epigenetic features of germ cells. Nature. 2005;434:583–9.
8. Bao J, Bedford MT. Epigenetic regulation of the histone-to-protamine transition during spermiogenesis. Reproduction. 2016;151:R55–70.
9. Goudarzi A, Shiota H, Rousseaux S, Khochbin S. Genome-scale acetylation-dependent histone eviction during spermatogenesis. J Mol Biol. 2014;426(20):3342–9.
10. Meyer-Ficca ML, Lonchar JD, Ihara M, Meistrich ML, Austin CA, Meyer RG. Poly(ADP-ribose) polymerases PARP1 and PARP2 modulate topoisomerase II beta (TOP2B) function during chromatin condensation in mouse spermiogenesis. Biol Reprod. 2011;84:900–9.
11. Gawecka JE, Ribas-Maynou J, Benet J, Ward WS. A model for the control of DNA integrity by the sperm nuclear matrix. Asian J Androl. 2015;17:610–5.
12. Gatewood JM, Cook GR, Balhorn R, Bradbury EM, Schmid CW. Sequence-specific packaging of DNA in human sperm chromatin. Science. 1987;236:962–4.
13. Jones EL, Zalensky AO, Zalenskaya IA. Protamine withdrawal from human sperm nuclei following heterologous ICSI into hamster oocytes. Protein Pept Lett. 2011;18:811–6.
14. Carrell DT, Hammoud SS. The human sperm epigenome and its potential role in embryonic development. Mol Hum Reprod. 2010;16:37–47.
15. Vavouri T, Lehner B. Chromatin organization in sperm may be the major functional consequence of base composition variation in the human genome. PLoS Genet. 2011;7(4):e1002036.
16. Rando OJ. Daddy issues: paternal effects on phenotype. Cell. 2012;151(4):702–8.
17. Jodar M, Oliva R. Protamine alterations in human spermatozoa. Adv Exp Med Biol. 2014;791:83–102.
18. Oliva R. Protamines and male infertility. Hum Reprod Update. 2006;12:417–35.
19. Castillo J, Amaral A, Azpiazu R, Vavouri T, Estanyol JM, Ballescà JL, et al. Genomic and proteomic dissection and characterization of the human sperm chromatin. Mol Hum Reprod. 2014;20:1041–53.
20. Balhorn R, Corzett M, Mazrimas JA. Formation of intraprotamine disulfides in vitro. Arch Biochem Biophys. 1992;296:384–93.
21. Björndahl L, Kvist U. Human sperm chromatin stabilization: a proposed model including zinc bridges. Mol Hum Reprod. 2010;16:23–9.
22. Balhorn R, Corzett M, Mazrimas J, Stanker LH, Wyrobek A. High-performance liquid chromatographic separation and partial characterization of human protamines 1, 2, and 3. Biotechnol Appl Biochem. 1987;9:82–8.
23. Nelson JE, Krawetz SA. Mapping the clonally unstable recombinogenic PRM1->PRM2->TNP2 region of human 16p13.2. DNA Seq. 1995;5:163–8.
24. Chirat F, Arkhis A, Martinage A, Jaquinod M, Chevaillier P, Sautière P. Phosphorylation of human sperm protamines HP1 and HP2: identification of phosphorylation sites. Biochim Biophys Acta. 1993;1203:109–14.
25. Castillo J, Estanyol JM, Ballescá JL, Oliva R. Human sperm chromatin epigenetic potential: genomics, proteomics, and male infertility. Asian J Androl. 2015;17:601–9.

26. Brunner AM, Nanni P, Mansuy IM. Epigenetic marking of sperm by post-translational modification of histones and protamines. Epigenetics Chromatin. 2014;7:1–12.
27. Pruslin FH, Imesch E, Winston R, Rodman TC. Phosphorylation state of protamines 1 and 2 in human spermatids and spermatozoa. Gamete Res. 1987;18:179–90.
28. Papoutsopoulou S, Nikolakaki E, Chalepakis G, Kruft V, Chevaillier P, Giannakouros T. SR protein-specific kinase 1 is highly expressed in testis and phosphorylates protamine 1. Nucleic Acids Res. 1999;27:2972–80.
29. Pirhonen A. Identification of phosphoseryl residues in protamines from mature mammalian spermatozoa. Biol Reprod. 1994;50:981–6.
30. de Mateo S, Ramos L, de Boer P, Meistrich M, Oliva R. Protamine 2 precursors and processing. Protein Pept Lett. 2011;18:778–85.
31. Luense LJ, Wang X, Schon SB, Weller AH, Lin Shiao E, Bryant JM, et al. Comprehensive analysis of histone post-translational modifications in mouse and human male germ cells. Epigenetics Chromatin. 2016;9:24.
32. Brykczynska U, Hisano M, Erkek S, Ramos L, Oakeley EJ, Roloff TC, et al. Repressive and active histone methylation mark distinct promoters in human and mouse spermatozoa. Nat Struct Mol Biol. 2010;17:679–87.
33. Carrell DT, Hammoud SS. The human sperm epigenome and its potential role in embryonic development. Mol Hum Reprod. 2009;16:37–47.
34. van der Heijden GW, Ramos L, Baart EB, van den Berg IM, Derijck AA, van der Vlag J, et al. Sperm-derived histones contribute to zygotic chromatin in humans. BMC Dev Biol. 2008;8:34.
35. Nanassy L, Liu L, Griffin JT, Carrell D. The clinical utility of the protamine 1/protamine 2 ratio in sperm. Protein Pept Lett. 2011;18:772–7.
36. Corzett M, Mazrimas J, Balhorn R. Protamine 1: protamine 2 stoichiometry in the sperm of eutherian mammals. Mol Reprod Dev. 2002;61:519–27.
37. Balhorn R, Reed S, Tanphaichitr N. Aberrant protamine 1/protamine 2 ratios in sperm of infertile human males. Experientia. 1988;44:52–5.
38. Simon L, Liu L, Murphy K, Ge S, Hotaling J, Aston KI, et al. Comparative analysis of three sperm DNA damage assays and sperm nuclear protein content in couples undergoing assisted reproduction treatment. Hum Reprod. 2014;29:904–17.
39. Hamad MF, Shelko N, Kartarius S, Montenarh M, Hammadeh ME. Impact of cigarette smoking on histone (H2B) to protamine ratio in human spermatozoa and its relation to sperm parameters. Andrology. 2014;2:666–77.
40. Aoki VW, Liu L, Jones KP, Hatasaka HH, Gibson M, Peterson CM, et al. Sperm protamine 1/protamine 2 ratios are related to in vitro fertilization pregnancy rates and predictive of fertilization ability. Fertil Steril. 2006;86:1408–15.
41. Torregrosa N, Domínguez-Fandos D, Camejo MI, Shirley CR, Meistrich ML, Ballescà JL, et al. Protamine 2 precursors, protamine 1/protamine 2 ratio, DNA integrity and other sperm parameters in infertile patients. Hum Reprod. 2006;21:2084–9.
42. Mengual L, Ballescà JL, Ascaso C, Oliva R. Marked differences in protamine content and P1/P2 ratios. J Androl. 2003;24:438–47.
43. Khara KK, Vlad M, Griffiths M, Kennedy CR. Human protamines and male infertility. J Assist Reprod Genet. 1997;14:282–90.
44. de Yebra L, Ballescà JL, Vanrell JA, Bassas L, Oliva R. Complete selective absence of protamine P2 in humans. J Biol Chem. 1993;268:10553–7.
45. de Mateo S, Gázquez C, Guimerà M, Balasch J, Meistrich ML, Ballescà JL, et al. Protamine 2 precursors (pre-P2), protamine 1 to protamine 2 ratio (P1/P2), and assisted reproduction outcome. Fertil Steril. 2009;91:715–22.
46. Carrell DT, Liu L. Altered protamine 2 expression is uncommon in donors of known fertility, but common among men with poor fertilizing capacity, and may reflect other abnormalities of spermiogenesis. J Androl. 2001;22:604–10.
47. Bach O, Glander HJ, Scholz G, Schwarz J. Electrophoretic patterns of spermatozoal nucleoproteins (NP) in fertile men and infertility patients and comparison with NP of somatic cells. Andrologia. 1990;22(3):217–24.

48. Lescoat D, Colleu D, Boujard D, Le Lannou D. Electrophoretic characteristics of nuclear proteins from human spermatozoa. Arch Androl. 1988;20:35–40.
49. Ribas-Maynou J, García-Peiró A, Martínez-Heredia J, Fernández-Encinas A, Abad C, Amengual MJ, et al. Nuclear degraded sperm subpopulation is affected by poor chromatin compaction and nuclease activity. Andrologia. 2015;47:286–94.
50. García-Peiró A, Martínez-Heredia J, Oliver-Bonet M, Abad C, Amengual MJ, Navarro J, et al. Protamine 1 to protamine 2 ratio correlates with dynamic aspects of DNA fragmentation in human sperm. Fertil Steril. 2011;95:105–9.
51. Castillo J, Simon L, de Mateo S, Lewis S, Oliva R. Protamine/DNA ratios and DNA damage in native and density gradient centrifuged sperm from infertile patients. J Androl. 2011;32:324–32.
52. Simon L, Castillo J, Oliva R, Lewis SEM. Relationships between human sperm protamines, DNA damage and assisted reproduction outcomes. Reprod BioMed Online. 2011;23:724–34.
53. Aoki VW, Emery BR, Liu L, Carrell DT. Protamine levels vary between individual sperm cells of infertile human males and correlate with viability and DNA integrity. J Androl. 2006;27:890–8.
54. Hammadeh ME, Hamad MF, Montenarh M, Fischer-Hammadeh C. Protamine contents and P1/P2 ratio in human spermatozoa from smokers and non-smokers. Hum Reprod. 2010;25:2708–20.
55. Nasr-Esfahani MH, Salehi M, Razavi S, Mardani M, Bahramian H, Steger K, et al. Effect of protamine-2 deficiency on ICSI outcome. Reprod BioMed Online. 2004;9:652–8.
56. Jodar M, Oriola J, Mestre G, Castillo J, Giwercman A, Vidal-Taboada JM, et al. Polymorphisms, haplotypes and mutations in the protamine 1 and 2 genes. Int J Androl. 2011;34:470–85.
57. Ni K, Spiess A-N, Schuppe H-C, Steger K. The impact of sperm protamine deficiency and sperm DNA damage on human male fertility: a systematic review and meta-analysis. Andrology. 2016;4:789–99.
58. Aoki VW. DNA integrity is compromised in protamine-deficient human sperm. J Androl. 2005;26:741–8.
59. Aoki VW, Liu L, Carrell DT. Identification and evaluation of a novel sperm protamine abnormality in a population of infertile males. Hum Reprod. 2005;20:1298–306.
60. Kouzarides T. Chromatin modifications and their function. Cell. 2007;128(4):693–705.
61. Ausió J. The shades of gray of the chromatin fiber. BioEssays. 2015;37:46–51.
62. Govin J, Caron C, Lestrat C, Rousseaux S, Khochbin S. The role of histones in chromatin remodelling during mammalian spermiogenesis. Eur J Biochem. 2004;271:3459–69.
63. Rajender S, Avery K, Agarwal A. Epigenetics, spermatogenesis and male infertility. Mutat Res. 2011;727:62–71.
64. Lin Q, Sirotkin A, Skoultchi AI. Normal spermatogenesis in mice lacking the testis-specific linker histone H1t. Mol Cell Biol. 2000;20:2122–8.
65. Fantz DA, Hatfield WR, Horvath G, Kistler MK, Kistler WS. Mice with a targeted disruption of the H1t gene are fertile and undergo normal changes in structural chromosomal proteins during spermiogenesis. Biol Reprod. 2001;64:425–31.
66. Martianov I, Brancorsini S, Catena R, Gansmuller A, Kotaja N, Parvinen M, et al. Polar nuclear localization of H1T2, a histone H1 variant, required for spermatid elongation and DNA condensation during spermiogenesis. Proc Natl Acad Sci. 2005;102:2808–13.
67. Tanaka H, Iguchi N, Isotani A, Kitamura K, Toyama Y, Matsuoka Y, et al. HANP1/H1T2, a novel histone H1-like protein involved in nuclear formation and sperm fertility. Mol Cell Biol. 2005;25:7107–19.
68. Fan Y, Sirotkin A, Russell RG, Ayala J, Skoultchi AI. Individual somatic H1 subtypes are dispensable for mouse development even in mice lacking the H10 replacement subtype. Mol Cell Biol. 2001;21:7933–43.
69. Changolkar LN, Costanzi C, Leu NA, Chen D, McLaughlin KJ, Pehrson JR. Developmental changes in histone macroH2A1-mediated gene regulation. Mol Cell Biol. 2007;27:2758–64.
70. Boulard M, Storck S, Cong R, Pinto R, Delage H, Bouvet P, et al. Histone variant macroH2A1 deletion in mice causes female-specific steatosis. Epigenetics Chromatin. 2010;3:8.

71. Celeste A, Petersen S, Romanienko PJ, Fernandez-Capetillo O, Chen HT, Sedelnikova OA, et al. Genomic instability in mice lacking histone H2AX. Science. 2002;296:922–7.
72. Faast R, Thonglairoam V, Schulz TC, Beall J, Wells JR, Taylor H, et al. Histone variant H2A.Z is required for early mammalian development. Curr Biol. 2001;11:1183–7.
73. Santoro SW, Dulac C, Banaszynski L, Allis C, Lewis P, Barski A, et al. The activity-dependent histone variant H2BE modulates the life span of olfactory neurons. Elife. 2012;1:662–74.
74. Tang MCW, Jacobs SA, Wong LH, Mann JR. Conditional allelic replacement applied to genes encoding the histone variant H3.3 in the mouse. Genesis. 2013;51:142–6.
75. Howman EV, Fowler KJ, Newson AJ, Redward S, MacDonald AC, Kalitsis P, et al. Early disruption of centromeric chromatin organization in centromere protein A (Cenpa) null mice. Proc Natl Acad Sci. 2000;97:1148–53.
76. Kalitsis P, Fowler KJ, Earle E, Griffiths B, Howman E, Newson AJ, et al. Partially functional Cenpa–GFP fusion protein causes increased chromosome missegregation and apoptosis during mouse embryogenesis. Chromosom Res. 2003;11:345–57.
77. Maze I, Noh K-M, Soshnev AA, Allis CD. Every amino acid matters: essential contributions of histone variants to mammalian development and disease. Nat Rev Genet. 2014;15:259–71.
78. Banaszynski LA, Allis CD, Lewis PW. Histone variants in metazoan development. Dev Cell. 2010;19:662–74.
79. Peterson CL, Laniel M-A. Histones and histone modifications. Curr Biol. 2004;14(14): R546–51.
80. Oliva R, Mezquita C. Histone H4 hyperacetylation and rapid turnover of its acetyl groups in transcriptionally inactive rooster testis spermatids. Nucleic Acids Res. 1982;10:8049–59.
81. Sonnack V, Failing K, Bergmann M, Steger K. Expression of hyperacetylated histone H4 during normal and impaired human spermatogenesis. Andrologia. 2002;34:384–90.
82. Govin J, Escoffier E, Rousseaux S, Kuhn L, Ferro M, Thévenon J, et al. Pericentric heterochromatin reprogramming by new histone variants during mouse spermiogenesis. J Cell Biol. 2007;176:283–94.
83. Oliva R, Bazett-Jones D, Mezquita C, Dixon GH. Factors affecting nucleosome disassembly by protamines in vitro. Histone hyperacetylation and chromatin structure, time dependence, and the size of the sperm nuclear proteins. J Biol Chem. 1987;262:17016–25.
84. Hazzouri M, Pivot-Pajot C, Faure AK, Usson Y, Pelletier R, Sèle B, et al. Regulated hyperacetylation of core histones during mouse spermatogenesis: involvement of histone deacetylases. Eur J Cell Biol. 2000;79:950–60.
85. Faure AK, Pivot-Pajot C, Kerjean A, Hazzouri M, Pelletier R, Péoc'h M, et al. Misregulation of histone acetylation in Sertoli cell-only syndrome and testicular cancer. Mol Hum Reprod. 2003;9:757–63.
86. Godmann M, Auger V, Ferraroni-Aguiar V, Di Sauro A, Sette C, Behr R, et al. Dynamic regulation of histone H3 methylation at lysine 4 in mammalian spermatogenesis. Biol Reprod. 2007;77(5):754–64.
87. Glaser S, Lubitz S, Loveland KL, Ohbo K, Robb L, Schwenk F, et al. The histone 3 lysine 4 methyltransferase, Mll2, is only required briefly in development and spermatogenesis. Epigenetics Chromatin. 2009;2:5.
88. Payne C, Braun RE. Histone lysine trimethylation exhibits a distinct perinuclear distribution in Plzf-expressing spermatogonia. Dev Biol. 2006;293:461–72.
89. Hammoud SS, Nix DA, Zhang H, Purwar J, Carrell DT, Cairns BR. Distinctive chromatin in human sperm packages genes for embryo development. Nature. 2009;460:473–8.
90. Krejčí J, Stixová L, Pagáčová E, Legartová S, Kozubek S, Lochmanová G, et al. Post-translational modifications of histones in human sperm. J Cell Biochem. 2015;116:2195–209.
91. Siklenka K, Erkek S, Godmann M, Lambrot R, McGraw S, Lafleur C, et al. Disruption of histone methylation in developing sperm impairs offspring health transgenerationally. Science. 2015;350(6261):aab2006.
92. Arpanahi A, Brinkworth M, Iles D, Krawetz SA, Paradowska A, Platts AE, et al. Endonuclease-sensitive regions of human spermatozoal chromatin are highly enriched in promoter and CTCF binding sequences. Genome Res. 2009;19:1338–49.

93. Samans B, Yang Y, Krebs S, Sarode GV, Blum H, Reichenbach M, et al. Uniformity of nucleosome preservation pattern in mammalian sperm and its connection to repetitive DNA elements. Dev Cell. 2014;30:23–35.
94. Royo H, Stadler MB, Peters AHFM, Arpanahi A, Brinkworth M, Iles D, et al. Alternative computational analysis shows no evidence for nucleosome enrichment at repetitive sequences in mammalian spermatozoa. Dev Cell Elsevier. 2016;37:98–104.
95. Zhong HZ, Lv FT, Deng XL, Hu Y, Xie DN, Lin B, et al. Evaluating γh2AX in spermatozoa from male infertility patients. Fertil Steril. 2015;104:574–81.
96. Zhang X, Gabriel MS, Zini A. Sperm nuclear histone to protamine ratio in fertile and infertile men: evidence of heterogeneous subpopulations of spermatozoa in the ejaculate. J Androl. 2006;27:414–20.
97. Zini A, Gabriel MS, Zhang X. The histone to protamine ratio in human spermatozoa: comparative study of whole and processed semen. Fertil Steril. 2007;87:217–9.
98. Zini A, Zhang X, Gabriel MS. Sperm nuclear histone H2B: correlation with sperm DNA denaturation and DNA stainability. Asian J Androl. 2008;10:865–71.
99. Singleton S, Zalensky A, Doncel GF, Morshedi M, Zalenskaya IA. Testis/sperm-specific histone 2B in the sperm of donors and subfertile patients: variability and relation to chromatin packaging. Hum Reprod. 2007;22:743–50.
100. Hammoud SS, Nix DA, Hammoud AO, Gibson M, Cairns BR, Carrell DT. Genome-wide analysis identifies changes in histone retention and epigenetic modifications at developmental and imprinted gene loci in the sperm of infertile men. Hum Reprod. 2011;26:2558–69.
101. Azpiazu R, Amaral A, Castillo J, Estanyol JM, Guimerà M, Ballescà JL, et al. High-throughput sperm differential proteomics suggests that epigenetic alterations contribute to failed assisted reproduction. Hum Reprod. 2014;29:1225–37.
102. de Mateo S, Castillo J, Estanyol JM, Ballescà JL, Oliva R. Proteomic characterization of the human sperm nucleus. Proteomics. 2011;11:2714–26.
103. Baker MA, Naumovski N, Hetherington L, Weinberg A, Velkov T, Aitken RJ. Head and flagella subcompartmental proteomic analysis of human spermatozoa. Proteomics. 2013;13:61–74.
104. Castillo J, Amaral A, Oliva R. Sperm nuclear proteome and its epigenetic potential. Andrology. 2014;2:326–38.

Chapter 3
Sperm Nuclear Architecture

W. Steven Ward

3.1 Introduction

We know a lot about sperm architecture in general, particularly the tail region, but in many ways the architecture of the sperm nucleus remains a mystery. The genetic material in the human sperm cell is condensed into a much smaller volume than in any other cell types [1–3]. When we try to examine the sperm nucleus by electron microscopy, we are often frustrated by the appearance of a solidly, electron dense mass that is impenetrable to visual assessment [4] (Fig. 3.1). Volume calculations of the sperm nucleus (mouse, in this case) have clearly shown that if the mouse sperm genome were packaged as mitotic chromosomes, the most tightly packaged form of DNA in a somatic cell cycle, it would not fit into the sperm nucleus [1–3]. As the first chapter discussed, the crystallization of sperm DNA into this very small volume is largely accomplished by the protamines. These protamines condense DNA into toroids with about 50 kb of DNA [5], suggesting that there would be at least 60,000 in the sperm nucleus. How these 60,000 protamine toroids are compacted so tightly that even transmission electron micrographs cannot resolve such chromatin structure in the fully condensed nucleus is the question that we will ponder in this chapter. There are many more questions than answers, but there are several important studies that point the way to a model for how it might be accomplished, revealing some insights into sperm chromatin function.

Sperm nuclear architecture remains an interesting mystery. The DNA that makes up the 23 human chromosomes is a little over 1 m in length. It is essentially crystallized and then efficiently folded into a volume barely larger than the DNA itself. It cannot be crystallized randomly. The process must be compliant with the needs of the embryo, which will unpackage this DNA into the active genome. However, this

W. Steven Ward (✉)
Institute for Biogenesis Research, John A. Burns School of Medicine,
University of Hawaii at Manoa, Honolulu, HI, USA
e-mail: wward@hawaii.edu

A. Zini, A. Agarwal (eds.), *A Clinician's Guide to Sperm DNA and Chromatin Damage*, https://doi.org/10.1007/978-3-319-71815-6_3

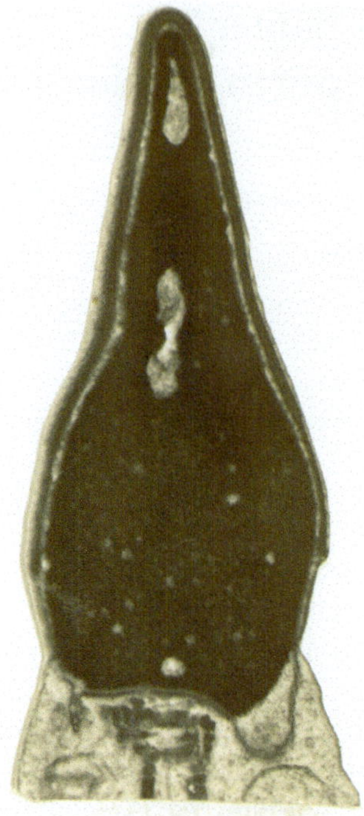

Fig. 3.1 Thin section transmission electron micrograph of a human sperm head (Courtesy of Dr. Ryuzo Yanagimachi)

crystallized DNA must still be viable. Moreover, there are epigenetic signals that must be incorporated into this compact chromatin that contribute to the instructions for the developing embryo's use of the paternal genome. Epigenetic signals are any chromatin-associated molecular change that does not change the DNA sequence. These include, but are not limited to, histone modifications, DNA methylation, and DNA attachment sites on the sperm nuclear matrix. Understanding how the 23 chromosomes are packaged in this "dark matter" requires a delicate unpackaging of this tightly wound knot of DNA strands, and several studies, discussed below, have made important contributions to our current models for sperm chromatin structure. However, they all suffer from the potential criticism that the original chromosome packaging was somewhat disrupted by the partial extraction procedures needed to visualize the structures. When it is unpackaged in the oocyte, it successfully transmits more than just the genetic information encoded in the base-pair sequences of the DNA but also epigenetic instructions for its use.

The first two chapters of this volume covered the best-known aspects of sperm chromatin structure, the protamines and histones that bind directly to the DNA and condense it at the molecular level. In this chapter, we will explore what is known about how the protamine/histone-bound chromosomes are folded into higher-order structures so that they can fit into the sperm nucleus and how these larger organizing features of sperm chromatin contribute to sperm function. Much of what is said in this chapter is our speculation based on the data we have so far. The difficult fact is that we do not yet have a strong model for how chromosomes are folded in the sperm nucleus. However, we do know many pieces of the puzzle, and some of these have important clinical applications.

3.2 A Model

We will start the discussion of this seemingly impregnable subject with a model for how chromosomes are folded into the human sperm nucleus. This is only a model, with many question marks still in place, and the evidence that supports various aspects of it will be discussed below (or, in some cases, has been mentioned in the previous two chapters of this volume). This model helps us to visualize the questions that remain to be answered in the context of what is known. To visualize the problem, let us start with a single chromosome which contains one strand of double helix DNA that is roughly 50,000 times as long as the sperm nucleus (remember, too, that the sperm nucleus accommodates 23 of these). Imagine that we were putting together the elements that fold this chromosome from a double helix into the condensed form that actually occupies in the sperm nucleus (in reality, of course, this is not the way chromosomes are folded during spermiogenesis, but this modeling helps to understand how it is condensed). The first step in this imaginary process would be to attach the DNA onto a structural component of the sperm nucleus termed the nuclear matrix [6–8] (Fig. 3.2). This compacts the DNA considerably, but not enough to make it fit into the sperm nucleus. The next step would be to condense each loop domain into a single protamine toroid [9] (Fig. 3.2c and discussed in Chap. 1). This is actually the most important step in "crystallizing" the sperm DNA. Protamines render the sperm DNA resistant to external assaults from nucleases [10] and mechanical shearing [11]. We do not really know, however, how these toroids are packaged together. We and others [12, 13] have proposed that the protamine toroids are stacked together like lifesavers, and this seems to be the most likely method of compacting toroids into the densest configuration possible. But this has not yet been demonstrated conclusively, and this part of the model remains a big question. It is also clear that some tracks of the DNA remain associated with histones. If all the DNA were packaged into toroids that were stacked together as shown in Fig. 3.2c, we have calculated that the 23 chromosomes would still be 700 times as long as the sperm nucleus. Thus, there must be a higher-order chromosome structure that folds these stacks of protamine toroids, but we do not yet have the information to propose a model for this. Lastly, several excellent publications from the Zalensky laboratory have shown that chromosomes from several mammalian species are configured so that their centromeres are positioned together in a chromocenter and their telomeres are together at the periphery of the nucleus (Fig. 3.2e). This orders the chromosomes themselves within the nucleus and can be considered the highest order of packaging of the entire genome.

3.3 Sperm Nuclear Matrix

The first step in reconstructing a sperm chromosome from the DNA strand would be to attach it to the sperm nuclear matrix in loop domains, as depicted in Fig. 3.2b. This has the practical effect of isolating the looped segments of DNA into topological domains. That means that because the DNA is tethered at either end on the

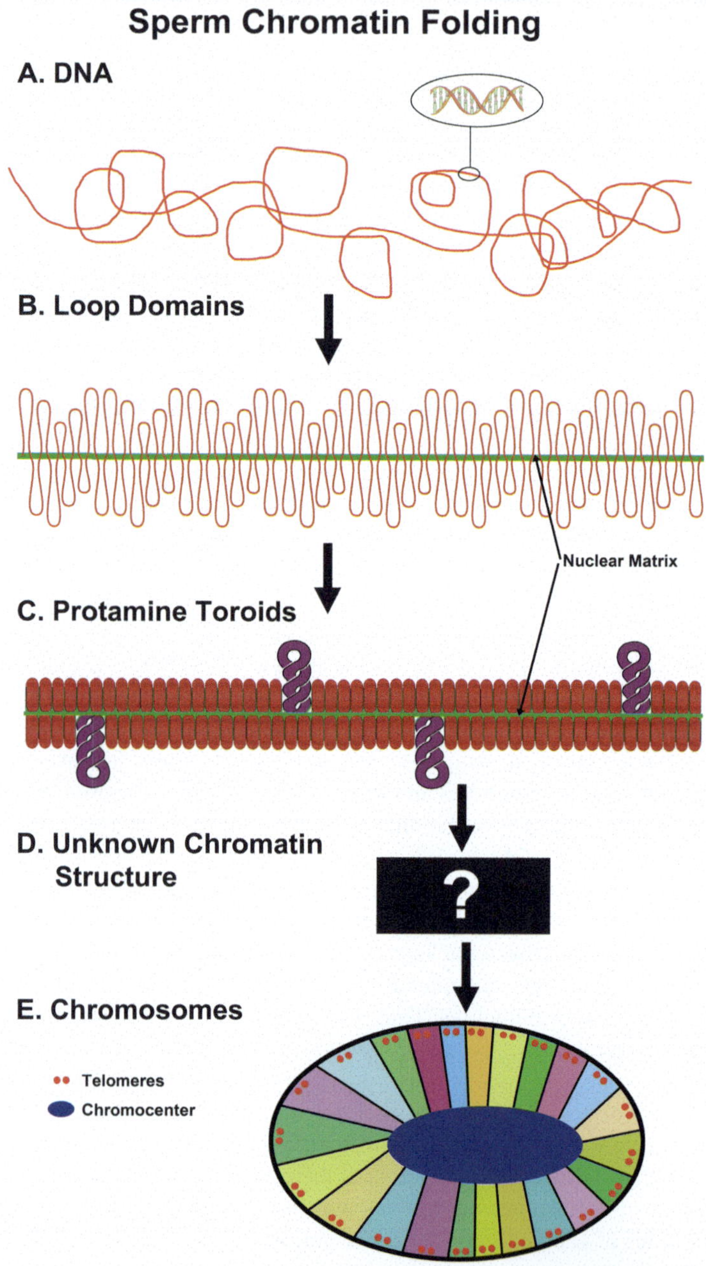

Fig. 3.2 Model for sperm chromatin packaging. This is a theoretical diagram of packaging chromatin into a sperm nucleus. (**a**) Each chromosome is made up of one long DNA double helix. (**b**) The DNA is organized into loop domains attached at their bases to the nuclear matrix (green). (**c**) Each DNA loop domain is condensed into a crystalline like toroid by protamines. These protamine toroids are probably stacked side by side. Some of the loop domains are packaged by the bulkier histones (purple loops). (**d**) A major unanswered question is how the stacked protamines are further coiled to fit into the sperm nucleus. (**e**) Evidence suggests that chromosomes occupy distinct domains in the sperm nucleus with the telomeres of each chromosome paired at the periphery and the centromeres all located in a chromocenter in the middle

nuclear matrix, if it is twisted or coiled in some way, it does not directly affect the neighboring loops. The first demonstration that vertebrate sperm DNA was actually arranged in topological domains came from the work of Risley and colleagues in 1986 [14] who showed that *Xenopus* sperm DNA could be supercoiled by ethidium bromide if the histones and protamines were removed. Three years later, we visualized these loop domains, directly, by using a technique which prepares sperm nuclear matrices with the DNA still attached as loop domains [6]. Since that time, several laboratories have verified that mammalian sperm DNA is organized into loop domains by the nuclear matrix [7, 15–17].

There are many questions about this particular level of sperm DNA organization. In somatic cells, the attachment sites for the loop domains, the so-called matrix attachment regions or MARs, are probably the sites where DNA replication begins in each replicon [18–21] and are probably the sites where DNA is transcribed into RNA [22–25]. Evidence supports the model that DNA is bound to the sperm nuclear matrix at specific sites [8, 26, 27], suggesting that there may be a physiological reason for this organization. Two possibilities exist: (i) that organization of sperm DNA by the nuclear matrix reflects chromatin functions that occur during spermiogenesis or (ii) that they provide epigenetic information for the embryo after fertilization. These two possibilities are, of course, not mutually exclusive, and neither has been definitively shown to be the case. We have provided evidence that the mouse sperm nuclear matrix is required for proper embryogenesis [28, 29] and, more specifically, that it is required for DNA replication of the paternal genome after fertilization [30] (Fig. 3.3b), supporting the second hypothesis. However, for the purposes of this discussion, either function of the sperm nuclear matrix organization, whether it be for proper spermiogenesis to form functional spermatozoa or to provide a matrix on which to replicate the DNA after fertilization, would impact clinical fertilization.

One important example of a sperm nuclear matrix function that may directly affect human fertility is its possible role in DNA integrity. We have shown that mouse [31], hamster [10], and human [32] sperm can be induced to digest their own DNA. This appears to be mediated by topoisomerase 2 at the bases of the DNA loop domains [33] (Fig. 3.3). This type of digestion of the chromatin is similar to apoptotic degradation of DNA in somatic cells, which begins with a reversible DNA double-stranded break at the base of the loop domains on the nuclear matrix and proceeds with an irreversible nuclease digestion of the chromatin. We have shown that there are two stages in sperm DNA digestion that mirror the two steps in somatic cell apoptosis [34, 35]. Using this mouse model for sperm DNA breaks, we have shown that in mouse sperm, this first, reversible double-stranded DNA breaks can be hidden by traditional methods that identify DNA breaks because the DNA remains attached to the nuclear matrix [36]. We have also shown that the single-stranded DNA breaks that occur in the second step are clearly identified by the SCSA assay and less efficiently by the TUNEL assay [34]. Though we are still in the process of linking the various DNA damage assays to the structural aberrations that each assay is thought to identify, it is already apparent that the different assays may detect particular types of chromosomal damage and that the different types of damage have different clinical implications [34].

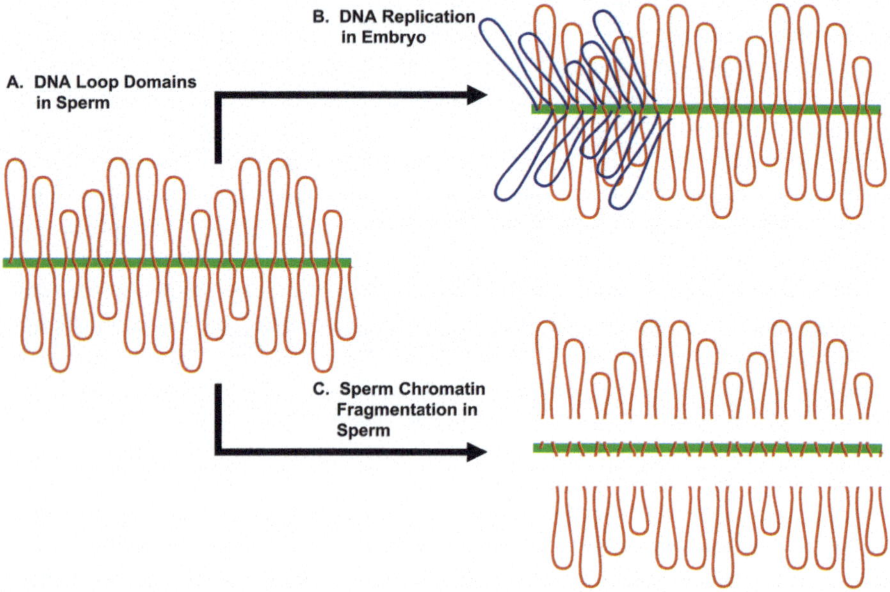

Fig. 3.3 Two functions of sperm DNA loop domain organization by the nuclear matrix. (**a**) Sperm DNA is organized into loop domains that serve two functions. (**b**) After fertilization, the paternal DNA is replicated on the sperm nuclear matrix. (**c**) In mature sperm cells, the nuclear matrix can be induced to cleave the DNA at the base of the loop domains. This suggests that the nuclear matrix may play a role as a checkpoint for sperm DNA integrity

3.4 Sperm Chromosomes

One question that has been difficult to answer is how the chromosomes are arranged in the nucleus as a whole. In somatic cells, numerous studies have shown that individual chromosomes occupy discrete domains that do not overlap [37], and similar studies in human sperm point to the same conclusion [38]. This suggests that in the compact human sperm nucleus, the chromosomes are packaged into discrete units—that is they are not wound around each other in a random fashion. In monotremes, the chromosomes appear to be ordered in a specific sequence indicating that there are clear rules for the packaging of sperm chromosomes [39]. There is also very good evidence for how the chromosomes are arranged spatially. The telomeres of each chromosome pair appear to be attached to each other in at least six different mammalian species, and they are located toward the periphery of the sperm nucleus [40–42]. The centromeres of all the chromosomes are located together in a chromocenter in the middle of the sperm nucleus [43–45]. This suggests a model diagramed in Fig. 3.2e showing an ordered packaging of the chromosomes with the telomeres pointed outward and the centromeres organized together in the center. This model is diagrammatic, only, as one would expect that many of the chromosomes would be stacked on top of each other in the thickest parts of the nucleus and not arranged side by side in a flat plane as shown.

3.5 Conclusions

We understand a lot about sperm chromatin structure, but there are still many more questions than answers at this point. One major unsolved riddle is the composition of the nuclear matrix, which remains a mystery because it is so complicated. At least one group has published a proteome of the rat sperm nuclear matrix showing 290 proteins [46]. Thus, we still do not know the major proteins that are responsible for organizing the sperm DNA into loop domains (Fig. 3.2b). Another complication is the mapping of the matrix attachment regions (MARs) and the chromosome points at which the DNA binds to the nuclear matrix. One group has made significant progress in this area [47, 48] and has concluded that there are sequences that appear to be enriched on the nuclear matrix. This suggests that either the attachment points are not rigidly defined or that our methods for identifying them have not yet been developed well enough. Finally, there is one level of sperm chromatin structure about which we have no idea. It is pretty clear that the protamine toroids must be stacked on top of each other as shown in Fig. 3.2c. But how these chromosomes are further folded or coiled to fit into the short space between the center of the nucleus and the periphery is still not known (Fig. 3.2d). We do not have any reasonable models for this level of sperm chromatin folding.

What is clear is that understanding sperm chromatin structure is crucial to our interpretations of what our various sperm DNA assays are telling us about the stability of the paternal genome. Different types of sperm DNA damage will have different effects on the outcome of ART, and a clearer understanding of how sperm is packaged will be important for fully understanding the clinical implications of these tests.

References

1. Wyrobek AJ, Meistrich ML, Furrer R, Bruce WR. Physical characteristics of mouse sperm nuclei. Biophys J. 1976;16(7):811–25. https://doi.org/10.1016/S0006–3495(76)85730-X.
2. Ward WS, Coffey DS. DNA packaging and organization in mammalian spermatozoa: comparison with somatic cells. Biol Reprod. 1991;44(4):569–74.
3. Yanagimachi R, Yanagimachi H, Rogers BJ. The use of zona-free animal ova as a test-system for the assessment of the fertilizing capacity of human spermatozoa. Biol Reprod. 1976;15(4):471–6.
4. Wolff HH, Schill WB. Ultrastructural study of human sperm acrosome during acetic acid extraction of acrosin. J Reprod Fertil. 1975;42(2):385–7.
5. Hud NV, Downing KH, Balhorn R. A constant radius of curvature model for the organization of DNA in toroidal condensates. Proc Natl Acad Sci U S A. 1995;92(8):3581–5.
6. Ward WS, Partin AW, Coffey DS. DNA loop domains in mammalian spermatozoa. Chromosoma. 1989;98(3):153–9.
7. Kalandadze AG, Bushara SA, Vassetzky YS Jr, Razin SV. Characterization of DNA pattern in the site of permanent attachment to the nuclear matrix located in the vicinity of replication origin. Biochem Biophys Res Commun. 1990;168(1):9–15.
8. Choudhary SK, Wykes SM, Kramer JA, Mohamed AN, Koppitch F, Nelson JE, et al. A haploid expressed gene cluster exists as a single chromatin domain in human sperm. J Biol Chem. 1995;270(15):8755–62.

9. Hud NV, Allen MJ, Downing KH, Lee J, Balhorn R. Identification of the elemental packing unit of DNA in mammalian sperm cells by atomic force microscopy. Biochem Biophys Res Commun. 1993;193(3):1347–54.
10. Sotolongo B, Lino E, Ward WS. Ability of hamster spermatozoa to digest their own DNA. Biol Reprod. 2003;69:2029–35.
11. Kuretake S, Kimura Y, Hoshi K, Yanagimachi R. Fertilization and development of mouse oocytes injected with isolated sperm heads. Biol Reprod. 1996;55(4):789–95.
12. Ward WS. Function of sperm chromatin structural elements in fertilization and development. Mol Hum Reprod. 2010;16(1):30–6. https://doi.org/10.1093/molehr/gap080.
13. Mudrak O, Chandra R, Jones E, Godfrey E, Zalensky A. Reorganisation of human sperm nuclear architecture during formation of pronuclei in a model system. Reprod Fertil Dev. 2009;21(5):665–71. https://doi.org/10.1071/RD08269.
14. Risley MS, Einheber S, Bumcrot DA. Changes in DNA topology during spermatogenesis. Chromosoma. 1986;94(3):217–27.
15. Barone JG, De Lara J, Cummings KB, Ward WS. DNA organization in human spermatozoa. J Androl. 1994;15(2):139–44.
16. Nadel B, de Lara J, Finkernagel SW, Ward WS. Cell-specific organization of the 5S ribosomal RNA gene cluster DNA loop domains in spermatozoa and somatic cells. Biol Reprod. 1995;53(5):1222–8.
17. Kramer JA, Krawetz SA. Nuclear matrix interactions within the sperm genome. J Biol Chem. 1996;271(20):11619–22.
18. Pardoll DM, Vogelstein B, Coffey DS. A fixed site of DNA replication in eucaryotic cells. Cell. 1980;19(2):527–36.
19. Berezney R. Visualizing DNA replication sites in the cell nucleus. Semin Cell Biol. 1991;2(2):103–15.
20. Dijkwel PA, Hamlin JL. Origins of replication and the nuclear matrix: the DHFR domain as a paradigm. Int Rev Cytol. 1995;162A:455–84.
21. Wilson RH, Coverley D. Relationship between DNA replication and the nuclear matrix. Genes Cells. 2013;18(1):17–31. https://doi.org/10.1111/gtc.12010.
22. Gerdes MG, Carter KC, Moen PT Jr, Lawrence JB. Dynamic changes in the higher-level chromatin organization of specific sequences revealed by in situ hybridization to nuclear halos. J Cell Biol. 1994;126(2):289–304.
23. Chang KS, Fan YH, Andreeff M, Liu J, Mu ZM. The PML gene encodes a phosphoprotein associated with the nuclear matrix. Blood. 1995;85(12):3646–53.
24. Ostermeier GC, Liu Z, Martins RP, Bharadwaj RR, Ellis J, Draghici S, et al. Nuclear matrix association of the human beta-globin locus utilizing a novel approach to quantitative real-time PCR. Nucleic Acids Res. 2003;31(12):3257–66.
25. Martins RP, Ostermeier GC, Krawetz SA. Nuclear matrix interactions at the human protamine domain: a working model of potentiation. J Biol Chem. 2004;279(50):51862–8.
26. Kaplan JG, Brown DL, Chaly N, Greer WL, Prasad KV, Severini A, et al. Structural and evolutionary implications of the packaging of DNA for differentiation and proliferation in the lymphocyte. J Mol Evol. 1987;26(3):173–9.
27. Ward WS, Coffey DS. Specific organization of genes in relation to the sperm nuclear matrix. Biochem Biophys Res Commun. 1990;173(1):20–5.
28. Ward WS, Kimura Y, Yanagimachi R. An intact sperm nuclear matrix may be necessary for the mouse paternal genome to participate in embryonic development. Biol Reprod. 1999;60(3):702–6.
29. Ward WS, Kishikawa H, Akutsu H, Yanagimachi H, Yanagimachi R. Further evidence that sperm nuclear proteins are necessary for embryogenesis. Zygote. 2000;8(1):51–6.
30. Shaman JA, Yamauchi Y, Ward WS. The sperm nuclear matrix is required for paternal DNA replication. J Cell Biochem. 2007;102:680–8.
31. Yamauchi Y, Shaman JA, Ward WS. Topoisomerase II mediated breaks in spermatozoa cause the specific degradation of paternal DNA in fertilized oocytes. Biol Reprod. 2007;76:666–72.

32. Sotolongo B, Huang TF, Isenberger E, Ward WS. An endogenous nuclease in hamster, mouse and human spermatozoa cleaves DNA into loop-sized fragments. J Androl. 2005;26(2):272–80.
33. Shaman JA, Prisztoka R, Ward WS. Topoisomerase IIB and an extracellular nuclease interact to digest sperm DNA in an apoptotic-like manner. Biol Reprod. 2006;75:741–8.
34. Gawecka JE, Boaz S, Kasperson K, Nguyen H, Evenson DP, Ward WS. Luminal fluid of epididymis and vas deferens contributes to sperm chromatin fragmentation. Hum Reprod. 2015;30(12):2725–36. https://doi.org/10.1093/humrep/dev245.
35. Yamauchi Y, Shaman JA, Boaz SM, Ward WS. Paternal pronuclear DNA degradation is functionally linked to DNA replication in mouse oocytes. Biol Reprod. 2007;77:407–15.
36. Ribas-Maynou J, Gawecka JE, Benet J, Ward WS. Double-stranded DNA breaks hidden in the neutral comet assay suggest a role of the sperm nuclear matrix in DNA integrity maintenance. Mol Hum Reprod. 2014;20(4):330–40. https://doi.org/10.1093/molehr/gat090.
37. Cremer M, von Hase J, Volm T, Brero A, Kreth G, Walter J, et al. Non-random radial higher-order chromatin arrangements in nuclei of diploid human cells. Chromosom Res. 2001;9(7):541–67.
38. Rives N, Wust S, David B, Duchesne V, Joly G, Mace B. Fluorescence in situ hybridization with chromosome paint probes: a novel approach to assess aneuploidy in human sperm nuclei. J Assist Reprod Genet. 1999;16(1):46–51.
39. Watson JM, Meyne J, Graves JA. Ordered tandem arrangement of chromosomes in the sperm heads of monotreme mammals. Proc Natl Acad Sci U S A. 1996;93(19):10200–5.
40. Meyer-Ficca M, Muller-Navia J, Scherthan H. Clustering of pericentromeres initiates in step 9 of spermiogenesis of the rat (Rattus norvegicus) and contributes to a well defined genome architecture in the sperm nucleus. J Cell Sci. 1998;111(Pt 10):1363–70.
41. Zalensky AO, Allen MJ, Kobayashi A, Zalenskaya IA, Balhorn R, Bradbury EM. Well-defined genome architecture in the human sperm nucleus. Chromosoma. 1995;103(9):577–90.
42. Zalensky AO, Tomilin NV, Zalenskaya IA, Teplitz RL, Bradbury EM. Telomere-telomere interactions and candidate telomere binding protein(s) in mammalian sperm cells. Exp Cell Res. 1997;232(1):29–41.
43. Zalensky AO, Breneman JW, Zalenskaya IA, Brinkley BR, Bradbury EM. Organization of centromeres in the decondensed nuclei of mature human sperm. Chromosoma. 1993;102(8):509–18.
44. Haaf T, Ward DC. Higher order nuclear structure in mammalian sperm revealed by in situ hybridization and extended chromatin fibers. Exp Cell Res. 1995;219(2):604–11.
45. Zalenskaya IA, Zalensky AO. Non-random positioning of chromosomes in human sperm nuclei. Chromosom Res. 2004;12(2):163–73.
46. Codrington AM, Hales BF, Robaire B. Chronic cyclophosphamide exposure alters the profile of rat sperm nuclear matrix proteins. Biol Reprod. 2007;77(2):303–11.
47. Schmid C, Heng HH, Rubin C, Ye CJ, Krawetz SA. Sperm nuclear matrix association of the PRM1—>PRM2—>TNP2 domain is independent of Alu methylation. Mol Hum Reprod. 2001;7(10):903–11.
48. Martins RP, Krawetz SA. Decondensing the protamine domain for transcription. Proc Natl Acad Sci U S A. 2007;104(20):8340–5. https://doi.org/10.1073/pnas.0700076104.

Part II
Laboratory Evaluation of Sperm Chromatin and DNA Damage

Chapter 4
Sperm Chromatin Structure Assay (SCSA®): Evolution from Origin to Clinical Utility

Donald P. Evenson

4.1 Origin, Standardization, and Verification of the SCSA Test as Marker of Male Sub-/Infertility

4.1.1 Origin of the SCSA Test

Thin section electron microscopy of ejaculated human sperm shows significant heterogeneity of nuclear chromatin structure between different men and within individuals [1]. Since sperm nuclear morphology is related to chromatin condensation and other nuclear phenomena occurring during spermatogenesis, it was hypothesized, as have others [2], that misshaped sperm nuclei have an altered chromatin structure. Furthermore, since the resistance of in situ DNA to thermal denaturation is related to counter ion and protein interactions with DNA [2, 3], it was further hypothesized that an altered chromatin structure would reflect in an abnormal DNA denaturation profile.

The hypothesis was introduced that if isolated and purified sperm nuclei were heated at 100 °C for 5 min, the denaturation of nuclear DNA would be heterogeneous between samples from high and low fertility humans and animals. Semen samples were obtained from three sources: (a) men of known fertility and men

This chapter is dedicated to the memory of Marcello Spano who died of a fatal heart attack in his ENEA lab in Rome, December, 2016. In 1979, Marcello invited me to his lab to set up the SCSA test. In 2000, he published a seminal paper, Sperm Chromatin Damage Impairs Human Fertility. The Danish First Pregnancy Planner Study Team. Fertil. Steril. 73:43-50. His frequent collaboration with Aleksander Giwercman and Mona Bungum in Sweden brought a wealth of valuable SCSA clinical data on sperm DNA fragmentation as related to male factor infertility. We are grateful for his excellent collaboration and warm friendship; he will be greatly missed.

D.P. Evenson (✉)
SCSA Diagnostics, Inc., Brookings, SD, USA
e-mail: don@scsatest.com

A. Zini, A. Agarwal (eds.), *A Clinician's Guide to Sperm DNA and Chromatin Damage*, https://doi.org/10.1007/978-3-319-71815-6_4

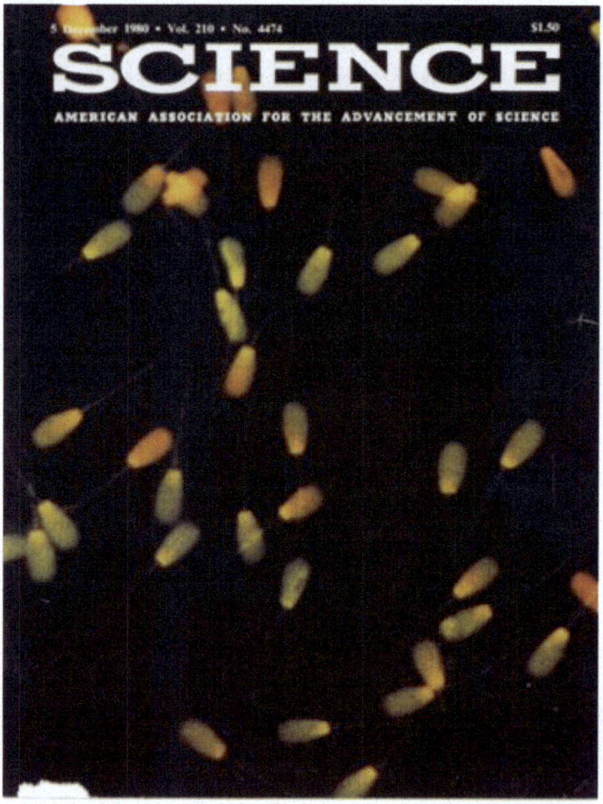

Fig. 4.1 Fluorescence photomicrograph of bull sperm nuclei heated and stained with acridine orange [4] (From Evenson et al. [4]; used with permission)

attending an infertility clinic, (b) bull semen from known fertile bulls and subfertile bulls, and (c) sperm from mice on a normal diet and diet of Zn^{+2} deficiency, a known factor required for intact sperm nuclear chromatin structure. Human and bull sperm from known subfertile donors as well as mice on a Zn^{+2}-deficient diet had two to four times greater red fluorescence (broken and denatured DNA) as seen by light microscopy (Fig. 4.1) and precisely quantitated by flow cytometry [4].

This new concept and solid data were the origin of the first publication [4] of flow cytometry-measured in situ sperm DNA denaturation as related to fertility both by men at an infertility clinic and bulls of known levels of high and low fertility. The ranking of the five bulls by their degree of sperm DNA denaturation was inversely the same as their ranking of field fertility by the Eastern Artificial Insemination Cooperative (Ithaca, NY).

Importantly, not only did the in situ DNA of misshaped sperm nuclei have significantly decreased resistance to thermal denaturation, but many morphologically normal nuclei derived from subfertile donors had abnormal susceptibility to in situ thermal denaturation of their DNA. This important point has been confirmed in various human clinical studies. For example, Avendaño et al. [5] found that in infertile men with moderate and severe teratozoospermia, the sperm with apparently normal morphology present in the motile fractions after swim-up may have broken DNA.

Studies by Wyrobek et al. [6] showed that sperm from genotoxin-exposed mice had high dose-response correlations with sperm head morphology. Studies, shown below, also demonstrated a very high dose-response correlation between abnormal sperm head morphology and SCSA data on sperm from genotoxin-exposed mice [7].

4.1.2 Standardization of the SCSA Test: Changes to the Finalized and Federal Registered Protocol

4.1.2.1 Problems with the Heated Sperm Nuclei Protocol

A high percentage of the nuclei stuck to the heated containers including surfaces of glass, plastic, polypropylene, siliconized surfaces, and others. Also, measuring whole sperm was equivalent to data on isolated nuclei [7]; thus, the time to prepare the samples was long and very technician unfriendly.

4.1.2.2 Low pH to Denature DNA at DNA Break Sites

Fortunately the two-step acid procedure used for somatic cells [3] gave the same results as the heat protocol [4, 7]. Technician time and effort were dramatically reduced. This procedure, as well as specific steps for preparation, measurement, and data processing, has been the FIXED SCSA® protocol for over three decades. Table 4.1 briefly outlines the protocol. Extensive details are published elsewhere [8–10].

Table 4.1 SCSA® Protocol

1. Prepare and measure one semen sample at a time
2. Transfer vial of frozen semen in LN2 tank near FCM to a 37° C water bath and immediately dilute with TNE buffer to ~1–2 × 10^6 sperm/ml
3. Acid (pH 1.20 for 30 s) denaturation (open up) DNA double helix at sites of ss or ds DNA breaks
4. AO staining of ss (red) and ds (green) DNA
5. Immediately place in flow cytometer and run sample/sheath for 1–2 min to establish fluidic equilibrium
6. Measure 5000 sperm by flow cytometry at rates <250/s
7. Computer calculations of data for clinical report
8. Send report to clinic by secure WEB site

Detailed protocol: ask for PDF (don@scsatest.com)

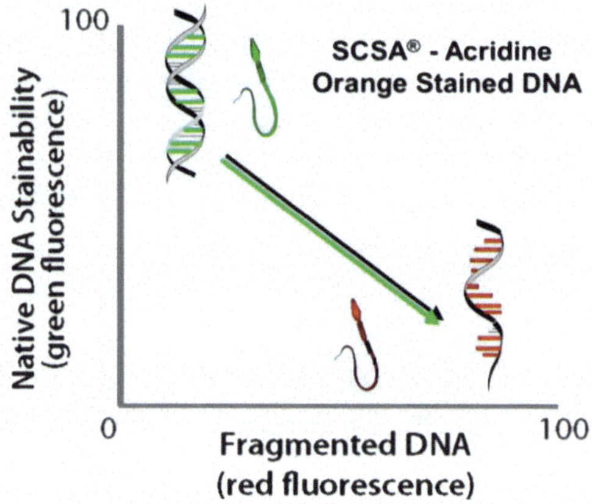

Fig. 4.2 Schematic of sperm nuclear DNA shift of staining from intact DNA (*green*) to high levels of DNA denaturation at sites of single-strand (ss) and double-strand (ds) DNA breaks (*red*)

4.1.3 Biochemistry of Acridine Orange (AO) and Sperm DNA Interactions of the SCSA Test

Figure 4.2 illustrates AO intercalated into dsDNA and stacked on ssDNA. At sites with ss or ds DNA strand breaks, the heat or acid locally denatures or "opens" the ds to ss DNA. AO stacks on the ssDNA that then collapses into a crystal and when exposed to blue laser light has a metachromatic shift to red fluorescence [3]. With an increasing number of DNA breaks, there is a concomitant decrease of green fluorescence and an increase of red fluorescence.

A very significant advantage of the SCSA test is that its marker for DNA strand breaks is the very small (MW 265), flat planer acridine orange (AO) molecule. Thus, AO likely penetrates the entire highly compact nuclear chromatin structure [11, 12]. In contrast, the TUNEL assay requires the large terminal deoxynucleotidyl transferase enzyme to label at sites of DNA strand breaks, except those breaks without a 3′OH end, and it is likely that the protamine toroid is not penetrable by this enzyme, thus reducing the efficiency of flow cytometric TUNEL testing by about 1/3 [11, 12]. Research from the lab of J Aitken [13] shows that the TUNEL assay consistently underestimates DNA damage in human spermatozoa and is influenced by DNA compaction and cell vitality. Efforts are described in using a S-S reducing agent (DTT: dithiothreitol) to open up the S-S compacted chromatin.

The light microscope TUNEL further reduces the %DFI from that measured by flow cytometry (FCM). Figure 4.3 illustrates the different potential staining sites by the SCSA and TUNEL tests.

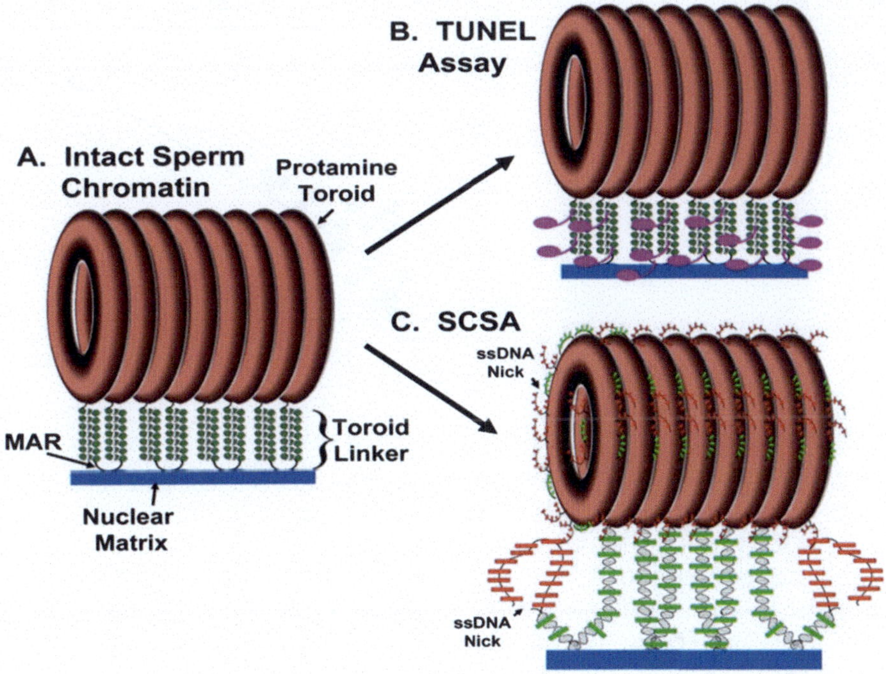

Fig. 4.3 SCSA vs. TUNEL accessibility to sperm chromatin for detection of DNA strand breaks. (**A**) Model of sperm chromatin, (**B**) TUNEL assay accessible sites, (**C**) SCSA accessible sites. SCSA = AO; TUNEL = TdTA + fluorochrome; TUNEL % DFI values 1/3 less than SCSA values [10, 11] (From Gawecka [11]; used with permission).

4.1.4 Does the SCSA Test Measure Potential or Existing Sperm DNA Strand Breaks?

Early publications of SCSA data stated that AO stained sites of decreased resistance to in situ denaturation leaving open any interpretation of mechanism [4]. The term "resistance to in situ denaturation" was later spoken of as sites of "sperm DNA fragmentation" leading to the expression "DNA fragmentation index" or % DFI, as adopted by users of other sperm DNA fragmentation (SDF) assays. A current expression is "sites of ss or ds DNA strand breaks" [12]. Previous literature often stated the concept that the TUNEL assay was a "direct" measure of DNA strand breaks, while the SCSA test was an "indirect test" measuring "potential DNA breaks." A recent review [14] stated that the "SCSA starts with an acid denaturation step and depends on the principle that abnormal DNA is more prone to further fragmentation by acid denaturation than intact DNA." Does that imply that the acid causes fragmentation, i.e., DNA strand breaks? No, all data to date strongly suggest

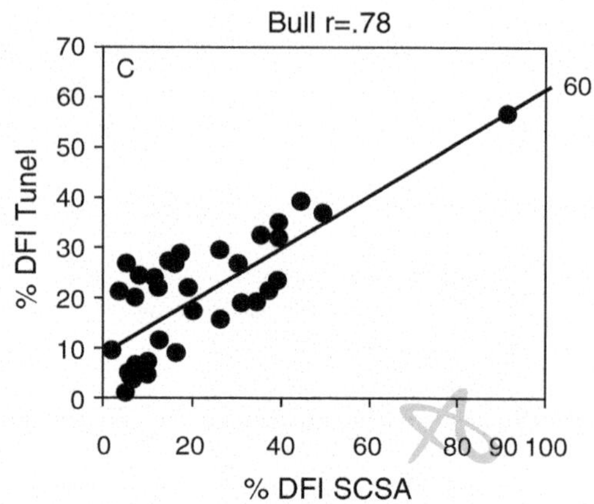

Fig. 4.4 Regression analysis depicting the relationship between %TdTA staining and % DFI staining of bull ($n = 38$) sperm. $r = 0.78$, $P < 0.001$ [16]. Note the top right dot at 60% DFI (TUNEL) vs. 90% DFI (SCSA) (From Sailer et al. [16]; used with permission)

that the function of the heat or pH 1.20 treatment for 30 s is to denature (open) the two DNA strands at the sites of *existing single or double DNA strand breaks*, i.e., "normal DNA" with single- or double-strand breaks.

Since neither heat (100 °C, 5 min) nor acid (pH 1.20/30 s) breaks the DNA phosphodiester backbone, both the TUNEL (listed as a "direct test") and the SCSA (listed as an "indirect test") are measuring existing DNA breaks *available* to each specific molecular probe. This view is supported by the following:

1. The first and likely foremost evidence needs to come from the co-founder, Z. Darzynkiewicz, of both the SCSA test [4] and TUNEL test [15]. These two tests, most importantly done by an expert in the same laboratory using the same flow cytometer, showed a correlation of $r = 0.87$; $P < 0.05$. This is a strong evidence suggesting that these two tests measure the same sites available to each specific probe.
2. Studies using bull semen samples showed a remarkably high correlation (0.99) between the TUNEL and SCSA tests for consecutive collections from a single bull [16]. However, the data suggest a one-third (60/90) less efficiency in labeling sites of DNA strand breaks using the TUNEL assay. Figure 4.4 shows data [16] on 38 bull semen samples measured by the SCSA and TUNEL tests ($r = 0.78$, $P < 0.001$). These data confirm the observations from Aitken's lab [13] that the TUNEL test underestimates DNA strand breaks.

4.1.5 Change in SCSA Terminology

The Sperm Chromatin Structure Assay (SCSA®) was named as such since it measures both *sperm DNA fragmentation* and *abnormal chromatin structure*. The major use of the SCSA test has been to determine the percentage of sperm with fragmented DNA. The original term for describing the percentage of sperm in a semen sample with fragmented DNA was cells outside the main population (COMP α_t).

Due to suggestions from human medical andrology interests that the acronym COMP α_t did not explain well what this meant, the COMP α_t terminology was changed to %DFI (DNA fragmentation index) [9]. Thus, the three equivalent values [(original): (new)] that describe the extent of DNA fragmentation are [%COMP α_t,]:(%DFI); [X α_t]:(X DFI); and [SD α_t]:(SD DFI). All of the other current sperm DNA fragmentation tests have now adopted the concept of %DFI expression of the percentage of sperm with fragmented DNA. However, in the animal andrology field, the original SCSA terms have been kept by most authors.

4.1.6 Clinical Report

Figure 4.5 shows typical SCSA clinical data on ejaculated sperm from men attending an infertility clinic. These raw and computer converted data are inserted into a clinical report that includes suggestions for clinical intervention.

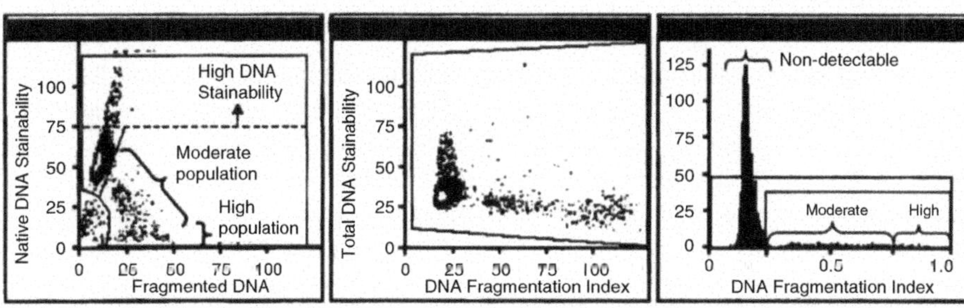

Patient	Date	Measurement	DFI	SD DFI	% DFI	% HDS
7272-87	####	1	213.5	111.6	6.8	5
		2	221.2	118.1	8.3	5.4
		mean	217.4	114.8	7.5	5.2
		sd	5.4	4.6	1.1	0.2

Fig. 4.5 SCSA test data. Top Box. Left panel. Raw data from a flow cytometer showing each of 5000 sperm as a single dot on a scattergram. *Y* axis = green fluorescence with 1024 gradations (channels) of DNA stainability. *X* axis = red fluorescence with 1024 gradations of red fluorescence (ss DNA). Axes shown are 1024/10. Dotted line at *Y* = 75 marks the upper boundary of DNA staining of normal sperm chromatin; above that line are sperm (dots) with uncondensed chromatin allowing more DNA stainability. Three levels of sperm DNA integrity: normal, moderate, and high levels of DNA fragmentation. Bottom left corner shows gating out of seminal debris. Middle panel. Raw data from left panels are converted by SCSAsoft® software (or equivalent) to red/red + green fluorescence. This transforms the angled normal sperm display in left panel to a vertical pattern that is often critical for accurately delineating the % of sperm with fragmented DNA. *Y* axis = total DNA stainability vs. *X* axis = red/red + green fluorescence (DFI). Right panel: Frequency histogram of data from middle panel showing computer gating into three categories: normal, moderate, and high DFI (moderate DFI + high DFI = total %DFI). Bottom box. SCSAsoft calculations of mean of two independent measures of mean and SD of DFI, SD DFI, and % DFI and %HDS

4.1.7 Relationship Between Sperm DNA Fragmentation Data and Classical Semen Parameters

Investigation of the male partner of infertile couples is traditionally based on the conventional WHO semen analysis, which includes an assessment of sperm count, motility, and normal sperm morphology. This analysis has, however, a limited value both as a diagnostic tool and as a guide to selection of the therapeutic procedure [17]. In numerous studies using the SCSA test, many investigators have recorded correlations between %DFI and the standard semen parameters. These stated correlations vary widely; however, the consensus is that the correlations are weak enough to conclude that the SCSA %DFI is a relatively independent parameter. The most highly correlated parameter is usually with motility. The rationale is that reactive oxygen species (ROS) activity breaks DNA and damages cellular membranes, including the mitochondrial membranes, likely inhibiting motility.

4.2 Biochemical Characteristics of SCSA-Defined Sperm Populations

Some investigators using other DNA fragmentation techniques that employ light microscopy have stated that their method advantageously analyzes single cells, while the SCSA measures groups of cells but not single cells. No, the very essence of flow cytometry is that every single cell is measured one at a time at a fast rate. Any single cell or cluster of cells can be characterized on a 1024 × 1024 grid on the computer monitor as seen in Fig. 4.5. As an example, a single cell, or cluster, may have a characteristic Y value of 540 nm green fluorescence (native DNA) and X value of 650 red fluorescence (broken DNA). Sperm with such values can be flow cytometry (FCM) sorted out for further morphological and biochemical characterization.

4.2.1 FCM Sorted SCSA Populations to Analyze Sperm Nuclear Morphology

A FACsort flow cytometer (Becton Dickenson, San Jose, CA) was used to separate four (normal, moderate DFI, high DFI, and HDS) SCSA populations [18]. Using the computer gates seen in Fig. 4.5, the sorted sperm were collected in tubes, spun down, resuspended, and then forced onto a glass microscope slide using a cytocentrifuge (Shandon Cytospin II, Minneapolis, MN) that concentrates the sperm into a small region of the glass slide.

For the first experiment, Feulgen-stained nuclei were photographed with a Nikon 800 light microscope interfaced to computer image analysis software. Three

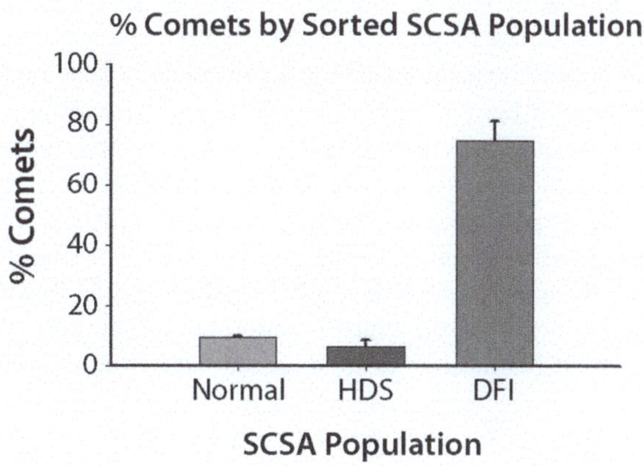

Fig. 4.6 Flow cytometry-sorted SCSA sperm populations of normal, HDS, and DFI populations. These sperm on glass slides were processed by the pH 10 (neutral) comet assay. Five hundred sperm per group were scored for the % with comets indicative of double-strand DNA breaks

measured slides/population for a total of 600 nuclei were analyzed for each sorted population. Of interest, both the SCSA normal population AND the moderate DFI population had nearly identical nuclear morphology images. Of clinical interest, these sperm may be picked up for ICSI due to their normal morphology, but they likely contain fragmented (broken) DNA.

In the second experiment [18], each of the four populations that was sorted onto glass slides was subjected to pH 10 (neutral) comet assay that identifies (a) sperm *without* dsDNA breaks and (b) sperm *with* dsDNA breaks having a pattern of an astrological comet. The main population and HDS population had few (background noise) comets. As seen in Fig. 4.6, about 75% of the sperm with moderate and high DNA fragmentation also had positive pH 10 comets indicative of dsDNA breaks, thus confirming the presence of dsDNA breaks measured by the SCSA test.

An alkaline comet assay was not run; it is hypothesized that both moderate and high %DFI fractions would show 100% alkaline comets, thus confirming SCSA measurements of *both ds and ssDNA breaks,* i.e., *breaks in the phosphodiester backbone of one or both of the DNA strands. This has also been described as DNA fragmentation* (Latin: *fragmentum*—a broken piece—thus, DNA with pieces of broken ss or ds DNA).

4.2.2 Characteristics of HDS Population: New Emphasis for the ART Lab

HDS sperm have abnormal nuclear proteins and/or other factors that prevent normal chromatin condensation thereby exposing more DNA to AO staining of ds DNA; this includes excess histones and other proteins such as unprocessed protamines [19]. Histone-complexed DNA has a 2.3 X greater AO staining than protamine-complexed DNA [20].

In a study by Zini et al. [21], samples from men ($n = 87$) attending an infertility clinic showed a significant relationship between sperm morphology defects according to strict criteria and SCSA parameters (%DFI and %HDS), i.e., normal sperm forms and both %HDS ($r = -0.40$) and sperm motility ($r = 0.32$). The observed relationship between sperm head defects and %HDS suggests that sperm head abnormalities may, in part, be due to incomplete sperm chromatin condensation.

Of importance, it is becoming clearer that a high %HDS is correlated with increased probability of early embryo-grown cessation and miscarriage [22–25]. The laboratory of Menezo [22] has been at the forefront in providing evidence on the importance of the decondensed chromatin population. Menezo's lab has called the %HDS fraction "DNA decondensation state index" (SDI) measured by aniline blue (AB) or by SCSA, which fortunately can simultaneously measure both DFI and HDS. Some gene families that are highly important for early embryo development are associated with histones in human spermatozoa [24]. "While it is well known that the oocyte can repair limited sperm DNA breaks, its capacity to improve tertiary structure is rather limited." Menezo's lab/clinical data [26] suggest that defective methylation linked to methylenetetrahydrofolate reductase (MTHFR) may contribute to sperm pathogenesis via increased %HDS (%SDI) [26].

The negative impact of high sperm chromatin decondensation (high HDS) may occur at the time of early developmental arrests up to miscarriages [23–25].

In a study of 1417 ART patients [26] where the man had an SCSA test, 77% had less than 20% HDS, 10% had 20 to <25% HDS, and 12% had >25% HDS. High %HDS values result in a large embryo loss at an approximate eight-cell stage. A very preliminary study at our SCSA diagnostic lab has seen ~80% embryo failure when HDS >35%, while the %DFI values were at acceptable levels.

It is of great interest that the negative influence of HDS on pregnancy outcomes follows closely to the curve shown in Fig. 4.7 for %DFI. Specifically, all is well with

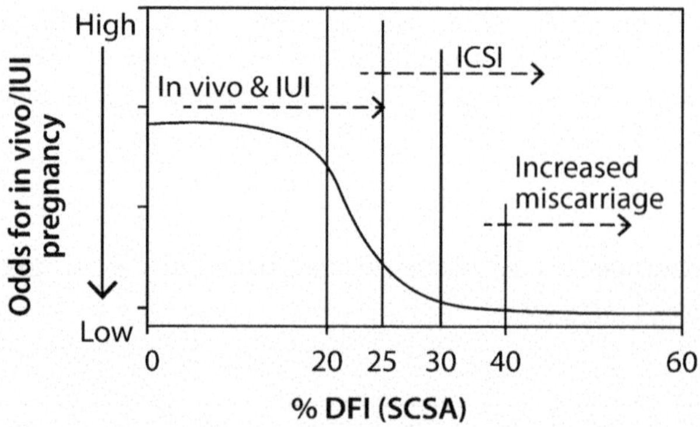

Fig. 4.7 Odds for in vivo/IUI/IFV pregnancy vs. % DFI. The curve was estimated from data from intercourse [8, 27], IUI [54] and IVF/ICSI [28] data. Below 15–20% DFI is without a known problem. Threshold for in vivo and IUI fertilization is 25%, and at that level ICSI should be considered. At ~40% DFI presents a high risk for no pregnancy and increased probability for miscarriage

<20% HDS. However, the outcomes become poorer from 20 % to 30% HDS, and at >30% HDS there is a high level of cessation of early embryo growth [25, 26].

Menezo's group have described how defective methylation linked to MTHFR may contribute to sperm pathogenesis via increased SDI (HDS). While the egg has repair capacity for broken sperm DNA, it has no capacity to fix the lack of organization found in the uncondensed chromatin (HDS) that may be critical to synthesizing the specific needed proteins for growth of the embryo.

4.3 Validation of SCSA Clinical Thresholds

4.3.1 Humans

The early SCSA human experiments suggested that the threshold for male factor subfertility via intercourse was ~25–27% DFI [8, 27]. Spano et al. [27] showed that pregnancy rate via intercourse *begins to drop* with >20% DFI [27]. Note that this represents TWO different statistical thresholds, namely, *20%DFI for the beginning level for fall off reproductive outcomes* and *25% as a statistical threshold for* in vivo *success*. Furthermore, a *third threshold is at >40%DFI* for very low success by any fertilization method and an increased level of miscarriages [27, 28]. The most common question asked by patients is "If 25% of my sperm have fragmented DNA, why can't the other 75% be sufficient for attaining a pregnancy?" More dramatically, the threshold for boars has repeatedly been shown to be 6%DFI [29]. An answer to this question is described as the "iceberg phenomena" [9]. The human threshold at 25% is equivalent to an iceberg with 25% of its mass above the water line. However, the 75% of the iceberg under the water line likely have sperm with negative factors such as pre-apoptotic sperm.

4.3.2 Animals

As stated by Barratt and De Jong [30], validation of sperm DNA fragmentation tests needs to include animal models where the breeding can be controlled to a much greater degree than for humans. To achieve this recommendation, known fertility data from bulls and boars were correlated with SCSA data.

4.3.2.1 Bulls

Perhaps the best way to eliminate many of the variables in potential female factor assessment of male fertility is to conduct heterospermic inseminations that are possible only in animal studies. Thus, e.g., if equal numbers of motile sperm from a black bull and a white bull are inseminated into 100 females, the ratio of black and

Table 4.2 Pearson correlation coefficients (r) of SCSA variables and fertility for 18 boars bred to 1867 females

	FR	APB
%DFI	−0.55[a]	−0.54[a]
SD DFI	−0.67[b]	−0.54[c]

[a]$p < 0.01$
[b]$p < 0.003$
[c]$p < 0.02$

white calves shows which bull has the greater fertility potential. SCSA test data [31] on sperm from nine bulls showed a very high correlation with a known fertility competitive index, measured by heterospermic performance (%DFI, −0.74, $P < 0.05$; SD DFI, −0.94, $P < 0.01$).

4.3.2.2 Boars

Heterospermic trial. Encouraged by the field [32] and heterospermic bull data [31], similar heterospermic experiments were done with boars [33]. Semen from six phenotypically different boars was mixed in equal motile sperm numbers in six three-way combinations and inseminated into at least three Duroc gilts per combination. The SCSA correctly predicted both the high and low fertility boars based on a ratio of offspring as deviated from the theoretical percentage. The "low fertility boars" had 3.0 times higher %DFI values than for the high fertility boars. The offspring of the high fertility boars were 4.8 times more than from the low fertility boars.

Multiparous animals. A great advantage for investigating not only fertility data on single-birth animals is to use multiparous animals that can help detect embryo loss in vivo as related to male factor.

Didion et al. [29] evaluated 18 sexually mature boars having fertility information. Boar fertility was defined by farrow rate (FR) and average total number of pigs born (ANB) per litter of gilts and sows mated to individual boars. Fertility data were compiled for 1867 matings across the 18 boars (Table 4.2).

The boar fertility rate had a high correlation with the %DFI ($r = -0.60$, $P < 0.01$) and SD DFI ($r = -0.68$, $P < 0.003$) [29]. It is of great interest to note the significant correlations between %DFI and SD DFI values and average number of piglets born (APB)/liter. Since oocytes do not discriminate against sperm with damaged DNA [34], these sperm with damaged DNA likely fertilize and the resulting embryo *implants* in the female only to be *lost later* when likely needed proteins are lacking due to a break in the DNA/gene required to supply that vital protein. Human data have clearly shown that DFI >30% are related to increased miscarriage rate [8, 27]. As stated by Borini et al. [35], high %DFI can compromise "embryo viability," resulting in pregnancy loss.

4.4 Validation of the SCSA Test for Precision and Accuracy

4.4.1 Invaluable Use of Flow Cytometry

Of critical importance for validation of any test is its precision and accuracy. Without a doubt flow cytometry is invaluable to achieve this requirement for the SCSA test. Flow cytometry (FCM) measuring of cells is highly rapid with exceptional *mechanical precision* that avoids human eye biases. Both TUNEL and SCSA tests are amenable for use with flow cytometry; SCSA has a significant advantage of being a dual parameter measurement. Thus, *each* sperm is characterized by 1024 × 1024 units (channels) of green vs. red fluorescence seen as a dot plot on the FCM monitor (Fig. 4.5). And for accuracy, i.e., the extent to which a given measurement agrees with the standard value for that measurement, it is near perfect for the SCSA test. Thus, EVERY SINGLE SPERM in a SCSA measurement can be characterized by the *exact extent* of DNA damage.

Figure 4.8 provides evidence for two important features of the SCSA test [36]: (1) lack of difference of %DFI between fresh and frozen samples and (2) the ability of setting up the flow cytometer for exact repeat measurements by the use of reference samples consisting of numerous frozen aliquots of a semen sample with about 10–15% DFI [9, 10]. These reference samples are used to set the mean green and red fluorescence values to the same exact (+ 5 channels) *X* and *Y* coordinates each time the FCM is set up for measuring samples.

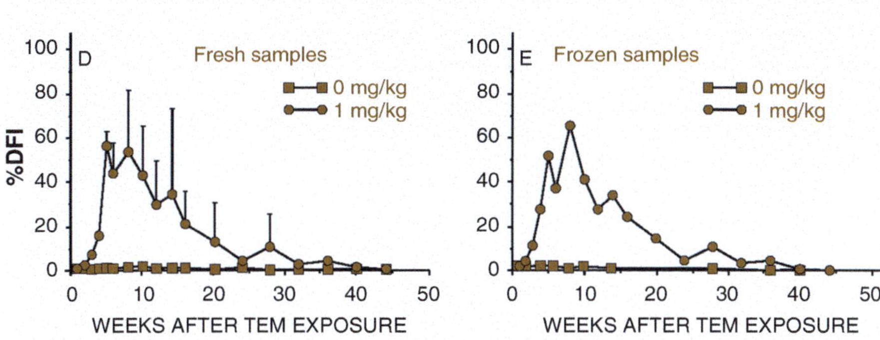

Fig. 4.8 Epididymal sperm from mice treated with triethylenemelamine (TEM) and over 45 weeks harvested with one fresh set measured by the SCSA test and a frozen aliquot measured months later by the SCSA test [36]

4.4.2 Repeatability of SCSA Data

4.4.2.1 Within Human Donors Over Time

It is well known that semen parameters such as count, motility, and morphology can vary widely over short periods of time [17]. For this reason, it is often recommended that a man has at least two classical semen tests over some weeks of time. In contrast, the evidence is strong that the SCSA test data are highly stable over months of time for healthy men [37] as seen in Fig. 4.9.

Note the consistent, unique cytogram patterns from month to month within individuals. Left column, excellent DNA integrity; middle column, poor DNA integrity with high % DFI; and right column, high %HDS and near absence of DNA breakage. Note that if the clinical report on the latter only listed %DFI, this would score as a very normal sample; however, the very high %HDS changes the clinical report to an increased probability of early embryo cessation of growth [22–26]. The CV of intra-individual eight monthly samples of 45 men was 10% [37].

Some studies have stated that the intra-individual CV for SCSA measures is as high as 30% [38]. This was a retrospective study of 282 consecutive patients referred for ART with repeated (2–5) SCSA measurements. The mean CV of DFI for repeated SCSA measurements was 29%. Thirty-seven percent of patients with DFI >30.0% in the first test had DFI <30.0% in the second test. Also, 27% of patients with 21–30% DFI values in the first test had DFI >30% in the second test. The authors concluded that with this high intra-individual variability in %DFI of repeated SCSA measurements, repeat SCSA measurements are recommended. *However*, a problem with this conclusion is that patients with an *initial value* of, e.g., 29.9% and a *follow-up value* of 30.1% would be scored as changing categories, while it is obvious that these two numbers are statistically the same.

To help resolve this problem, a new study [39] was done in which SCSA analyses were performed on 616 samples from men between 18 and 66 years of age. A calculation was performed using an interval of 29–31% instead of the 30.0% cutoff value (switch from <29 to >31% or vice versa). "When the DFI interval 29–31% was used instead of the 30% cut-off level, 12% of the subjects switched categories. Thus, in the clear majority of the subjects, repeated SCSA testing does not result in a switch in DFI category, in relation to the clinical cut-off level of 30%. This repeatability adds to the utility of the SCSA %DFI as a valuable tool in the investigation of men from infertile couples." There is a highly likely reason why the CV of % DFI is greater in patients than what is seen in non-patient donors. When a man at an infertility clinic has a high % DFI with the realization that pregnancy would be more easily obtained with a lower % DFI, the patient is often encouraged to ingest antioxidants [40], keep the testes cool [41], lower BMI values, avoid some medications (e.g., selective serotonin reuptake inhibitors (SSRIs) [42], reduce stress, fix large varicoceles [43, 44], and overall move to a healthier lifestyle. Many of the changes are known to reduce %DFI by a significant amount. And consequently,

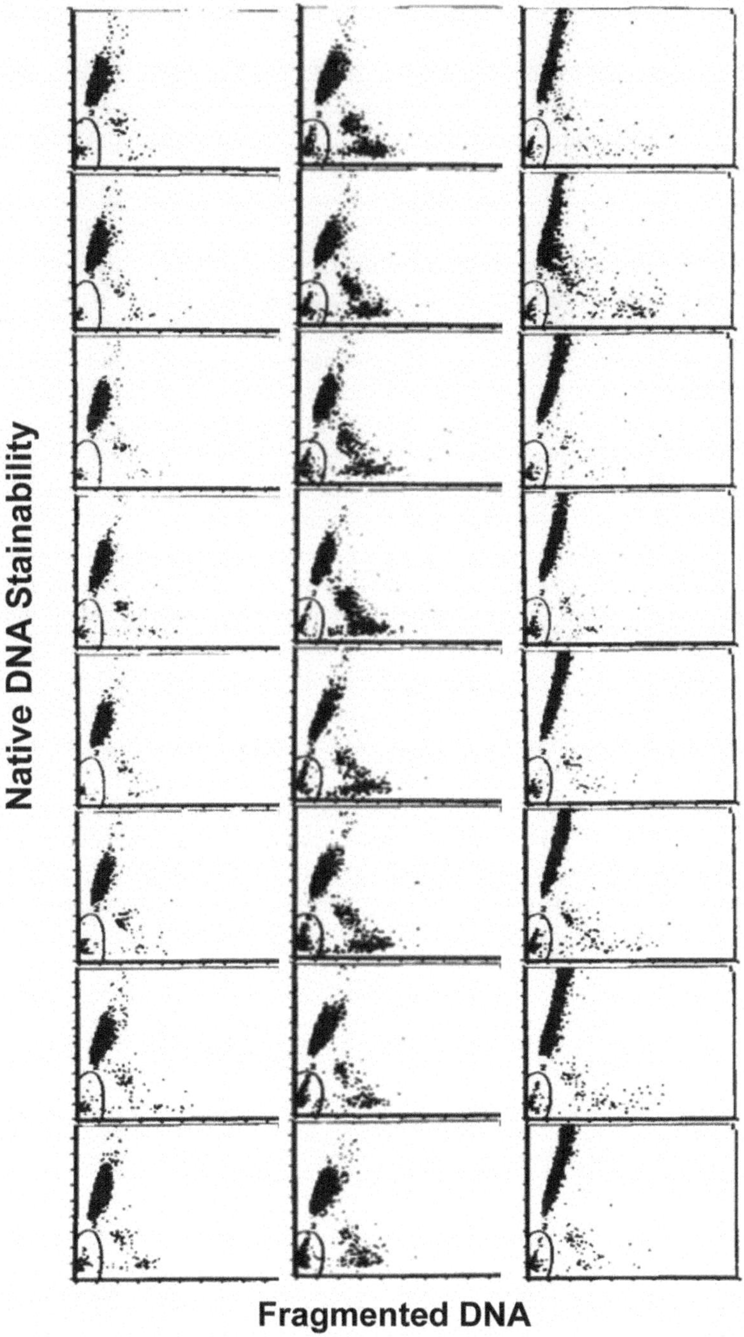

Fig. 4.9 Repeatability of SCSA measures of donor sperm over time. Shown here are semen samples from three donors obtained for eight consecutive months. Note the highly consistent patterns for each man despite a significant difference between the men shown [37] (From Evenson et al. [37]; used with permission)

there is often a greater CV for repeat measurements due to the patient and not the SCSA test.

Data on repeatability of %DFI in a single non-smoking fertile donor over 10 years (age 40–50) showed that semen parameters and sperm DNA integrity remained normal, and no trend was observed over the study period. Of interest, the %DFI was less than 20% [45].

4.4.2.2 SCSA Data Using Different Flow Cytometers Internationally on Sperm from Eight Different Mammalian Species

Now that flow cytometers are available in numerous laboratories and medical institutions around the world, it is very important to know whether multiple types of flow cytometers are compatible to measure with exacting results for the two sperm DNA fragmentation assays that use flow cytometry, namely, the SCSA and TUNEL tests. For the SCSA test, it has long been known that measurements on different flow cytometers produce the same results when using the SCSAsoft®, or equivalent, software for clinical output. In 1995, Evenson and ten collaborators in seven centers on two continents made comparative SCSA %DFI measurements of aliquots of the same frozen semen aliquots from human, mouse, rat, turkey, bull, ram, boar, and stallion [46]. Both epi-illumination and orthogonal optic flow cytometers were compared. Even with the great difference in the shape of the cytograms between FCMs with orthogonal vs. epi-illumination optics, using software equivalent to SCSAsoft showed the near exact same level of %DFI (26% and 25% DFI) (Table 4.3).

Of great importance, the overall %DFI values for the total 132 samples had correlations of 0.9886 ($P < 0.001$). This number solidly demonstrates that the crucial SCSA measurements around the world on very different flow cytometers produced with SCSAsoft (or equivalent red/red + green fluorescence) the near exact same results.

Table 4.3 Correlations between the same SCSA variables measured on the PCP22A and Cytofluorograf 30 FCM

Species	Bull (n = 23)	Rams (n = 18)	Boars (n = 28)	Stallions (n = 39)	Mice (n = 14)	Humans (n = 10)	Overall (n = 132)
%DFI	0.9788	0.9816	0.9952	0.9864	0.9961	0.9833	0.9871
SD DFI	0.9902	0.9934	0.9983	0.9909	0.9998	0.9241	0.9886

4.4.2.3 Comparisons Between Measurements of Aliquots of Human Patient Semen Samples on Three Continents

A near exact level of reproducibility is seen (Fig. 4.10) with aliquots of human semen samples shared between SCSA Diagnostics, Inc. and SCSA certified laboratories in Denmark and India. Similar correlations between international labs using the same FCM and the TUNEL assay have been reported [47].

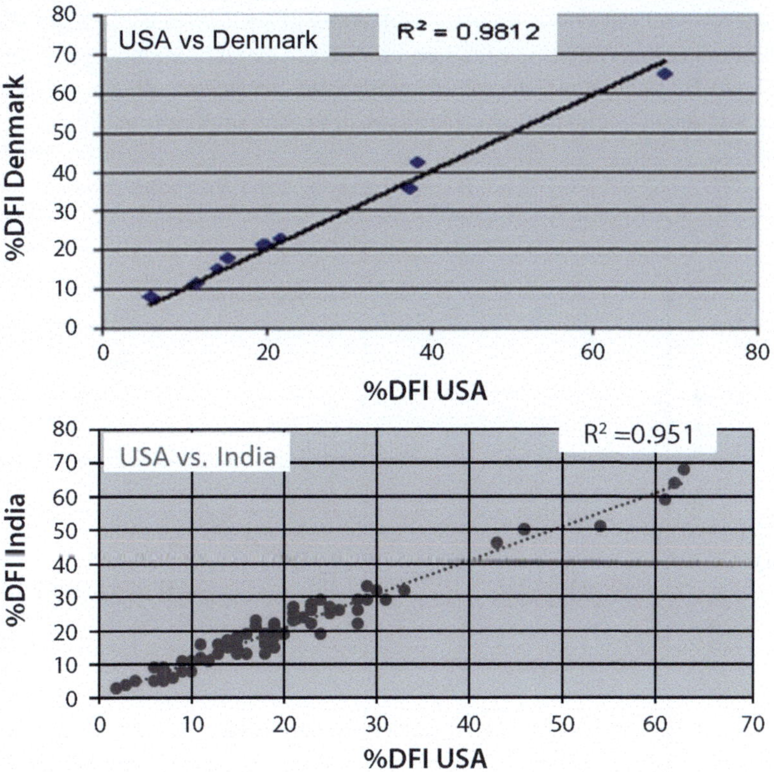

Fig. 4.10 Correlations between SCSA data obtained on three continents. Upper box. Correlation between SCSA %DFI on ten frozen/thawed human samples on two different brands of flow cytometers (Cytofluorograf 30; Ortho Diagnostics) at SCSA Diagnostics, Inc. in South Dakota. USA and (FACScan, Beckton Dickenson) at the University of Copenhagen, Denmark. (Correlation: R2 = 0.961). Lower box. Correlation between SCSA %DFI on 57 frozen/thawed human samples on two different brands of flow cytometers (Cytofluorograf 30; Ortho Diagnostics) at SCSA Diagnostics, Inc. in South Dakota and a Beckman Coulter flow cytometer in the Andrology Lab, Coimbatore, India. (Correlation: R2 = 0.9812)

4.5 SCSA Data as Related to Male Age, a Very Important Infertility Issue

While the age of females seeking pregnancy has received vast amounts of coverage in medical and laymen publications, very little has been said about the effects of the man's age on male factor infertility. Data in Fig. 4.11 show that above age 45, the man's sperm DNA integrity deteriorates more rapidly with increasing %DFI.

Both healthy donors [48] and men attending infertility clinics (n = 3026) [49] show a significant increase of %DFI at about age >45 and a decreasing %HDS. These data have been hypothesized to relate to the data in a Swedish study that followed the consequences on offspring of fathers conceiving a child after the age of 40 [49]. Sperm DNA fragmentation becoming significantly elevated at >40 age is consistent with the significantly elevated psychiatric birth defects of offspring [50].

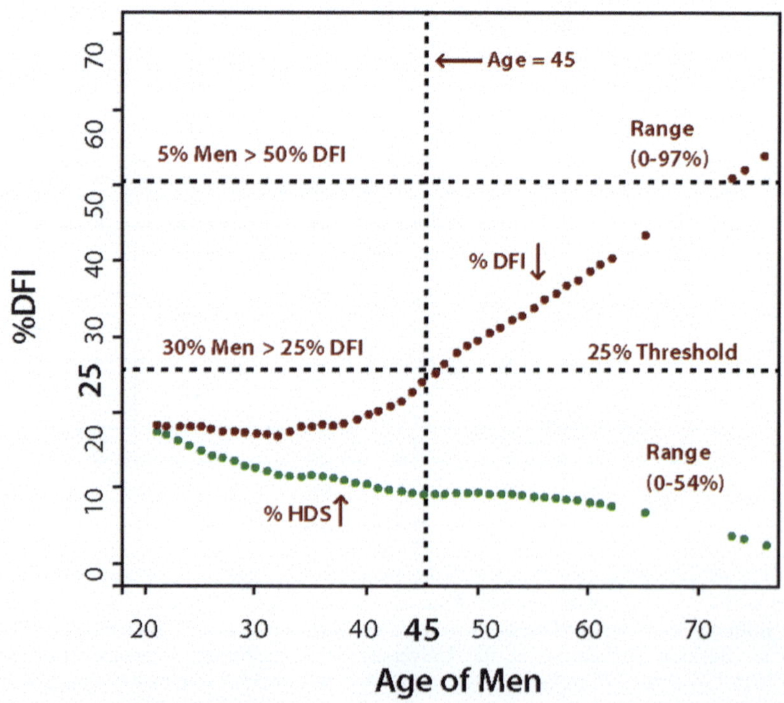

Fig. 4.11 Data on 3026 men attending fertility clinics and sending semen samples to SCSA Diagnostics showing %DFI and %HDS

4.6 SCSA Data Are Predictive of Male Infertility Via Intercourse, IUI, IVF, and ICSI

4.6.1 Pioneer In Vivo Male Factor Study

The 1980 *Science* paper [4] showed the first flow cytometric comparison of sperm DNA fragmentation between known fertile men and men attending an infertility clinic. The mean sperm DNA fragmentation score for men seeking their fertility status was nearly twice as high as the score for men of known fertility [4]. These human data were complemented with clear results (as seen above) of data on bulls and boars of known varying fertility.

The first well-executed in vivo study correlating sperm DNA integrity with pregnancy outcome was done in collaboration with Mike Zinaman at Georgetown University [8]. The SCSA test was used to measure human semen samples from 165 presumably fertile couples wishing to achieve pregnancy over 12 menstrual cycles. Any woman with female infertility factors was excluded. SCSA data from the male partners of 73 couples (group 1) achieved pregnancy during months 1–3 were compatible with "high fertility." These SCSA values were significantly different from those of 40 couples (group 3) achieving pregnancy in months 4–12 ($P < 0.01$) and of those male partners of 31 couples (group 4) not achieving pregnancy ($P < 0.001$). Group 2 contained couples who had a miscarriage. "Based on logistic regression, the level of %DFI was the best predictor for whether a couple would not achieve pregnancy." Some 84% of males in Group 1 had <15% DFI; no couples achieved pregnancy in Group 1 with >30% DFI. Using selected cutoff values for chromatin integrity, the SCSA data predicted 7 of 18 miscarriages (39%).

Shortly after the above publication, Spano et al. [27] published a time to natural pregnancy on 215 "Danish first pregnancy planners" with no previous knowledge of their fertility status. Data was obtained on 1301 cycles (838 cycles, months 1–6; 463 cycles, months 7–24). The probability of pregnancy in a menstrual cycle across the entire range of SCSA values obtained from the initial semen samples is incorporated into the drawing in Fig. 4.7 that also includes pregnancy estimates from IUI and IVF/ICSI studies [8, 27, 28, 51–54].

At 20% DFI, fecundability started dropping and became very small for values of 30–40%. Thus, the probability of producing a healthy pregnancy via intercourse sharply declined beginning at 20% DFI and was negligible when this fraction added up to 40%. As stated by the authors, "this level 'makes this individual a good candidate' not to conceive." The results of both above studies [8, 27] are consistent with the finding that sperm chromatin structure is reflective of fertility potential, which significantly deteriorates when %DFI is >30%. As stated, SCSA data is highly indicative of male subfertility, regardless of the number, the motility, and the morphology of the spermatozoa [27].

The publications of the two above studies remained for many years as the only two papers showing odds ratios (ORs) via intercourse on semen samples measured by the SCSA. These ORs of 7–8 were confirmed by independent meta-analysis [51, 52].

In contrast to the data presented in these two above studies, the 2006 (and subsequent years) American Society for Reproductive Medicine Compendium of Practice Report found no significant effects of elevated sperm DNA fragmentation by using a 30% DNA fragmentation index (DFI) threshold for natural fertilization and SCSA data (odds ratio, 1.07; 95% confidence interval, 0.39–2.93) [51]. In an independent meta-analysis [51, 52], it was shown that these two in vivo studies showed significant odds ratios of 6.54 (95% confidence interval, 1.71, 24.91) and 7.58 (95% confidence interval, 2.54, 22.67), which resulted in the conclusion that the pregnancy rates are statistically significantly higher for the group with DFI below the thresholds of 30% and 40%, respectively.

4.6.2 *ART Clinic*

4.6.2.1 IUI

A SCSA study including IUI couples was done by Bungum et al. [54] in 2007. Of great interest was the observation that when the SCSA %DFI value was greater than 30%, the pregnancy rate was a dramatically low 1.5% in contrast to those with <30% that had a successful pregnancy rate of 19.0%. These data strongly suggested that men with a DFI of >30% had a very low chance with both natural and IUI conception and should move to ICSI. These IUI data are also incorporated into the clinical interventions as seen in Fig. 4.7.

Figure 4.7 shows the very significant drop in successful pregnancies as the %DFI falls from the 20 % to 30%. The threshold for IUI and natural fertility has been set at ~25% DFI [8, 27, 54].

4.6.2.2 IVF/ICSI

Bungum et al. [54] analyzed a total of 998 cycles (387 IUI, 388 IVF, and 223 ICSI). No statistical difference between the outcomes of IVF versus ICSI was observed in the group with DFI ≤27%. In the DFI >27% group, however, the results of ICSI were significantly better than those of IVF. Comparing ICSI with IVF, the OR (95% CI) for BP was 26 (1.9–350). The IVF and ICSI fertilization rates were not statistically different between high- and low-DFI groups. More men with >15% HDS had lower (<25% and <50%) IVF fertilization rates. Men with >30% DFI were at risk for low blastocyst rates (<30%) and no ongoing pregnancies. Thus, the authors proposed that "all infertile men should be tested with SCSA as a supplement to the standard semen analysis. When DFI exceeds 30%, ICSI should be the method of choice."

A recent study by Oleszczuk et al. [28] was based on 1633 IVF or ICSI cycles. DFI values were categorized into four intervals: DFI ≤ 10% (reference group), 10% < DFI ≤ 20%, 20% < DFI ≤ 30%, and DFI > 30%. For the three latter intervals, the following outcomes of IVF/ICSI procedures were analyzed in relation to the reference group: fertilization, good quality embryo, pregnancy, miscarriage, and live births. In the standard IVF group, a significant negative association between DFI and fertilization rate was found. When calculated per ovum pickup (OPU), odds ratios (ORs) for at least one good quality embryo (GQE) were significantly lower in the standard IVF group if DFI > 20%. OR for live birth calculated per OPU was significantly lower in standard IVF group if DFI > 20% (OR 0.61; 95% CI: 0.38–0.97; $p = 0.04$). No such associations were seen in the ICSI group. OR for live birth by ICSI compared to IVF was statistically significantly higher for DFI > 20% (OR 1.7; 95% CI: 1.0–2.9; $p = 0.05$). OR for miscarriage was significantly increased for DFI > 40% (OR 3.8; 95% CI: 1.2–12; $p = 0.02$). *The results suggest that ICSI might be a preferred method of* in vitro *treatment in cases with high DFI.*

4.7 Conclusions

Now after nearly four decades of basic and clinical research with an estimated > ~150,000 animal and human sperm samples measured by the SCSA, it can be stated with confidence that the *SCSA test is well suited for testing in the human clinic. Specifically:*

- A 0–20% DFI is considered excellent DNA integrity. However, for the man with one or more abnormal WHO semen parameters, the OR significantly decreases for a successful pregnancy.
- From 20% to 30% DFI, a continuous falling off odds for a successful pregnancy by in vivo and IUI.
- HDS >25% [22–26] and certainly >35% leads to very poor embryo development, few blastocysts, and embryos arresting at about eight-cell stage.
- When SCSA %DFI is above 20–30%, there are data to support moving from standard IVF treatment to ICSI.
- Above 40–50% DFI, the odds for pregnancy are very low by any means of fertilization and with increased odds for miscarriages. Consideration may be made to use testicular sperm/ICSI (TESE) [55].
- Men above the age of 45 seeking to father a child should have sperm analyzed by SCSA since these men are at increased risk of sperm DNA damage and this is the point of age at which the mean %DFI is indicative of poorer pregnancy outcomes.
- It is a small cost, relative to many other male and female infertility tests, to take a SCSA test that may indicate the male as the prime factor in lack of a pregnancy. Such SCSA reports become highly valuable to *both* the patient and the clinic's interests.
- A recent review by Agarwal et al. [56] outlined the evolution of sperm DNA fragmentation (SDF] tests from their origin to current utility in the urology and infertility clinics and recognize that SDF has been generally acknowledged as a

valuable tool for male fertility evaluation. These authors [56] note that the latest American Urological Association (AUA) and the European Association of Urology (EWAU) have acknowledged the importance of DNA fragmentation in sperm as guidelines on male infertility. The authors conclude their review with the statement: "SDF testing should be included in the evaluation of male factor fertility along with the standard semen analysis. Any couple that fails to obtain a pregnancy within a year would gain a valuable insight into the potential that couple infertility may be due to sperm DNA fragmentation and, if so, to proceed with the recommendation to reduce SDF by lifestyle changes or select an ART procedure in part determined by the results of a SDF test."

- SCSA testing can be done at any lab that follows the precise published protocol on all known flow cytometers when using SCSAsoft, or equivalent, software for clinical reports; alternatively, most continents have labs with commercial SCSA testing, including North America (www.scsatest.com), London (www.tdlpathology.com), India (www.andrologycenter.in), Brazil (www.androscience.com), and Sweden (www.med.lu.se), and other sites may become available.

References

1. Evenson DP, Witkin S, de Harven E, Bendich A. Ultrastructure of partially decondensed human spermatozoal chromatin. J Ultrastruct Res. 1978;63:178–87.
2. Ringertz NR, Gledhill BL, Darzynkiewicz Z. Changes in deoxyribonucleoprotein during spermiogenesis in the bull. Sensitivity of DNA to heat denaturation. Exp Cell Res. 1970;62:204–18.
3. Darzynkiewicz Z, Traganos F, Sharpless T, Melamed MR. Thermal denaturation of DNA in situ as studied by acridine orange staining and automated cytofluorometry. Exp Cell Res. 1975;90:411–28.
4. Evenson DP, Darzynkiewicz Z, Melamed MR. Relation of mammalian sperm chromatin heterogeneity to fertility. Science. 1980;210:131–3.
5. Avendaño C, Franchi A, Taylor S, Morshedi M, Bocca S, Oehninger S. Fragmentation of DNA in morphologically normal human spermatozoa. Fertil Steril. 2009;91:1077–84.
6. Wyrobek AJ. Changes in mammalian sperm morphology after x-ray and chemical exposure. Genetics. 1975;92:105–19.
7. Evenson DP, Higgins PH, Grueneberg D, Ballachey B. Flow cytometric analysis of mouse spermatogenic function following exposure to ethylnitrosourea. Cytometry. 1985;6:238–53.
8. Evenson DP, Jost LK. Utility of the sperm chromatin structure assay as a diagnostic and prognostic tool in the human fertility clinic. Hum Reprod. 1999;14:1039–49.
9. Evenson DP, Larson K, Jost LK. The sperm chromatin structure assay (SCSATM): clinical use for detecting sperm DNA fragmentation related to male infertility and comparisons with other techniques. Andrology Lab Corner. J Androl. 2002;23:25–43.
10. Evenson D. Sperm Chromatin Structure Assay (SCSA®): detailed protocol. In: Zini A, Agarwal A, editors. Sperm chromatin: biological and clinical applications in male infertility and assisted reproduction. New York: Springer Sciences; 2011. Chapter 35:487–97. PDF available: don@scsa.com.
11. Gawecka JE, Boaz S, Kasperson K, Nguyen H, Evenson DP, Ward WS. Luminal fluid of epididymis and vas deferens contributes to sperm chromatin fragmentation. Hum Reprod. 2015;30:2725–36.

12. Evenson DP. The Sperm Chromatin Structure Assay (SCSA®) and other sperm DNA fragmentation tests for evaluation of sperm nuclear DNA integrity as related to fertility. Anim Reprod Sci. 2016;169:56–75.
13. Mitchell LA, De Iuliis GN, Aitken RJ. The TUNEL assay consistently underestimates DNA damage in human spermatozoa and is influenced by DNA compaction and cell vitality: development of an improved methodology. Int J Androl. 2011;34:2–13.
14. Vu Bach P, Schlegel PN. Sperm DNA damage and its role in IVF and ICSI. Basic Clin Androl J. 2016;26:15. Review
15. Gorczyca W, Traganos F, Jesionowska H, Darzynkiewicz Z. Presence of DNA strand breaks and increased sensitivity of DNA in situ to denaturation in abnormal human sperm cells: analogy to apoptosis of somatic cells. Exp Cell Res. 1993;207:202–5.
16. Sailer BL, Jost LK, Evenson DP. Mammalian sperm DNA susceptibility to in situ denaturation associated with the presence of DNA strand breaks as measured by the terminal deoxynucleotidyl transferase assay. J Androl. 1995;16:80–7.
17. Jequier AM. Clinical andrology-still a major problem in the treatment of infertility. Hum Reprod. 2004;19:1245–9.
18. Evenson D, Tritle D. SCSA is a direct measure of sperm DNA fragmentation. Abstract. ASRM Elsevier; 2004.
19. Evenson DP, Jost LK, Corzett M, Balhorn R. Characteristics of human sperm chromatin structure following an episode of influenza and high fever: a case study. J Androl. 2000;21:739–46.
20. Evenson DP, Darzynkiewicz Z, Jost L, Janca F, Ballachey B. Changes in accessibility of DNA to various fluorochromes during spermatogenesis. Cytometry. 1986;7:45–53.
21. Zini A, Phillips S, Courchesne A, Boman JM, Baazeem A, Bissonnette F, Kadoch IJ, San GM. Sperm head morphology is related to high deoxyribonucleic acid stainability assessed by sperm chromatin structure assay. Fert Steril. 2009;91:2495–500.
22. Hamidi J, Frainais C, Amar E, Bailly E, Clément P, Menezo Y. A double-blinded comparison of in situ TUNEL and aniline blue versus flow cytometry acridine orange for the determination of sperm DNA fragmentation and nucleus decondensation state index. Zygote. 2015;23:556–62.
23. Hammoud SS, Nix DA, Zhang H, et al. Distinctive chromatin in human sperm packages genes for embryo development. Nature. 2009;460:473–8.
24. Kazerooni T, Asadi N, Jadid L, et al. Evaluation of sperm's chromatin quality with acridine orange test, chromomycin A3 and aniline blue staining in couples with unexplained recurrent abortion. J Assist Reprod Genet. 2009;26:591–6.
25. Cornet D, Cohen M, Clement A, Amar E, Fournols L, Clement P, Neveux P, Ménézo Y. Association between the MTHFR-C677T isoform and structure of sperm DNA. J Assist Reprod Genet 2017. https://doi.org/10.1007/s10815-017-1015-2. [Epub ahead of print].
26. Menezo Y, Clement P, Amar E. Evaluation of sperm DNA structure, fragmentation and decondensation: an essential tool in the assessment of male infertility. Transl Androl Urol. 2016;5:935–50.
27. Spano M, Bonde JP, Hjollund HI, Kolstad HA, Cordelli E. Leter G sperm chromatin damage impairs human fertility. The Danish First Pregnancy Planner Study Team. Fertil Steril. 2000;73:43–50.
28. Oleszczuk A, Giwercman A, Bungum M. Sperm chromatin structure assay in prediction of in vitro fertilization outcome. Andrology. 2016;4:290–6.
29. Didion BA, Kasperson KM, Wixon R, Evenson DP. Boar fertility and sperm chromatin structure status: a retrospective report. J Androl. 2009;30:655–60.
30. Barratt CL, De Jonge CJ. Clinical relevance of sperm DNA assessment: an update. Fertil Steril. 2010;94:1958–9.
31. Ballachey BE, Saacke RG, Evenson DP. The sperm chromatin structure assay: relationship with alternate tests of sperm quality and heterospermic performance of bulls. J Androl. 1988;9:109–15.
32. Ballachey BE, Hohenboken WD, Evenson DP. Heterogeneity of sperm nuclear chromatin structure and its relationship to fertility of bulls. Biol Reprod. 1987. 1987;36:915–25.

33. Evenson DP, Thompson L, Jost L. Flow cytometric evaluation of boar semen by the sperm chromatin structure assay as related to cryopreservation and fertility. Theriogenology. 1994;41:637–51.
34. Ahmadi A, Ng SC. Fertilizing ability of DNA-damaged spermatozoa. J Exp Zool. 1999;284:696–704.
35. Borini A, Tarozzi N, Bizzaro D, Bonu MA, Fava L, Flamigni C, Coticchio G. Sperm DNA fragmentation: paternal effect on early post-implantation embryo development in ART. Hum Reprod. 2006;21:2876–81.
36. Evenson DP, Baer RK, Jost LK. Long term effects of triethylenemelamine exposure on mouse testis cells and sperm chromatin structure assayed by flow cytometry. Environ Mol Mutagen. 1989;14:79–89.
37. Evenson DP, Jost L, Baer R, Turner T, Schrader S. Individuality of DNA denaturation patterns in human sperm as measured by the sperm chromatin structure assay. Reprod Toxicol. 1991;5:115–25.
38. Erenpreiss J, Bungum M, Spano M, et al. Intra-individual variation in sperm chromatin structure assay parameters in men from infertile couples: clinical implications. Hum Reprod. 2006;21:2061–4.
39. Oleszczuk K, Giwercman A, Bungum M. Intra-individual variation of the sperm chromatin structure assay DNA fragmentation index in men from infertile couples. Hum Reprod. 2011;26:3244–8.
40. Aitken RJ, Gibb Z, Baker MA, Drevet J, Gharagozloo P. Causes and consequences of oxidative stress in spermatozoa. Reprod Fertil Dev. 2016;28:1–10.
41. Karabinus DS, Vogler CJ, Saacke RG, Evenson DP. Chromatin structural changes in bovine sperm after scrotal insulation of Holstein bulls. J Androl. 1997;18:549–55.
42. Tanrikut C, Feldman AS, Altemus M, Paduch DA, Schlegel PN. Adverse effect of paroxetine on sperm. Fertil Steril. 2010;94:1021–6.
43. Werthman P, Wixon R, Kasperson K, Evenson DP. Significant decrease in sperm deoxyribonucleic acid fragmentation after varicocelectomy. Fertil Steril. 2008;90:1800–4.
44. Alhathal N, San Gabriel M, Zini A. Beneficial effects of microsurgical varicocoelectomy on sperm maturation, DNA fragmentation, and nuclear sulfhydryl groups: a prospective trial. Andrology. 2016;4:1204–8.
45. Sergerie M, Mieusset R, Daudin M, Thonneau P, Bujan L. Ten-year variation in semen parameters and sperm deoxyribonucleic acid integrity in a healthy fertile man. Fertil Steril. 2005;84:356–64.
46. Evenson DP, Jost L, Gandour D, Rhodes L, Stanton B, Clausen OP, DDe Angelis P, Coico R, Daley AA, Becker K, Yopp T. Comparative sperm chromatin structure assay measurements on epiillumination and orthogonal axes flow cytometers. Cytometry. 1995;19:295–303.
47. Sharma R, Ahmad G, Esteves SC, Agarwal A. Terminal deoxynucleotidyl transferase dUTP nick end labeling (TUNEL) assay using bench top flow cytometer for evaluation of sperm DNA fragmentation in fertility laboratories: protocol, reference values, and quality control. J Assist Reprod Genet. 2016;33:291–300.
48. Wyrobek AJ, Eskenazi B, Young S, Arnheim N, Tiemann-Boege I, Jabs EW, Glaser RL, Pearson F, Evenson D. Advancing age in healthy men has differential effects on DNA strand damage, chromatin integrity, gene mutations, aneuploidies and diploidies in sperm. Proc Natl Acad Sci U S A. 2006;103:9601–6.
49. Evenson DP, Brannian J., Hansen K, Kasperson K, Christianson J. Relationships between sperm DNA fragmentation, age of donors and patients and children with psychiatric disorders. ASRM abstract; 2004.
50. D'Onofrio BM, Rickert ME, Frans E, et al. Paternal age at childbearing and offspring psychiatric and academic morbidity. JAMA Psychiatry. 2014;71:432–8.
51. Evenson D, Wixon R. Meta-analysis of sperm DNA fragmentation using the sperm chromatin structure assay. Reprod Biomed Online. 2006;12:466–72.

52. Evenson D, Wixon R. Data analysis of two in vivo fertility studies using SCSA derived DNA fragmentation index (DFI) vs pregnancy outcome. Fertil Steril. 2008;90:1229–31.
53. Collins JA, Barnhart KT, Schlegel PN. Do sperm DNA integrity tests predict pregnancy with in vitro fertilization? Fertil Steril. 2008;89:823–31.
54. Bungum M, Humaidan P, Axmon A, Spano M, Bungum L, Erenpreiss J, Giwercman A. Sperm DNA integrity assessment in prediction of assisted reproduction technology outcome. Hum Reprod. 2007;22:174–9.
55. Bernie AM, Mata DA, Ramasamy R, Schlegel PN. Comparison of microdissection testicular sperm extraction, conventional testicular sperm extraction, and testicular sperm aspiration for nonobstructive azoospermia: a systematic review and meta-analysis. Fertil Steril. 2015;104:1099–103.
56. Agarwal A, Majzoub A, Esteves SC, et al. Clinical utility of sperm DNA fragmentation testing: practice recommendations based on clinical scenarios. Transl Androl Urol. 2016;5:935–50.

Chapter 5
TUNEL Assay

Monica Muratori and Elisabetta Baldi

5.1 Introduction

Routine semen parameter evaluation is the cornerstone analysis in a male fertility workup and helps the clinician in choosing the suitable assisted reproductive technique (ART) treatment of infertile couples. However, routine semen analysis cannot reveal many sperm traits necessary to successfully fertilize the oocyte and deliver an intact paternal genome [1] and thus shows a limited value for diagnosis of male infertility. The poor predictive ability of routine semen analysis is further worsened by the high technical (intra- and interassay [2, 3]) variability and the poor individual stability over time of semen parameters [4, 5]. Several sperm markers have been investigated in the last decades to discriminate between fertile and infertile subjects, and DNA integrity appears to be one of the most promising sperm traits. High levels of sperm DNA damage negatively impact human reproduction by delaying natural pregnancy [6–8] and increasing the miscarriage rate [9, 10]. Many studies also report a negative impact on ART outcomes, even if other investigations have failed to establish a clear relationship between sperm DNA damage and the success of fertilization, embryo development, and achievement of pregnancy in couples treated by in vitro fertilization/intracytoplasmic sperm injection (IVF/ICSI) [11, 12]. Such controversy derives likely from a great heterogeneousness of the characteristics of the studies [13], including couple selection criteria and the different techniques used to assess sperm DNA integrity. Regarding the latter point, among the available techniques, the most popular are sperm chromatin structure assay (SCSA), single-cell gel electrophoresis assay (known as *comet*), terminal deoxynucleotidyl transferase (TdT) dUTP nick-end labeling (TUNEL), and the sperm chromatin dispersion

M. Muratori (✉) • E. Baldi
Center of Excellence DeNothe, University of Florence, Florence, Italy

Experimental and Clinical Biomedical Sciences, University of Florence, Florence, Italy
e-mail: monica.muratori@unifi.it; elisabetta.baldi@unifi.it

A. Zini, A. Agarwal (eds.), *A Clinician's Guide to Sperm DNA and Chromatin Damage*, https://doi.org/10.1007/978-3-319-71815-6_5

(SCD, also known as Halosperm) test. These techniques largely differ in many features including the type, the amount, and the manner of expressing the detected DNA damage, the degree of access into the compacted sperm nuclei, and the specificity and sensitivity of the measurements. Given all these aspects, it is not surprising that also the clinical correlates of sperm DNA damage can be different depending on the technique used [9, 12].

The variability of the measurements of sperm DNA damage occurs also within the same method, since most procedures lack the necessary standardization to minimize the technical variation of sperm DNA damage assessment and to compare the results among different laboratories.

Two recent studies employed different techniques to reveal sDF and its impact on reproduction in the same patient cohort, thus blunting the variability due to the study design and couple recruitment. Ribas-Maynou et al. [14] employed TUNEL, SCSA, SCD, and alkaline and neutral comet assays, to compare the ability to differentiate between fertile and infertile subjects, and reported that all techniques, except neutral *comet*, successfully predicted male fertility. TUNEL and alkaline comet assay showed the best performance, confirmed by a recent meta-analysis [15]. In addition, Simon et al. [16] reported that both TUNEL and *comet*, but not FCCE (flow cytometric chromatin evaluation, a method similar to SCSA), successfully predicted pregnancy in couples treated with IVF/ICSI. However, only large, multicenter standardized studies would be able to solve the old-standing problem of establishing, if any, the gold standard method of revealing sDF in the clinical setting [9, 12].

Here, we will revise briefly the main differences among the available versions of the TUNEL technique used to detect sDF and introduce the TUNEL/PI assay currently used in our laboratory.

5.2 Versions of TUNEL Assay

TUNEL is one of the most popular techniques used to detect sperm DNA breakage, since it is rapid and easy to perform as it can be revealed also by fluorescence microscope besides flow cytometry. The TUNEL assay detects sperm DNA fragmentation (sDF) as it labels single- and double-DNA strand breaks using modified dUTP nucleotides (dUTPs) that are incorporated into DNA by the TdT enzyme. The modified dUTPs can be directly fluorescent or revealed by secondary detection (indirect system). The TdT enzyme possesses the unusual property of incorporating nucleotides in a primer and template-independent manner; thus, it is able to label double-stranded fragments at the 3′OH ends (i.e., blunt-ended or 5′ recessed DNA fragments), as well as single-stranded fragments [17]. The access of TUNEL reagents into sperm chromatin appears to be limited by the high degree of compactness of sperm nuclei. Indeed, TUNEL measures increase in samples treated with dithiothreitol, which breaks the disulfide bridges between adjacent protamine molecules and thus relaxes sperm chromatin [18, 19]. The sensitivity of TUNEL appears further reduced when indirect revealing systems are used, such as that incorporating 5-bromo-2′-deoxyuridine-5′-triphosphate (BrdUTP) into DNA fragments subsequently revealed with a fluorescent antibody anti-BrdUTP (Forte et al., unpublished results).

As mentioned, fluorescent dUTPs can be revealed by both a fluorescence microscope and a flow cytometer [20]. Flow cytometry is an objective, highly reproducible technology and guarantees measurements based on large numbers of cells, unlike procedures using a microscope. On the other hand, flow cytometry requires skilled operators and appropriate strategies to recognize and separate spermatozoa from signals of other cells/elements present in the sample which, conversely, can be easily recognized using fluorescence microscopy.

Since the first studies employing TUNEL to label DNA breaks [21, 22], many versions of the assay have been developed, differing in one or more steps of the procedure, all affecting the measurements of sDF [23]. One of the major sources of variability is represented by the use of two types of instrumentation to measure the percentage of TUNEL-positive spermatozoa, i.e., flow cytometry and fluorescence microscopy [24]. With flow cytometry, the percentage of TUNEL-positive spermatozoa is usually determined in a test sample (labeled in the presence of TdT), using a negative (TdT omitted) or, less frequently, a positive (DNA fragmentation induced by treatment with DNase) control [25] as a reference. The measurements taken with a microscope rely on scoring brilliant spermatozoa [20] and result in about half of those obtained by flow cytometry [24] suggesting limited sensitivity for the microscopic evaluation.

An often neglected and poorly standardized feature of the TUNEL technique regards storing after the fixing procedure and before processing the semen samples. We found that fixation with paraformaldehyde modified the amount of sDF during prolonged storage at 4 °C [23]; thus, in the procedure currently used in our laboratory, labeling of DNA breaks immediately follows the fixation step. At our knowledge, no data have been reported about the effect of storing conditions in samples fixed with other reagents.

As a result of the employment of many versions of the TUNEL assay, average percentages of DNA-fragmented spermatozoa in semen of subfertile men can vary from a few points (for instance, in [26]) to more than 40% (for instance, in [27]). In the absence of a standardized procedure to which adheres to measuring sDF by TUNEL assay, each laboratory must build up its own threshold value to be used in the diagnosis of male infertility.

One advantage of TUNEL is the possibility to detect simultaneously, by flow cytometry, DNA fragmentation and other cell parameters, thus allowing us to quantitatively study several characteristics of sperm with DNA fragmentation. TUNEL-positive sperm can also be recovered by cell sorting and further analyzed for features nondetectable by flow cytometry [19]. Other available tests detecting sDF do not use flow cytometry and/or rely on partial or complete cell destruction, preventing the simultaneous detection of other cell traits. Recently, our group has used TUNEL to study, at a single-cell level, the association between sDF and (i) caspase activity and cleaved poly ADP-ribose polymerase, (ii) creatine phosphokinase, and (iii)

8-hydroxy-2′-deoxyguanosine and malondialdehyde, in order to investigate the role of apoptosis, defects in maturation, and oxidative attack in the origin of sperm DNA breakage [19]. The role of incomplete maturation was further investigated in sorted TUNEL-positive sperm by staining with aniline blue, a dye revealing the excess of residual histones [19]. Another interesting example of simultaneous detection of TUNEL with other cell characteristics is the dual staining procedure for sDF and sperm vitality, the latter revealed by a fluorescent reagent that binds to dead cells in the fresh sample in a stable manner, hence remaining after the washing and fixation steps required by the TUNEL procedure. With this novel version of TUNEL assay, Mitchell et al. [18] showed that a great amount of DNA-fragmented sperm in the ejaculate is nonviable. In addition, the same authors later investigated whether sDF in the viable sperm fraction (the one taking part to the oocyte fertilization) improved the ability of the assay to discriminate between fertile and infertile men, failing however to increase the diagnostic performance with this novel version of TUNEL [27]. Finally, coupling TUNEL to sperm nuclear staining as in TUNEL/PI assay (see below) allowed us to ameliorate the accuracy of flow cytometric measures of sDF and unveiled the existence of two different sperm populations [28].

5.2.1 TUNEL/PI Assay

Our group has been long using TUNEL assay coupled to flow cytometry for sDF detection. As mentioned before, flow cytometric analysis of fluorescent cells needs a strategy to identify the cell population of interest, and this is particularly true when analyzing human semen which is a very complex biological matrix. For flow cytometry identification of spermatozoa, the usual gating strategy based on size and internal complexity properties is not sufficient, due to the presence in semen of apoptotic bodies that partially locate in the same FSC/SSC region (FR) of spermatozoa [29, 30] (Fig. 5.1a). Semen apoptotic bodies (Fig. 5.1b) were first described in our laboratory as round anucleate elements massively occurring in poor-quality semen samples [29, 30] and provoking a heavy underestimation of TUNEL measures of sDF if they are not excluded from the flow cytometric analysis [28] (Fig. 5.2). Since apoptotic bodies do not or poorly contain chromatin, staining semen samples with a nuclear dye (such as propidium iodide (PI)) and gating the events that simultaneously locate in the FR region and stain with PI guarantee the exclusion of every non-sperm element (somatic and immature germ cells and apoptotic bodies) present in semen (Fig. 5.1). Recently, it has been demonstrated that this gating strategy includes all spermatozoa present in the sample, as the sperm number obtained by scoring PI-stained events in the FR region overlaps with the number of sperm counted in the analyzed sample by routine methods, indicating that the gated spermatozoa are representative of the entire ejaculate [31]. The TUNEL/PI version of TUNEL shows good precision (intra-assay coefficient of variation <5%, [23]) and is currently used for the clinical service of sDF determination and for research purposes in our laboratory. A scheme of TUNEL/PI assay is shown in Fig. 5.3.

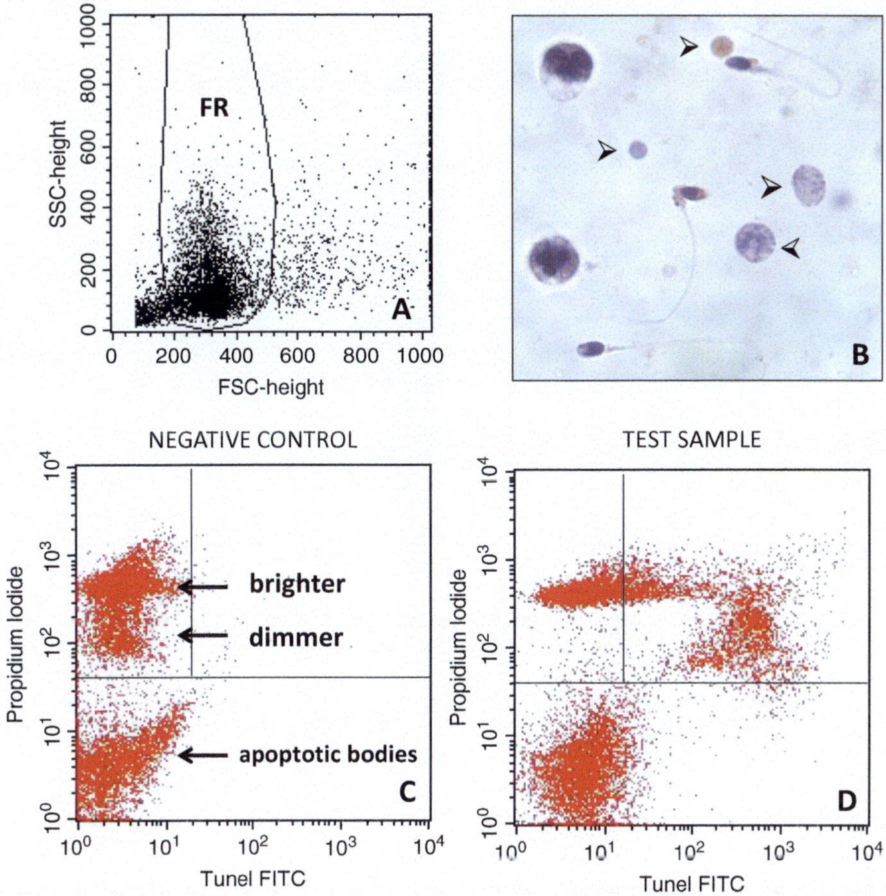

Fig. 5.1 (**a**) Image of a semen sample after smearing and staining with May-Grunwald Giemsa. Note that apoptotic bodies (➢) can have a similar size to sperm heads. (**b**) FSC/SSC dot plot of a semen sample. FR region excludes debris and large cells and includes apoptotic bodies and spermatozoa. (**c**, **d**) TUNEL/PI dot plots depicting the events of FR region in the negative control (**c**) and in the test sample (**d**). After exclusion of apoptotic bodies, a vertical marker is set in the negative control and then translated to the test sample for determination of the percentage of sDF. Note that PI staining separates apoptotic bodies from spermatozoa and brighter and dimmer populations within spermatozoa

The clinical usefulness of a biological parameter also depends on its stability over time in one individual. SDF shows an average intraindividual coefficient of variation (i-i CV) around 10–30%, when assessed by both SCSA [32, 33] and TUNEL [34]. By using TUNEL/PI assay, when sDF determination was repeated within 90 days or 1 year, we found an average i-i CV of, respectively, 9.2 ± 8.6% ($n = 25$) and 12.9 ± 12.7% ($n = 53$) which resulted lower than that of any conventional semen parameter [35]. The lower intraindividual variability of sDF found in our study with respect to previous ones could be explained by the exclusion of patients

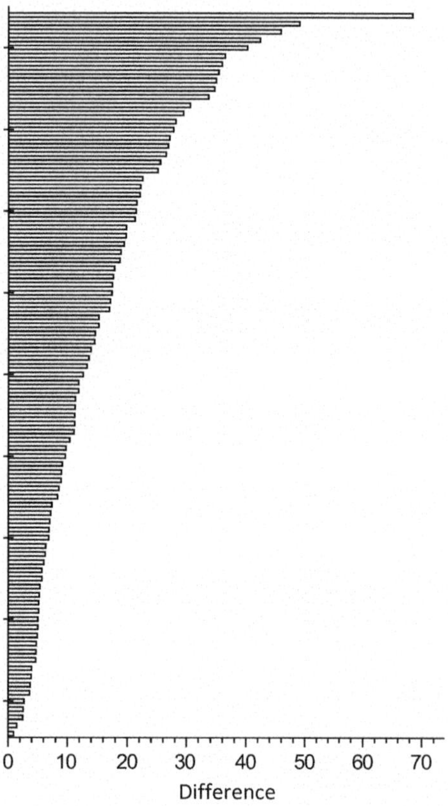

Fig. 5.2 Differences between the percentages of sDF calculated by TUNEL/PI and TUNEL assay (respectively, excluding and including semen apoptotic bodies from flow cytometric analysis of sDF) in 89 patients

presenting any conditions known to affect sDF (for instance, treatment with antibiotics or high fever [36, 37]). In addition, the exclusion of semen apoptotic bodies, highly correlating to poor semen parameters, might render sDF values more independent from semen quality, thus decreasing the variability of the percentages of DNA-fragmented sperm.

5.2.2 *Brighter and Dimmer Sperm Populations*

Staining semen samples after fixation for TUNEL/PI assay unveiled the occurrence of two sperm populations, differing for the intensity of PI staining and thus indicated as PI dimmer and PI brighter populations [28]. These two sperm populations show many other differences, and, from the beginning, we suspected that they could have also a different clinical meaning. PI dimmer sperm are all dead [38] and DNA fragmented [28], whereas the brighter population contains both live and dead [38] and both fragmented and not fragmented sperm [28]. Recently, we also found that the origin of sDF can be different in the two populations [19]. Indeed, DNA

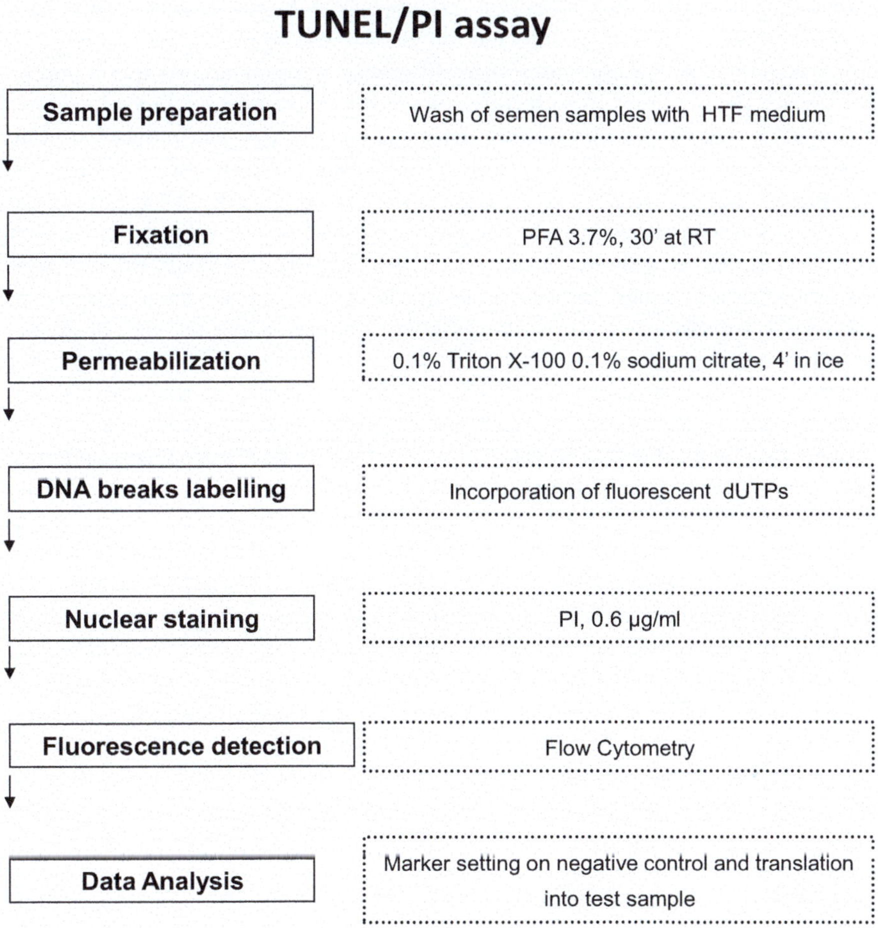

Fig. 5.3 Scheme of the procedure of TUNEL/PI assay. *HTF* human tubal fluid, *PFA* paraformaldehyde, *PI* propidium iodide

breakage in the dimmer and in the dead brighter sperm appears to derive mainly from apoptotic processes occurring in the testis [19]. Conversely, the fraction of live DNA-fragmented sperm in the brighter population can be attributed to oxidative attack, possibly occurring during the transit through the male genital tracts [19]. This finding suggests that the brighter fraction is a more focused target than total sDF for testing the ability of antioxidant therapies to decrease the amount of DNA damage in infertile patients [19]. Originally, the lower staining of PI-dimmer sperm seemed to be caused by the loss of chromatin fragments following the apoptotic DNA cleavage [31]; however, the two sperm populations cannot be more distinguished after a sharp nuclear decondensation, indicating that a similar DNA content occurs in dimmer and brighter spermatozoa (Forte et al., unpublished results). A super compacted status of chromatin, possibly due to the apoptotic process generating sDF in this population [19, 39], appears to be responsible for the hampered access of nuclear dyes into the nuclei of these spermatozoa (Forte et al., unpublished results). Another interesting difference between the two sperm populations regards the relationship with conventional semen parameters. Indeed, whereas dimmer sDF sharply correlates with abnormal morphology and reduced motility and sperm count, brighter sDF is completely independent from semen quality [28]. This finding suggests that the weak association between sperm DNA damage and conventional semen parameters reported by many studies [40–42] is driven by dimmer sDF and that the brighter fraction of sDF is the one that could provide additional information on male fertility status in addition to routine semen analysis.

Recently, we evaluated sDF in the brighter, dimmer, and total (i.e., brighter + dimmer) sperm population in 86 subjects of proven fertility and 348 male partners of infertile couples attending our clinic to perform routine semen analysis [35]. Since this type of patient cohort could include up to 40% of fertile men [43], we could not establish a true sDF threshold for discrimination between fertile and infertile men; however, we could compare the ability to predict male fertility status in the three fractions of sDF. We found that all the fractions of sDF showed greater median values in patients (total, 43.9[33.0–55.7]%; brighter, 24.4[17.7–32.4]%; dimmer, 15.4[10.0–25.4]%) than in fertile men (total, 28.9[23.1–39.6]%; brighter, 17.0 [12.3–23.3]%; dimmer, 10.8[7.1–17.0]%) and discriminated the two groups of subjects [35]. However, after matching fertile men and patients for conventional semen parameters and age, dimmer fraction completely lost its predictive ability, unlike the brighter fraction [35]. This finding indicates that the predictive ability of dimmer sDF depends on the poorer semen quality and older age of patients, whereas the predictive power of brighter sDF is independent from these confounding variables [35]. After matching, it was observed that, at high values of total sDF, the brighter fraction is a better predictor of male fertility status than total sDF [35]. Such finding can be explained by the different contribution of brighter and dimmer populations to total sDF, in patients and fertile men. Whereas in the latter, the high values of sDF were mainly due to the dimmer spermatozoa (i.e., those ones that do not participate in the fertilization process as they are all dead), in the former, brighter and dimmer spermatozoa contributed equally to the total sDF (Fig. 5.4). As a consequence, the brighter sDF is able to still discriminate between fertile men and patients with similar age and semen parameters, even in the case that they exhibited equal amounts of total sDF [35].

TUNEL/PI assay was recently used to investigate the effect of sperm selection with density gradient centrifugation (DGC) on DNA damage and on pregnancy rate in infertile couples treated by IVF/ICSI [44]. We found that in about 45% of patients, DGC is associated with an increased level of DNA damage and subsequently reduced probability of pregnancy (50% lower than those subjects where DNA damage induction does not occur following DGC) (OR = 3.12; 95% CI, 1.05–9.27; $p = 0.041$, after adjustment for female factor, female and male age, and female BMI) [44]. In this study, we used brighter sDF to evaluate the variation of DNA damage during DGC as the results are more sensitive than the total fraction in detecting the increases of sDF when it occurs [44]. Indeed, brighter sDF is not affected by the

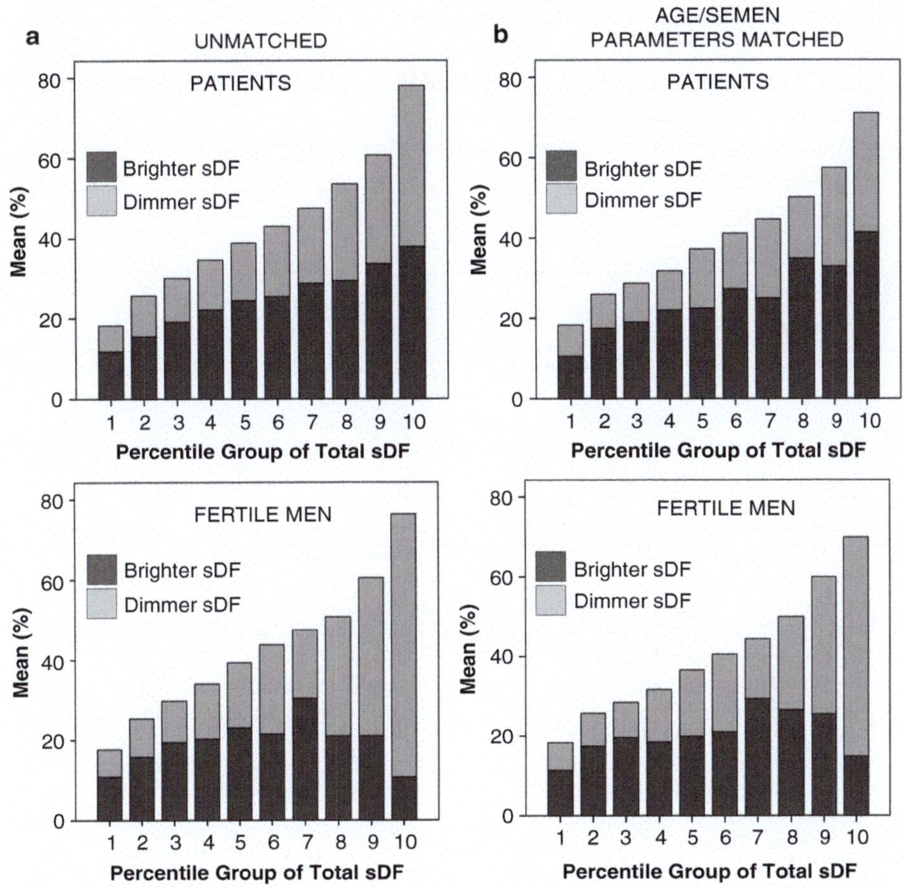

Fig. 5.4 Contribution of brighter and dimmer fractions to total values of sDF in fertile men and patients. Percentage of total sDF levels in (**a**) unmatched and (**b**) age- and semen parameter-matched fertile men (bottom) and patients (top) are expressed as deciles (With permission from Muratori et al. [35])

decrease of sDF due to elimination of dead and DNA-fragmented sperm of the dimmer population during sperm selection [28, 38, 44].

5.3 Concluding Remarks

TUNEL is a popular method used to detect sDF, as it is rapid and easy to execute. However, many variants of this assay make TUNEL results difficult to compare among studies. One major advantage of TUNEL is the possibility to be detected by flow cytometry, adding statistical robustness to the measurements, and to be coupled with the detection of other cell features. In particular, the TUNEL/PI version improves the accuracy of the sDF measurements with flow cytometry and distinguishes sDF in two fractions, brighter and dimmer. Detecting sDF in the brighter fraction appears more accurate and sensitive in identifying fertile/infertile subjects and in revealing those patients undergoing an increase of DNA damage during sperm selection by DGC with respect to the evaluation of the total TUNEL-positive sperm population.

References

1. Muratori M, Marchiani S, Tamburrino L, Forti G, Luconi M, Baldi E. Markers of human sperm functions in the ICSI era. Front Biosci (Landmark Ed). 2011;16:1344–63.
2. Filimberti E, Degl'Innocenti S, Borsotti M, Quercioli M, Piomboni P, Natali I, et al. High variability in results of semen analysis in andrology laboratories in Tuscany (Italy): the experience of an external quality control (EQC) programme. Andrology. 2013;1:401–7. https://doi.org/10.1111/j.2047-2927.2012.00042.x.
3. World Health Organization. WHO laboratory manual for the examination and processing of human semen. 5th ed. Geneva: World Health Organization; 2010.
4. Alvarez C, Castilla JA, Martínez L, Ramírez JP, Vergara F, Gaforio JJ. Biological variation of seminal parameters in healthy subjects. Hum Reprod. 2003;18:2082–8.
5. Keel BA. Within- and between-subject variation in semen parameters in infertile men and normal semen donors. Fertil Steril. 2006;85:128–34.
6. Evenson DP, Jost LK, Marshall D, Zinaman MJ, Clegg E, Purvis K, et al. Utility of the sperm chromatin structure assay as a diagnostic and prognostic tool in the human fertility clinic. Hum Reprod. 1999;14:1039–49.
7. Spanò M, Bonde JP, Hjøllund HI, Kolstad HA, Cordelli E, Leter G. Sperm chromatin damage impairs human fertility. The Danish First Pregnancy Planner Study Team. Fertil Steril. 2000;73:43–50.
8. Giwercman A, Lindstedt L, Larsson M, Bungum M, Spano M, Levine RJ, et al. Sperm chromatin structure assay as an independent predictor of fertility in vivo: a case-control study. Int J Androl. 2010;33:e221–7. https://doi.org/10.1111/j.1365-2605.2009.00995.x.
9. Robinson L, Gallos ID, Conner SJ, Rajkhowa M, Miller D, Lewis S, et al. The effect of sperm DNA fragmentation on miscarriage rates: a systematic review and meta-analysis. Hum Reprod. 2012;27:2908–17. https://doi.org/10.1093/humrep/des261.
10. Zhao J, Zhang Q, Wang Y, Li Y. Whether sperm deoxyribonucleic acid fragmentation has an effect on pregnancy and miscarriage after in vitro fertilization/intracytoplasmic sperm injection: a systematic review and meta-analysis. Fertil Steril. 2014;102:998–1005.e8. https://doi.org/10.1016/j.fertnstert.2014.06.033.
11. Tamburrino L, Marchiani S, Montoya M, Elia Marino F, Natali I, Cambi M, et al. Mechanisms and clinical correlates of sperm DNA damage. Asian J Androl. 2012;14:24–31. https://doi.org/10.1038/aja.2011.59.
12. Simon L, Zini A, Dyachenko A, Ciampi A, Carrell DT. A systematic review and meta-analysis to determine the effect of sperm DNA damage on in vitro fertilization and intracytoplasmic sperm injection outcome. Asian J Androl. 2016. https://doi.org/10.4103/1008-682X.182822.
13. Zini A. Are sperm chromatin and DNA defects relevant in the clinic? Syst Biol Reprod Med. 2011;57:78–85. https://doi.org/10.3109/19396368.2010.515704. Epub 2011 Jan 6
14. Ribas-Maynou J, García-Peiró A, Fernández-Encinas A, Abad C, Amengual MJ, Prada E, et al. Comprehensive analysis of sperm DNA fragmentation by five different assays: TUNEL assay, SCSA, SCD test and alkaline and neutral Comet assay. Andrology. 2013;1:715–22. https://doi.org/10.1111/j.2047-2927.2013.00111.x.

15. Cui ZL, Zheng DZ, Liu YH, Chen LY, Lin DH, Lan F-H. Diagnostic accuracies of the TUNEL, SCD, and Comet based sperm DNA fragmentation assays for male infertility: a meta-analysis study. Clin Lab. 2015;61:525–35.
16. Simon L, Liu L, Murphy K, Ge S, Hotaling J, Aston KI, et al. Comparative analysis of three sperm DNA damage assays and sperm nuclear protein content in couples undergoing assisted reproduction treatment. Hum Reprod. 2014;29:904–17. https://doi.org/10.1093/humrep/deu040.
17. Manicardi GC, Tombacco A, Bizzaro D, Bianchi U, Bianchi PG, Sakkas D. DNA strand breaks in ejaculated human spermatozoa: comparison of susceptibility to the nick translation and terminal transferase assays. Histochem J. 1998;30:33–9.
18. Mitchell LA, De Iuliis GN, Aitken RJ. The TUNEL assay consistently underestimates DNA damage in human spermatozoa and is influenced by DNA compaction and cell vitality: development of an improved methodology. Int J Androl. 2011;34:2–13. https://doi.org/10.1111/j.1365-2605.2009.01042.x.
19. Muratori M, Tamburrino L, Marchiani S, Cambi M, Olivito B, Azzari C, et al. Investigation on the origin of sperm DNA fragmentation: role of apoptosis, immaturity and oxidative stress. Mol Med. 2015;21:109–22. https://doi.org/10.2119/molmed.2014.00158.
20. Domınguez-Fandos D, Camejo MI, Ballesca JL, Oliva R. Human sperm DNA fragmentation: correlation of TUNEL results as assessed by flow cytometry and optical microscopy. Cytometry A. 2007;71A:1011–8.
21. Ausubel MF, Brent R, Kingston RE, Moore DD, Seidman JG, Smith JA, et al. Short protocols in molecular biology. 2nd ed. New York: Greene Publishing Association and Wiley; 1992.
22. Gorczyca W, Traganos F, Jesionowska H, Darzynkiewicz Z. Presence of DNA strand breaks and increased sensitivity of DNA in situ to denaturation in abnormal human sperm cells: analogy to apoptosis of somatic cells. Exp Cell Res. 1993;207:202–5.
23. Muratori M, Tamburrino L, Tocci V, Costantino A, Marchiani S, Giachini C, et al. Small variations in crucial steps of TUNEL assay coupled to flow cytometry greatly affect measures of sperm DNA fragmentation. J Androl. 2010;31:336–45. https://doi.org/10.2164/jandrol.109.008508.
24. Muratori M, Tamburrino L, Marchiani S, Guido C, Forti G, Baldi E. Critical aspects of detection of sperm DNA fragmentation by TUNEL/flow cytometry. Syst Biol Reprod Med. 2010;56:277–85. https://doi.org/10.3109/19396368.2010.489660.
25. Sharma R, Masaki J, Agarwal A. Sperm DNA fragmentation analysis using the TUNEL assay. Methods Mol Biol. 2013;927:121–36.
26. Younglai EV, Holt D, Brown P, Jurisicova A, Casper RF. Sperm swim-up techniques and DNA fragmentation. Hum Reprod. 2001;16:1950–3.
27. Aitken RJ, De Iuliis GN, Finnie JM, Hedges A, McLachlan RI. Analysis of the relationships between oxidative stress, DNA damage and sperm vitality in a patient population: development of diagnostic criteria. Hum Reprod. 2010;25:2415–26. https://doi.org/10.1093/humrep/deq214.
28. Muratori M, Marchiani S, Tamburrino L, Tocci V, Failli P, Forti G, et al. Nuclear staining identifies two populations of human sperm with different DNA fragmentation extent and relationship with semen parameters. Hum Reprod. 2008;23:1035–43. https://doi.org/10.1093/humrep/den058.
29. Muratori M, Porazzi I, Luconi M, Marchiani S, Forti G, Baldi E. AnnexinV binding and merocyanine staining fail to detect human sperm capacitation. J Androl. 2004;25:797–810.
30. Marchiani S, Tamburrino L, Maoggi A, Vannelli GB, Forti G, Baldi E, et al. Characterization of M540 bodies in human semen: evidence that they are apoptotic bodies. Mol Hum Reprod. 2007;13:621–31.
31. Marchiani S, Tamburrino L, Olivito B, Betti L, Azzari C, Forti G, et al. Characterization and sorting of flow cytometric populations in human semen. Andrology. 2014;2:394–401. https://doi.org/10.1111/j.2047-2927.2014.00208.x.

32. Erenpreiss J, Bungum M, Spano M, Elzanaty S, Orbidans J, Giwercman A. Intraindividual variation in sperm chromatin structure assay parameters in men from infertile couples: clinical implications. Hum Reprod. 2006;21:2061–4.
33. Oleszczuk K, Giwercman A, Bungum M. Intra-individual variation of the sperm chromatin structure assay DNA fragmentation index in men from infertile couples. Hum Reprod. 2011;26:3244–8.
34. Sergerie M, Laforest G, Boulanger K, Bissonnette F, Bleau G. Longitudinal study of sperm DNA fragmentation as measured by terminal uridine nick end–labelling assay. Hum Reprod. 2005;20:1921–7.
35. Muratori M, Marchiani S, Tamburrino L, Cambi M, Lotti F, Natali I, et al. DNA fragmentation in brighter sperm predicts male fertility independently from age and semen parameters. Fertil Steril. 2015;104:582–90.e4. https://doi.org/10.1016/j.fertnstert.2015.06.005.
36. Sergerie M, Mieusset R, Croute F, Daudin M, Bujan L. High risk of temporary alteration of semen parameters after recent acute febrile illness. Fertil Steril. 2007;88:970.e1–7.
37. Evenson DP, Jost LK, Corzett M, Balhorn R. Characteristics of human sperm chromatin structure following an episode of influenza and high fever: a case study. J Androl. 2000;21:739–46.
38. Marchiani S, Tamburrino L, Giuliano L, Nosi D, Sarli V, Gandini L, et al. Sum01-ylation of human spermatozoa and its relationship with semen quality. Int J Androl. 2011;34:581–93. https://doi.org/10.1111/j.1365-2605.2010.01118.x.
39. Sakkas D, Seli E, Bizzaro D, Tarozzi N, Manicardi GC. Abnormal spermatozoa in the ejaculate: abortive apoptosis and faulty nuclear remodelling during spermatogenesis. Reprod Biomed Online. 2003;7:428–32.
40. Oosterhuis GJ, Mulder AB, Kalsbeek-Batenburg E, Lambalk CB, Schoemaker J, et al. Measuring apoptosis in human spermatozoa: a biological assay for semen quality? Fertil Steril. 2000;74:245–50.
41. Irvine DS, Twigg JP, Gordon EL, Fulton N, Milne PA, Aitken RJ. DNA integrity in human spermatozoa: relationships with semen quality. J Androl. 2000;21:33–44.
42. Saleh RA, Agarwal A, Nada EA, El-Tonsy MH, Sharma RK, Meyer A, Nelson DR, Thomas AJ. Negative effects of increased sperm DNA damage in relation to seminal oxidative stress in men with idiopathic and male factor infertility. Fertil Steril. 2003;79:1597–605. https://doi.org/10.1016/j.rbm0.2013.06.014.
43. Lewis SE, John Aitken R, Conner SJ, Iuliis GD, Evenson DP, Henkel R, et al. The impact of sperm DNA damage in assisted conception and beyond: recent advances in diagnosis and treatment. Reprod Biomed Online. 2013;27:325–37. https://doi.org/10.1016/j.rbm0.2013.06.014.
44. Muratori M, Tarozzi N, Cambi M, Boni L, Iorio AL, Passaro C, et al. Variation of DNA fragmentation levels during density gradient sperm selection for assisted reproduction techniques: a possible new male predictive parameter of pregnancy? Medicine (Baltimore). 2016;95:e3624. https://doi.org/10.1097/MD.0000000000003624.

Chapter 6
TUNEL Assay by Benchtop Flow Cytometer in Clinical Laboratories

Rakesh Sharma, Zeynep Cakar, and Ashok Agarwal

6.1 Introduction

Infertility is described as the inability of a sexually active couple to get pregnant within a year of unprotected sex. Up to 12–15% of couples are considered infertile, of which approximately 35% is due to female factors, 30% due to male factors, 20% due to a combination of both male and female factors, and 15% unexplained [1]. When encountering male infertility, routine semen analysis is the first step for laboratory evaluations. Almost 15% of infertile men who undergo this test display semen parameters that are within normal reference range [2]. Thus, assessing an individual's fertility not only depends on physical parameters of spermatozoa but also on their functional capability. Numerous studies have reported that sperm DNA fragmentation (SDF) is linked to reduced fertilization rate. Several hypotheses have been proposed in order to understand the origin of sperm DNA fragmentation [3]. The first is characterized by endonuclease-mediated DNA cleavage, also called abortive apoptosis. This occurs when sperm with damaged DNA escape from normal programmed cell death [4]. The second hypothesis is DNA strand breaks induced by oxidative stress [5]. The third hypothesis is that during spermiogenesis, the increase in torsional stress can increase the activity of endogenous endonucleases, which may stimulate DNA fragmentation [4].

R. Sharma • Z. Cakar
American Center for Reproductive Medicine, Cleveland Clinic, Cleveland, OH, USA

A. Agarwal (✉)
American Center for Reproductive Medicine, Glickman Urological and Kidney Institute, Cleveland Clinic, Cleveland, OH, USA
e-mail: agarwaa@ccf.org

A. Zini, A. Agarwal (eds.), *A Clinician's Guide to Sperm DNA and Chromatin Damage*, https://doi.org/10.1007/978-3-319-71815-6_6

6.2 DNA Fragmentation and Male Infertility

Infertile males have more sperm DNA fragmentation compared to males of proven fertility [6, 7]. As the male contributes to half the genetic material of the embryo, increased DNA damage in human spermatozoa may compromise embryonic development [8].

Many intrinsic and extrinsic factors can cause sperm DNA damage, specifically via DNA fragmentation such as single-strand and double-strand DNA breaks. Some of these intrinsic factors include oxidative stress [9], endogenous endonuclease and caspase activation [10], alterations to chromatin remodeling during spermiogenesis, [11] and apoptosis of germ cells at the beginning of meiosis [12]. Extrinsic factors include radiotherapy, chemotherapy, and environmental toxicants [13–16].

A number of sperm function tests have been introduced to assess sperm DNA integrity. It is becoming increasingly important to define which DNA damage test is the most appropriate for clinical screening purposes. Sperm chromatin structure assay (SCSA), comet assay, sperm chromatin dispersion (halo) test (SCD), and terminal deoxynucleotidyl transferase dUTP nick end labeling (TUNEL) assay are the main tests that are currently used to measure sperm DNA fragmentation (Table 6.1). SCSA measures the susceptibility of sperm DNA to acid-induced DNA denaturation in situ [17, 18]. The comet assay can detect either single- or both double-strand breaks. The principle of this assay is based on the concept that DNA fragments have different mobility in the electrophoretic field depending on their size [16], whereas the SCD test detects sperm with fragmented DNA based on the fact that they do not produce the characteristic halos of DNA strands after acid denaturation and removal of nuclear proteins [19]. The TUNEL assay is used for identifying DNA fragmentation that results from apoptotic signaling cascades. Mechanism of TUNEL assay depends on the presence of nicks in the DNA that can be recognized by terminal deoxynucleotidyl transferase or TdT, an enzyme that catalyzes the addition of dUTPs secondarily labeled with a marker [18].

TUNEL assay can be further analyzed either with flow cytometry or fluorescence microscopy. Flow cytometry is a robust and widely used technique to analyze multiple parameters of individual cells within heterogeneous populations [20]. Currently SCSA is considered the gold standard; however, there is a lack of standardized protocols for other tests [21]. TUNEL assay is an efficient tool that provides objective and reproducible analysis for andrology lab and male infertility [22].

Two earlier studies reported TUNEL cutoff values in an attempt to quantify the amount of DNA fragmentation that can appropriately distinguish fertile and infertile male populations. A study by Sergerie et al. reported a cutoff value of 20% [23], whereas, Sharma et al. reported a cutoff of 19.25% obtained by comparing male infertility patients and controls with proven and unproven fertility [24]. Recently, these authors described a detailed protocol and quality control steps for measurement of TUNEL assay using benchtop flow cytometry on a large cohort of patient and controls with proven and unproven fertility. A reference value of 16.8% was

Table 6.1 Tests for measurement of DNA fragmentation

Assay	Advantages	Disadvantages
SCSA		
For single-stranded DNA 1. Mild acid treatment denatures DNA with single-strand (SS) or double-strand (DS) breaks 2. Acridine orange binds to DNA 3. Double-stranded DNA (non-denatured) fluoresces green, single-stranded DNA (denatured) fluoresces red 4. Flow cytometry counts 10,000 cells 5. DNA fragmentation index (DFI)—the percentage of sperm with a ratio of red to (red+green) fluorescence greater than the main cell population	1. Direct and objective 2. Established clinical thresholds 3. Many cells rapidly examined 4. High repeatability 5. Fresh or frozen samples 6. Most published studies and is reproducible	1. Proprietary method 2. Not available in commercial kits 3. Expensive equipment 4. Acid-induced denaturation 5. Small variations in lab conditions affect results 6. Calculations involve qualitative decisions 7. Very few labs conduct this assay
COMET		
For single- and double-stranded DNA 1. Electrophoresis of single sperm cells 2. DNA fragments form tail 3. Intact DNA stays in head Alkaline COMET 1. Alkaline conditions, denatures all DNA 2. Identifies both DS and SS breaks Neutral COMET 1. Does not denature DNA 2. Identifies DS breaks	1. Indirect assay, subjective 2. Poor repeatability 3. High sensitivity 4. Fresh samples only 5. Correlates with seminal parameters 6. Small number of cells required 7. Versatile (alkaline or neutral)	1. Variable protocols 2. Unclear thresholds 3. Not available in commercial kits 4. Time and labor intensive 5. Small number of cells assayed 6. Subjective 7. Lacks correlation with fertility 8. Requires special imaging software
SCD test		
1. Individual cells immersed in agarose 2. Denatured with acid then lysed 3. Normal sperm produce halo	1. Easy 2. Can use bright-field microscopy	1. Thresholds for SCD are not clearly established for men with unexplained infertility 2. Low-density nucleoids are faint and produce less contrasting images 3. Few studies have shown correlation between sperm DNA damage and ART outcome 4. Cannot discriminate the type of DNA fragmentation or quantify the amount of DNA damage at the spermatozoa level

(continued)

Table 6.1 (continued)

Assay	Advantages	Disadvantages
TUNEL		
1. Adds labeled nucleotides to free DNA ends 2. Individual template 3. Labels SS and DS breaks 4. Measures percent cells with labeled DNA	1. Direct objective 2. Performed on few sperm (10,000) 3. High repeatability 4. Objective, high sensitivity (flow cytometry) 5. Fresh or frozen samples 6. Indicative of apoptosis 7. Correlates with semen parameters 8. Associated with fertility 9. Available in commercial kits	1. Thresholds not standardized 2. Variable assay protocols 3. Not designed specifically for spermatozoa 4. Need for special equipment (flow cytometer) 5. Template independent 6. Requires proper controls

identified [2]. In this chapter, we describe the protocol for the measurement of DNA fragmentation using the TUNEL assay in conjunction with Accuri C6 benchtop flow cytometer (Fig. 6.1a).

6.3 Principle of the TUNEL Assay

DNA fragmentation occurs when endonucleases are activated during apoptosis. These nucleases degrade the higher order sperm chromatin structure into fragments ~30 kb in length and then subsequently into smaller DNA pieces. This fragmented DNA can be detected by the TUNEL (terminal deoxynucleotidyl transferase dUTP nick end labeling) assay. It is a single-step staining method that labels DNA breaks with FITC-dUTP; flow cytometry is then used to identify the sites of the strand breaks. TUNEL utilizes a template-independent DNA polymerase called terminal deoxynucleotidyl transferase (TdT) that non-preferentially adds deoxyribonucleotides to 3′ hydroxyl (OH) single- and double-stranded DNA. Deoxyuridine triphosphate (dUTP) is the substrate that is added by the TdT enzyme to the free 3′-OH break-ends of DNA (Fig. 6.1b). The more DNA strand break sites are present, the more labels are incorporated within a cell. The assay kit used in this protocol is the APO-DIRECT™ Kit (BD Pharmingen, Catalog #556381). It consists of the following components:

- Negative control cells
- Positive control cells
- Rinse buffer
- Wash buffer
- Reaction buffer
- FITC-dUTP

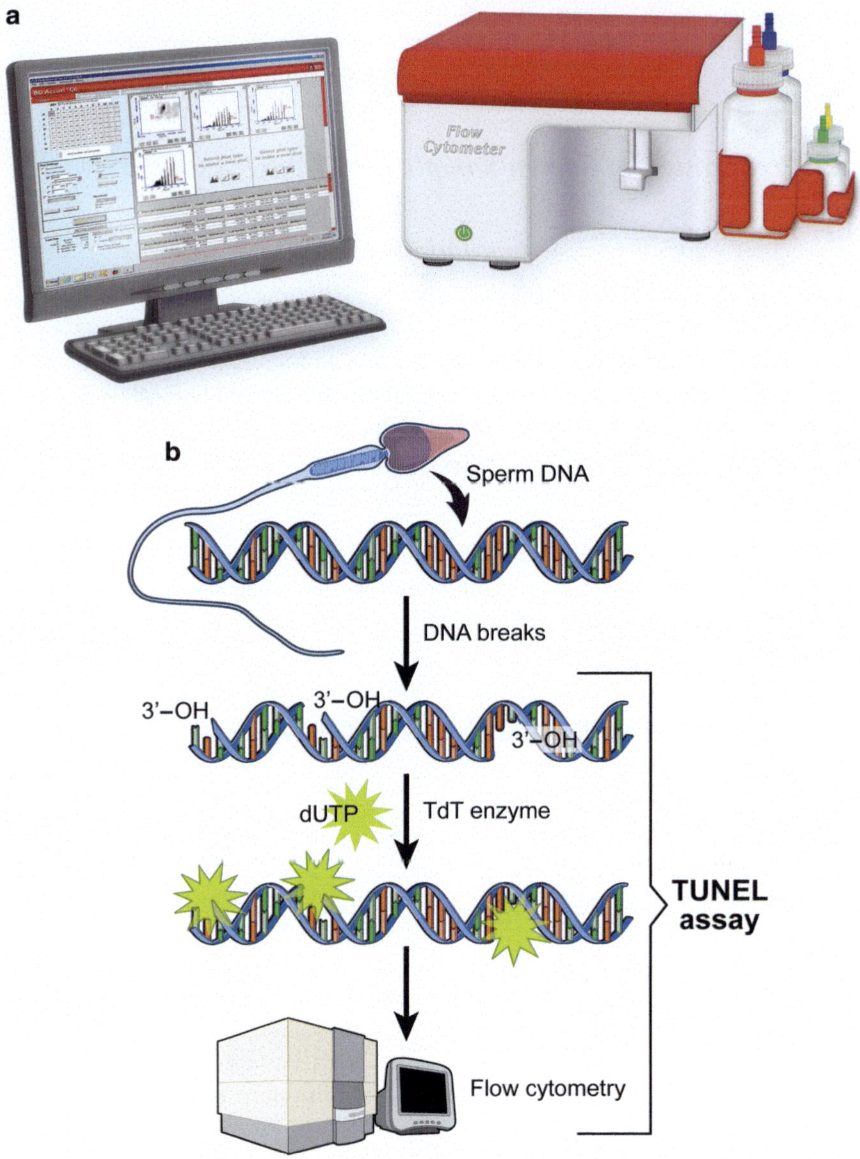

Fig. 6.1 (**a**) Schematic of the TUNEL assay; (**b**) benchtop flow cytometer

- TdT enzyme
- PI/RNase staining buffer

6.3.1 *Preparation of Semen Sample for TUNEL Assay*

6.3.1.1 Specimen Collection

1. Ideally, the sample will be collected after a minimum of 2–3 days of sexual abstinence.
2. Following liquefaction, evaluate semen specimens for volume, round cell concentration, sperm concentration, total cell count, motility, and morphology.
3. Adjust the sperm concentration to 2.5×10^6/mL.

   Label each tube with the following information:

- TUNEL
- Patient name
- Medical record number
- Date

6.3.2 *Preparation of Test and Negative Control*

1. Label two tubes as "test sample" and two as "negative sample."
2. Add the required amount of seminal ejaculate into the tube. Centrifuge the sample at 400 g for 7 min and remove seminal plasma. Resuspend the pellet in 1 mL of phosphate buffer saline (PBS).

6.3.3 *Preparation of Positive Control*

1. Prepare a 2% hydrogen peroxide solution (1:14 dilution) from the 30% stock solution.
2. Resuspend the spermatozoa in 1 mL of the diluted H_2O_2 solution.
3. Place the tube in heating block at 50 °C for 1 h.
4. Centrifuge for 7 min at 400 g.
5. Remove the supernatant and replace with 1 mL of PBS.
6. Centrifuge for 7 min at 400 g.
7. Remove the supernatant and replace with 1 mL of PBS.
8. Together with the test and the negative samples, centrifuge for 7 min at 400 g.
9. Remove the supernatant and proceed to fixation and permeabilization.

6.3.4 *Fixation and Permeabilization*

1. Prepare paraformaldehyde 3.7% solution by diluting the 10 mL stock formaldehyde 37% solution in 90 mL of PBS.
2. After removing the supernatant from the samples and spermatozoa controls, add 1 mL of 3.7% paraformaldehyde solution. Incubate at room temperature for 15 min.
3. Centrifuge for 4 min at 400 g.
4. Remove the paraformaldehyde and add 1 mL of PBS.
5. Centrifuge for 4 min at 400 g, remove the supernatant, and replace with 1 mL of ice cold ethanol (70%).

6.3.5 *Preparation for TUNEL Staining*

6.3.5.1 Preparation of Kit Controls and Test Samples

Vortex the negative (Cat# 6553LZ; White cap) and positive (Cat# 6552LZ; Brown cap) samples provided in the kit.

Note Verify the catalog numbers and the cap color to match each vial.

1. Mix the contents of each vial by vortexing. Remove 2 mL aliquots of the control cell suspensions (approximately 1×10^6 cells/mL), and place in 12×75 mm centrifuge tubes.
2. Return the vials to −20 °C.
3. Include three to four samples with known DNA damage along with the kit controls.
4. Centrifuge at 400 g for 7 min and discard the supernatant.
5. Centrifuge the control cell suspensions for 5 min at 400 g, and remove the 70% (v/v) ethanol by aspiration, being careful to not disturb the cell pellet.
6. To the control and test samples, add 1.0 mL of "wash buffer" (6548AZ) (blue cap) and vortex. Centrifuge as before and discard the supernatant.
7. Repeat the "wash buffer" treatment. Centrifuge and discard the supernatant.
8. Number the tubes consecutively beginning with "negative" and "positive kit controls," "test samples," and negative and positive test controls.

6.3.5.2 Staining for TUNEL Assay

1. Check the number of tubes that will be required for the TUNEL assay. It is helpful to prepare the stain for an additional three to five tubes.
2. Remove the reaction buffer from 4 °C and the TdT and FITC-dUTP from −20 °C, and place them at 37 °C for 20 min to warm.
3. Prepare the stain and calculate the required volumes.

Note The preparation of the stain and all subsequent steps must be carried out in the dark.

4. For the negative controls, omit the TdT enzyme from the staining solution.
5. Return the stains to appropriate storage temperature.

Note The staining solution is active for approximately 24 h at 4 °C.

6. Resuspend the pellet in each tube in 50 μL of the staining solution.

Note The same tip can be used to add the stain as long as the stain is added on the side of the tube and the tip does not come in contact with the solution.

7. Incubate the sperm in the staining solution for 60 min at 37 °C. Cover the tubes with aluminum foil.

Note Record the incubation time on the aluminum foil.

8. At the end of the incubation time, add 1.0 mL of "rinse buffer" to each tube, and centrifuge at 400 g for 7 min. Discard the supernatant.
9. Repeat the cell rinsing with 1.0 mL of the "rinse buffer," repeat centrifugation, and discard the supernatant.
10. Resuspend the cell pellet in 0.5 mL of the "PI/RNase staining buffer."
11. Incubate the cells in the dark for 30 min at room temperature.
12. Number the tubes according to the sample list. Cap the tubes and carefully cover the tubes with aluminum foil. The tubes are now ready for analysis.

Note The cells must be analyzed within 3 h of staining. Cells may begin to deteriorate if left overnight before analysis.

6.3.5.3 General Setup

All boxes are deselected or "unchecked" before selecting the box as "checked."

1. Open the software by double-clicking the "BD Accuri C6 software" icon on desktop.
2. Check the fluid levels in all bottles. The waste bottle must be empty and the sheath, cleaner, and decontamination bottles full.
3. Pull the sample stage forward underneath the Sheath Injection Port (SIP).

Note The sample stage accommodates any brand of 12×75 mm tube and most microcentrifuge tubes. Be careful not to bend or catch the SIP when inserting tubes.

4. Place a tube with 0.22 μm-filtered deionized water.

Note A tube of 0.22 μm-filtered deionized (DI) water is placed on the SIP at all times to keep the SIP from drying out—before use, during use, and even after the machine is shut down.

5. Firmly press the power button on the front of the cytometer unit.
6. While starting up the BD Accuri software, "traffic light" will turn yellow and the pumps will start to run.
7. Wait 5 min for the machine to flush the fluidics line with sheath fluid.

Warning Do not open the lid of the cytometer during this time. This will disrupt the laser warm-up process.

8. The BD Accuri software "traffic light" will turn green and displays "C6 is connected and ready" when complete.
9. To remove bubbles from the system, place a tube of 0.22 μm-filtered DI water on the SIP.
10. Select "run with limits" and set to 15 min.
11. Select "fluidics" speed to "fast" and click the "RUN" button.
12. Leave tube on SIP.

Note Validate the performance of the cytometer using the 8-Peak Validation Beads for FL1-FL3 (Spherotech, Catalog # 653144) and 6-Peak Validation Beads for FL4 (Spherotech, Catalog # 653145, BD Bioscience) according to the manufacturer's instructions before processing any samples.

6.3.6 *Shutting Down and Ending the Run*

1. Place a tube with 2 mL of bleach (diluted decontamination solution) on the SIP, and select an empty "data well" in the collect tab of the BD Accuri software.
2. Set a time limit of "2 min" and set fluidics speed to "fast" and click the "RUN" button.
3. Once the run is finished, remove the tube from the SIP, and place a new tube with 0.22 μm-filtered DI water on the SIP.
4. Select another empty "data well" in the BD Accuri software and repeat #2 and #3.
5. Press the power button to start the shutdown cycle. The cycle will take 15 min to complete then the cytometer will automatically shut down.

Note The automatic shutdown cycle can be bypassed by pressing down the power button for 5 s. However, the cytometer will take additional time to recover and return to the steady state if it is shut down in this manner. The BD Accuri software will display the following message if the machine is shut down using this method. It is unnecessary to shut down the software or computer during the shutdown process.

6. Maintenance and Troubleshooting: Follow the instructions provided in the BD Accuri C6 Flow Cytometer Instrument Manual.
7. Instrument validation is done by using 8-peak and 6-peak beads provided by the company, BD.
8. Running Kit Controls

Note Kit controls are run under the "collect" tab.

1. Double-click “Kit Control Template.”
2. All data will be saved in folder.
3. Save the workspace.
4. Select well “A1” (move to adjacent cell if occupied).
5. In field “A1” type “kit negative-date-tech initials.”
6. Set the run parameters as follows:

   - “Run with limits”: 10,000 events; in ungated samples
   - “Fluidics” speed: slow
   - Threshold: 80,000 on FSC-H. If it does not show, click Threshold and enter the number 80,000.

7. Remove tube of DI water from the SIP.
8. Vortex and place negative control on the SIP.
9. Click “RUN” button.
10. Run will finish after collecting 10,000 events.
11. Data will populate in plots 1–4.

    - Plot 1: FSC-A/SSC-A
    - Plot 2: FSC-A/FL2-A
    - Plot 3: FL2-A/FL2-H
    - Plot 4: FL1-A/FL2-A

12. Select well “A2” and repeat steps #4 – #9.
13. Remove negative kit control from SIP/stage.
14. Clean the SIP with a lint-free wipe.
15. Put a positive control tube on the SIP.
16. Click well “A3.”
17. Name “A03” as “kit positive-date-tech initials.”
18. Repeat steps #4 – #9.
19. Select well “A4” and repeat steps for positive control run (steps #15 and #16).

6.3.7 Data Acquisition

6.3.7.1 Running Kit Controls (Kit Control Template)

Note Maintain a written record of all results.

1. Under the collect tab, click on well A1 for the first negative kit control.
2. Observe the graph for the negative control.
3. The last plot is a quadrant: lower left (Q-LL), lower right (Q-LR), upper left (Q-UL), and upper right (Q-UR).
4. Observe only the percent positive (FITC+) value in the upper right quadrant (Q-UR).
5. Click on well A2 and follow steps #2 – #4 for the second negative kit control.
6. Click on well A3 and A4 for the positive kit controls.

6.3.7.2 Running Patient Samples

Note Samples are run under the "collect" tab. All data should be saved in folder.

1. Double-click on the "Assay template" under folder.
2. Wait for the software to load.
3. Check each well to ensure no data already exists inside.
4. Select well "A5."
5. Begin with tube #5 (first test sample).
6. Remove DI water from the SIP.
7. Vortex the tube (test sample) and place on the SIP.
8. Set the run parameters as follows:
   - "Run with limits": 10,000 events
   - "Fluidics" speed: slow
   - Gate P1 in P3
   - Threshold: 80,000 on FSC-H
9. Click the "RUN" button to start the collection.
10. After 10,000 events the run will finish.
11. Remove tube from SIP and clean the SIP with a lint-free.
12. Vortex and place the subsequent tube on the SIP.
13. Select the next well (A6 and so on) for the new sample.
14. Repeat steps #5–#13 until all samples have been processed.
15. Remove final tube and place the "bleach tube" on the SIP.
16. Set the parameters as follows:
    - "Run with limits": 2 min
    - "Fluidics" speed: fast
    - Threshold: 80,000 on FSC-H
17. Click the "RUN" tab.
18. When the run is finished, wipe SIP.
19. Remove tube and replace with DI water tube.
20. Repeat steps steps #17–#19 with DI water.
21. Proceed to shutdown step.

6.3.8 Data Analysis

The following strategies will be used for data analysis.

1. Alignment strategy and data analysis in "Collect tab": use a standard acquisition file of a sperm sample that is tested negative for DNA fragmentation to align all the samples. This strategy is done in the "Collect tab."
2. Data analysis in the "Analyze tab": align each sample, to its respective "Negative control." This strategy is used in the "Analyze tab."

6.3.8.1 Alignment Strategy and Data Analysis in "Collect Tab"

1. Click on File, open Workspace or template (Fig. 6.2).
2. Click on the well where the standard is to be imported. It is important to have an internal standard with a known amount of DNA damage. In the analyze tab, the quadrant will be adjusted to coincide with this DNA damage.
3. Go to the standard template and select it and click on the file import.
4. Click on the workspace.
5. Go to the Results folder, click on your recent TUNEL results.
6. Select the negative peak of the standard sample as the standard to be applied to all samples.
7. Click on F1 well.
8. Click on the histogram.
9. Change the X-axis parameter from FSC-A to FL2-A (Fig. 6.2).
10. Change the gate to P3 in P1 for plot 5. This gate is the same as plot 4, which is a quadrant gate (Fig. 6.2).
11. Select the vertical line icon at the bottom left of the histogram plot (Fig. 6.3A).

    i. Align the selected red line to the center of the histogram to obtain 50% cell population on either side
    ii. Note: Zoom on the histogram for easy alignment of the red bar in the middle of the peak.

12. Right click on the X-axis and click on virtual gain (Fig. 6.3A).
13. Align the blue line to the center of the peak of the histogram plot (Fig. 6.3B).
14. Next pick the sample to be aligned, for example, A5 (Fig. 6.3C).
15. Align the blue line to the center of the peak of the sample (Fig. 6.3D).
16. Click on the "Preview," "Apply" (Fig. 6.3E).
17. Chose option "Apply" to this sample only and close.

Note Do not change any of the settings in the four plots.

18. The plots in which Virtual Gain applied will appear with an asterisk in the FL1 axis.
19. Go to file and save the changes (save workspace as a result and analysis file).

6.3.8.2 Data Analysis in Analyze Tab

It is necessary to create a new set of three plots for each sample.

1. The analysis of the data acquired is done using the Accuri C6 Software in the Analyze tab.
2. When the Analyze tab is opened for the first time, the workspace is empty.

Note The plots are automatically selected from the original template. Make sure the original gates are used.
To close the plot, do not click on the X at the corner but click in the box with a horizontal line.

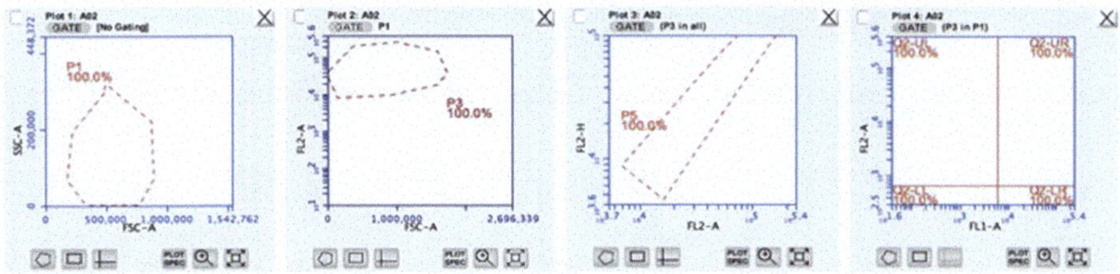

Fig. 6.2 Template for the analysis of sperm for TUNEL assay showing gating of the spermatozoa with expected size

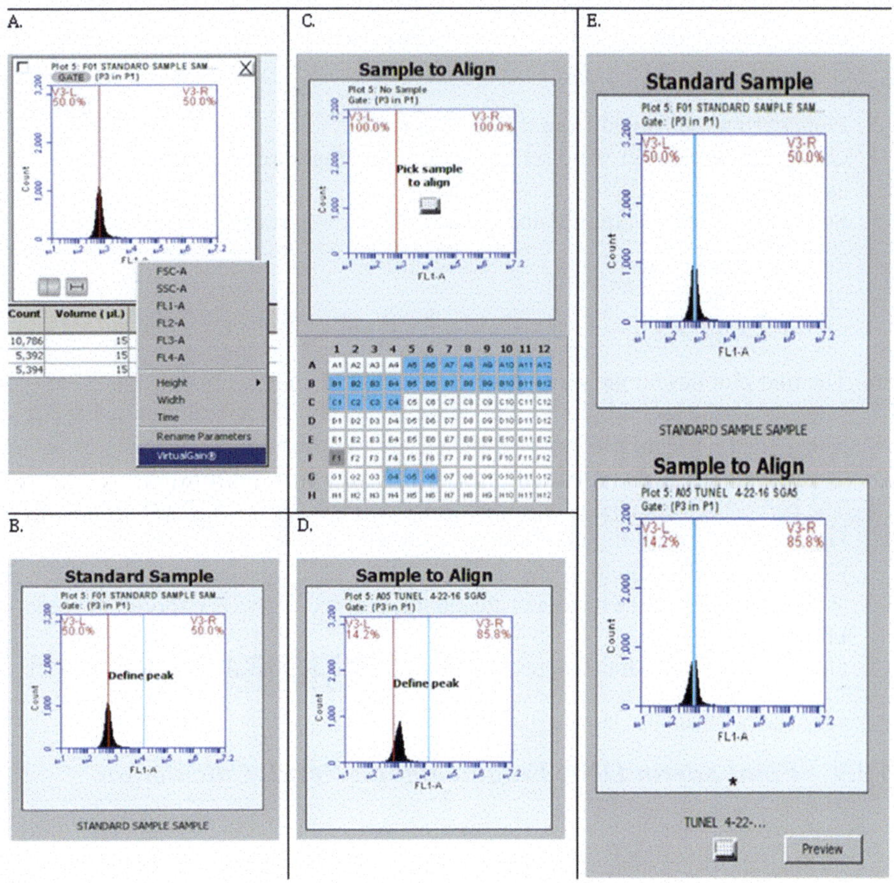

Fig. 6.3 Steps showing application of the virtual gain selection for the histogram plot and alignment of test sample to the standard sample

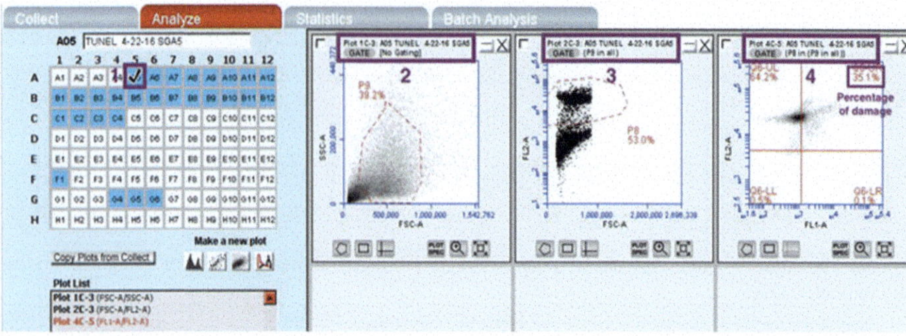

Fig. 6.4 Representative plot in the analyzed mode showing the percentage of DNA damage

3. Plots need to be copied from the Collect tab.
4. Gating strategies that were set up in the collect tab are applied in Analyze tab as well.
5. Select the samples acquired and create a three plot group for each sample:
   i. FSC-A/SSC-A
   ii. FSC-A/FL2-A
   iii. FL1-A/FL2-A
6. The first plot has no gating and the cell population is P9.
7. The gate in the second plot will be P9 in all events. The population is P8.
8. The gate in the third plot will be P8 in P9 (in all events) (Fig. 6.4).
9. The adjustment is recorded only in the BD Accuri C6 Software file.
10. The percentage damage is recorded from the FL1-A/FL2-A PLOT (Fig. 6.4).
11. For more information about how to apply virtual gain, consult the BD Accuri C6 Software User Guide.
12. Write the preliminary results of the analysis in the TUNEL Laboratory Report Form.
13. Go to file and save the changes (save workspace as a result and analysis file).

6.3.9 Final Sperm DNA Fragmentation Result Calculation

1. Calculate the average negative sample value for each sample.
2. The average value of the negative samples of each sample has to be subtracted from the average value obtained from the data analysis. This is done to subtract the autofluorescence in the sample.

6.3.10 Validation of TUNEL Test

To confirm that the TUNEL test was correctly performed and that the DNA fragmentation was accurately detected, two conditions have to be fulfilled:

i. The percentage of spermatozoa positive for TUNEL in the spermatozoa-positive control sample has to be higher than the percentage for the non-control spermatozoa samples.
ii. The percentage of cells positive for TUNEL in the kit positive control cells has to be higher than 30%.

If both these conditions are verified, the assay is considered correct.

6.3.11 Reference Values

A cutoff of 17% with >95% specificity can differentiate infertile men with DNA damage from healthy men. The high sensitivity and specificity makes this an ideal test.

6.3.12 Factors Affecting the Assay Results

Several factors are important to consider when performing this assay:

1. Accessibility of the DNA
2. Sperm preparation
3. Presence of dead cells
4. Number of cells examined
5. Interobserver and intraobserver as well as inter-assay and intra-assay variations.

6.4 Conclusion

The TUNEL assay is an efficient protocol that allows for objective analysis of sperm DNA fragmentation with validated thresholds for the evaluation of male infertility.

References

1. Esteves SC, Schattman GL, Agarwal A. Definitions and relevance of unexplained infertility in reproductive medicine. In: Unexplained infertility. New York: Springer Science + Business Media; 2015. p. 3–5.
2. Sharma R, Ahmad G, Esteves SC, Agarwal A. Terminal deoxynucleotidyl transferase dUTP nick end labeling (TUNEL) assay using bench top flow cytometer for evaluation of sperm

DNA fragmentation in fertility laboratories: protocol, reference values, and quality control. J Assist Reprod Genet. 2016;33(2):291–300.
3. Sharma RK, Agarwal A. Laboratory evaluation of sperm chromatin: TUNEL assay. In: Zini A, Agarwal A, editors. Sperm chromatin: biological and clinical applications in male infertility and assisted reproduction. New York: Springer Science + Business Media; 2012. p. 201–15.
4. Palermo GD, Neri QV, Cozzubbo T, Rosenwaks Z. Perspectives on the assessment of human sperm chromatin integrity. Fertil Steril. 2014;102(6):1508–17.
5. Aitken RJ, Smith TB, Joblings MS, Baker MA, De Iuliis GN. Oxidative stress and male reproductive health. Asian J Androl. 2014;16(1):31–8.
6. Schulte RT, Ohl DA, Sigman M, Smith GD, Sperm DNA. damage in male infertility: etiologies, assays, and outcomes. J Assist Reprod Genet. 2010;27(1):3–12.
7. Zini A, Albert O, Robaire B. Assessing sperm chromatin and DNA damage: clinical importance and development of standards. Andrology. 2014;2(3):322–5.
8. Aitken R, Bronson R, Smith TB, De Iuliis GN. The source and significance of DNA damage in human spermatozoa; a commentary on diagnostic strategies and straw man fallacies. Mol Hum Reprod. 2013;19(8):475–85.
9. Aitken RJ, De Iuliis GN. Origins and consequences of DNA damage in male germ cells. Reprod BioMed Online. 2007;14(6):727–33.
10. Maione B, Pittogi C, Achene L, Lorenzini R, Spadafora C. Activation of endogenous nucleases in mature sperm cells upon interaction with exogenous DNA. DNA Cell Biol. 1997;16(9):1087–97.
11. Carrell DT, Emery BR, Hammoud S. Altered protamine expression and diminished spermatogenesis: what is the link? Hum Reprod Update. 2007;13(3):313–27.
12. Sakkas D, Seli E, Manicardi GC, Nijs M, Ombelet W, Bizzaro D. The presence of abnormal spermatozoa in the ejaculate: did apoptosis fail? Hum Fertil (Camb). 2004;7(2):99–103.
13. Sailer BL, Sarkar LJ, Bjordahl JA, Jost LK, Evenson DP. Effects of heat stress on mouse testicular cells and sperm chromatin structure. J Androl. 1997;18(3):294–301.
14. Evenson DP, Wixon R. Environmental toxicants cause sperm DNA fragmentation as detected by the Sperm Chromatin Structure Assay (SCSA). Toxicol Appl Pharmacol. 2005;207(2 Suppl):532–7.
15. Rubes J, Selevan SG, Evenson DP, Zudova D, Vozdova M, Zudova Z, et al. Episodic air pollution is associated with increased DNA fragmentation in human sperm without other changes in semen quality. Hum Reprod. 2005;20(10):2776–83.
16. Lewis SE. Sperm DNA fragmentation and base oxidation. In: Baldi E, Muratori M, editors. Genetic damage in human spermatozoa, advances in experimental medicine and biology. New York: Springer + Business Media; 2014. p. 103–16.
17. Mitchell LA, De Iuliis G, Aitken RJ. The TUNEL assay consistently underestimates DNA damage in human spermatozoa and is influenced by DNA compaction and cell vitality: development of an improved methodology. Int J Androl. 2011;34(1):2–13.
18. Sharma R, Masaki J, Agarwal A. Sperm DNA fragmentation analysis using the TUNEL assay. Methods Mol Biol. 2013;927:121–36.
19. Fernandez JL, Muriel L, Rivero MT, Goyanes V, Vazquez R, Alvarez JG. The sperm chromatin dispersion test: a simple method for the determination of sperm DNA fragmentation. J Androl. 2003;24(1):59–66.
20. Agarwal A, Gupta S, Sharma R. Andrological evaluation of male infertility: a laboratory guide. New York: Springer; 2016.
21. Practice Committee of the American Society of Reproductive Medicine. The clinical utility of sperm DNA integrity testing: a guideline. Fertil Steril. 2013;99(3):673–7.
22. Mahfouz RZ, Said TM, Agarwal A. The diagnostic and therapeutic applications of flow cytometry in male infertility. Arch Med Sci. 2009;5(1A):S99–108.
23. Sergerie M, Laforest G, Bujan L, Bissonnette F, Bleau G. Sperm DNA fragmentation: threshold value in male fertility. Hum Reprod. 2005;20(12):3446–51.
24. Sharma RK, Sabanegh E, Mahfouz R, Gupta S, Thiyagarajan A, Agarwal A. TUNEL as a test for sperm DNA damage in the evaluation of male infertility. Urology. 2010;76(6):1380–6.

Chapter 7
The Comet Assay

Elva I. Cortés-Gutiérrez, Martha I. Dávila-Rodríguez, and Carmen López-Fernández

7.1 Introduction

The main difference between a damaged DNA molecule in somatic and germ line cells is that while in somatic cells the DNA damage can be partially repaired, the DNA damage present in the germ line cells (this is true especially in spermatozoa, cells that possess a nonorthodox DNA molecule) cannot be repaired due to the absence of DNA repair mechanisms and a highly condensed chromatin structure. Repair of sperm DNA damage occurs within the oocyte after fertilization. There are four possible mechanisms that have been identified to play a role in the pathophysiology of sperm DNA damage: (i) abortive apoptosis: spermatozoa with defective DNA escape the physiological apoptotic pathway during meiosis I resulting in the ejaculate [1]; (ii) defective chromatin condensation during spermatogenesis: DNA breaks occur as a result of inappropriate protamination and insufficient chromatin packaging [2]; (iii) oxidative stress resulting from an imbalance between reactive oxygen species (ROS) production and antioxidant capacity [3]; and (iv) the existence of endogenous sperm nucleases that cleave the DNA into loop-sized fragments of about 50 kB [4]. This activity, in fact, resembles that of several nucleases in somatic cells that cleave the DNA into similar sizes during the activation of apoptosis [5–9]. The function of these nucleases in the mature spermatozoa is to carry the DNA to the oocyte without any damage. In humans, the nature of damaged DNA that occurs within certain patient populations is still poorly understood [10, 11].

E.I. Cortés-Gutiérrez (✉) • M.I. Dávila-Rodríguez
Department of Genetics, Centro de Investigación Biomédica del Noreste, Instituto Mexicano del Seguro Social, IMSS, Monterrey, Mexico

Unit of Genetics, Department of Biology, Universidad Autónoma de Madrid, Madrid, Spain
e-mail: elvacortes@cibinmty.net; marthadavila@cibinmty.net

C. López-Fernández
Unit of Genetics, Department of Biology, Universidad Autónoma de Madrid, Madrid, Spain
e-mail: mariadelcarmen.lopez@uam.es

A. Zini, A. Agarwal (eds.), *A Clinician's Guide to Sperm DNA and Chromatin Damage*, https://doi.org/10.1007/978-3-319-71815-6_7

One of the key aspects that needs to be investigated concerning the problem of cellular DNA damage is the discrimination between the presence of single-strand DNA breaks (SSBs) and double-strand DNA breaks (DSBs) or both affecting the same DNA thread. This is mainly related to the origin of the DNA damage. The causes of sperm DNA damage resulting in SSBs or DSBs are extremely variable and include exposure to adverse environmental factors such as pesticides, radiation, smoking, or pathological conditions such as cancer, varicocele, and infection (bacterial, viral) [12]. These and presumably other causes of sperm DNA breakage are mediated through one or a combination of the mechanisms mentioned above. With respect to the putative origin of DNA fragmentation in the sperm cells, we might also expect different types of DNA lesion that could possibly be predictive or diagnostic in nature. For example, nucleases, either endogenous or exogenous, usually produce SSBs and/or DSBs, whereas DNA breaks produced by chromatin remodeling during spermiogenesis appear to correspond to DSBs produced by topoisomerase II and SSBs produced by topoisomerase I [13]. On the other hand, we have ROS and other radical molecules such as those derived from nitric oxide which generate SSBs associated with the creation of abasic sites or the presence of 8-hydroxyguanine [14, 15]. It has been reported that more than 20 damaged DNA base lesions can be present in a cell exposed to oxidative stress [16].

The comet assay, also known as single-cell gel electrophoresis (SCGE), was developed in 1984 [17] and is known for its ability to detect DNA damage at a single-cell level. The rationale of the technique is very simple. The assay requires detergents to first lyse the cells embedded in an inert agarose matrix on a slide. A high salt concentration results in deproteinized nuclei recognized as nucleoids. Following this, DNA is electrophoresed. The idea of the technique is that nuclei containing DNA segments that are detached from the original chromosome migrate toward the anodes, resulting in an image resembling a comet that can be observed under the microscope. The comet is formed by a part of the original nucleoid retaining a large part of undamaged DNA and an emerging tail that putatively accumulates a large part of the DNA that presented DNA breaks (Fig. 7.1a, original image, and 7.1b, digitally enhanced images). Most of the DNA retained in the head consists of intact DNA that is not recognized by the technique, whereas the tail is made up of broken DNA or strands with heterogeneous molecular weights. The intensity of the comet represents the proportion of DNA that has been broken off, and the distance traveled by the comet relates to the relative size of the DNA fragments.

The comet assay commonly utilizes commercially available software programs to evaluate the extent of DNA damage at the single-cell level. These programs provide a large number of measurement outcomes, i.e., tail length (the length of the tail measured from the leading edge of the head), tail DNA percentage (the percentage of DNA in the tail compared to the percentage in the "head" or unfragmented DNA), and olive tail moment (OTM). OTM is the percentage of tail DNA × tail moment length (tail DNA percentage = 100 × tail DNA intensity/cell; the tail moment length is measured from the center of the head to the center of the tail). The OTM is expressed in arbitrary units. Each of these parameters describes endogenous DNA damage corresponding to DNA strand breakage and/or alkali-labile sites (ALSs). In

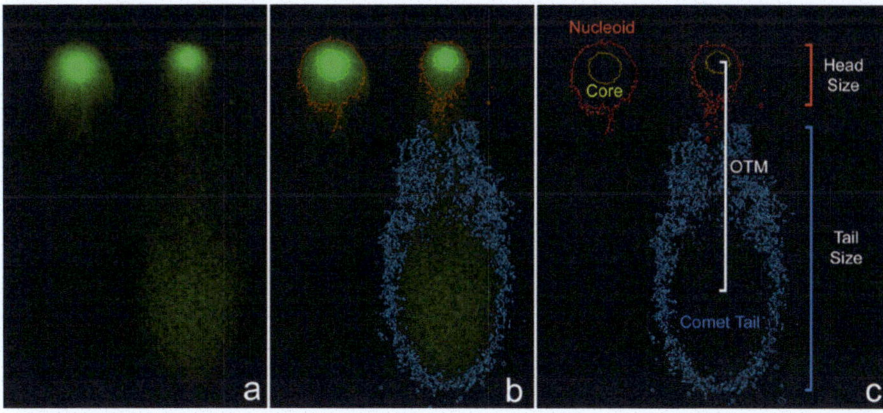

Fig. 7.1 Original (**a**) and image after application of a common electronic filter showing the comet head (consists of intact DNA) and emerging tail which possesses DNA breaks (**b**), features that are important for comet assay analysis (**c**)

the optimization of the alkaline comet for use with sperm, tail DNA was found to be the most reproducible parameter [18]; therefore, sperm DNA damage is expressed as tail DNA (Fig. 7.1c, digitally enhanced images).

The formation of a tail provides information on two important issues related to DNA damage concerning (i) the amount of DNA damage present in the original nucleoid and (ii) the type of DNA damage affecting the orthodox double-strand DNA conformation. For (i), it is generally assumed that the larger the tail and/or the higher the DNA density in the tail, the greater is the extent of DNA damage. For (ii), the presence of ssDNA breaks or dsDNA breaks or both affecting the same DNA thread is of crucial importance for understanding the images produced by the comet assay.

There are three types of comet assay techniques: (i) The neutral comet assay [18], in which DNA stretches originated from DSBs migrate under a neutral buffer according to the size of the DNA fragment. The larger the fragment, the lower the migration distance. (ii) The alkaline comet assay [19], in which DNA stretches containing both DSBs and SSBs migrate under alkaline conditions. Because alkaline conditions produce DNA denaturation, single-strand DNA threads resulting from DNA denaturation starting from the 5′ to 3′ free ends at the place of the DNA break migrate to the anode. (iii) The two-dimensional or two-tailed comet (2T-comet) assay combines the ability of the neutral and alkaline comet assay, allowing the differentiation within the same cell of the presence of DSB and SSB at the original nucleoid [20, 21].

These three techniques can be used on somatic cells, as well as in spermatozoa to assess DNA damage. However, as explained in detail later, given that the DNA is complexed with different proteins (histones, protamines, or both), depending on the cell type or cell activity, a general protocol does not exist to produce equivalent results on different cells and the basic methodology requires technical adaptations to obtain the best results.

7.2 Neutral Comet Assay

DSBs are considered to be the most biologically lethal lesions affecting somatic and sperm DNA mainly because they are difficult to repair and often lead to genome instability even after being repaired by nonhomologous chromosome rejoining [22, 23].

The rationale of the technique is very simple, since is based on the principle that a naturally charged DNA molecule migrates when subjected to an electrophoretic field. Subsequently, identification of DNA damage is simple. Basically, when lysed cells with no DNA fragmentation are subjected to an electric field and by using a buffer under non-denaturing conditions, no substantial comet tails will be formed (Fig. 7.2a). In contrast, those spermatozoa containing sperm with a damaged DNA molecule tend to show an extensive migration of DNA fragments emerging from the original sperm nucleoid (Fig. 7.2b, c). These migrating DNA fragments are associated with the presence of DSBs at the origin, but it is not possible to know if the DNA threads that distribute along the comet tail contain SSBs.

Confirmation that comets visualized under neutral conditions are indeed large DNA molecules containing DSBs is based on the observation that similar comets can be produced after incubation with classic double-strand DNA cutters such as restriction endonucleases [24].

Double-stranded breaks may be a male infertility factor. Understanding its mechanism and its identification in different clinical groups (such as asthenoteratozoospermic (ATZ) with or without varicocele, oligoasthenoteratozoospermic (OAT), balanced chromosome rearrangements, and fertile donors) may be useful for determining the prognosis of male infertility associated with these conditions. Double-stranded DNA damage is also related to a higher risk of male factor-associated miscarriage, possibly due to the failure of repair of sperm DSB breaks by the oocyte [23].

7.3 Alkaline Comet Assay

The technical aspect of this version of the comet assay is similar to the previous methodology described with the principle based on the fact that DNA stretches containing 3′ 5′ free ends denaturize when the protein-depleted nuclei are subjected to an alkaline environment producing single-strand free threads of DNA. The alterations found in DNA such as strand breaks (single or double) result in the extension of DNA loops from lysed and salt-extracted nuclei; these in turn form a comet-like

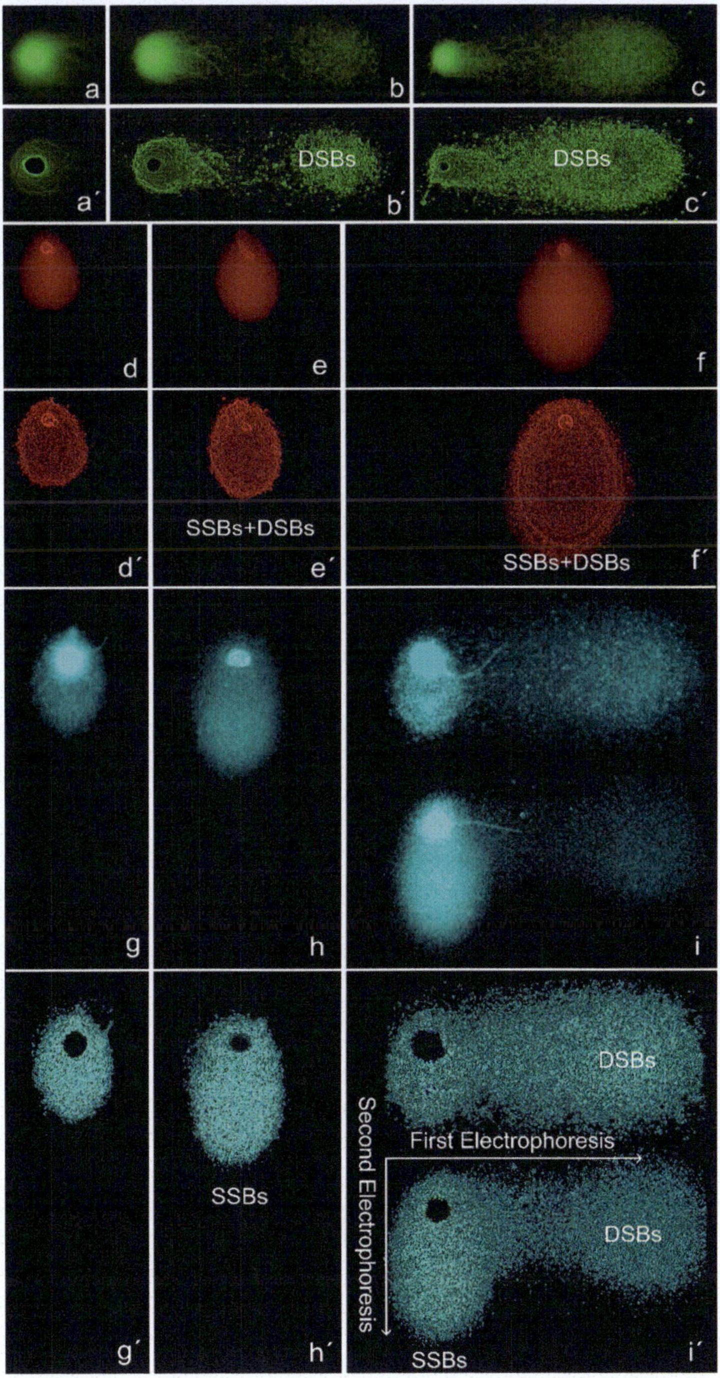

Fig. 7.2 Nonfragmented (**a**, **d**, and **g**) and fragmented spermatozoa (**b**, **c**, **e**, **f**, and **i**) in alkaline (**a–c**), neutral (**d–f**), and 2T-comet assays (**g–i**). Different levels of sperm DNA damage are shown for spermatozoa (SYBR® Green staining). The 2T-comet assay detected simultaneous DNA SSBs and DSBs in human spermatozoa. Undamaged (**g**) single-stranded DNA breaks (SSBs) (**h**), double-stranded DNA breaks (DSBs) (**i**), and SSBs/DSBs in the same cell (**i**). (**a′–i′**) Images after application of a common electronic filter scale

tail after alkaline electrophoresis, indicating global DNA damage identifying both single- (SSBs) and double-strand breaks (DSBs) [18, 25, 26].

DNA breaks are the starting points for alkaline DNA unwinding due to the disruption of hydrogen bonds between purines and pyrimidines. Moreover, mutagens may induce DNA base loss, and deoxyribose lesions may be transformed into SSBs by alkaline conditions, being designated as alkali-labile sites (ALS). Remarkably, when the spermatozoa of mammalian species are subjecting to denaturant alkaline conditions and electrophoresed, they exhibit a prominent comet tail (Fig. 7.2d–f) [25, 26]. Probably, the need of a highly compacted DNA molecule at the spermatozoa is favored by the presence of these ALS.

ALS can also be detected using DNA breakage detection-fluorescence in situ hybridization (DBD-FISH). This technique quantifies putative DNA breaks and ALS in situ within a single cell. It has the added advantage that it may also be utilized to scan the whole-genome or specific DNA sequences in sperm cells that have been embedded within an inert agarose matrix on a specifically prepared microscope slide [27]. The cells are then lysed to remove the membranes and proteins, and the resulting nucleoids are exposed to a controlled denaturation step using alkaline buffers. The alkali gives rise to ssDNA stretches starting from the 5′ to 3′ free DNA ends or from highly sensitive DNA motifs to alkaline conditions. These ssDNA threads may then be detected by hybridization with specific or whole-genome fluorescent DNA probes. Because DNA breaks increase in a target region, additional ssDNA are produced and further DNA probes are hybridized, resulting in a more intense FISH signal as additional ssDNA is produced (Fig. 7.3e, f). The resulting hybridized signal in the whole genome can be quantified using image analysis systems. The DBD-FISH signal obtained in the absence of exogenous DNA-damaging agents reflects the background level of ALS present in a genome (Fig. 7.3d) [28].

DNA damage detected by the comet assay suggests a possible high density of short unpaired DNA stretches that could act as origins of denaturation for alkaline treatment in the DBD-FISH procedure [28].

This same result has been seen in the large pericentromeric interstitial telomeric repeat sequence blocks from Chinese hamster cell lines. These short unpaired DNA segments could be a consequence of torsional stress of DNA loops during the process of chromatin packing, as they were initially found to be abundant in the chromatin of condensing mitotic chromosomes [29].

The comet assay is found to be a more sensitive technique in the evaluation of sperm DNA damage and fragmentation compared to the conventional TUNEL (Terminal deoxynucleotidyl transferase dUTP nick end lebeling), the sperm chromatin dispersion test, or flow cytometry [30]. Particularly, the alkaline comet assay has been tested in vitro and in vivo in a wide variety of mammalian cells [19, 31, 32] employing a number of different genotoxic stimuli including UV radiation, carcinogens, radiotherapy, and chemotherapy [33]. It has been shown to be rapid [33, 34], reproducible [35], and with higher sensitivity than alkaline elution or nick translation assays, even with prior chromatin decondensation [36, 37]. The alkaline comet

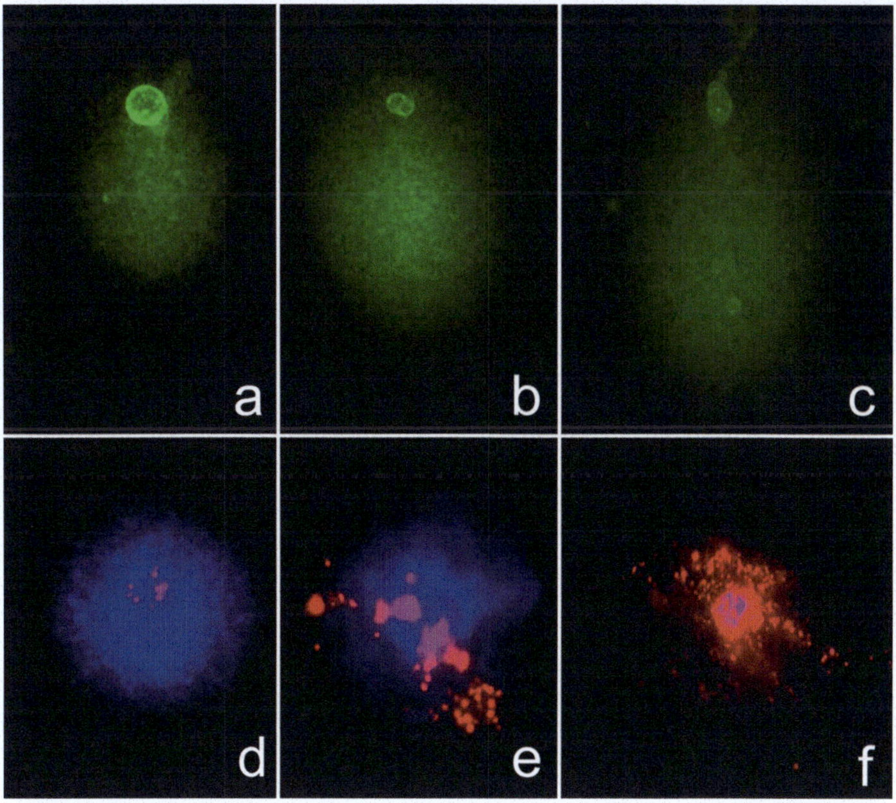

Fig. 7.3 Sperm cell classification according to DNA damage levels after alkaline comet assay (**a**–**c**) and DBD-FISH (**d**–**f**). Sperm with a "structural comet" or without DNA damage (**a**) exhibit a slightly fluorescent signal, (**d**) and nuclei with a prominent comet tail (**b** and **c**) result in a more intense FISH signal after DBD-FISH (**e** and **f**)

assay can detect damage equivalent to as few as 50 single-strand breaks (SSBs) per cell. One of its unique and powerful features is the ability to characterize the responses of a heterogeneous population of cells by measuring DNA damage within an individual (Fig. 7.2d), cells as opposed to just one overall measure of damaged cells versus undamaged (Fig. 7.2e, f).

Evaluation of sperm DNA damage by the alkaline comet assay is a more promising diagnostic test for male infertility as well as prognostic test for assisted reproductive technology (ART) outcomes. It has been shown to be closely associated with numerous fertility outcomes including negative relationships with fertilization, embryo quality, implantation, and positive relationships with miscarriage and childhood diseases [38].

7.4 Two-Tailed (2T)-Comet Assay

A modification of the original comet assay has been developed for the simultaneous evaluation of DNA SSBs and DSBs in human spermatozoa. The 2T-comet assay is a relatively fast, sensitive, and reliable technique for the quantification and characterization of whole DNA damage in spermatozoa [39–41].

In this protocol, cells are subject to an electrophoretic field under non-denaturing conditions to mobilize isolated free discrete DNA fragments produced from DSBs. This is similar to the neutral comet as explained above. Following mobilization of the DNA containing DSBs, a second electrophoresis which runs perpendicular to the first one but under alkaline conditions is performed to produce DNA denaturation. This process exposes both SSBs and DSBs existing in the comet head and tail formed during the first neutral electrophoresis. The result is a two-dimensional comet tail emerging from the core where SSBs and DBBs can be simultaneously discriminated (Fig. 7.2g–i). Three different comet figures may be produced (i) small comet representing a sperm free of DNA damage, resulting from the presence of large alkali-labile sites at each sperm (displacement at Y-axis) (Fig. 7.2g) (ii) comet at the Y-axis with equivalent size to the previous one but presenting additionally DNA displacement at the X-axis (Fig. 7.2i): this image is interpreted as a spermatozoa presenting DSBs at the origin and (iii) comet presenting displacement at the X- and Y-axis: in this case, the presence of SSBs is integrated at the Y-axis comet, while DSBs are mostly placed at the X-axis (Fig. 7.2i). The tail DNA produced after the first electrophoresis is formed because of the presence of DSBs at the origin but may contain SSBs distributed along the DNA threads. After denaturation, single-stranded DNA threads mobilize at the Y-axis, parallel to the migrating DNA remaining at the original comet head.

The 2T-comet assay is an innovative method for assessing whole sperm DNA integrity, which has not been extensively used for diagnostic purposes related to male infertility [39–42]. The technique can be used to assess highly damaged sperm DNA characterized by the presence of extensive presence of single- and double-strand breaks in some clinical situations such as Kartagener's syndrome [41] or in varicocele patients [40, 42].

7.5 The Clinical Relevance of the Comet Assay

Sperm DNA damage assays are important in assisting in the diagnosis of male infertility [36, 43–50] and may serve as prognostic tests for predicting ART outcomes. High levels of damaged DNA in the ejaculate of patients have been shown to have negative relationships with fertilization, embryo quality, and implantation failures and positive relationships with miscarriage and childhood diseases [38]. However, the optimal sperm DNA test and the value of these tests as predictors of reproductive outcomes still remain debatable.

The comet assay can be considered a reliable tool to assess sperm DNA damage, but most laboratories find it more difficult to perform compared to the Sperm Chromatin Structure Assay (SCSA), the TUNEL, or the Sperm Chromatin Dispersion (SCD) test. It is true that a standardized protocol with high quality controls for reproducibility is necessary in order to produce consistent and comparable results among different laboratories. With these limitations in mind, our experience using this technique is positive allowing a fine definition on the nature of the DNA break (SSBs or DSBs) present in the ejaculate. We must bear in mind that the presence of high level of DSBs in fertilizing spermatozoa shall be practically unrepairable at the oocyte with highly negative results on the embryo development even during the first stage [51, 52].

All types of comet assays have been used to assess different aspects of DNA quality in human sperm in order to find any possible correlation with pregnancy. However, as mentioned above, the alkaline comet assay has the capacity to visualize SSBs, DSBs, and additionally all constitutive alkali-labile sites present in the mammalian sperm. The proponents of the alkaline comet assay suggest that this assay is the most powerful to assess all DNA damage present in cells because it is based on the full capacity to denature the DNA when free 5–3′ breaks are present along the DNA molecule [53]. The neutral comet assay has not been used as widely as the alkaline comet assay but may be of relevance at the time of evaluating massive presence of DSBs. The 2T-comet assay is the least used methodology to assess sperm DNA damage, but important aspects on the nature of the DNA damage, such as the assessment of the relative presence of DSBs versus SSBs, are possible, and its relevance in fertility remains to be evaluated.

With respect to the neutral comet assay indicating the relative amount of DSBs affecting a certain proportion of the whole sperm population, some interesting information can be derived from published studies. Thus, SDF assessed by neutral comet has been found to be quite variable among different patient groups, with different sperm qualities [54]. While in normozoospermic individuals, Sperm DNA Fragmentation (SDF) values were around 10.5%, they were higher in other groups such as asthenozoospermic (15.2%), oligoteratozoospermic (18.3%), asthenoteratozoospermic (17.5%), or oligoasthenoteratozoospermic (21.3%). These results suggest that a single threshold value of SDF is probably not representative of the sperm's fertilizing capacity in achieving pregnancy, and the value needs to be tailored according to the type of patient under study.

Using the neutral comet assay, Ribas-Maynou et al. [55] studied the presence of DSBs and SSBs in sperm samples of patients with asthenoteratozoospermia (ATZ) with or without varicocele, oligoasthenoteratozoospermia (OAT), or balanced chromosome rearrangements. All of these patient groups were compared to fertile donors. The results revealed different sperm DNA damage profiles. Fertile donors presented low values for DSBs as well as for SSBs. OAT, ATZ, and ATZ presenting with an additional varicocele had higher SSB and DSB percentage compared with normozoospermic individuals. Interestingly in rearranged chromosome carriers, they presented with two different profiles: a high-equivalent comet assay profile, which could be compatible with a bad prognosis, and a nonequivalent comet assay profile, which was found in three fertile donors. These results support the theory that a neutral comet assay profile applied to different clinical groups may be useful for characterizing different male infertility groups.

The predictive value of the neutral comet assay in pregnancy loss has also been reported [23]. The study included 25 fertile donors and 20 recurrent pregnancy loss (RPL) patients with at least two unexplained first-trimester miscarriages. SDF values were analyzed using both alkaline and neutral comet assays. The unexplained RPL patients showed a low SSB and high DSB profile. This profile was observed in 85% of unexplained RPL and 33% of fertile donors, suggesting that DSBs can be associated with a male factor-related RPL. Receiver operating characteristic (ROC) curve analysis done with respect to recurrent miscarriage set the cutoff value at 77.50% of DSBs.

The alkaline comet assay has been shown to have a significant clinical value in male reproductive health and in predicting the success of ART [56]. Although the assay is not included in routine infertility tests, some studies recognize this experimental approach as an advanced, accurate, and reliable test for analyzing all DNA damage affecting a genome. When the alkaline comet assay is used to assess human semen quality and sperm DNA damage in infertile and fertile males, a significantly lower sperm concentration, sperm viability, and sperm motility were observed in all of the infertile subjects presenting with a high level of SDF [57].

The alkaline comet assay is also suitable for obtaining information about the level of SDF present after density gradient centrifugation. This is crucial as the sperm selection for IVF influences the chances of achieving pregnancy. It was found that men with SDF higher than 25% had a high risk of infertility (OR, 117.33; 95% confidence interval [CI], 12.72–2731.84; RR, 8.75) [56]. Fertilization rates and embryo quality decreased as SDF increased in semen and in density gradient centrifugation sperm. These results suggest that the risk of failure to achieve a pregnancy increased when SDF exceeded a prognostic threshold value of 52% for semen (OR, 76.00; CI, 8.69–1714.44; RR, 4.75) and 42% for density gradient centrifugation sperm (OR, 24.18; CI, 2.89–522.34; RR, 2.16). In a different study, the alkaline comet assay was used to assess SDF in neat semen samples and in spermatozoa following density gradient centrifugation. In this case, 203 couples undergoing In Vitro Fertlization (IVF) and 136 couples undergoing ICSI were included to establish any relationship existing between SDF level and live-birth rate after IVF and intracytoplasmic sperm injection (ICSI). Following IVF, couples with <25% SDF had a live-birth rate of 33%. In contrast, couples with >50% SDF had a much lower live-birth rate of 13% following IVF. Following ICSI, there were no significant differences in levels of sperm DNA damage between any groups of patients [58].

Sperm DNA damage evaluated by an alkaline comet assay was also associated with implantation and embryo quality [59]. In a cross-sectional study of 215 men from infertile couples undergoing ART, the paternal effect of sperm DNA damage was observed at each stage of early embryonic development. In both the early and late paternal effect stages, the low DNA damage group had a higher percentage of good-quality embryos ($P < 0.05$) and a lower percentage of poor-quality embryos ($P < 0.05$) compared with the high DNA damage group. Implantation was lower in the high DNA damage (33.33%) group compared with intermediate DNA damage (55.26%; $P < 0.001$) and low DNA damage (65.00%; $P < 0.001$) groups.

The implications of genomic damage in spermatozoa of type 1 diabetic patients were evaluated by alkaline comet assay [60] by comparing the SDF and the levels of oxidative DNA modifications with nondiabetic men. Spermatozoa from 11 patients with type 1 diabetes showed significantly higher levels of DNA fragmentation (44% versus 27%; $P < 0.05$) and concentrations of 8-OHdG (3.6 versus 2.0 molecules of 8-OHdG per 10(5) molecules of deoxyguanosine; $P < 0.05$) compared to 12 patients without diabetes. Furthermore, a positive correlation (rs = 0.7; $P < 0.05$) was observed between DNA fragmentation and concentration of 8-OHdG.

By using the alkaline comet assay, the actual damage load of small cohorts of sperm may be measured. As the alkaline comet only requires 100 cells for analysis, it has also been particularly useful for studies involving DNA of testicular sperm and for men with low sperm concentrations [61]. This is of importance as in addition to the low number of spermatozoa present in these samples, they are also contaminated with somatic cells. Other methodologies such as the SCSA are not operative in these cases. Using the alkaline comet assay, the apoptotic indices and SDF were compared in sperm collected after ejaculation from vasectomized men and fertile men undergoing vasectomy. Testicular biopsies from vasectomized ($n = 26$) and fertile men ($n = 46$) were used to calculate sperm/gram and also formalin-fixed to determine the numbers of developing sperm and incidence and intensities of testicular FasL, Fas, Bax, and Bcl-2. Increased intensities of FasL and Bax staining were observed in the seminiferous tubules of vasectomized men. FasL positivity also increased in Sertoli cells, and both FasL and Fas positivity increased in primary spermatocytes and round spermatids of vasectomized men [62]. These results demonstrate that SDF can be considered an end point marker of apoptosis with significantly higher sperm SDF in vasectomized men compared to fertile men. Another study [63] concluded that an inverse relationship between pregnancy and SDF is observed for both testicular and ejaculated sperm. However, no relationships were observed between SDF and fertilization rates.

According to the information we have summarized previously, it seems that a high level of SDF in the ejaculate or in the selected sample for fertilization purposes is negatively correlated with reproductive outcomes. However, it is not only the amount of detected damaged DNA but also the nature of the DNA breaks that is of importance in explaining certain reproductive outcome failures [39, 40]. In this scenario, the 2T-comet assay may provide additional information not provided by the neutral or alkaline comets regarding the nature of the DNA damage. This methodology may provide important and singular information understanding a part of andrological pathology as is the case for Kartagener's syndrome [41].

Some studies have obtained interesting results using the 2T-comet assay. Enciso et al. [21] studied the frequency of sperm cells containing SSBs and DSBs in the ejaculates of a group of ten infertile patients with abnormal semen parameters such as volume, concentration, and sperm motility and compared them with those obtained in a group of ten normozoospermic fertile men. The infertile patient group had a significantly higher percentage of spermatozoa containing DSBs, compared to the group of fertile subjects. Nevertheless, no significant differences were found in the percentage of spermatozoa with SSBs between infertile patients and fertile men.

In another study, Gosálvez et al. [41] established SSB and DSB profiles in infertile patients with varicocele and compared them to fertile normozoospermic subjects by 2T-comet assay. In this study, the authors analyzed a particular sperm class observed after applying the sperm chromatin dispersion test that was referred to as "degraded" sperm because they showed relatively low amounts of chromatin remaining in the nucleoid after protein removal when compared to normal or even sperm containing fragmented DNA. The 2T-comet assay demonstrated that degraded sperm containing both massive double- and single-strand DNA breaks coexist in the same spermatozoa. Recently, it has been reported that these types of spermatozoa, also present in the ejaculate of normal individuals, are fully covered with ALS which can be used as another indication of the presence of sperm DNA damage [27]. These "degraded" spermatozoa, a distinctive subpopulation in varicocele patients (six times more than fertile men), probably occur due to the fact that both DNA and protein fractions are affected by intratesticular oxidative stress. The 2T-comet assay has been also used to assess SSBs and DSBs in one patient with Kartagener's syndrome with four failures of fertilization after ISCI using testicular sperm obtained with testicular sperm aspiration [41]. The authors concluded that in addition to a failure of sperm motility, this patient was infertile because of a high level of unrepairable DBSs (85.2%) present in the ejaculate.

The clinical implication of the information provided by the comet assay in fertilization and embryo development depends on the balance between the DNA damage in sperm and the oocyte's repair capacity. Moreover, the type and/or complexity of DNA lesions in the different sperm can vary, and this would influence the embryonic development. After penetration into the oocyte, sperm with extensive DSBs, associated with apoptotic-like processes, will lead to a delayed paternal DNA replication, paternal DNA degradation, and arrest of embryo development if this exceeds the repair capacity of the oocyte [63]. Conversely, when sperm DNA damage is composed mainly of a low level of DSBs, SSBs, abasic sites, and/or DNA base modifications, the oocyte's various specific DNA repair pathways are likely to be more effective, resulting in functional male pronucleus DNA and normal early embryonic development. Nevertheless, some misrepaired or unrepaired DNA lesions could still potentially lead to mutations or chromosome aberrations. Unrepaired SSBs or other lesions types may also result in DSBs when DNA is replicating, leading to structural chromosomal abnormalities [64]. If these chromosome aberrations are unstable, they are more likely to affect the normal mitotic segregation of chromosomes, resulting in genomic instability and cell death, and thereby adversely affect embryo development [65]. When DNA repair is complete, the morula and blastocyst stages can be achieved. In contrast, if the repair processes are defective, blastocyst arrest or spontaneous abortion may then result [66]. SDF can lead to congenital malformations and genetic illnesses, as well as potentially increase the risk of certain cancers in related offspring [67]. The long-term consequences on development and behavior of mice generated by ICSI with fragmentation sperm were investigated [66]. Anatomopathological analysis of animals at

Table 7.1 Types of comet assay and their clinical importance

Comet assay		
Type	DNA break detected	Clinical relevance
Neutral	DSBs	DSBs have been associated with male infertility [54, 55] and pregnancy loss [23]. The identification of DSBs has biological importance at the sperm because of deficiency of DNA damage reparation mechanisms. Standardization, reproducibility, and validation of this technique are necessary
Alkaline	SSBs + DSBs + ALS	Clinical relevance in infertility [38], embryo quality [58, 59], implantation [59], and miscarriage [66] pregnancy [56].Used to assess SDF in obstructive azoospermia [61], varicocele [40, 55] vasectomy [62], chromosomal abnormalities [64], childhood diseases cancer [66], and diabetes mellitus [60]. The methodology is not included in routine infertility tests
Two-tailed comet (neutral + alkaline)	Discrimination of DSBs and SSBs	An innovative method to assess the simultaneous presence of DSB + SSB profiles within the same cell. It has been used to assess infertility [39], varicocele [40], and in a case of Kartagener's syndrome [41]. This methodology may provide important and singular information to understand a part of human fertility and andrological associated problems

SSBs single-strand breaks, *DSBs* double-strand breaks, *ALS* alkali-labile sites, *SDF* sperm DNA fragmentation

16 months of age showed that 33% of females produced with fragmented sperm presented some solid tumors in the lungs and the dermis of the back or neck.

The comet assay, in its different versions, offers the possibility of discriminating between single- and double-strand breaks, and this aspect is of relevance in predicting the fate of the embryo prior to implantation. However, further studies are necessary to understand the mechanisms of paternal DNA damage as a cause of early loss of developmental stages and congenital malformations. The technical problems inherent to the comet assay represent the only bottleneck that limits its wide use in reproduction. In Table 7.1 we have summarized the different types of comet assay and the main clinical relevance associated with each one.

7.6 Conclusions

(i) Assessment of DNA damage (DSBs) can be obtained using a neutral comet assay; whole (SSBs and DSBs) sperm DNA damage can be performed using an alkaline comet assay; the study of whole DNA damage and discrimination between SSBs and DSBs is possible using a 2T-comet assay. (ii) DNA damage evaluation by comet assay – or alternative strategies – as a predictor of male fertility is highly appreciated to assist in the diagnosis of recurrent spontaneous abortions or failures in ART. However, until we demonstrate with certainty which is the best protocol to assess sperm DNA damage, the acceptability and widespread application of any version of the comet assay will limit the application of this test as a research tool.

References

1. Sakkas D, Moffatt O, Manicardi GC, Mariethoz E, Tarozzi N, Bizzaro D. Nature of DNA damage in ejaculated human spermatozoa and the possible involvement of apoptosis. Biol Reprod. 2002;66:1061–7.
2. Marcon L, Boissonneault G. Transient DNA strand breaks during mouse and human spermiogenesis: new insights in stage specificity and link to chromatin remodelling. Biol Reprod. 2004;70:910–8.
3. Agarwal A, Saleh RA, Bedaiwy MA. Role of reactive oxygen species in the pathophysiology of human reproduction. Fertil Steril. 2003;79:829–43.
4. Sotolongo B, Lino E, Ward WS. Ability of hamster spermatozoa to digest their own DNA. Biol Reprod. 2003;69:2029–35.
5. Li TK, Chen AY, Yu C, Mao Y, Wang H, Liu LF. Activation of topoisomerase II-mediated excision of chromosomal DNA loops during oxidative stress. Genes Dev. 1999;13:1553–60.
6. Yakovlev AG, Wang G, Stoica BA, Boulares HA, Spoonde AY, Yoshihara K, Smulson ME. A role of the Ca21/Mg21-dependent endonuclease in apoptosis and its inhibition by Poly(ADP-ribose) polymerase. J Biol Chem. 2000;275:21302–8.
7. Boulares AH, Zoltoski AJ, Sherif ZA, Yakovlev AG, Smulson ME. The Poly (ADP-ribose) polymerase-1-regulated endonuclease DNAS1L3 is required for etoposide-induced internucleosomal DNA fragmentation and increases etoposide cytotoxicity in transfected osteosarcoma cells. Cancer Res. 2002;62:4439–44.
8. Boulares AH, Zoltoski AJ, Contreras FJ, Yakovlev AG, Yoshihara K, Smulson ME. Regulation of DNAS1L3 endonuclease activity by poly (ADP-ribosyl)ation during etoposide-induced apoptosis. Role of poly (ADP-ribose) polymerase-1 cleavage in endonuclease activation. J Biol Chem. 2002;277:372–8.
9. Solovyan VT, Bezvenyuk ZA, Salminen A, Austin CA, Courtney MJ. The role of topoisomerase II in the excision of DNA loop domains during apoptosis. J Biol Chem. 2002;277:21458–67.
10. Ribas-Maynou J, García-Peiró A, Martínez-Heredia J, Fernández-Encinas A, Abad C, Amengual MJ, Navarro J, Benet J. Nuclear degraded sperm subpopulation is affected by poor chromatin compaction and nuclease activity. Andrologia. 2015;47:286–94.
11. Sotolongo B, Huang TT, Isenberger E, Ward WS. An endogenous nuclease in hamster, mouse, and human spermatozoa cleaves DNA into loop-sized fragments. J Androl. 2005;26:272–80.
12. Cortés-Gutiérrez EI, López-Fernández C, Fernández JL, Dávila-Rodríguez MI, Johnston SD, Gosálvez J. Interpreting sperm DNA damage in a diverse range of mammalian sperm by means of the two-tailed comet assay. Front Genet. 27. 2014;5:404.
13. Laberge RM, Boissonneault G. On the nature of DNA strand breaks in elongating spermatids. Biol Reprod. 2005;73:289–96.
14. Reiter TA. NO∗ chemistry: a diversity of targets in the cell. Redox Rep. 2006;11:194–206.
15. Dizdaroglu M. Oxidative damage to DNA in mammalian chromatin. Mutat Res. 1992;275:331–42.
16. Cooke MS, Evans MD, Dizdaroglu M, Lunec J. Oxidative DNA damage: mechanisms, mutation, and disease. FASEB J. 2003;17:1195–214.
17. Ostling O, Johanson KJ. Microelectrophoretic study of radiation-induced DNA damages in individual mammalian cells. Biochem Biophys Res Commun. 1984;123:291–8.
18. Olive PL, Wlodek D, Banath JP. DNA double-strand breaks measured in individual cells subjected to gel electrophoresis. Cancer Res. 1991;51:4671–6.
19. Singh NP, McCoy MT, Tice RR, Schneider EL. A simple technique for quantitation of low levels of DNA damage in individual cells. Exp Cell Res. 1988;175:184–91.
20. Fernández JL, Muriel L, Rivero MT, Goyanes V, Vazquez R, Alvarez JG. The sperm chromatin dispersion test: a simple method for the determination of sperm DNA fragmentation. J Androl. 2003;24:59–66.
21. Enciso M, Sarasa J, Agarwal A, Fernández JL, Gosálvez J. A two-tailed comet assay for assessing DNA damage in spermatozoa. Reprod BioMed Online. 2009;5:609–16.

22. McMillan TJ, Tobi S, Mateos S, Lemon C. The use of DNA double-strand break quantification in radiotherapy. Int J Radiat Oncol Biol Phys. 2001;49:373–7.
23. Ribas-Maynou J, García-Peiró A, Abad C, Amengual MJ, Navarro J, Benet J. Alkaline and neutral comet assay profiles of sperm DNA damage in clinical groups. Hum Reprod. 2012;27:652–8.
24. Brooks JE. Properties and uses of restriction endonucleases. Methods Enzymol. 1987;152:113–29.
25. Singh NP, Stephens RE. X-ray induced DNA double-strand breaks in human sperm. Mutagenesis. 1998;13:75–9.
26. Cortés-Gutiérrez EI, Dávila-Rodríguez MI, López-Fernández C, Fernández JL, Crespo F, Gosálvez J. Localization of alkali-labile sites in donkey (Equus asinus) and stallion (Equus caballus) spermatozoa. Theriogenology. 2014;81:321–5.
27. Fernández JL, Vázquez-Gundin F, Delgado A, Goyanes VJ, Ramiro-Díaz J, de la Torre J, Gosálvez J (2000) DNA breakage detection-FISH (DBD-FISH) in human spermatozoa: technical variants evidence different structural features. Mutat Res 453:77–82.
28. López-Fernández C, Arroyo F, Fernández JL, Gosálvez J. Interstitial telomeric sequence blocks in constitutive pericentromeric heterochromatin from *Pyrgomorpha conica* (Orthoptera) are enriched in constitutive alkali-labile sites. Mutat Res. 2006;599:36–44.
29. Rivero MT, Mosquera A, Goyanes V, Slijepcevic P, Fernández JL. Differences in repair profiles of interstitial telomeric sites between normal and DNA double-strand break repair deficient Chinese hamster cells. Exp Cell Res. 2004;295:161–72.
30. Evenson DP, Kasperson K, Wixon RL. Analysis of sperm DNA fragmentation using flow cytometry and other techniques. Soc Reprod Fertil. 2007;65:93–113.
31. Tice RR, Andrews PW, Singh NP. The single cell gel assay: a sensitive technique for evaluating intercellular differences in DNA damage and repair. Basic Life Sci. 1990;53:291–301.
32. Olive PL, Johnston PJ, Banath JP, Durand RE. The alkaline comet assay: a new method to examine heterogeneity associated with solid tumours. Nat Med. 1998;4:103–5.
33. Fairbairn DW, Olive PL, O'Neill KL. The alkaline comet assay: a comprehensive review. Mutat Res. 1995;339:37–59.
34. McKelvey-Martin VJ, Green MH, Schmezer P, Pool-Zobel BL, De Meo MP, Collins A. The single cell gel electrophoresis assay (alkaline comet assay): a European review. Mutat Res. 1993;288:47–63.
35. Hughes CM, Lewis SE, McKelvey-Martin VJ, Thompson W. Reproducibility of human sperm DNA measurements using the alkaline single cell gel electrophoresis assay. Mutat Res. 1997;374:261–8.
36. Irvine DS, Twigg JP, Gordon EL, Fulton N, Milne PA, Aitken RJ. DNA integrity in human spermatozoa: relationships with semen quality. J Androl. 2000;21:33–44.
37. Leroy T, Van Hummelen P, Anard D, Castelain P, Kirsch Volders M, Lauwerys R, Lison D. Evaluation of three methods for the detection of DNA single-strand breaks in human lymphocytes: alkaline elution, nick translation and single-cell gel electrophoresis. J Toxicol Environ Health. 1996;47:409–22.
38. Lewis SE, Simon L. Clinical implications of sperm DNA damage. Hum Fertil. 2010;13:201–7.
39. Enciso M, Sarasa J, Agarwal A, Fernàndez JL, Gosálvez J. A two-tailed comet assay for assessing DNA damage in spermatozoa. Reprod BioMed Online. 2009;18:609–16.
40. Gosálvez J, Rodríguez-Predreira M, Mosquera A, López Fernández C, Esteves SC, Agarwal A, Ferández JL. Characterisation of a subpopulation of sperm with massive nuclear damage, as recognised with the sperm chromatin dispersion test. Andrologia. 2014;46:602–9.
41. Nuñez R, López-Fernández C, Arroyo F, Caballero P, Gosálvez J. Characterization of sperm DNA damage in Kartagener's syndrome with recurrent fertilization failure: case revisited. Sex Reprod Health. 2010;1:73–5.
42. Esteves SC, Gosálvez J, López-Fernández C, Núñez-Calonge R, Caballero P, Agarwal A, Fernández JL. Diagnostic accuracy of sperm DNA degradation index (DDSi) as a potential noninvasive biomarker to identify men with varicocele-associated infertility. Int Urol Nephrol. 2015;47:1471–7.

43. Gatewood JM, Cook GR, Balhorn R, Schmid CW, Bradbury EM. Isolation of four core histones from human sperm chromatin representing a minor subset of somatic histones. J Biol Chem. 1990;265:20662–6.
44. Hughes CM, Lewis SE, McKelvey-Martin VJ, Thompson W. A comparison of baseline and induced DNA damage in human spermatozoa from fertile and infertile men, using a modified comet assay. Mol Hum Reprod. 1996;2:613–9.
45. Evenson DP, Jost LK, Marshall D, Zinaman MJ, Clegg E, Purvis K, de Angelis P, Claussen OP. Utility of the sperm chromatin structure assay as a diagnostic and prognostic tool in the human fertility clinic. Hum Reprod. 1999;14:1039–49.
46. Spano M, Bonde JP, Hjollund HI, Kolstad HA, Cordelli E, Leter G. Sperm chromatin damage impairs human fertility. The Danish First Pregnancy Planner Study Team. Fertil Steril. 2000;73:43–50.
47. Carrell DT, Liu L. Altered protamine 2 expression is uncommon in donors of known fertility, but common among men with poor fertilizing capacity, and may reflect other abnormalities of spermiogenesis. J Androl. 2001;22:604–10.
48. Zini A, Bielecki R, Phang D, Zenzes MT. Correlations between two markers of sperm DNA integrity, DNA denaturation and DNA fragmentation, in fertile and infertile men. Fertil Steril. 2001;75:674–7.
49. Zini A, Fischer MA, Sharir S, Shayegan B, Phang D, Jarvi K. Prevalence of abnormal sperm DNA denaturation in fertile and infertile men. Urology. 2002;60:1069–72.
50. Zhang X, San Gabriel M, Zini A. Sperm nuclear histone to protamine ratio in fertile and infertile men: evidence of heterogeneous subpopulations of spermatozoa in the ejaculate. J Androl. 2006;27:414–20.
51. Marchetti F, Bishop JB, Cosentino L, Moore D 2nd, Wyrobek AJ. Paternally transmitted chromosomal aberrations in mouse zygotes determine their embryonic fate. Biol Reprod. 2004;70:616–24.
52. Nanassy L, Carrell DT. Paternal effects on early embryogenesis. J Exp Clin Assist Reprod. 2008;5:2.
53. Lewis SEM, Agbaje IM. Using the alkaline comet assay in prognostic tests for male infertility and assisted reproductive technology outcomes. Mutagenesis. 2008;23:163–70.
54. Chi HJ, Chung DY, Choi SY, Kim JH, Kim GY, Lee JS, Lee HS, Kim MH, Roh SI. Integrity of human sperm DNA assessed by the neutral comet assay and its relationship to semen parameters and clinical outcomes for the IVF-ET program. Clin Exp Reprod Med. 2011;38:10–7.
55. Ribas-Maynou J, Gardía-Peiró A, Fernández-Encinas A, Amengual MJ, Prada E, Cortés P, Navarro J, Benet J. Double stranded sperm DNA breaks, measured by comet assay, are associated with unexplained recurrent miscarriage in couples without a female factor. PLoS One. 2012;7:e44679.
56. Simon L, Lutton D, McManus J, Lewis SE. Sperm DNA damage measured by the alkaline comet assay as an independent predictor of male infertility and in vitro fertilization success. Fertil Steril. 2011;95:652–7.
57. Ramzan MH, Ramzan M, Khan MM, Ramzan F, Wahabb F, Khan MA, Jillani M, Shah M. Human semen quality and sperm DNA damage assessed by comet assay in clinical groups. Turk J Med Sci. 2015;45:729–37.
58. Simon L, Proutski I, Stevenson M, Jennings D, McManus J, Lutton D, Lewis SE. Sperm DNA damage has negative association with live-birth rates after IVF. Reprod BioMed Online. 2012;26:68–78.
59. Simon L, Murphy K, Shamsi MB, Liu L, Emery B, Aston KI, Hotaling J, Carrell DT. Paternal influence of sperm DNA integrity on early embryonic development. Hum Reprod. 2014;29:2402–12.
60. Agbaje IM, Rogers DA, McVicar CM, McClure N, Atkinson AB, Mallidis C, Lewis SE. Insulin dependant diabetes mellitus: implications for male reproductive function. Hum Reprod. 2007;22:1871–7.
61. Dalzell LH, McVicar CM, McClure N, Lutton D, Lewis SE. Effects of short and long incubations on DNA fragmentation of testicular sperm. Fertil Steril. 2004;82:1443–5.

62. O'Neill DA, McVicar CM, McClure N, Maxwell P, Cookie I, Pogue KM, Lewis SE. Reduced sperm yield from testicular biopsies of vasectomized men is due to increase apoptosis. Fertil Esteril. 2007;87:834–41.
63. Fatehi AN, Bevers MM, Schoevers E, Roelen BA, Colenbrander B, Gadella BM. DNA damage in bovine sperm does not block fertilization and early embryonic development but induces apoptosis after the first cleavages. J Androl. 2006;27:176–88.
64. Marchetti F, Essers J, Kanaar R, Wyrobek KJ. Disruption of DNA repair increases sperm derived chromosomal aberrations. Proc Natl Acad Sci U S A. 2007;104:17725–9.
65. Gawecka JE, Marh J, Ortega M, Yamauchi Y, Ward MA, Ward WS. Mouse zygotes respond to severe sperm DNA damage by delaying paternal DNA replication and embryonic development. PLoS One. 2013;8:e56385.
66. Fernandez-Gonzalez R, Moreira PN, Perez-Crespo M, Sanchez-Martin M, Ramirez MA, Pericuesta E, Bilbao A, Bermejo-Alvarez P, de Dios Hourcade J, de Fonseca FR, Gutiérrez-Adán A. Long-term effects of mouse intracytoplasmic sperm injection with DNA-fragmented sperm on health and behavior of adult offspring. Biol Reprod. 2008;78:761–72.
67. Hales BF. DNA repair disorders causing malformations. Curr Opin Genet Dev. 2005;15:234–40.

Chapter 8
Sperm Chromatin Dispersion (SCD) Assay

José Luis Fernández, Stephen Johnston, and Jaime Gosálvez

8.1 Introduction

The essential function of a spermatozoon is the transmission of a haploid genome from the male to the female oocyte. Nevertheless, current spermiogram appears primarily centered on the carrier of the DNA package and not in the content [1]; indeed, in the past, many andrologists were primarily interested in sperm motility, a sperm characteristic with little importance in the context of ICSI. In contrast, the relevance of sperm DNA integrity in the classical spermiogram is typically regarded with a lower level of interest and importance in many centers. This occurs as the focus has been given to sperm motility instead, based on the assumption that motile spermatozoa must contain a normal DNA molecule. If this were to be true, a simple swim-up procedure would not only eliminate non-motile spermatozoa but also sperm with DNA damage. However, this is not the case. In every isolated subpopulation obtained from a swim-up, it is possible to find spermatozoa with evidence of fragmented DNA [2, 3]. Furthermore, given the logical relevance of sperm DNA integrity to completion of the diploid zygote and normal embryonic development, the assessment of this parameter should be incorporated as part of the fundamental component of conventional semen analysis [4–7].

J.L. Fernández (✉)
Unidad de Genética, Complejo Hospitalario Universitario A Coruña (CHUAC), Instituto de Investigación Biomédica de A Coruña (INIBIC), 15006, As Xubias, 84, A Coruña 15006, Spain

Laboratorio de Genética Molecular y Radiobiología, Centro Oncológico de Galicia, A Coruña, 15009 Spain
e-mail: Jose.Luis.Fernandez.Garcia@sergas.es

S. Johnston
School of Agriculture and Food Sciences, The University of Queensland, Gatton, Australia

J. Gosálvez
Unidad de Genética, Facultad de Biología, Universidad Autónoma de Madrid, Spain

A. Zini, A. Agarwal (eds.), *A Clinician's Guide to Sperm DNA and Chromatin Damage*, https://doi.org/10.1007/978-3-319-71815-6_8

Although all mammalian species that have been examined to date have shown evidence of some proportion of the ejaculate containing sperm with fragmented DNA, the occurrence of this phenomenon appears to be both species-specific and varies interindividually [8, 9]. In humans, it has been well established that infertile males and poor sperm quality samples (according to the standard seminal analysis) tend to have a higher proportion of spermatozoa with fragmented DNA [10–12]. Even some individuals with normal standard parameters may show elevated levels of sperm with DNA fragmentation (SDF) [13]. Furthermore, studies performed on semen samples subjected to assisted reproductive technology (ART) have demonstrated that increased SDF in the processed sample negatively affect the fertilization rate, embryo quality, blastocyst rate, implantation rate, and the pregnancy outcome [14–17]. Additionally, the assessment of sperm DNA integrity has also been shown to have relevance or be associated with common andrological pathologies, such as varicocele [18], genital infections [19], cancer [20], and toxicogenetics [21].

Several techniques have been applied to analyze DNA fragmentation in spermatozoa, including sperm chromatin structure assay (SCSA), terminal deoxynucleotidyl transferase-mediated nick end labeling (TUNEL), in situ nick translation (ISNT) assay, single-cell gel electrophoresis (SCGE), and comet assay [14, 22–24]. These procedures are all useful and reliable when adequately performed. Nevertheless, they are comparatively complex to perform on a routine basis as they are difficult to implement, time-consuming, technically demanding, relatively expensive, and requiring skilled personnel. In many cases, sperm samples need to be delivered offsite to a specialized center to be processed. Consequently, most of these procedures are not ideal to be performed routinely in the conventional semen analysis laboratory. The sperm chromatin dispersion (SCD) test overcomes some of these limitations, offering a user-friendly procedure that is cost-effective and easy to conduct in routine evaluation of SDF.

8.2 The SCD Test: DNA Denaturation Coupled with Controlled Nuclear Protein Depletion

The human SCD assay is a simple yet elegant scientific concept, consisting of three main steps: (1) embedding of the sperm cells in an inert microgel matrix, (2) sequential incubation in an acid and a species-specific lysing solution, and (3) staining for visualization [25].

Firstly, the native unfixed spermatozoa are immersed in an agarose matrix on a microscope slide, which provides an inert suspension-like substrate to manipulate the cells. Secondly, the cells are incubated in an acid DNA unwinding solution followed by a lysing solution. The acid solution is a soft DNA denaturant, which "melts" the DNA double helix only when it contains massive DNA breakage. These DNA breaks behave as starting points of denaturation which subsequently move along the DNA helix [26, 27]. If the sperm DNA molecule is massively broken, most of the genome will be denatured, whereas non-fragmented DNA will remain intact. Having said that, stronger denaturants can also affect the non-fragmented sperm DNA; therefore, precise incubation with the acid solution for an appropriate length of time allows a better discrimination between the two.

Secondly, the sperm are immersed in a specific lysing solution to remove nuclear proteins, especially the protamines. These highly basic proteins strongly pack the DNA loops together within the sperm nucleus. Protamine removal results in spreading of DNA loops into the surrounding microgel, in a phenomenon akin to what happens in the nucleus of somatic cells after the removal of histones [28]; these deproteinized nuclei are known as nucleoids, whereby the dispersed loops constitute a peripheral halo of DNA-chromatin emerging from a central core or residual nuclear area. Accordingly, nucleoids of sperm without fragmented DNA (i.e., without significant denatured DNA by the previous acid treatment) show large halos of dispersed DNA. Conversely, when lysis is performed on sperm nucleoids with massively broken DNA, which are susceptible to denaturation, dispersal of DNA in microgel is not observed or occurs only to a limited extent; these nucleoids therefore appear without a halo or possess only a very small halo. This particular behavior is likely related to the characteristic sperm chromatin structure.

Finally, after a brief wash and dehydration in increasing ethanol baths, the sperm nucleoids are stained for visualization under bright-field microscopy using the Wright stain or the Diff-Quik (Fig. 8.1a). Alternatively, they can also be observed using the fluorescence microscope after staining with any suitable DNA fluorochrome (Fig. 8.1b). Occasionally, some nucleoids without halos may also appear faintly or irregularly stained; these nucleoids as revealed by the SCD test are designated as "degraded" and are associated with more severe nuclear damage affecting both DNA and the proteinaceous matrix. Spermatozoa with fragmented DNA therefore correspond to those with a small halo, no halo, or degraded. Microscopic visualization of these different nucleoid categories is easy to differentiate (Figs. 8.1 and 8.2). An important element of the SCD test is that the species-specific lysing solution also preserves the morphology of sperm tail which can be stained with the bright-field dye or using fluorochromes for proteins like the 2.7-dibrom-4-hydroxy-mercury-fluorescein [29]. Using these fluorochromes, the tail or any residual proteins in the core will fluoresce green, whereas the nucleoid may be contrasted in red or blue fluorescence using GelRed (Biotium, Hayward, CA, USA) or 4′,6-diamidino-2-phenylindole (DAPI), respectively. The visualization of the tail helps to discriminate sperm from other cell types presented in the ejaculate or testicular biopsy.

The SCD test is available as a kit (Halosperm®), which provides all the reagents of the assay to ensure easy technical operation and provide repeatable and consistent results in different clinical laboratories. The technical procedure is simple, can be completed in 45 min, and does not require any costly equipment. Furthermore, the nucleoid scoring process is also very fast: 500 sperm may be categorized under the microscope in 5–10 min, depending on the sperm concentration. While it is possible to employ a microscope with a motorized stage and a digital camera for image

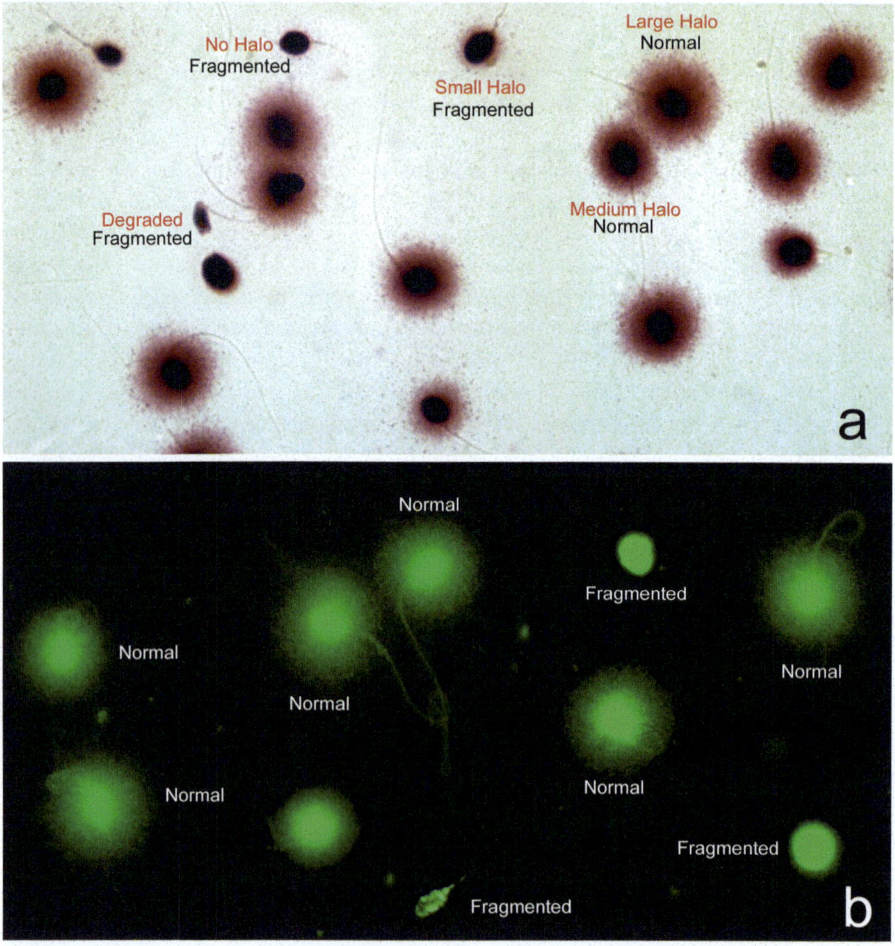

Fig. 8.1 Bright-field (**a**) and fluorescence microscope (**b**) images of human sperm processed by the SCD test. Sperm showing big- and medium-sized halos of chromatin dispersion contain non-fragmented DNA, whereas those showing small or no halos carry fragmented DNA. Degraded sperm have fragmented DNA, showing no halo and irregular or faint stain of the core

capture coupled to specifically validated image analysis software to automate scoring, analysis using the naked eye is equally as effective.

Evaluation under the microscope also allows for simultaneous identification of the presence of cells other than sperm, including spermatogonia, spermatocytes, leukocytes, epithelial cells, and even bacteria. High proportions of these cells could potentially confound the results in non-morphological-based assays of sperm DNA fragmentation. For the same reason, the SCD test is ideal for the assessment of samples with very few sperm such as in oligospermic patients or in testicular biopsies.

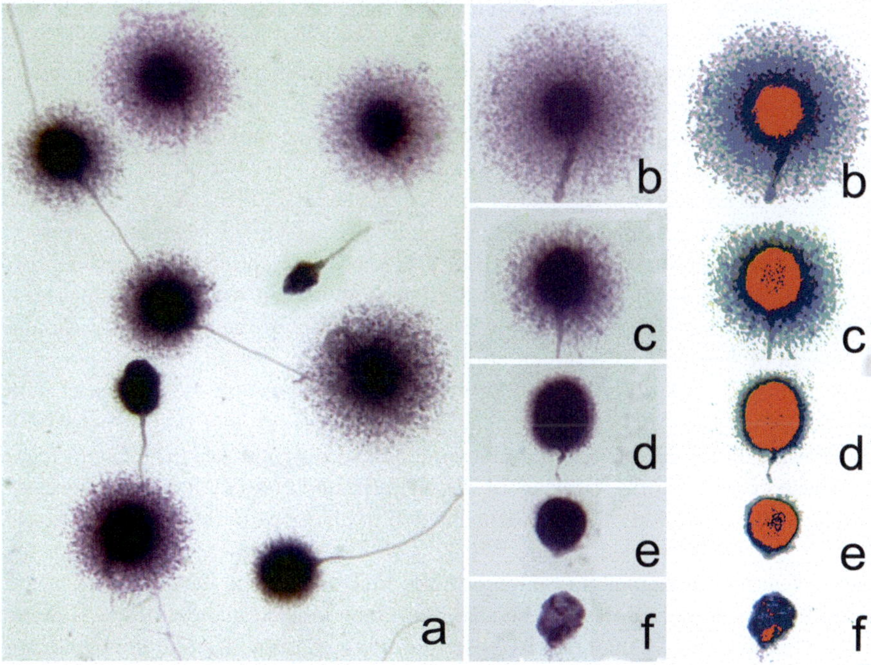

Fig. 8.2 Human sperm processed by the SCD test and visualized under the bright-field microscope (**a**). Representative sperm with big halo (**b**), medium-sized halo (**c**), small halo (**d**), no halo (**e**), and degraded (**f**). (**b′**–**f′**) Electronically filtering to enhance domains of the halo (*blue*) and the core (*red*)

8.3 The SCD Test: Validated by Different Sequential In Situ Assays

The SCD test has been extensively validated with a range of different but complementary approaches. The sperm nucleoids obtained after the SCD test are also amenable to be processed to determine DNA breaks using other in situ procedures. DNA breakage detection-fluorescence in situ hybridization (DBD-FISH) is a powerful technique for detecting DNA breaks and, in fact, has some similarity in its concept and application to that of the SCD assay [30, 31]. In DBD-FISH, cells embedded in the microgel are exposed to a DNA denaturant solution that transforms DNA breaks into single-stranded DNA motifs starting from the end of the breaks. These single-strand regions are targets for hybridization of fluorescent-labeled DNA probes. Using dose-dependent ionizing radiation to artificially induce DNA breaks and the subsequent unwinding of single-stranded DNA motifs, it is possible to demonstrate a corresponding dose-dependent greater hybridization of the probe, reflected in intensity of the fluorescence that is measured. The DBD-FISH is a reliable technique that allows determination of DNA breakage within a specific sequence or chromatin area; different sequence regions may also be compared for DNA breakage density by hybridizing differentially labeled DNA probes [31, 32]. The SCD procedure also makes use of the DNA unwinding and lysis steps, so that before dehydration and staining, the sperm nucleoids can be incubated with the fluorescent-labeled human whole-genome DNA probe. This probe then hybridizes with the single-stranded DNA produced from DNA breaks by the unwinding acid solution. When this microgel preparation is DNA counterstained, it reveals only those sperm nucleoids with a small or no halo to be labeled by the DBD-FISH assay; in fact, this is the basis of the original development of the SCD test [33, 34]. Given the complex and time-consuming nature of the DBD-FISH procedure and the near perfect correlation between halo size and hybridization of the nucleoid with the DNA probe, it is much more cost-, labor-, and time-efficient to employ the SCD assay for the assessment of sperm DNA fragmentation.

The nucleoids resulting from SCD processing may not only be incubated with labeled DNA probes but also with enzymes such as terminal deoxynucleotidyl transferase (TdT) or the Klenow fragment of the DNA polymerase I from *Escherichia coli*. These enzymes form the basis of the TUNEL and end-labeling procedures as they allow incorporation of fluorescent-labeled nucleotides to the free 3′-hydroxyl group of the DNA break [22, 23, 35]. *E. coli* DNA polymerase I may also be employed in a similar manner, extending the nicks along the DNA duplex in the 5–3′ direction while replacing these sites with new labeled nucleotides, following the ISNT assay [23, 35]; again, only those sperm nucleoids with small or no halo are labeled by the enzymatic assays. The SCD test is the only SDF assay which has been systematically validated in situ with other breakage labeling procedures performed on the same sperm cell [34, 36].

Several conventional strategies have confirmed the reliability of the SCD test. Treatment of sperm with DNase I that produces single- and double-strand DNA breaks specifically with 3′-hydroxyl ends results in nucleoids without halo after SCD processing [37]. The same result occurs with restriction endonucleases that produce double-strand DNA breaks. Moreover, incubation of sperm with increasing concentrations of sodium nitroprusside (SNP), a nitric oxide (NO) donor, also results in a progressive increase of the proportion of nucleoids with small or no halo [36, 37]. NO reacts with molecular oxygen producing nitrous anhydride and with the superoxide radical yielding peroxynitrite, a potent oxidant that induces DNA damage [38]. Furthermore, treatment with hydrogen peroxide, which decomposes into highly reactive hydroxyl radicals that leads to DNA damage including single-strand breaks with chemically modified ends, also results in sperm nucleoids with small halo or without a halo [37]. These experiments with different DNA damaging agents provide convincing evidence that the SCD test is able to detect both single- and double-strand DNA breaks, either with "clean" or with chemically altered ends.

Finally, a strong correlation has been obtained when the same sperm samples were processed with different DNA fragmentation assays like the TUNEL, comet, or SCSA, in human and in different animal species [39, 40].

8.4 The SCD Test: A Versatile Methodology for Basic and Clinical Research

The nucleoids obtained after acid and lysis incubation can be processed with other techniques to obtain further information on chromatin structure and packaging or that can be directly correlated with the presence or absence of DNA fragmentation in specific individual spermatozoa; this allows the technique to be used for both basic and applied forms of research activity. The combination of SCD with other techniques has already been demonstrated in the previous section of this chapter with regard to the sequential use of DBD-FISH or enzymatic labeling of DNA breaks. For example, conventional FISH can be performed on dehydrated sperm nucleoids obtained by the SCD procedure [41]. For such purpose, DNA is denatured and hybridized with a range of locus-specific DNA probes. It should be noted that the denaturation process mentioned here must not be confused with that of the acid treatment; as the denaturation is now performed in all nucleoids, so the DNA probe hybridizes in all of them.

It is also important to understand that nucleoids are very delicate; the halos may be lost by the action of strong denaturation, long incubation with DNA probe, and washing steps. Consequently, sperm without fragmented DNA (i.e., those with large halos) may then resemble those with DNA fragmentation if conditions are not carefully controlled [42]. As such, sperm halos should be scored both before and after denaturation and hybridization. Nucleoid denaturation with preservation of halos can be achieved by formaldehyde fixation and a very brief incubation with NaOH for a few seconds. After incubation with the DNA probes, the washing steps in formamide solution should not be higher than 44°C and long incubation times should be avoided. Only those slides with well-preserved halos (with categories of SCD nucleoids comparable to that of the control undenatured slide and similar before and after treatment) should be analyzed. Using this approach, aneuploidies and DNA fragmentation can be assessed simultaneously in each sperm as it has been demonstrated that sperm with fragmented DNA, with small or without halos, contain a significant higher proportion of chromosomal aneuploidies [41]. The possibility that could explain this is that the sperm with an abnormal genome as a consequence of meiotic failure could be genetically inactivated inducing DNA fragmentation.

Denatured sperm nucleoids may also be incubated with antibodies against specific DNA lesions or modifications. Using an antibody against 8-oxoguanosine (8-oxoG), this base lesion has been identified in sperm with fragmented DNA (those with small or without halos) [37]. Since 8-oxoG is a product of oxidative stress, such finding infers that DNA fragmentation is likely linked to oxidative damage. As another example, SCD nucleoids can be incubated with antibodies against 5-methylcytosine so that DNA fragmentation and DNA methylation levels can be simultaneously evaluated.

As previously indicated, fluorescence microscopy allows the synchronous use of different fluorochromes for evaluation of different targets. Thus, besides DNA dyes, proteins can be stained by the green emission fluorochrome 2.7-dibrom-4-hydroxy-mercury-fluorescein to observe the residual nuclear matrix of lysed sperm as well as the tail [29]. Somatic cells such as leukocytes could also be present in the ejaculate and be processed through the SCD procedure. Despite the lysis, these cells retain the histone proteins as a consequence of the previous acid treatment; therefore, they do not produce halos and show strong green fluorescence by the fluorochrome. The concurrent staining of DNA with a red emission fluorochrome results in a yellow fluorescence in a double band-pass filter, in which leukocytes can be easily discriminated.

8.5 The SCD Test: Its Diagnostic Value for Predicting ART Outcome

SDF cannot be overlooked as an irrelevant neutral characteristic of sperm. The SCD test was performed on 210 sperm donors and a random cohort of 775 males attending an infertility clinic and revealed that donor sperm had a mean SDF (10.7 ± 8.7) that was significantly lower than the random cohort (29.2 ± 17.6). A SDF cutoff value of 16% discriminated both cohorts of individuals with a sensitivity of 85% and a specificity of 75% [12]. Initial studies using the SCD assay revealed a significant correlation between SDF and (1) oocyte fertilization rate, (2) embryo quality, (3) blastocyst rate, and (4) implantation rate but not with pregnancy rate [16, 43]. The lack of strong relationship between SDF and clinical pregnancy rate could be due to two reasons. Firstly, following ICSI, embryos fertilized by sperm containing fragmented DNA may not be selected for transfer, decreasing the predictive value. Many studies performed in animals, where embryos are not selected, have shown a clear influence of SDF on pregnancy [44, 45]. A second and very important factor is the variability of the moment when the SDF procedure is determined, since SDF may increase with time after ejaculation. This, in fact, may be the explanation for the lack of convincing results in an old IUI study [46] as well as in other reports using different SDF techniques. SDF is not a static phenomenon, and iatrogenic DNA damage progresses over time after in vitro incubation prior to ART and is dependent on the laboratory conditions and processing of the individual sample. Under these uncontrolled circumstances, SDF assessment is unlikely to be meaningful.

Many recent reports corroborate the value of the SCD test in human fertility assessment and in predicting pregnancy outcome. For example, in a cohort study of 152 infertile couples, SDF was found more informative than using high magnification assessment of detailed sperm morphology. The predictive cutoff for pregnancy established using the SCD test was 25.5% of sperm DNA fragmentation, with a negative predictive value of 72.7% [47]. Time-lapse recording of embryos produced following ICSI (n = 165) has shown that higher SDF levels correlated with an increase in the period of time to achieve the blastocyst stage and decreased pregnancy rates [48].

As expected, female factor infertility may accentuate the adverse effect of SDF on reproductive outcome [49]. As a matter of fact, the impact of SDF was found to be more significant in women with a lower ovarian reserve. In a study of 2865 couples undergoing IVF-ICSI, Jim et al. [50] determined that a cutoff value of SDF at 27.3% could help predict the clinical pregnancy rate in the group of women with reduced ovarian reserve. Above this SDF threshold, live-birth and implantation rates were significantly decreased. Moreover, the risk of early abortion was also increased in the group of women with normal ovarian reserve when SDF was above the same cutoff. Regarding the relationship between SDF and miscarriage, it has been reported that SDF was higher in men from couples with idiopathic recurrent spontaneous abortion, unlike Y microdeletion frequency [51]. The influence of SDF in abortion was also confirmed when using testicular sperm for ICSI instead of ejaculated sperm, in oligozoospermic males with high SDF levels in the ejaculated sample ($n = 147$ couples). In this study, it was evidenced that testicular sperm decreased SDF from 40.7 to 8.3%, and the miscarriage rate dramatically dropped from 34.4 to 10.0%, so the live-birth rate increased from 26.4 to 46.7% [52].

To control for the DNA repair capacity of the oocytes, a prospective study using high-quality donor oocytes was performed in 70 couples to examine on the effects of SDF on reproductive outcomes. The SCD procedure was conducted in both the raw and the swim-up processed sperm sample subsequently employed for ICSI and at equivalent time period to account for any adverse iatrogenic-induced DNA damage. The swim-up procedure usually decreases SDF in comparison with the original neat sample. Whereas the cutoff value for pregnancy in the neat semen of this study was 24.8%, a 17% threshold SDF value for established pregnancy was determined for the swim-up processed aliquot, with 77.8% sensitivity and 71.1% specificity [53]. Then, the SDF from the selected highly motile sperm fraction maintains the predictive significance but at a lower threshold number [54]. It is possible that the SFD value sometimes could be indicative of some unrecognized damage in the rest of the sperm population [14, 17].

8.6 The SCD Test: Provides Complementary Information in Andrological Assessment

SDF can be increased in the ejaculates of males with a range of andrological pathologies, providing additional relevant information that can be used to complement standard seminal analysis. For example, sperm from individuals with varicocele tend to show elevated SDF values in comparison with fertile subjects, similar to those samples from infertile patients [18]. Interestingly, the subpopulations of sperm with fragmented DNA from individuals with varicocele also tend to possess a higher proportion of "degraded" sperm subcategory. The faint or irregular staining of DNA in these spermatozoa could be the result of extreme nuclear damage, in both DNA and proteins [55]. The proportion of "degraded" sperm in the whole population of sperm with fragmented DNA has been termed as the sperm DNA degradation index (SDDI) [55, 56]. After analysis of 593 semen samples from donors and patients with different pathologies, sperm samples from individuals with varicocele diagnosed as either clinical or subclinical showed a remarkable elevated SDDI; a SDDI value >0.33 was able to predict varicocele patients with an accuracy of 94% [56]. It has been speculated that this extreme nuclear damage could be a consequence of a higher than normal level of testicular oxidative stress associated with poor thermoregulation of the testis and epididymis. From a practical point of view, when performing a SDF evaluation using the SCD test, if one out of three sperm with fragmented DNA is degraded, this is likely to be associated with the presence of a clinical or subclinical varicocele. In addition, detection of lower levels of SDDI would also be of great value in the follow-up of any successful treatment of this pathology.

The SCD test has also been used to linked elevated SDF levels to urogenital infections. This was demonstrated in vitro after incubation of sperm samples with farnesol, a quorum-sensing molecule released to the medium by the yeast *Candida albicans* in order to inhibit the transition to the filamentous growth form. Farnesol induces sperm DNA fragmentation in a dose-dependent way, and it is possible that yeast infection could also influence host fertility [57]; such a phenomenon could easily be explored using the SDF test, as it could also be used to test the cytotoxic effects of range of pathogens.

Patients with urogenital infection with *Chlamydia trachomatis* and *Mycoplasma* ($n = 143$) showed a 3.2-fold increase in the frequency of spermatozoa with fragmented DNA with respect to fertile controls, whereas standard seminal parameters were scarcely affected [19]. A higher incidence of sperm DNA damage associated with chlamydiosis or the inflammation associated with the disease could explain the subfertility of the infected patients. Furthermore, antibiotic treatment of patients in this study reversed the high incidence of SDF in the majority of the 95 patients examined 3 months following treatment [19]. Consequently, the determination of sperm DNA fragmentation may not only have value in disease detection but also in assessing the efficacy of therapies designed to treat the disease or inflammation.

Even before any therapy, the presence of some forms of cancer can elevate the incidence of SDF to a magnitude similar to that found in most infertile subjects; Meseguer et al. [20] found that 35.8% of cryopreserved samples from 50 patients presenting with lymphoma, leukemia, testicular tumors, and other cancers had elevated levels of SDF. The increase in SDF was considered independent of the origin of the neoplasia and perhaps could be an underlying cause of transient infertility. Therefore, we maintain that SDF should be evaluated in the sperm samples to be frozen before therapy in order to select those most adequate cells for preservation.

SDF is of great interest in reproductive toxicology as it can be used to reveal and evaluate the adverse effect of different endogenous or environmental agents on the germ line. For example, the SCD test has been used to detect an increase of SDF in samples from smokers, when sperm were selected by swim-up [21]. Moreover, a SDF dynamic assay may enhance the detection of sperm damage associated with reproductive toxicology that might otherwise go undetected. Following this approach, the sample is incubated in vitro at 36–37°C and SDF is determined for consecutive periods of time and the SDF increases progressively at a particular rate. This dynamic procedure can be easily accomplished using the Dyn-Halosperm® kit and accurate statistical analysis is performed using the Kaplan-Meier survival curves. When sperm samples are transiently exposed to damaging agents like SNP or high temperature or low pH, they may not show a significant variation in SDF when immediately assessed. However, if these same sperm samples are evaluated dynamically, it may be possible to elucidate a higher rate of SDF with respect to the control untreated samples [58]. This is a proof of concept that the dynamic assay may unmask cryptic sperm damage initially not evident. The damage may be initially induced at different targets, DNA, proteins, or membranes, and is later expressed by triggering processes that lead to DNA fragmentation which can then be detected.

In the clinical laboratory, possible cryptic iatrogenic damage induced to sperm during sample processing ex vivo can also be demonstrated using the dynamic SDF assay, for example, during storage or centrifugation [59]. In this study, the rate of SDF following thawing of cryopreserved samples from five donors was found to be 4.3% per hour after 6 h of incubation. This velocity was on average three times higher than that found in fresh samples of the same semen, 1.6% per hour [60], and clearly emphasizes the necessity of the rapid use of the thawed sperm. The dynamic SDF assay is a powerful tool for quality control of the procedures of sperm handling.

8.7 The SCD Test: Easy Assessment of Sperm DNA Longevity

SDF increases with time after ejaculation in vitro and therefore most likely does the same in vivo within the female genital tract. As a consequence, different times of examination for different samples make the comparisons of SDF inappropriate and the correlations with the different fertility parameters inaccurate. This may be one explanation as to the disparity of results in some clinical studies as the time dimension must be taken into account when reporting the SDF value from a sample, especially if a frozen-thawed semen sample is being evaluated.

SDF dynamics varies between species and individuals [8, 9]. The differences in "DNA longevity" of the different sperm can be consequence of cryptic damage in different biochemical sperm components, which precipitate the subsequent DNA fragmentation, as described above [58]. Interestingly, oral antioxidant treatment for 3 months in a cohort of 20 infertile asthenoteratozoospermic patients not only decreased the basal SDF but also increased the DNA stability as demonstrated with the dynamic SCD test [61].

Furthermore, chromatin architecture deeply influences DNA stability. A thorough comparison of sets of 10 samples from 11 animal species points to protamination-related packing as a significant factor. Species with higher sperm DNA longevity like bull and boar contain strongly packed chromatin with only one protamine type (P1) with a high level of cysteine residues and disulfide bonds between them. Otherwise, mouse and human sperm, which includes two protamine types, P1 and P2, and less disulfide bonding show a less stable chromatin. Consequently, abnormal protamination or poor chromatin packing could decrease sperm DNA stability [9]. In fact, human patients exhibiting unbalanced P1/P2 ratios show a higher rate of SDF [62].

The rate of SDF damage for cryopreserved human spermatozoa samples after incubation in vitro at 36°C (temperature of the female genital tract) has been shown to be habitually faster during the first 4 h after thawing. Nevertheless, one individual may show a rapid SDF increase per hour, whereas another exhibits a slow increase [8]. If the first sample is used for IUI or IVF, the prolonged time required for fertilization either in vivo or in vitro would result in a much higher SDF than that obtained after ejaculation. Accordingly, some studies on IVF have recommended only short periods of co-incubation with the oocyte to achieve better rates of fertilization [63]. This would also happen if there is a significant delay between collection or thawing of the cryopreserved sample and the ICSI procedure. The information on the SDF dynamics of an individual patient may help to improve the strategy of how to handle the sperm prior to the IVF or ICSI procedure. Besides evaluation of the treatment efficacy in individual patients [61], dynamic SDF studies are also relevant to donor sperm banks in order to select those individuals exhibiting the highest DNA stability.

8.8 Conclusion

DNA transmission from one individual to the next is the fundamental basis of successful reproduction, so that it would seem pertinent and logical that any standard seminogram should also include systematic evaluation of sperm DNA quality. While there are a variety of techniques which have been used to determine sperm DNA damage, we have presented in this review evidence for the utility of the sperm chromatin dispersion test in terms of its validation, its use in fundamental and applied clinical research, and its efficacy as a cost-effective simple user-friendly assay. We have also demonstrated how the assay can be applied in dynamic assessment of sperm DNA fragmentation and how this paradigm might be used to explore in vitro incubation as a model for what happens to the sperm in the female reproductive tract and to prevent and/or improve clinical practice associated with iatrogenic-induced DNA pathology.

References

1. Makhlouf AA, Niederberger C. DNA integrity tests in clinical practice: it is not a simple matter of black and white (or red and green). J Androl. 2006;27:316–23.
2. Younglai EV, Holt D, Brown P, Jurisicova A, Casper RF. Sperm swim-up techniques and DNA fragmentation. Hum Reprod. 2001;16:1950–3.
3. Santiso R, Tamayo M, Gosálvez J, Meseguer M, Garrido N, Fernández JL. Swim-up procedure selects spermatozoa with longer telomere length. Mutat Res. 2010;688:88–90.
4. Agarwal A, Allamaneni SS. Sperm DNA damage assessment: a test whose time has come. Fertil Steril. 2005;84:850–3.
5. Zini A, Sigman M. Are test of sperm DNA damage clinically useful? Pros and cons. J Androl. 2009;30:219–29.
6. Lewis SE, Aitken JR, Conner SJ, Iuliis GD, Evenson DP, Henkel R, et al. The impact of sperm DNA damage in assisted conception and beyond: recent advances in diagnosis and treatment. Reprod BioMed Online. 2013;27:325–37.
7. Lewis SE. Should sperm DNA fragmentation testing be included in the male fertility work-up? Reprod BioMed Online. 2015;31:134–7.
8. Gosálvez J, Elva C, López-Fernández C, Fernández JL, Caballero P, Nuñez R. Sperm DNA fragmentation dynamics in fertile donors. Fertil Steril. 2009;92:170–3.
9. Gosálvez J, López-Fernández C, Fernández JL, Gouraud A, Holt WW. Relationships between the dynamics of iatrogenic DNA damage and genomic design in mammalian spermatozoa from eleven species. Mol Reprod Dev. 2011;78:951–61.
10. Agarwal A, Said TM. Role of sperm chromatin abnormalities and DNA damage in male infertility. Hum Reprod Update. 2003;9:331–45.
11. Tesarik J, Mendoza-Tesarik R, Mendoza C. Sperm nuclear damage: update on the mechanism, diagnosis and treatment. Reprod BioMed Online. 2006;12:715–21.
12. Gosálvez J, Fernández JL, Yaniz J, de la Casa M, López-Fernández C, Johnston SA. Comparison of sperm DNA damage in the neat ejaculate of sperm donors and males presenting for their initial seminogram. Austin J Reprod Med Infertil. 2015;2:1014.
13. Oleszczuk K, Augustinsson L, Giwercman A, Bungum M. Prevalence of high DNA fragmentation index in male partners of unexplained infertile couples. Andrology. 2013;1:357–60.
14. Evenson DP, Larson KJ, Jost LK. Sperm chromatin structure assay: its clinical use for detecting sperm DNA fragmentation in male infertility and comparisons with other techniques. J Androl. 2002;23:25–43.
15. Virro MR, Larson-Cook KL, Evenson DP. Sperm chromatin structure assay (SCSA®) parameters are related to fertilization, blastocyst development, and ongoing pregnancy in in vitro fertilization and intracytoplasmic sperm injection cycles. Fertil Steril. 2004;81:1289–95.
16. Muriel L, Garrido N, Fernández JL, Remohí J, Pellicer A, de los Santos MJ, et al. Value of the sperm deoxyribonucleic acid fragmentation level, as measured by the sperm chromatin dispersion test, in the outcome of in vitro fertilization and intracytoplasmic sperm injection. Fertil Steril. 2006;85:371–83.
17. Evenson DP, Wixon R. Clinical aspects of sperm DNA fragmentation detection and male infertility. Theriogenology. 2006;15:979–91.
18. Enciso M, Muriel L, Fernández JL, Goyanes V, Segrelles E, Marcos M, et al. Infertile men with varicocele show a high relative proportion of sperm cells with intense nuclear damage level, evidenced by the sperm chromatin dispersion (SCD) test. J Androl. 2006;27:106–11.
19. Gallegos G, Ramos B, Santiso R, Goyanes V, Gosalvez J, Fernández JL. Sperm DNA fragmentation in infertile men with genitourinary infection by chlamydia trachomatis and mycoplasma sp. Fertil Steril. 2008;90:328–34.
20. Meseguer M, Santiso R, Garrido N, Fernández JL. The effect of cancer on sperm DNA fragmentation measured by the sperm chromatin dispersion (SCD) test. Fertil Steril. 2008;90:225–7.

21. Viloria T, Garrido N, Fernández JL, Remohí J, Pellicer A, Meseguer M. Sperm selection by swim-up in terms of DNA fragmentation as measured by the sperm chromatin dispersion (SCD) test is altered in heavy smokers. Fertil Steril. 2007;88:523–5.
22. Gorczyca W, Traganos F, Jesionowska H, Darzynkiewicz Z. Presence of DNA strand breaks and increased sensitivity of DNA in situ to denaturation in abnormal human sperm cells: analogy to apoptosis of somatic cells. Exp Cell Res. 1993;207:202–5.
23. Muriel L, Segrelles E, Goyanes V, Gosálvez J, Fernández JL. Structure of human sperm DNA and background damage, analyzed by in situ enzymatic treatment and digital image analysis. Mol Hum Reprod. 2004;10:203–9.
24. Baumgartner A, Cemeli E, Anderson D. The comet assay in male reproductive toxicology. Cell Biol Toxicol. 2009;25:81–98.
25. Fernández JL, Cajigal D, Gosálvez J. Assessing sperm DNA fragmentation with the sperm chromatin dispersion (SCD) test. Methods Mol Biol. 2011;682:291–301.
26. Rydberg B. The rate of strand separation in alkali of DNA of irradiated mammalian cells. Radiat Res. 1975;61:274–87.
27. Ahnström G. Techniques to measure DNA strand breaks in cells: a review. Int J Radiat Biol. 1998;54:695–707.
28. Cook PP, Brazell IA. Spectrofluorometric measurement of the binding of ethidium to superhelical DNA from cell nuclei. Eur J Biochem. 1978;84:465–77.
29. Santiso R, Muriel L, Goyanes V, Segrelles E, Gosálvez J, Fernández JL. Evidence of modified nuclear protein matrix in human spermatozoa with fragmented deoxyribonucleic acid. Fertil Steril. 2007;87:191–4.
30. Fernández JL, Goyanes VJ, Ramiro-Díaz J, Gosálvez J. Application of FISH for in situ detection and quantification of DNA breakage. Cytogenet Cell Genet. 1998;2:251–6.
31. Fernández JL, Gosálvez J. Application of FISH to detect DNA damage: DNA breakage detection-FISH (DBD-FISH). Methods Mol Biol. 2002;203:203–16.
32. Vázquez-Gundín F, Rivero MT, Gosálvez J, Fernández JL. Radiation-induced DNA breaks in different human satellite DNA sequence areas, analyzed by DNA breakage detection-fluorescence in situ hybridisation. Radiat Res. 2002;157:711–20.
33. Fernández JL, Vázquez-Gundín F, Delgado A, Goyanes VJ, Ramiro-Díaz J, de la Torre J, et al. DNA breakage detection-FISH (DBD-FISH) in human spermatozoa: technical variants evidence different structural features. Mutat Res. 2000;453:77–82.
34. Fernández JL, Muriel L, Rivero MT, Goyanes V, Vázquez R, Alvarez JG. The sperm chromatin dispersion test: a simple method for the determination of sperm DNA fragmentation. J Androl. 2003;24:59–66.
35. Dierendonck JH. DNA damage detection using DNA polymerase I or its Klenow fragment: applicability, specificity, limitations. Methods Mol Biol. 2002;203:81–108.
36. Fernández JL, Muriel L, Goyanes V, Segrelles E, Gosálvez J, Enciso M, et al. Simple determination of human sperm DNA fragmentation with an improved sperm chromatin dispersion (SCD) test. Fertil Steril. 2005;84:833–42.
37. Santiso R, Tamayo M, Gosálvez J, Meseguer M, Garrido N, Fernández JL. Simultaneous determination in situ of DNA fragmentation and 8-oxoguanine in human sperm. Fertil Steril. 2010;93:314–8.
38. Burney S, Caulfield JL, Niles C, Whishnok JS, Tannenbaum SR. The chemistry of DNA damage from nitric oxide and peroxynitrite. Mutat Res. 1999;424:37–49.
39. Chohan KR, Griffi JT, Lafromboise M, de Jonge CJ, Carrell DT. Comparison of chromatin assays for DNA fragmentation evaluation in human sperm. J Androl. 2006;27:53–9.
40. Ribas-Maynou J, García-Peiró A, Fernández-Encinas A, Abad C, Amengual MJ, Prada E, et al. Comprehensive analysis of sperm DNA fragmentation by five different assays: TUNEL assay, SCSA, SCD test and alkaline and neutral comet assay. Andrology. 2013;1:715–22.
41. Muriel L, Goyanes V, Segrelles E, Gosálvez J, Alvarez JG, Fernández JL. Increased aneuploidy rate in sperm with fragmented DNA as determined by the sperm chromatin dispersion (SCD) test and FISH analysis. J Androl. 2007;28:38–49.

42. Balasuriya A, Speyer B, Serhal P, Doshi A, Harper JC. Sperm chromatin dispersion test in the assessment of DNA fragmentation and aneuploidy in human spermatozoa. Reprod BioMed Online. 2011;22:428–36.
43. Velez de la Calle JF, Muller A, Walschaerts M, Clavere JL, Jimenez C, Wittemer C, et al. Sperm deoxyribonucleic acid fragmentation as assessed by the sperm chromatin dispersion test in assisted reproductive technology programs: results of a large prospective multicenter study. Fertil Steril. 2008;90:1792–9.
44. Gosálvez J, López-Fernández C, Hermoso A, Fernández JL, Kjelland ME. Sperm DNA fragmentation in zebrafish (Danio rerio) and its impact on fertility and embryo viability—implications for fisheries and aquaculture. Aquaculture. 2014;433:173–82.
45. Johnston SD, López-Fernández C, Arroy F, Gosálvez A, Gutierrez-Cortés E, Fernández JL, et al. Reduced sperm DNA longevity is associated with an increased incidence of still born; evidence form a multi-ovulating sequential artificial insemination animal model. J Assist Reprod Genet. 2016;33:1231–8.
46. Muriel M, Meseguer M, Fernández JL, Alvarez JG, Remohí J, Pellicer A, et al. Value of the sperm chromatin dispersion (SCD) test in predicting pregnancy outcome in intrauterine insemination: a blind prospective study. Hum Reprod. 2006;21:738–44.
47. López G, Lafuente R, Checa MA, Carreras R, Brassesco M. Diagnostic value of sperm DNA fragmentation and sperm high-magnification for predicting outcome of assisted reproduction treatment. Asian J Androl. 2015;15:790–4.
48. Wdowiak A, Bakalczuk S, Bakalczuk G. The effect of sperm DNA fragmentation on the dynamics of the embryonic development in intracytoplasmatic sperm injection. Reprod Biol. 2015;15:94–100.
49. Meseguer M, Santiso R, Garrido N, García-Herrero S, Remohí J, Fernández JL. Effect of sperm DNA fragmentation on pregnancy outcome depends on oocyte quality. Fertil Steril. 2011;95:124–8.
50. Jin J, Pan C, Fei Q, Ni W, Yang X, Zhang L, Huang X. Effect of sperm DNA fragmentation on the clinical outcomes for in vitro fertilization and intracytoplasmic sperm injection in women with different ovarian reserves. Fertil Steril. 2015;103:910–6.
51. Bellver J, Meseguer M, Muriel L, García-Herrero S, Barreto MA, Garda AL, et al. Y chromosome microdeletions, sperm DNA fragmentation and sperm oxidative stress as causes of recurrent spontaneous abortion of unknown etiology. Hum Reprod. 2010;25:1713–21.
52. Esteves SC, Sánchez-Martín F, Sánchez-Martín P, Schneider DT, Gosálvez J. Comparison of reproductive outcome in oligozoospermic men with high sperm DNA fragmentation undergoing intracytoplasmic sperm injection with ejaculated and testicular sperm. Fertil Steril. 2015;104:1398–405.
53. Núñez-Calonge R, Caballero P, López-Fernández C, Guijarro JA, Fernández JL, Jonhston S, et al. An improved experimental model for understanding the impact of sperm DNA fragmentation on human pregnancy following ICSI. Reprod Sci. 2012;19:1163–8.
54. Gosálvez J, Caballero P, López-Fernández C, Andrés J, Fernández JL, Johnston S, et al. Can DNA fragmentation of neat or swim-up spermatozoa be used to predict pregnancy following ICSI of fertile oocyte donors? Asian J Androl. 2013;15:812–8.
55. Gosálvez J, Rodríguez-Pedreira M, Mosquera A, López-Fernández C, Esteves SC, Agarwal A, et al. Characterization of a subpopulation of sperm with massive nuclear damage, as recognized with the sperm chromatin dispersion (SCD) test. Andrologia. 2014;46:602–9.
56. Esteves SC, Gosálvez J, López-Fernández C, Núñez-Calonge R, Caballero P, Agarwal A, et al. Diagnostic accuracy of sperm DNA degradation index (DDSi) as a potential noninvasive biomarker to identify men with varicocele-associated infertility. Int Urol Nephrol. 2015;47:1471–7.
57. Rennemeier C, Frambach T, Hennicke F, Dietl J, Staib P. Microbial quorum-sensing molecules induce acrosome loss and cell death in human spermatozoa. Infect Immun. 2009;77:4990–7.

58. Santiso R, Tamayo M, Gosálvez J, Johnston S, Mariño A, Fernández C, et al. DNA fragmentation dynamics allows the assessment of cryptic sperm damage in human: evaluation of exposure to ionizing radiation, hyperthermia, acidic pH and nitric oxide. Mutat Res. 2012;734:41–9.
59. Gosálvez J, Johnston S, López-Fernández C, Gosálbez A, Arroyo F, Fernández JL, et al. Sperm fractions obtained following density gradient centrifugation in human ejaculates show differences in sperm DNA longevity. Asian Pacific J Reprod. 2014;3:116–20.
60. Gosálvez J, Núñez R, Fernández JL, López-Fernández C, Caballero P. Dynamics of sperm DNA damage in fresh versus frozen-thawed and gradient processed ejaculates in human donors. Andrologia. 2011;43:373–7.
61. Abad C, Amengual MJ, Gosálvez J, Coward K, Hannaoui N, Benet J, et al. Effects of oral antioxidant treatment upon the dynamics of human sperm DNA fragmentation and subpopulations of sperm with highly degraded DNA. Andrologia. 2013;45:211–6.
62. García-Peiró A, Martínez-Heredia J, Oliver-Bonet M, Abad C, Amengual MJ, Navarro J, et al. Protamine 1 to protamine 2 ratio correlates with dynamic aspects of DNA fragmentation in human sperm. Fertil Steril. 2011;95:105–9.
63. Bungum M, Bungum L, Humaidan P. A prospective study, using sibling oocytes, examining the effect of 30 seconds versus 90 minutes gamete co-incubation in IVF. Hum Reprod. 2006;21:518–23.

Chapter 9
Cytochemical Tests of Sperm Chromatin Maturity

Juris Erenpreiss and Ksenija Zubkova

9.1 Introduction

Infertility affects approximately 15% of couples trying to conceive, and a male cause is believed to be a sole or contributing factor in approximately half of these cases [1]. In clinical practice, the traditional, manual-visual light microscopic methods for evaluating semen quality maintain their central role in assessment of male fertility potential. However, often a definitive diagnosis of male fertility cannot be made as a result of basic semen analysis due to the overlap of sperm concentration, motility, and morphology between fertile and infertile men [2].

It has been demonstrated that abnormalities in the male genome, characterized by disturbed chromatin packaging and damaged sperm DNA may be a cause for male infertility regardless of routine semen parameters [3, 4]. Focus on the chromatin maturity and integrity of the male gamete has been intensified by the growing concern about transmission of damaged DNA through assisted reproductive techniques (ARTs), especially by means of intracytoplasmic sperm injection (ICSI) that bypasses processes of natural selection during sperm-oocyte interaction, which are still present in conventional in vitro fertilization (IVF). There are concerns relating to potential chromosomal abnormalities, congenital malformations, and developmental abnormalities in ICSI-born progeny [5–8]. Accumulated evidence suggests a negative relationship between abnormal sperm chromatin structure and the fertility potential of spermatozoa both in vivo and in vitro [9–13].

Abnormalities in the sperm chromatin organization may be indicative of male infertility regardless of normal semen parameters [3, 4]. Evaluation of sperm chromatin structure is an independent measure of sperm quality that provides good prognostic and diagnostic capabilities. Therefore, it may be considered a reliable predictor of a couple's inability to conceive.

J. Erenpreiss (✉) • K. Zubkova
Riga Stradins University, Riga, Latvia
e-mail: jerenpreiss@gmail.com

A. Zini, A. Agarwal (eds.), *A Clinician's Guide to Sperm DNA and Chromatin Damage*, https://doi.org/10.1007/978-3-319-71815-6_9

Many techniques have been described for evaluation of the chromatin status and maturity. There is a group of methods based on the ability of some stains to test the conformation of sperm chromatin, which in turn depends on sperm DNA breaks and DNA interaction with proteins. These assays, often referred to as "cytochemical," include acidic aniline blue (AAB), toluidine blue (TB), and chromomycin A3 tests.

9.2 Cytochemical Properties of Human Sperm Chromatin

In many mammals, spermatogenesis leads to the production of highly homogenous spermatozoa. For example, mouse sperm nuclei contain more than 95% protamines in their nucleoprotein component [14]. This allows the mature sperm nuclei to adopt a volume 40 times less than that of normal somatic nuclei [15]. The final, very compact packaging of the primary sperm DNA filament is produced by DNA-protamine complexes, which contrary to nucleosomal organization in somatic cells provided by histones approach the physical limits of molecular compaction [16]. Human sperm nuclei, however, contain considerably fewer protamines (around 85%) than sperm nuclei of bull, stallion, hamster, and mouse [17, 18]. Human sperm chromatin, therefore, is less regularly compacted and frequently contains DNA strand breaks [19, 20].

To achieve this uniquely condensed state, sperm DNA must be organized in a specific manner, which differs substantially from that of somatic cells [15]. The fundamental packaging unit of mammalian sperm chromatin is a toroid containing 50–60 kb of DNA. Individual toroids represent the DNA loop domains highly condensed by protamines and fixed at the nuclear matrix; toroids are cross-linked by disulfide bonds, formed by oxidation of sulfhydryl groups of cysteine present in the protamines [16, 21]. Thus, each chromosome represents a garland of toroids, while all 23 chromosomes are clustered by centromeres into a compact chromocenter positioned well inside the nucleus with telomere ends united into dimers exposed to the nuclear periphery [22, 23]. This condensed, insoluble, and highly organized nature of sperm chromatin acts to protect genetic integrity during transport of the paternal genome through the male and female reproductive tracts. It also ensures that the paternal DNA is delivered in the form that sterically allows the proper fusion of two gametic genomes, their centromeric rings, and enables the developing embryo to correctly express the genetic information [23–25].

In comparison with other species [26], human sperm chromatin packaging is exceptionally variable. This variability has been mostly attributed to its basic protein component. The retention of 15% histones, which are less basic than protamines, leads to the formation of less compact chromatin structure [16]. Moreover, human spermatozoa contain two types of protamines, P1 and P2, with a second type deficient in cysteine residues [27]. This results in diminished disulfide cross-linking responsible for more stable packaging as compared to species containing P1 alone [28].

Chromatin structural probes using aromatic cationic dyes allow to analyze chromatin structure in terms of protein packaging correctness and disulfide cross-linking density. These probes are both sensitive and simple to use and therefore attractive for clinical use. However, their cytochemical background is rather complex. Several factors influence the staining of the chromatin by planar ionic dyes: (1) secondary structure of DNA, (2) regularity and density of chromatin packaging, and (3) binding of DNA to chromatin proteins.

9.2.1 DNA Secondary Structure and Conformation

Fragmented DNA is easily denatured [29]. However, even a single DNA strand break causes conformational transition of the DNA loop domain from a supercoiled state to a relaxed state. Supercoiled DNA avidly takes up intercalating dyes (like acridine orange) because this reduces the free energy of torsion stress. In contrast, the affinity for intercalation is low in relaxed DNA and is lost in fragmented DNA. In this case, an external mechanism of dye binding to DNA phosphate residues and dye polymerization (metachromasy) is favored [30, 31]. Nevertheless, fragmentation of DNA is not the only factor affecting the determination between metachromatic and orthochromatic staining. Chromatin packaging density also influences this balance.

9.2.2 Chromatin Packaging Density

If the chromatin is regularly arranged and sufficiently densely packed, dye coplanar polymerization providing metachromatic shift (change of color) is favored [32, 33]. However, if the chromatin is packaged even more densely (as in normal sperm), the polymerization of the dye is hindered [34] and may even prevent dye binding, especially by large, bulky dyes at an unfavorable pH. The latter case is seen with aniline blue at low pH where it stains basic proteins loosely associated with DNA and is unable to bind to the chromatin of normal sperm, which is very densely packaged and low charged. Binding of protamine molecules to DNA facilitates DNA condensation and toroid formation [35]. Substitution of histones for more basic protamines occurring during spermiogenesis neutralizes the DNA negative charge and decreases the accessibility of DNA-specific cationic dyes. Thus, the fluorescence staining intensity of a haploid sperm is much lower than the fluorescence intensity of a haploid round spermatid. However, after removal of nuclear proteins (e.g., by acid extraction), increase in sperm DNA stainability can vary depending on the chemical structure of the dye and the binding type the dye forms with the DNA substrate [36].

9.2.3 Chromatin Proteins

Chromatin proteins affect the binding of DNA dyes in the way that they themselves bind differently to relaxed (fragmented) or supercoiled DNA. DNA supercoiling requires covalent binding of some nuclear matrix proteins and tighter ionic interactions between DNA and chromatin proteins to support negative supercoils [37]. Relaxed and fragmented DNA has looser ionic interactions with chromatin proteins, which can be more easily displaced from the DNA, thus favoring external metachromatic binding of the dye to DNA phosphate groups. Both mechanisms of dye binding, external and intercalating, compete within each constraint loop domain (toroid) depending on its conformational state.

9.3 Sperm Chromatin Structural Probes

Chromatin proteins in sperm nuclei with the impaired DNA appear to be more accessible to binding with the acidic dye, as found by the AAB test [38, 39]. An increase in the ability to stain sperm by AAB indicates a looser chromatin packaging and increased accessibility of the basic groups of the nucleoprotein. This is due to the presence of residual histones [40]. Chromomycin A3 (CMA3) is another staining technique, which has been used as a measure of sperm chromatin condensation anomalies. CMA3 is a fluorochrome specific for GC-rich sequences and is believed to compete with protamines for association with DNA. The extent of staining is therefore related to the degree of protamination of mature spermatozoa [41, 42]. In turn, phosphate residues of sperm DNA in nuclei with loosely packed chromatin and/or impaired DNA will be more liable to binding with basic dyes. Such conclusions were also deduced from the results of staining with basic dyes, such as TB, methyl green, and Giemsa stain [43, 44].

9.3.1 Acidic Aniline Blue

The AAB stain discriminates between lysine-rich histones and arginine/cysteine-rich protamines. This technique provides a specific positive reaction for lysine and reveals differences in the basic nuclear protein composition of human spermatozoa. Histone-rich nuclei of immature spermatozoa are rich in lysine and will consequently take up the blue stain. On the contrary, protamine-rich nuclei of mature spermatozoa are rich in arginine and cysteine and contain relatively low levels of lysine, which means they will not take up the stain [45].

Technique: slides are prepared by making a smear of 5 μl of either raw or washed semen sample. The slides are air-dried and fixed for 30 min in 3% glutaraldehyde in phosphate-buffered saline (PBS). The smear is dried and stained for 5 min in 5%

aqueous AB solution (pH 3.5). Sperm heads containing immature nuclear chromatin stain blue and those with mature nuclei do not. The percentage of spermatozoa stained with AB is determined by counting 200 spermatozoa per slide under bright-field microscopy [46].

A strong association between the results of AAB staining and male infertility has been shown [47]. It has been reported by some studies that chromatin condensation as visualized by the AAB staining is predictive for IVF outcome [48], but it was not a case for ICSI. Other studies, in turn, have reported an association also with the ICSI outcomes: fertilization and cleavage rate [49, 50]. Also, an association of poor chromatin condensation as detected by the AAB test with the abortion rates following the IUI cycles has been reported [51].

9.3.2 Toluidine Blue Stain Assay

TB is a basic planar nuclear dye used for metachromatic and orthochromatic staining of the chromatin. The phosphate residues of sperm DNA in nuclei with loosely packed chromatin and/or impaired DNA become more liable to binding with TB, providing a metachromatic shift due to coplanar dimerization of the dye molecules from light-blue to purple-violet color [38, 52]. This stain is a sensitive structural probe for DNA structure and packaging.

Technique: thin smears were prepared on pre-cleaned defatted slides and then air-dried for 30 min. Dried smears are fixed with freshly made 96% ethanol-acetone (1:1) at 40 °C for 30 min to 12 h and air-dried. Hydrolysis is performed with 0.1 N HCl at 40C for 5 min followed by three changes of distilled water, 2 min each. Toluidine blue (0.05% in 50% McIlvaine's citrate phosphate buffer at pH 3.5) is applied for 5 min. The slides are rinsed briefly in distilled water, dehydrated in tertiary butanol and xylene (both two times for 3 min) at room temperature, and mounted with DPX.

The results of the TB test are estimated using oil-immersion light microscopy. Sperm heads with good chromatin integrity stain light blue, and those with diminished integrity stain violet (purple) [53]. The proportion of cells with violet heads (high optical density) is calculated based on 200 sperm cells examined per sample. Based on the different optical densities of sperm cells stained by the TB, the image analysis cytometry test had been elaborated [54].

TB staining may be considered a fairly reliable method for assessing sperm chromatin. Abnormal nuclei (purple-violet sperm heads) have been shown to correlate with counts of red-orange sperm heads as revealed by the acridine orange test [38]. Also, correlations between the results of the TB test, sperm chromatin structure assay (SCSA), and terminal deoxynucleotidyl transferase dUTP nick-end labeling (TUNEL) tests have been demonstrated [53]. A threshold for proportion of sperm cells with abnormal sperm chromatin structure (violet staining) was set at 45%, providing 92% specificity and 42% sensitivity for infertility detection [55]. The association between the TB test and the outcome of IVF/ICSI cycles has not been investigated.

TB staining is simple and inexpensive and has advantage of providing permanent preparations for use with an ordinary microscope. However, these methods may have the inherent limits of repeatability dictated by a limited number of cells, which can be reasonably scored.

It has been shown that sperm chromatin maturity as demonstrated both by AAB and TB tests is associated by zygote development following ICSI [56].

9.3.3 Chromomycin A3 Assay

Chromomycin A3 is a fluorochrome that specifically binds to guanine-cytosine DNS sequences. It reveals chromatin that is poorly packed in spermatozoa by visualization of protamine-deficient DNA. Chromomycin A3 and protamines compete for the same binding sites in the DNA. Therefore, high CMA3 fluorescence is an indicator of the low protamination state of the chromatin of spermatozoa [41].

Technique: for CMA3 staining, semen smears are first fixed in methanol-glacial acetic acid (3:1) at 40C for 20 min and are then allowed to air-dry at room temperature for 20 min. The slides are treated for 20 min with 100 μl of CMA3 solution that consists of 0.25 mg/mL CMA3 in Mcllvaine's buffer (pH 7.0) supplemented with 10 mmol/L $MgCl_2$. The slides are rinsed in buffer and mounted with 1:1 v/v PBS-glycerol. The slides are then kept at 40C overnight. Fluorescence is evaluated using a fluorescence microscopy. A total of 200 spermatozoa are randomly evaluated on each slide. CMA3 staining is evaluated by distinguishing spermatozoa that stain bright yellow (CMA3 positive) from those that stain dull yellow (CMA3 negative) [41].

CMA3 staining has demonstrated a sensitivity of 73% and specificity of 75% for the IVF success (>50% oocytes fertilized) [57]. It appears that semen samples with high CMA3 positivity (>30%) may have significantly lower fertilization rates if used for ICSI, and poor chromatin packaging can contribute to a failure in the decondensation process and reduced fertility [58, 59].

The CMA3 assay yields reliable results as it is strongly correlated with other assays used in the evaluation of sperm chromatin. The sensitivity and specificity of the CMA3 stain (75% and 82%, respectively) are comparable with those of the AAB stain (60% and 91%, respectively) if used to evaluate the chromatin status in infertile men.

It has been shown that the results of the AAB and TB tests (both detecting chromatin condensation and conformation) are well correlated [60, 61]. However, the results of the CMA3 test differ from these two in some specific biological conditions, for example, after induced sperm capacitation [61], providing another evidence not only for the complexity of the cytochemical background behind these assays as described above but also for the complexity of sperm chromatin biology. It also shows the complexity of sperm chromatin remodeling during sperm functioning processes like sperm capacitation when the change of sperm chromatin conformation (or condensation) can be detected by assays like AAB and TB, but assays like CMA3 (competing with protamines) or sperm chromatin structure assay (SCSA, targeting the susceptibility of abnormal sperm chromatin for in situ denaturation) do not detect any change in sperm chromatin [61].

A relationship between poor sperm chromatin maturity and integrity is detected by means of all three methods (AAB, TB, and CMA3), and recurrent spontaneous pregnancy loss has been shown [62, 63]. Regarding the utility of these methods in context of the ART, there is still inconsistency regarding the published data whether sperm chromatin maturity and integrity as tested by these cytochemical methods are related to the outcome of the IVF and ICSI. For example, some studies have shown an association between CMA3 test and fertilization rates following ICSI, failing to demonstrate the same associations for the AAB test [59], while other studies are showing such a relationship between the AAB test and ICSI outcome [64]. Some studies do not find any association between the results of all three tests (AAB, TB, and CMA3) and the outcome of ICSI [65]. Therefore, unlike the good predictive power of these tests for in vivo fertility capacity of men, their utility in IVF/ICSI cycles is still debatable.

9.4 Conclusion

Cytochemical sperm chromatin assays described here (AAB, TB, and CMA3 assays) are simple, inexpensive to perform, and sensitive tests for the evaluation of sperm chromatin structure, although their cytochemical backgrounds and targeting tools in sperm chromatin are different. They are reliable methods for the more refined diagnosis of male in vivo fertility and are also shown to be predictive of in vitro fertilization processes, although the accumulation of more evidence for the relationship between the results of these methods and in vitro fertilization is needed. A very robust reproducibility of these assays might be their weak point because of the assessment of the limited numbers of sperm cells (usually 200–300) under the bright-field or fluorescence microscopy. On the other hand, the acquisition of the permanent preparations by the AAB and TB assays must be mentioned as the strength of these tests.

References

1. Oehninger S. Strategies for the infertile man. Semin Reprod Med. 2001;19:231–7.
2. Guzick DS, Overstreet JW, Factor-Litvak P, National Cooperative Reproductive Medicine Network, et al. Sperm morphology, motility, and concentration in fertile and infertile men. N Engl J Med. 2001;345:1388–93.
3. Lopes S, Jurisicova A, Sun JG, Casper RF. Reactive oxygen species: potential cause for DNA fragmentation in human spermatozoa. Hum Reprod. 1998;13:896–900.

4. Sakkas D, Tomlinson M. Assessment of sperm competence. Semin Reprod Med. 2000;18:133–9.
5. Hansen M, Kurinczuk JJ, Bower C, Webb S. The risk of major birth defects after intracytoplasmic sperm injection and in vitro fertilization. N Engl J Med. 2002;346:725–30.
6. Schieve LA, Meikle SF, Ferre C, Peterson HB, Jeng G, Wilcox LS. Low and very low birth weight in infants conceived with use of assisted reproductive technology. N Engl J Med. 2002;346:731–7.
7. Moll AC, Imhof SM, Cruysberg JR, Schouten-van Meeteren AY, Boers M, van Leeuwen FE. Incidence of retinoblastoma in children born after in-vitro fertilisation. Lancet. 2003;361:309–10.
8. Orstavik KH, Eiklid K, van der Hagen CB, Spetalen S, Kierulf K, Skjeldal O, Buiting K. Another case of imprinting defect in a girl with Angelman syndrome who was conceived by intracytoplasmic semen injection. Am J Hum Genet. 2003;72:218–9.
9. Aitken RJ, de Iuliis GN. Origins and consequences of DNA damage in male germ cells. Reprod BioMed Online. 2007;14:727–33.
10. Zini A, Sigman M. Are tests of sperm DNA damage clinically useful? Pros and cons. J Androl. 2009;30:219–29.
11. Zini A, Jamal W, Cowan L, Al-Hathal N. Is sperm DNA damage associated with IVF embryo quality? A systematic review. J Assist Reprod Genet. 2011;28:391–7.
12. Zini A. Are sperm chromatin and DNA defects relevant in the clinic? Syst Biol Reprod Med. 2011;57:78–85.
13. Simon L, Zini A, Dyachenko A, Ciampi A, Carrell DT. A systematic review and meta-analysis to determine the effect of sperm DNA damage on in vitro fertilization and intracytoplasmic sperm injection outcome. Asian J Androl. 2017;19(1):80–90.
14. Bellve AR, McKay DJ, Renaux BS, Dixon GH. Purification and characterization of mouse protamines P1 and P2. Amino acid sequence of P2. Biochemistry. 1988;27:2890–7.
15. Ward WS, Coffey DS. DNA packaging and organization in mammalian spermatozoa: comparison with somatic cells. Biol Reprod. 1991;44:569–74.
16. Fuentes-Mascorro G, Serrano H, Rosado A. Sperm chromatin. Arch Androl. 2000;45:215–25.
17. Gatewood JM, Cook GR, Balhorn R, Bradbury EM, Schmid CW. Sequence-specific packaging of DNA in human sperm chromatin. Science. 1987;236:962–4.
18. Bench GS, Friz AM, Corzett MH, Morse DH, Balhorn R. DNA and total protamine masses in individual sperm from fertile mammalian subjects. Cytometry. 1996;23:263–71.
19. Sakkas D, Mariethoz E, Manicardi G, Bizzaro D, Bianchi PG, Bianchi U. Origin of DNA damage in ejaculated human spermatozoa. Rev Reprod. 1999;4:31–7.
20. Irvine DS, Twigg JP, Gordon EL, Fulton N, Milne PA, Aitken RJ. DNA integrity in human spermatozoa: relationships with semen quality. J Androl. 2000;21:33–44.
21. Ward WS. Deoxyribonucleic acid loop domain tertiary structure in mammalian spermatozoa. Biol Reprod. 1993;48:1193–201.
22. Zalensky AO, Allen MJ, Kobayashi A, Zalenskaya IA, Balhorn R, Bradbury EM. Chromosoma. 1995;103:577–90.
23. Solov'eva L, Svetlova M, Bodinski D, Zalensky AO. Nature of telomere dimers and chromosome looping in human spermatozoa. Chromosom Res. 2004;12:817–23.
24. Ward WS, Zalensky AO. The unique, complex organization of the transcriptionally silent sperm chromatin. Crit Rev Eukaryot Gene Expr. 1996;6:139–47.
25. De Jonge CJ. Paternal contributions to embryogenesis. Reprod Med Rev. 2000;8:203–14.
26. Lewis JD, Song Y, de Jong ME, Bagha SM, Ausio J. A walk through vertebrate and invertebrate protamines. Chromosoma. 1999;111:473–82.
27. Corzett M, Mazrimas J, Balhorn R. Protamine 1 : protamine 2 stoichiometry in the sperm of eutherian mammals. Mol Reprod Dev. 2002;61:519–27.
28. Jager S. Sperm nuclear stability and male infertility. Arch Androl. 1990;25:253–9.
29. Darzynkiewicz Z. Acid-induced denaturation of DNA in situ as a probe of chromatin structure. Methods Cell Biol. 1994;41:527–41.

30. Erenpreisa EA, Zirne RA, Zaleskaia ND, S'iakste TG. Effect of single-stranded breaks on the ultrastructural organization and cytochemistry of the chromatin in tumor cells. Biull Eksp Biol Med. 1988;106:591–3. [Article in Russian].
31. Erenpreisa EA, Sondore OI, Zirne RA. Conformational changes in the chromatin of tumor cells and the phenomenon of nuclear achromasia. Eksp Onkol. 1988;10:54–7. [Article in Russian].
32. Sculthore HH. Metachromasia. Med Lab Sci. 1978;35:365–70.
33. Erenpreisa J, Zaleskaya N. Effect of triton X-100 on cytochemical and ultrastructural pattern of chromatin. Acta Morphol Hung. 1983;31:387–93.
34. Erenpreisa J, Freivalds T, Selivanova G. Influence of chromatin condensation on the absorption spectra of nuclei stained with toluidine blue. Acta Morphol Hung. 1992;40:3–10.
35. Brewer LR, Corzett M, Balhorn R. Protamine-induced condensation and decondensation of the same DNA molecule. Science. 1999;286:120–3.
36. Evenson D, Darzynkiewicz Z, Jost L, Janca F, Ballachey B. Changes in accessibility of DNA to various fluorochromes during spermatogenesis. Cytometry. 1986;7:45–53.
37. Benyajati C, Worcel A. Isolation, characterization, and structure of the folded interphase genome of Drosophila melanogaster. Cell. 1976;9:393–407.
38. Erenpreiss J, Bars J, Lipatnikova V, Erenpreisa J, Zalkalns J. Comparative study of cytochemical tests for sperm chromatin integrity. J Androl. 2001;22:45–53.
39. Auger J, Mesbah M, Huber C, Dadoune JP. Aniline blue staining as a marker of sperm chromatin defects associated with different semen characteristics discriminates between proven fertile and suspected infertile men. Int J Androl. 1990;13:452–62.
40. Terquem T, Dadoune JP. Aniline blue staining of human spermatozoa chromatin. Evaluation of nuclear maturation. In: Adre J, editor. The sperm cell. The Hague: Martinus Nijhoff Publishers; 1983. p. 249–52.
41. Manicardi GC, Bianchi PG, Pantano S, Azzoni P, Bizzaro D, Bianchi U, Sakkas D. Presence of endogenous nicks in DNA of ejaculated human spermatozoa and its relationship to chromomycin A3 accessibility. Biol Reprod. 1995;52:864–7.
42. Bianchi PG, Manicardi GC, Bizzaro D, Bianchi U, Sakkas D. Effect of deoxyribonucleic acid protamination on fluorochrome staining and in situ nick-translation of murine and human mature spermatozoa. Biol Reprod. 1993;49:1083–8.
43. Mello ML. Induced metachromasia in bull spermatozoa. Histochemistry. 1982;74:387–92.
44. Andreetta AM, Stockert JC, Barrera C. A simple method to detect sperm chromatin abnormalities: cytochemical mechanism and possible value in predicting semen quality in assisted reproductive procedures. Int J Androl. 1995;18(1):23–8.
45. Hammadeh ME, Zeginiadov T, Rosenbaum P, et al. Predictive value of sperm chromatin condensation (aniline blue staining) in the assessment of male fertility. Arch Androl. 2001;46:99–104.
46. Baker H, Liu D. Assessment of nuclear maturity. In: Acosta A, Kruger T, editors. Human spermatozoa in assisted reproduction. London: CRC Press; 1996. p. 193–203.
47. Foresta C, Zorzi M, Rossato M, Varotto A. Sperm nuclear instability and staining with aniline blue: abnormal persistence of histones in spermatozoa in infertile men. Int J Androl. 1992;15:330–7.
48. Hammadeh ME, Stieber M, Haidl G, Schmidt W. Association between sperm cell chromatin condensation, morphology based on strict criteria, and fertilization, cleavage and pregnancy rates in an IVF program. Andrologia. 1998;30:29–35.
49. Irez T, Sahmay S, Ocal P, Goymen A, Senol H, Erol N, Kaleli S, Guralp O. Investigation of the association between the outcomes of sperm chromatin condensation and decondensation tests, and assisted reproduction techniques. Andrologia. 2015;47:438–47.
50. Asmarinah, Syauqy A, Umar LA, Lestari SW, Mansyur E, Hestiantoro A, Paradowszka-Dogan A. Sperm chromatin maturity and integrity correlated to zygote development in ICSI program. Syst Biol Reprod Med. 2016;62:309–16.

51. Mohamed EE, Mohamed MA. Effect of sperm chromatin condensation on the outcome of intrauterine insemination in patients with male factor infertility. J Reprod Med. 2012;57:421–6.
52. Sato S, Matsumoto S, Freivalds T, Erenpreisa J. Consideration on the metachromatic spectra of toluidine blue dimers formed on DNA oligomers. Bull Chem Soc Jpn. 2010;83(10):1216–22.
53. Erenpreiss J, Jepson K, Giwercman A, Tsarev I, Erenpreisa J, Spano M. Toluidine blue cytometry test for sperm DNA conformation: comparison with the flow cytometric sperm chromatin structure and TUNEL assays. Hum Reprod. 2004;19:2277–82.
54. Erenpreisa J, Erenpreiss J, Freivalds T, Slaidina M, Krampe R, Butikova J, Ivanov A, Pjanova D. Toluidine blue test for sperm DNA integrity and elaboration of image cytometry algorithm. Cytometry. 2003;52:19–27.
55. Tsarev I, Bungum M, Giwercman A, Erenpreisa J, Ebessen T, Ernst E, Erenpreiss J. Evaluation of male fertility potential by toluidine blue test for sperm chromatin structure assessment. Hum Reprod. 2009;24:1569–74.
56. Esterhuizen AD, Franken DR, Lourens JG, Prinsloo E, van Rooyen LH. Sperm chromatin packaging as an indicator of in-vitro fertilization rates. Hum Reprod. 2000;15:657–61.
57. Sakkas D, Urner F, Bianchi PG, Bizzaro D, Wagner I, Jaquenoud N, Manicardi G, Campana A. Sperm chromatin anomalies can influence decondensation after intracytoplasmic sperm injection. Hum Reprod. 1996;11:837–43.
58. Sakkas D, Urner F, Bizzaro D, Manicardi G, Bianchi PG, Shoukir Y, Campana A. Sperm nuclear DNA damage and altered chromatin structure: effect on fertilization and embryo development. Hum Reprod. 1998;13(4):11–9.
59. Iranpour FG. Impact of sperm chromatin evaluation on fertilization rate in intracytoplasmic sperm injection. Adv Biomed Res. 2014;3:229.
60. Kim HS, Kang MJ, Kim SA, Oh SK, Kim H, Ku SY, Kim SH, Moon SY, Choi YM. The utility of sperm DNA damage assay toluidine blue and aniline blue staining in routine semen analysis. Clin Exp Reprod Med. 2013;40:23–8.
61. De Lamirande E, San Gabriel MC, Zini A. Human sperm chromatin undergoes physiological remodeling during in vitro capacitation and acrosome reaction. J Androl. 2012;33:1025–35.
62. Talebi AR, Vahidi S, Aflatoonian A, Ghasemi N, Ghasemzadeh J, Firoozabadi RD, Moein MR. Cytochemical evaluation of sperm chromatin and DNA integrity in couples with unexplained recurrent spontaneous abortions. Romanian J Morphol Embryol. 2011;52:645–51.
63. Kazerooni T, Asadi N, Jadid L, Kazerooni M, Ghanadi A, Ghaffarpasand F, Kazerooni Y, Zolghadr J. Evaluation of sperm's chromatin quality with acridine orange test, chromomycin A3 and aniline blue staining in couples with unexplained recurrent abortion. J Assist Reprod Genet. 2009;26:591–6.
64. Simon L, Liu L, Murphy K, Ge S, Hotaling J, Aston KI, Emery B, Carrell DT. Comparative analysis of three sperm DNA damage assays and sperm nuclear protein content in couples undergoing assisted reproduction treatment. Hum Reprod. 2014;29:904–17.
65. Sadeghi MR, Lakpour N, Heidari-Vala H, Hodjat M, Amirjannati N, Hossaini Jadda H, Binaafar S, Akhondi MM. Relationship between sperm chromatin status and ICSI outcome in men with obstructive azoospermia and unexplained infertile normozoospermia. Andrologia. 2012;44(1):462–70.

Chapter 10
Is There an Optimal Sperm DNA Test?

Michelle M. Kim and Cigdem Tanrikut

10.1 Overview of Common Sperm DNA Assays

Assessment of sperm DNA integrity has become a common part of the male fertility evaluation. It provides additional information to the standard semen analysis, potentially identifying male factor issues and predicting outcomes for assisted reproductive technology (ART) [1, 2]. There are several tests now available to measure sperm DNA damage as reviewed in more detail by the preceding chapters (see Table 10.1). These tests are classified as either direct or indirect DNA assays. Direct tests assess DNA fragmentation by incorporating probes at sites of damage, thus directly detecting DNA strand breaks. Indirect assays measure the susceptibility of DNA to denaturation and damage. This chapter will briefly present the various tests commonly used, review correlations and comparisons among the assays, and contend whether there may be an ideal assay for determination of sperm DNA integrity.

M.M. Kim
Urology Resident, Department of Urology, Massachusetts General Hospital,
Harvard Medical School, Boston, MA, USA

C. Tanrikut (✉)
MGH Fertility Center, Massachusetts General Hospital, Harvard Medical School,
Boston, MA, USA
e-mail: ctanrikut@partners.org

A. Zini, A. Agarwal (eds.), *A Clinician's Guide to Sperm DNA and Chromatin Damage*, https://doi.org/10.1007/978-3-319-71815-6_10

Table 10.1 Summary of DNA assays

Method	Assay	Measurement
Direct	TUNEL	Measures % cells with labeled DNA
		Detects single- and double-stranded DNA breaks
	Comet	Measures % sperm with long tails resembling a "comet"
		Alkaline: detects all single- and double-stranded DNA breaks
		Neutral: detects double-stranded and some single-stranded DNA breaks
	In situ nick translation assay	Measures % cells with incorporated dUTP
		Detects single-stranded DNA breaks
Indirect	Sperm chromatin structure assay	Measures DNA fragmentation index (red/red+green), susceptibility to acidic denaturation
		Detects single-stranded DNA and double-stranded DNA
	Sperm chromatin dispersion test	% Normal spermatozoa that produce halo characteristic of DNA decondensation
	Staining assays	
	Acridine orange	Denatures double-stranded and single-stranded DNA with breaks, binds to DNA
	Aniline blue	Impaired sperm DNA denoted with increased staining
	Toluidine blue	Incorporates stain into damaged dense chromatin
	Chromomycin A3	Indirect visualization of nicked, denatured DNA

10.1.1 Direct Tests

10.1.1.1 TUNEL Assay

The terminal deoxynucleotidyl transferase-mediated (TdT) deoxyuridine triphosphate (dUTP) nick end labeling (TUNEL) assay is a direct test that quantifies sperm DNA breaks. It incorporates fluorescing dUTP into strand defects via a reaction catalyzed by the template-independent enzyme TdT. Single- and double-stranded breaks can then be assessed using fluorescent microscopy, light microscopy, or flow cytometry. Sperm are categorized as TUNEL positive or negative based on the percentage of total sperm in population. [For more detail regarding TUNEL assays, please refer to Chaps. 5 and 6.]

10.1.1.2 Comet Assay

The comet assay is a sperm DNA test that derives its name from the DNA fragments that move through the electrophoresis gel, resembling a comet's tail [3, 4]. DNA damage is quantified using decondensed sperm suspended in an agarose gel, which is then subjected to either alkaline or neutral conditions to identify DNA breaks [5, 6]. Alkaline tests detect both single- and double-stranded DNA breaks, whereas the neutral test detects single-stranded DNA breaks and some double-stranded DNA breaks. The longer and denser the tail, the more DNA damage present. [For more detail regarding the comet assay, please refer to Chap. 7.]

10.1.1.3 In Situ Nick Translation Assay

In situ nick translation (ISNT) incorporates biotinylated dUTP at single-stranded DNA (ssDNA) breaks using template-dependent DNA polymerase I [7]. The number of fluorescent sperm with incorporated dUTP is measured.

10.1.2 Indirect Tests

10.1.2.1 Sperm Chromatin Structure Assay

The Sperm Chromatin Structure Assay (SCSA®) is the oldest test in use to evaluate sperm DNA integrity [8]. This assay measures the susceptibility of sperm DNA to denaturation after exposure to heat or acidic conditions. Acridine orange (AO) binding determines the fraction of denatured DNA by changing "good" sperm from green to red as measured by flow cytometry. Acridine orange (AO) binding determines the fraction of sperm with double-stranded DNA (dsDNA—emits green fluorescence) to that with single-stranded DNA (ssDNA—emits red fluorescence), and this can be measured by flow cytometry. The denatured fraction of sperm DNA is reported as a percentage of total sperm in the sample and referred to as the DNA fragmentation index (DFI). [For more detail regarding SCSA®, please refer to Chap. 4].

10.1.2.2 Sperm Chromatin Dispersion Test

The sperm chromatin dispersion (SCD) test is a simple and inexpensive assay for sperm DNA testing [9]. Sperm are treated with a denaturing acid or alkaline solution to remove nuclear proteins and to generate ssDNA from DNA breaks. When treated with a lysis buffer, this produces nucleoids with a central core and a peripheral halo of dispersed DNA loops. Sperm with fragmented DNA fail to produce a halo of dispersed DNA loops that is characteristic of non-fragmented DNA. [For more detail regarding the SCD test, please refer to Chap. 8.]

10.1.2.3 Acridine Orange

Acridine orange is a nucleic acid-specific fluorescent cationic dye which measures the amount of DNA denaturation with a mild acid treatment [10]. AO binds to double-stranded DNA (dsDNA) to produce green fluorescence, while binding of AO to ssDNA produces red fluorescence. The change in fluorescence approximates the DNA sperm damage. The AO assay uses a fluorescence microscope to detect DNA denaturation.

10.1.2.4 Aniline Blue

Aniline blue (AB) is an acidic dye which measures sperm chromatin integrity [11]. Immature spermatozoa have a higher proportion of residual histones, leading to looser chromatin packing. This, in turn, allows increased aniline blue staining of the basic groups of the nucleoproteins.

10.1.2.5 Toluidine Blue

Toluidine blue (TB) evaluates sperm chromatin integrity by staining the phosphate residue of sperm DNA. When the stain attaches to lysine-rich regions of the histone, it produces violet-blue coloration, indicating loosely packed sperm chromatin. The sample can be analyzed with an ordinary light microscope. Flow cytometry can also be used for assessment [12].

10.1.2.6 Chromomycin A3

Chromomycin A3 (CMA3) is a fluorochrome specific for guanine-cytosine-rich sequences and interacts with DNA at the same site at which protamine binds DNA [13]. The extent of staining is related to the degree of protamination of mature sperm. Greater intensity of staining indicates protamine deficiency or aberrant chromatin packing.

10.2 Correlation Among Sperm DNA Assays

The available sperm DNA assays measure different aspects of DNA integrity but, overall, provide comparable results in assessing sperm DNA integrity and ART outcomes [9, 12, 14–18]. The following section will review the literature on correlations among sperm DNA assays.

10.2.1 Assessment of Sperm DNA Integrity

Sperm DNA integrity has been extensively studied using many of the available assays. While the SCSA® was the first and most commonly studied DNA assay, many studies have compared the SCSA® to other tests to assess sperm DNA integrity. SCSA® has been most commonly compared to the TUNEL assay and has been shown to be highly correlated in several studies [15, 16, 19, 20]. Comparisons of TUNEL found similar results to the SCSA® data ($r = 0.859$, $p < 0.001$; $r = 0.63$, $p = 0.005$) [15, 19]. This held true for other animals including bulls ($r = 0.78$,

$p < 0.001$), stallions ($r = 0.65$, $p < 0.001$), and rams ($r = 0.84$, $p < 0.001$) [20]. Spano et al. also found that both the TUNEL assay and SCSA® showed increased levels of DNA abnormalities in sperm from men who have poor semen parameters [16].

Among fertile and infertile men, Chohan et al. found a strong correlation among the SCSA®, TUNEL, and SCD assays with respect to detection of DNA fragmentation [14]. This degree of concordance was not observed between SCSA® and the AO test for DNA fragmentation in assessing infertile men and fertile donors [14]. Garcia-Peiro et al. similarly studied sperm DNA fragmentation for TUNEL, SCSA®, and SCD and found no difference in the estimation of DNA damage across the three assays with note of strong correlation among the assays ($r > 0.75$) [21]. Ribas-Maynou et al. compared correlations among various sperm DNA fragmentation assays performed in infertile patients [22]. Strong correlations were noted between SCD and SCSA® ($r = 0.71$; $p < 0.001$), as well as SCSA® and TUNEL ($r = 0.79$, $p < 0.001$).

DNA fragmentation index measured by SCSA® and the percentage of sperm cells with fragmented DNA measured by SCD had significant concordance between the two tests ($r = 0.85$) [9]. SCD had a slightly higher sensitivity for detecting sperm DNA fragmentation than SCSA®, but both were deemed interchangeable. Irvine et al. compared the comet and two ISNT assays (one with and one without chemical decondensation) in normozoospermic men without reproductive difficulty and men seeking treatment at a fertility center. Control subjects had lower levels of DNA damage detected by comet only [23]. However, ISNT assays were more salient in detecting semen quality when assessing efficiency of DNA compaction and damage. Zini et al. found significantly higher rates of DNA denaturation and fragmentation in infertile men compared to fertile men when using both AO and TUNEL assays [24]. DNA denaturation was also significantly negatively correlated with sperm motility, morphology, and concentration.

Other staining assays such as AO, toluidine blue, AB, and CM3 also correlate well with SCSA®, TUNEL, and with each other [12]. Erenpreiss et al. found that toluidine blue correlated strongly with the proportion of abnormal cells detected by SCSA® and TUNEL assays ($r = -0.84$, $r = -0.80$, $p < 0.001$) [15]. The assays also showed significant negative correlations with sperm concentration, motility, and normal morphology. The TB assay had higher positive abnormal cells than those for SCSA® and TUNEL assays. DNA chromatin packaging was negatively correlated with CMA3 ($r = 0.40$; $p = 0.001$) and with AB ($r = 0.33$; $p = 0.001$).

10.2.2 Assessment of Sperm Chromatin Structure in Fertility Evaluations

Sperm chromatin structure has been shown to be associated with male fertility. Evenson et al., in creating the SCSA®, examined human and bull sperm DNA and found that the spermatozoa of fertile subjects had less heat-induced DNA fragmentation than subfertile subjects [8]. Their subsequent work in boars also showed that the degree of DNA fragmentation was highly correlated with pregnancy outcome ($r \leq 0.93$, $p < 0.01$) [25]. Human studies have corroborated the animal studies, showing a strong correlation between infertile men and higher levels of DNA denaturation and fragmentation and ART outcomes [26, 27].

As the first sperm DNA assay, SCSA® has been researched extensively. Most studies have indicated that DFI levels >30% were associated with poorer fertility in vivo or in vitro, despite the results of standard semen parameters [16, 27, 28]. Other sperm DNA assays have shown similar results in predicting fertility. Using the comet assay, a higher risk of infertility has been demonstrated in men with sperm DNA fragmentation greater than 25% (OR, 117.33; 95% confidence interval [CI], 12.72–2731.84) [29]. As DNA fragmentation increases, embryo quality and fertility rates decrease. Other assays using TUNEL, SCD, and aniline blue as the testing modalities have also demonstrated that high levels of DNA labeling in infertile men are associated with poorer fertility outcomes [30–37].

Comparisons of these assays have shown that the alkaline comet assay was superior in predicting male infertility, followed by TUNEL, SCD, and SCSA®, whereas the neutral comet assay did not have predictive power [22]. IUI outcomes investigating sperm DNA quality on intrauterine insemination (IUI) outcomes using TUNEL and AO found that they were moderately correlated ($r = 0.22–0.33$; $p < 0.01$) [38]. Other studies examined less commonly used assays, ISNT and CMA3, to determine the impact of sperm DNA quality on fertilization rates in conventional in vitro fertilization (IVF) [39]. ISNT and CMA3 were significantly correlated with fertilization rates.

Defects in sperm chromatin structure have also raised concerns about ART outcomes [27, 30, 38, 40–42]. Furthermore, it has been questioned whether ART is able to compensate for poor sperm DNA quality [27, 28, 40]. Evenson et al. performed meta-analyses of the association of sperm chromatin defects with ART outcomes using SCSA® [43]. They found that a DFI threshold of <30% was associated with increased likelihood of IVF-associated pregnancy but did not show an association with pregnancy employing intracytoplasmic sperm injection (ICSI). Zini et al. also conducted a meta-analysis of sperm DNA damage and pregnancy loss after conventional IVF or IVF-ICSI [1]. They found that sperm DNA damage was significantly associated with an increased risk of miscarriage. Specifically, they reviewed those studies that had used SCSA® or TUNEL to evaluate DNA damage. The meta-regression analysis in their study demonstrated a significant difference in the odds ratio estimates between the TUNEL and the SCSA® studies ($p = 0.012$). Similarly, Collins et al. conducted a meta-analysis of sperm DNA integrity and ART outcomes reviewing studies that had measured SCSA® or TUNEL [44]. While they found that the DNA integrity estimates in SCSA® and TUNEL studies were similar, both tests were poor in their predictive capacities for ART outcomes.

Along these lines, more recent meta-analyses have demonstrated significant, albeit modest, relationships between sperm DNA damage and reproductive outcomes after IVF-ICSI [45, 46]. Specifically, sperm DNA damage has been associated with poorer IVF-ICSI pregnancy rates and an increased risk of pregnancy loss. These studies provide a clinical consideration for assessment of sperm DNA damage prior to ART in order to elucidate the association between sperm DNA integrity and pregnancy loss [1].

10.3 Comparisons of Sperm DNA Assays

Each test that assesses DNA integrity has advantages and disadvantages that should be considered when selecting which test to pursue (see Table 10.2). It is especially important to determine what each test measures and whether data link the test results to semen parameters and/or fertility outcomes.

10.3.1 Direct Tests

10.3.1.1 TUNEL Assay

The TUNEL assay, while not a standardized test like SCSA ®, can provide meaningful clinical information by measuring both single- and double-stranded DNA fragmentation. It is an inexpensive, less technically demanding test that can be

Table 10.2 Comparison of DNA assays

Method	Assay	Pros	Cons
Direct	TUNEL	Few sperm needed	Variable protocols across different labs
		Inexpensive	Non-standardized thresholds
		Detects single- and double-stranded DNA breaks	
		Not technically demanding	
	Comet	Measures DNA damage in individual cells	Labor intensive, need experienced lab technicians
		Can detect heterogeneity	
		Few sperm needed	Interobserver variation
		Standardized	Non-standardized protocols
			Requires imaging software
		Alkaline: identifies all DNA breaks	Alkaline: identifies some clinically irrelevant DNA breaks
		Neutral: identifies mostly clinically relevant DNA breaks	Neutral: may not identify all DNA breaks
	In situ nick translation assay	Simple	Only quantifies single-stranded DNA breaks
		Inexpensive	Thresholds not determined
Indirect	Sperm chromatin structure assay	Standardized	Expensive
		Precise	
	Sperm chromatin dispersion test	Inexpensive	Non-standardized
		Simple, does not require expensive equipment	Interobserver variation
	Staining assays	Simple, does not require expensive equipment	Heterogeneity of staining and coloring of slide
	Acridine orange		Interlab and observer variation
	Aniline blue		Lack of reproducibility
	Toluidine blue		Rapid color fading
	Chromomsycin A3		

conducted in various labs with fewer sperm cells. However, this also leaves room for varying protocols, making comparisons challenging. While thresholds may differ between laboratories due to the variation in practices, there may be consensus within the same laboratory [47].

Previous versions of the assay did not have a lysis step which prevented accessibility of the TdT to the entire DNA structure [48]. Recent improvements to the assay, including cell lysis, allow for relaxation of the whole chromatin structure, thus providing TdT access to all defects [49]. If DNA fragmentation is >10% as detected by TUNEL, low rates of fertilization have been demonstrated [38, 42]. A meta-analysis of IVF outcomes has shown that the clinical pregnancy rate decreased significantly with higher degrees of sperm DNA damage (RR 0.68, 95% CI 0.54–0.85, $p = 0.0006$). A negative correlation has also been demonstrated between sperm DNA fragmentation rate and quality of embryo development [50].

10.3.1.2 Comet Assay

The comet assay is unique in that it measures DNA damage within an individual cell rather than reporting an aggregate measure of damage as do the TUNEL assay and SCSA®. This allows for sperm DNA heterogeneity to be uncovered [12]. The comet assay only uses 5000 sperm, allowing remaining sperm to be reserved for clinical use, if needed. Comet is standardized by manipulating various conditions such as pH, temperature, salinity, and electrophoresis time in order to reduce protocol variants with different sensitivities. This manipulation requires experienced laboratory technicians to perform the comet assay. As such, this labor intensive process with significant interobserver variability imposes a major limitation to wide use of this test [12]. Men with a DNA fragmentation of greater than 25% as measured by comet assay have a higher risk of infertility. Clinical thresholds for diagnosis with the comet assay have been established to predict successful IVF cycles; the risk of failure to achieve pregnancy increased when sperm DNA fragmentation exceeded a threshold of 52% [29]. In addition, inverse relationships have been shown between comet length and embryo quality [41].

10.3.1.3 In Situ Nick Translation Assay

ISNT is a simple, inexpensive test which only requires a fluorescent microscope. The major limitation is that it uses a template-dependent polymerase and it can only quantify single-stranded DNA breaks, potentially leading to underestimation of DNA fragmentation [12]. Studies have shown that ISNT staining is negatively correlated with sperm concentration, motility, and morphology [13, 39]. The numbers of ISNT-stained (DNA-damaged) spermatozoa was significantly higher in infertile men [39].

10.3.2 *Indirect Tests*

10.3.2.1 Sperm Chromatin Structure Assay

SCSA®, one of the original sperm DNA tests, is a standardized test performed by a single primary reference laboratory (SCSA® Diagnostics, Brookings, SD) or its approved centers. Semen is batched and shipped to the primary lab and analyzed using its dedicated flow cytometer. Given the strict conditions under which this test is performed, it has high statistical robustness and is considered by some to be the most precise and repeatable DNA fragmentation assay [12, 51]. The SCSA® classifies DNA fragmentation as low (<15%), moderate (15–30%), and high (>30%); these values have been shown to have a strong association with fertility-related outcomes. Men with a DFI between 10% and 20% had an increased risk of infertility in comparison to men with a DFI <10% (OR, 2.5; 95% CI, 1.0–6.1) [52]. Men with a DFI >20% (OR, 8.4; 95% CI, 3.0–23) also had a higher incidence of infertility.

The probability of ongoing pregnancy or live birth with natural conception or IUI is near zero if the proportion of sperm cells with DFI >30% is detected by SCSA®. Similarly, IVF outcomes are poorer as DFI increases [16, 27, 28, 53].

10.3.2.2 Sperm Chromatin Dispersion Test

The SCD assay is an inexpensive test that is simple and does not require complex instrumentation. SCD, like the comet assay, requires that sperm be embedded in an agarose gel but without employing electrophoresis, thus making it comparatively faster and easier [12]. Light microscopy can be used if staining is done by eosin and azure B solution; otherwise, a fluorescence microscope is needed if fluorochromes are used for DNA detection. Interobserver subjectivity to categorize the halos limits this technique—an otherwise reasonable assay for DNA damage quantification. Infertile men have been found to have a high percentage of DNA fragmentation compared to fertile men with this test [9, 12, 14]. Specifically, a DNA fragmentation rate <18% was a significant predictor of oocyte fertilization [33].

10.3.2.3 Staining Assays

The AO, toluidine blue, aniline blue, and CMA3 staining assays are all inexpensive tests that can be conducted with a light microscope. All of these tests suffer from heterogeneity of staining and coloring on the slide as well as interlab and interobserver variation and lack of reproducibility [12, 15, 54]. One study found that the sensitivity and specificity values for CMA3 and AB were 75% and 82%, and 60% and 91%, respectively.

10.4 Ideal Sperm DNA Test

Several advancements in sperm DNA testing have occurred over the past 30 years and have led to a burgeoning area of research and clinical interest. Many mechanisms have been proposed for male infertility as reflected by abnormalities in sperm DNA quality related to intrinsic and extrinsic factors [2]. These include apoptosis in the seminiferous tubule epithelium, defects in chromatin remodeling during spermiogenesis, post-testicular DNA fragmentation induced by oxygen free radicals, DNA fragmentation induced by endogenous endonucleases, and DNA damage as a consequence of exposures to radiotherapy, chemotherapy, and environmental toxins [31]. As a result, test development has moved toward understanding and targeting these mechanisms for diagnosis.

Current technology for sperm DNA testing exhibits limitations in its ability to diagnose and predict male infertility [1, 44]. Sperm DNA tests focus on measuring global sperm DNA incompetence such as DNA fragmentation and strand breaks that may or may not be clinically significant. SCSA® and TUNEL, two of the mainstays of sperm DNA testing, are among the most commonly used studies. The SCSA® is the original sperm DNA test. It is an expensive standardized test, which reduces interlab and observer variability, leading to robust and consistent results. This is in contrast to TUNEL, which is less expensive and requires fewer sperm but is lab dependent, introducing some variability to the results. Other tests also have pros and cons as previously discussed. Yet even with the varying characteristics, all of these tests fare poorly in their predictive capacity for determining male fertility and ART outcomes. As a result of the many of the studies publishing equivocal fertility outcomes, the American Society for Reproductive Medicine does not endorse routine sperm DNA testing in the evaluation of the infertile male [55].

As the popularity of sperm DNA testing grows in conjunction with increased use of assisted reproductive therapies, new tests will be developed to better understand and measure sperm DNA integrity. These tests should be designed to be simple, inexpensive, and easy to interpret. But more importantly, they must provide a level of standardization that allows accuracy with a high sensitivity and specificity. This would allow detection of infertile patients with positive tests and fertile patients with negative tests [2, 56].

Furthermore, DNA tests should better define specific DNA parameters associated with poor fertilization, embryo quality, and pregnancy rates [56]. Tests should answer questions about the quality and location of the DNA defects, as well as define thresholds for determining fertility potential. Current tests may show that an infertile patient has elements of DNA damage, but the degree to which this matters still is not completely clear. Lastly, tests should be geared to cost-effectiveness, as infertility evaluation and treatment may not be accessible to the general public due to high costs and variable insurance coverage.

10.5 Conclusion

Male factor infertility is a multifaceted problem that requires a thorough evaluation. Recent advances have improved the diagnosis and treatment of male factor infertility. Among these advances are sperm DNA tests which evaluate sperm chromatin quality and DNA fragmentation. These tests have shed light on the association between sperm DNA abnormalities and male factor infertility as well as failed ARTs [42, 44, 57]. Since the advent of SCSA®, the first sperm DNA test, many more tests have been developed including the TUNEL, comet, and SCD assays. Each of these tests has advantages and disadvantages and may be used as an adjunct to the standard infertility work-up. However, there has yet to be a single test that best diagnoses and predicts male infertility. Further research will aim to develop a more predictive test that is cost-effective and broadly accessible.

References

1. Zini A, Boman JM, Belzile E, Ciampi A. Sperm DNA damage is associated with an increased risk of pregnancy loss after IVF and ICSI: systematic review and meta-analysis. Hum Reprod. 2008;23:2663–8.
2. Zini A, Sigman M. Are tests of sperm DNA damage clinically useful? Pros and cons. J Androl. 2009;30:219–29.
3. Klaude M, Eriksson S, Nygren J, Ahnström G. The comet assay: mechanisms and technical considerations. Mutat Res/DNA Repair. 1996;363:89–96.
4. Baumgartner A, Cemeli E, Anderson D. The comet assay in male reproductive toxicology. Cell Biol Toxicol. 2009;25:81–98.
5. Singh NP, McCoy MT, Tice RR, Schneider EL. A simple technique for quantitation of low levels of DNA damage in individual cells. Exp Cell Res. 1988;175:184–91.
6. Cortés-Gutiérrez EI, López-Fernández C, Fernández JL, Dávila-Rodríguez MI, Johnston SD, Gosálvez J. Interpreting sperm DNA damage in a diverse range of mammalian sperm by means of the two-tailed comet assay. 30 years of the Comet Assay: an overview with some new insights. 2015:123.
7. Gorczyca W, Melamed MR, Darzynkiewicz Z. Apoptosis of S-phase HL-60 cells induced by DNA topoisomerase inhibitors: detection of DNA strand breaks by flow cytometry using the in situ nick translation assay. Toxicol Lett. 1993;67:249–58.
8. Evenson D, Darzynkiewicz Z, Melamed M. Relation of mammalian sperm chromatin heterogeneity to fertility. Science. 1980;210:1131–3.
9. Fernández JL, Muriel L, Goyanes V, Segrelles E, Gosálvez J, Enciso M, LaFromboise M, De Jonge C. Simple determination of human sperm DNA fragmentation with an improved sperm chromatin dispersion test. Fertil Steril. 2005;84:833–42.
10. Tejada RI, Mitchell JC, Norman A, Marik JJ, Friedman S. A test for the practical evaluation of male fertility by acridine orange (AO) fluorescence. Fertil Steril. 1984;42:87–91.
11. Dadoune J, Mayaux M, Guihard-Moscato M. Correlation between defects in chromatin condensation of human spermatozoa stained by aniline blue and semen characteristics. Andrologia. 1988;20:211–7.
12. Shamsi MB, Imam SN, Dada R. Sperm DNA integrity assays: diagnostic and prognostic challenges and implications in management of infertility. J Assist Reprod Genet. 2011;28:1073–85.

13. Manicardi GC, Tombacco A, Bizzaro D, Bianchi U, Bianchi PG, Sakkas D. DNA strand breaks in ejaculated human spermatozoa: comparison of susceptibility to the nick translation and terminal transferase assays. Histochem J. 1998;30:33–9.
14. Chohan KR, Griffin JT, Lafromboise M, Jonge CJ, Carrell DT. Comparison of chromatin assays for DNA fragmentation evaluation in human sperm. J Androl. 2006;27:53–9.
15. Erenpreiss J, Jepson K, Giwercman A, Tsarev I, Erenpreisa J, Spano M. Toluidine blue cytometry test for sperm DNA conformation: comparison with the flow cytometric sperm chromatin structure and TUNEL assays. Hum Reprod. 2004;19:2277–82.
16. Spanò M, Bonde JP, Hjøllund HI, Kolstad HA, Cordelli E, Leter G. Danish first pregnancy planner study team. Sperm chromatin damage impairs human fertility. Fertil Steril. 2000;73:43–50.
17. Aravindan G, Bjordahl J, Jost L, Evenson D. Susceptibility of human sperm to in situ DNA denaturation is strongly correlated with DNA strand breaks identified by single-cell electrophoresis. Exp Cell Res. 1997;236:231–7.
18. Donnelly ET, O'Connell M, McClure N, Lewis SEM. Differences in nuclear DNA fragmentation and mitochondrial integrity of semen and prepared human spermatozoa. Hum Reprod. 2000;15:1552–61.
19. Gorczyca W, Gong J, Darzynkiewicz Z. Detection of DNA strand breaks in individual apoptotic cells by the in situ terminal deoxynucleotidyl transferase and nick translation assays. Cancer Res. 1993;53:1945–51.
20. Sailer B, Jost L, Evenson D. Mammalian sperm DNA susceptibility to in situ denaturation associated with the presence of DNA strand breaks as measured by the terminal Deoxynucleotidyl transferase assay. J Androl. 1995;16:80–7.
21. García-Peiró A, Oliver-Bonet M, Navarro J, Abad C, Guitart M, Amengual M, Gosálvez J, Benet J. Dynamics of sperm DNA fragmentation in patients carrying structurally rearranged chromosomes. Int J Androl. 2011;34:e546–53.
22. Ribas-Maynou J, García-Peiró A, Fernández-Encinas A, Abad C, Amengual M, Prada E, Navarro J, Benet J. Comprehensive analysis of sperm DNA fragmentation by five different assays: TUNEL assay, SCSA, SCD test and alkaline and neutral comet assay. Andrology. 2013;1:715–22.
23. Irvine D, Twigg J, Gordon E, Fulton N, Milne P, Aitken R. DNA integrity in human spermatozoa: relationships with semen quality. J Androl. 2000;21:33–44.
24. Zini A, Bielecki R, Phang D, Zenzes MT. Correlations between two markers of sperm DNA integrity, DNA denaturation and DNA fragmentation, in fertile and infertile men. Fertil Steril. 2001;75:674–7.
25. Evenson D, Thompson L, Jost L. Flow cytometric evaluation of boar semen by the sperm chromatin structure assay as related to cryopreservation and fertility. Theriogenology. 1994;41:637–51.
26. Zini A, Fischer MA, Sharir S, Shayegan B, Phang D, Jarvi K. Prevalence of abnormal sperm DNA denaturation in fertile and infertile men. Urology. 2002;60:1069–72.
27. Larson KL, DeJonge CJ, Barnes AM, Jost LK, Evenson DP. Sperm chromatin structure assay parameters as predictors of failed pregnancy following assisted reproductive techniques. Hum Reprod. 2000;15:1717–22.
28. Evenson DP, Jost LK, Marshall D, Zinaman MJ, Clegg E, Purvis K, de Angelis P, Claussen OP. Utility of the sperm chromatin structure assay as a diagnostic and prognostic tool in the human fertility clinic. Hum Reprod. 1999;14:1039–49.
29. Simon L, Lutton D, McManus J, Lewis SEM. Sperm DNA damage measured by the alkaline comet assay as an independent predictor of male infertility and in vitro fertilization success. Fertil Steril. 2011;95:652–7.
30. Lopes S, Sun J, Jurisicova A, Meriano J, Casper RF. Sperm deoxyribonucleic acid fragmentation is increased in poor-quality semen samples and correlates with failed fertilization in intracytoplasmic sperm injection. Fertil Steril. 1998;69:528–32.
31. Sakkas D, Alvarez JG. Sperm DNA fragmentation: mechanisms of origin, impact on reproductive outcome, and analysis. Fertil Steril. 2010;93:1027–36.

32. Høst E, Lindenberg S, Smidt-jensen S. DNA strand breaks in human spermatozoa: correlation with fertilization in vitro in oligozoospermic men and in men with unexplained infertility. Acta Obstet Gynecol Scand. 2000;79:189–93.
33. Velez de la Calle JF, Muller A, Walschaerts M, Clavere JL, Jimenez C, Wittemer C, Thonneau P. Sperm deoxyribonucleic acid fragmentation as assessed by the sperm chromatin dispersion test in assisted reproductive technology programs: results of a large prospective multicenter study. Fertil Steril. 2008;90:1792–9.
34. Muriel L, Garrido N, Fernández JL, Remohí J, Pellicer A, de los Santos MJ, Meseguer M. Value of the sperm deoxyribonucleic acid fragmentation level, as measured by the sperm chromatin dispersion test, in the outcome of in vitro fertilization and intracytoplasmic sperm injection. Fertil Steril. 2006;85:371–83.
35. Hammadeh ME, al-Hasani S, Stieber M, Rosenbaum P, Kupker D, Diedrich K, Schmidt W. The effect of chromatin condensation (aniline blue staining) and morphology (strict criteria) of human spermatozoa on fertilization, cleavage and pregnancy rates in an intracytoplasmic sperm injection programme. Hum Reprod. 1996;11:2468–71.
36. Haidl G, Schill W. Assessment of sperm chromatin condensation: an important test for prediction of IVF outcome. Arch Androl. 1994;32:263–6.
37. Hammadeh M, Stieber M, Haidl G, Schmidt W. Association between sperm cell chromatin condensation, morphology based on strict criteria, and fertilization, cleavage and pregnancy rates in an IVF program. Andrologia. 1998;30:29–35.
38. Duran EH, Morshedi M, Taylor S, Oehninger S. Sperm DNA quality predicts intrauterine insemination outcome: a prospective cohort study. Hum Reprod. 2002;17:3122–8.
39. Tomlinson MJ, Moffatt O, Manicardi GC, Bizzaro D, Afnan M, Sakkas D. Interrelationships between seminal parameters and sperm nuclear DNA damage before and after density gradient centrifugation: implications for assisted conception. Hum Reprod. 2001;16:2160–5.
40. Morris ID, Ilott S, Dixon L, Brison DR. The spectrum of DNA damage in human sperm assessed by single cell gel electrophoresis (Comet assay) and its relationship to fertilization and embryo development. Hum Reprod. 2002;17:990–8.
41. Tomsu M, Sharma V, Miller D. Embryo quality and IVF treatment outcomes may correlate with different sperm comet assay parameters. Hum Reprod. 2002;17:1856–62.
42. Benchaib M, Braun V, Lornage J, Hadj S, Salle B, Lejeune H, Guerin JF. Sperm DNA fragmentation decreases the pregnancy rate in an assisted reproductive technique. Hum Reprod. 2003;18:1023–8.
43. Evenson D, Wixon R. Meta-analysis of sperm DNA fragmentation using the sperm chromatin structure assay. Reprod BioMed Online. 2006;12:466–72.
44. Collins JA, Barnhart KT, Schlegel PN. Do sperm DNA integrity tests predict pregnancy with in vitro fertilization? Fertil Steril. 2008;89:823–31.
45. Cissen M, van Wely M, Scholten I, Mansell S, de Bruin JP, Mol BW, Braat D, Repping S, Hamer G. Measuring sperm DNA fragmentation and clinical outcomes of medically assisted reproduction: a systematic review and meta-analysis. PLoS One. 2016;11:e0165125.
46. Simon L, Zini A, Dyachenko A, Ciampi A, Carrell DT. A systematic review and meta-analysis to determine the effect of sperm DNA damage on in vitro fertilization and intracytoplasmic sperm injection outcome. Asian J Androl. 2017;19:80–90.
47. Henkel R, Kierspel E, Hajimohammad M, Stalf T, Hoogendijk C, Mehnert C, Menkveld R, Schill W, Kruger TF. DNA fragmentation of spermatozoa and assisted reproduction technology. Reprod BioMed Online. 2003;7:477–84.
48. Tesarik J, Mendoza-Tesarik R, Mendoza C. Sperm nuclear DNA damage: update on the mechanism, diagnosis and treatment. Reprod BioMed Online. 2006;12:715–21.
49. Mitchell LA, De Iuliis GN, Aitken RJ. The TUNEL assay consistently underestimates DNA damage in human spermatozoa and is influenced by DNA compaction and cell vitality: development of an improved methodology. Int J Androl. 2011;34:2–13.
50. Sun JG, Jurisicova A, Casper RF. Detection of deoxyribonucleic acid fragmentation in human sperm: correlation with fertilization in vitro. Biol Reprod. 1997;56:602–7.

51. Bungum M, Bungum L, Giwercman A. Sperm chromatin structure assay (SCSA): a tool in diagnosis and treatment of infertility. Asian J Androl. 2011;13:69–75.
52. Giwercman A, Lindstedt L, Larsson M, Bungum M, Spano M, Levine RJ, Rylander L. Sperm chromatin structure assay as an independent predictor of fertility in vivo: a case–control study. Int J Androl. 2010;33:e221–7.
53. Venkatesh S, Singh A, Shamsi MB, Thilagavathi J, Kumar R, Mitra DK, Dada R. Clinical significance of sperm DNA damage threshold value in the assessment of male infertility. Reprod Sci. 2011;18:1005–13.
54. Schulte RT, Ohl DA, Sigman M, Smith GD. Sperm DNA damage in male infertility: etiologies, assays, and outcomes. J Assist Reprod Genet. 2010;27:3–12.
55. Practice Committee of the American Society for Reproductive Medicine. The clinical utility of sperm DNA integrity testing. Fertil Steril. 2006;86:S35–7.
56. Agarwal A, Allamaneni SS. Sperm DNA damage assessment: a test whose time has come. Fertil Steril. 2005;84:850–3.
57. Simon L, Brunborg G, Stevenson M, Lutton D, McManus J, Lewis SEM. Clinical significance of sperm DNA damage in assisted reproduction outcome. Hum Reprod. 2010;25:1594–608.

Part III
Etiology of Sperm DNA Damage: Biological and Clinical Factors

Chapter 11
Oxidative Stress

Ralf Henkel and Michael Solomon

11.1 Introduction

According to the International Committee for Monitoring Assisted Reproductive Technology (ICMART) and the World Health Organization (WHO), infertility is clinically defined as "a disease of the reproductive system defined by the failure to achieve a clinical pregnancy after 12 months or more of regular unprotected sexual intercourse" [1]. As such, this condition affects almost 50 million couples worldwide [2] rendering it an important health and social concern, particularly in African and Asian countries where the onus of reproduction rather rests on the female partner [3]. Reported prevalence rates are between 9% [2] and 15% [4, 5] with about 50% of the causes for couple infertility being associated with the male [3, 6, 7], which represents about 7.5% of male partners affected by infertility during their reproductive lifetime. Thus, the prevalence of male infertility is even higher than for diabetes mellitus types I and II, which are considered as common diseases [8].

Male factor infertility is a multifactorial disorder, and patients clinically present with low or absent sperm counts or nonfunctional spermatozoa [9]. Despite increasing research efforts with relevant results during the past decades, this condition remains largely idiopathic with a wide variety of different causes including dysfunctions along the hypothalamic-pituitary-gonadal axis, hypogonadism, Kallmann syndrome, varicocele, cryptorchidism, infections (e.g., epididymitis) [10], environmental, chemical, and lifestyle (e.g., poor nutrition, alcohol, smoking) exposures, or iatrogenic causes (e.g., chemotherapy, radiotherapy) [11–14]. A major component of the pathophysiological mechanism of many of the conditions causing male infertility is the so-called oxidative stress [15]. Oxidative stress is a concept that was coined and introduced into redox biology and medicine by Helmut Sies in 1985 [16] and "denotes a shift in the prooxidant/antioxidant balance in favor of the former" [17].

R. Henkel (✉) • M. Solomon
Department of Medical Bioscience, University of the Western Cape, Bellville, South Africa
e-mail: rhenkel@uwc.ac.za

A. Zini, A. Agarwal (eds.), *A Clinician's Guide to Sperm DNA and Chromatin Damage*, https://doi.org/10.1007/978-3-319-71815-6_11

Considering that oxidative stress is involved in the pathogenesis of many conditions ranging from infections, inflammations, obesity, and cancer to male factor infertility, the general prevalence of this condition can be expected to be very high. Even in the aging process, oxidative stress is involved [18]. This is also reflected by the high number of almost 154,000 PubMed entries for a general search for "oxidative stress" and 1741 entries for the combination "oxidative stress" and "sperm" in July 2016. For oxidative stress contributing to sperm damage, prevalence rates between 30% and 80% have been reported in infertile men [19–23]. The prevalence of male genital tract infections in this patient group ranges from 35% up to 45% [24, 25]. The feature of this condition is that it is caused either by an excessive production of reactive oxygen species (ROS) or a deficiency in the antioxidative defenses of the body [26, 27]. Therefore, it is important to understand not only the pathophysiology and biochemistry of the respective medical condition, as well as the consequences and treatment options.

11.2 Reactive Oxygen Species (ROS)

Since cyanobacteria started producing oxygen in the process called photosynthesis about 2.4 billion years ago, the atmospheric oxygen concentration rose to about 2–4% [28, 29] corresponding to 20–40 μM dissolved oxygen in the surrounding water, which is close to the oxygen partial pressure in most mammalian tissues at the ends of capillary beds and to the saturation midpoint (P50) of hemoglobin [30]. In contrast, at the site of the oxygen consumption, cytochrome c, in modern mitochondria the oxygen P50 is with 0.3 μM [31] about 150 times lower than outside the cell [32]. Over time, atmospheric oxygen level increased to 20% that we see nowadays. Nevertheless, most metabolic pathways including fatty acid oxidation and synthesis, heme synthesis, glutathione metabolism, or the Krebs cycles that we know today relate back to the chemistry of life of about 3.5 billion years ago when the earth was anaerobic (an atmosphere without oxygen) [33, 34]. Since these times, life adapted to these increased oxygen levels and many organisms developed protective mechanisms against this primary toxic and unsafe element, oxygen, as this element is highly reactive.

From a chemical point of view, atmospheric and dissolved oxygen is not a single atom, but molecular as O_2. Although the electronic structure with its even number of electrons in the triplet ground state explains the relative kinetic inertness of molecular oxygen (O_2), molecular oxygen has two unpaired electrons in its outer molecular orbitals. Radicals are highly reactive compounds and are defined as atoms or molecules having one or more unpaired electrons in the outer valence molecular orbital. Considering that molecular oxygen has two unpaired electrons, this renders this element a biradical. The two free, unpaired electrons have the same spin quantum number. If molecular oxygen oxidizes other atoms or molecules, the two new electrons must have parallel spin, which imposes significant restrictions on the oxidation process by molecular oxygen as normally an electron pair in an atom

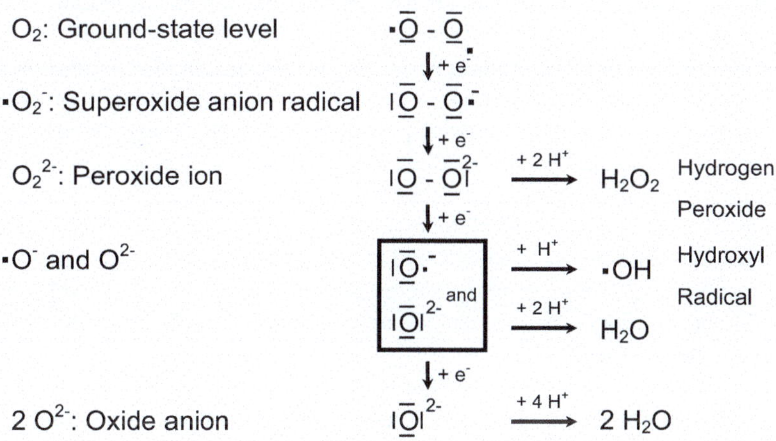

Fig. 11.1 Oxidation forms of oxygen. If molecular oxygen, which is a biradical with two unpaired electrons, is reduced, it acquires four electrons and water (H_2O) is formed. The dashes around the oxygen (O) represent paired electrons; the points represent unpaired electrons

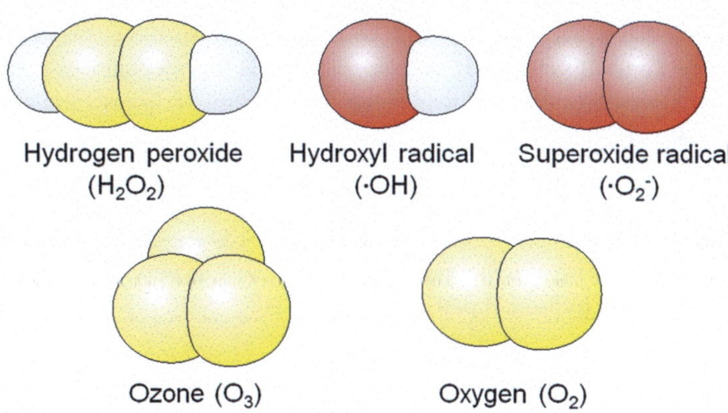

Fig. 11.2 Some examples of reactive oxygen species (ROS) with respective half-life times and specific features

or molecular orbital has antiparallel spins [35]. As a result, only one electron at a time can be transferred in this process (Fig. 11.1). Three types of reactions can take place leading to superoxide radical ($.O_2-$) and related species, peroxyl radicals (ROO.), and singlet oxygen ($^1O_2$).

For these reasons, ROS are chemically unstable and exhibit half-life times between nanosecond (10^{-9} s) (·OH; hydroxyl radicals) and a few seconds (RO·; 7 s), depending on the specific oxygen derivative (Fig. 11.2). Due to this highly reactive nature, ROS are commonly said to have detrimental effects on cells. However, in biological systems, these compounds not only cause damage but also have physiological functions in terms of triggering essential physiological events. In spermatozoa, these physiological events include hyperactivation, capacitation, and acrosome reaction [36–39].

With regard to their intracellular energy production, spermatozoa are principally not different from other cells, and energy as ATP is largely aerobically produced in the mitochondria by means of oxidative phosphorylation and oxidation of hydrogen in the form of nicotinamide adenine dinucleotide (NADH). This process of cellular energy production involving the mitochondrial electron transfer chain is affected by taking up of four electrons by elementary oxygen (O_2) whereby highly reactive intermediate products as free radicals and eventually water (H_2O) are generated. In addition, spermatozoa also produce chemical energy in the form of ATP via glycolysis. However, this is species-specific and dependent on the demands set in the female genital tract [40].

In the midpiece of the flagellum, sperm contains a specific NADPH-dependent oxidoreductase (diaphorase) [41, 42]. Furthermore, mitochondria in somatic cells have been shown to possess at least nine sites capable of producing superoxide radicals (Eq. 11.1) [43], of which the Complex I (NADH dehydrogenase) and Complex III (coenzyme Q: cytochrome c—oxidoreductase) have been demonstrated in spermatozoa [44, 45]. Disruption of the mitochondrial electron transfer chain and subsequent electron leakage leads to ROS production from Complex I or III [18, 45]. This is a normal process which results in about 1–5% of the consumed oxygen being converted into ROS [46, 47]. ROS produced via this mechanism are regarded as cytotoxic by-products that are involved in the etiology of disease and aging [48].

$$NADH + 2O_2 \rightarrow 2 \cdot O_{2^-} NAD^+ + H^+ \quad (11.1)$$

The superoxide that is produced dismutates into H_2O_2 by the action of superoxide dismutase (SOD) (Eq. 11.2) rendering spermatozoa as very competent producers of superoxide and hydrogen peroxide.

$$2 \cdot O_{2^-} + 2H^+ \xrightarrow{SOD} O_2 + H_2O_2 \quad (11.2)$$

In vivo, these two reactions are coupled in the Fenton and Haber-Weiss reaction which are accelerated by other cofactors as well as transition metal ions such as Fe^{2+}/Fe^{3+}.

$\cdot O_2^- + Fe^{3+} \rightarrow Fe^{2+} + O_2$	*Fenton reaction*
$Fe^{2+} + H_2O_2 \rightarrow Fe^{3+} + \cdot OH + OH^-$	
$\cdot O_{2^-} + H_2O_2 \xrightarrow{Fe^{2+}} O_2 + OH^- + \cdot OH$	*Haber-Weiss reaction*

In intact systems such as in other somatic cells, the production of these highly reactive compounds is counter-regulated by scavenging enzymes like manganese superoxide dismutase (MnSOD), copper/zinc superoxide dismutase (Cu/ZnSOD), glutathione peroxidase (GPx), and catalase (CAT).

Considering that normal functional spermatozoa have only very little cytoplasm, they lack such protective enzymes. Yet, immature germ cells where the cytoplasm is not removed by the Sertoli cells during spermiogenesis and spermatozoa with poor morphology are deemed to generate excessive amounts of ROS [49–51] as this process is then excessively fueled by the sperm cells' own cytoplasmic glucose-6-phosphate dehydrogenase [49].

11.3 What Is Oxidative Stress?

Under normal physiological circumstances, cells are functioning rather in a chemically reduced state. Therefore, cellular production of ROS and their relevant scavengers need to be in a finely balanced equilibrium in order for spermatozoa to fertilize oocytes [52]. These scavengers can be categorized as enzymatic antioxidants like glutathione peroxidase or catalase, nonenzymatic antioxidants such as vitamins A, C, or E, glutathione or L-carnitine, as well as other antioxidants like ubiquinol, albumin, or carotenes [53]. On the other hand, the principles of the antioxidant mechanisms can be categorized in three processes, namely, (i) prevention, (ii) interception, and (iii) repair [54]. Prevention refers to two mechanisms, whereby either ROS are not releases by the enzymes involved or where metal chelation is a major means of controlling lipid peroxidation. The interception process can be achieved by scavenging the radicals that are produced, either enzymatically or non-enzymatically. Lastly, in case the aforementioned processes are not sufficient or as the last chance of cells to counteract the damaging influence of oxidative stress, cells have the ability to repair damages to DNA oxidized proteins and lipids. Hence, cells are constantly facing the dilemma between the oxidative and reductive status. In cases where this steady state derails for whatever reason, an imbalance in favor of oxidants is created, which can then potentially cause cellular or genetic damage. This condition is called "oxidative stress" [16], and the relevant biochemical and clinical consequence includes infertility or the induction of cancer (Fig. 11.3). The latter would then develop due to the fact that DNA damage cannot be repaired because of the shutdown of apoptotic caspases which would normally eliminate badly damaged or necrotic cells. As a result, these damaged cells will survive and cause injury to neighboring areas.

Oxidative stress is particularly detrimental for spermatozoa as the male germ cell is especially sensitive to this condition because of (i) the lack of cytoplasm and therefore a lack of protective enzymes and (ii) the extraordinary high content of polyunsaturated fatty acids (PUFAs) in their plasma membrane [55–57].

On the other hand, an uncontrolled and nonphysiologic shift of the redox status from the normal physiologic zone into the reduced state is also highly problematic for cells in general and spermatozoa in particular, as then the trigger function of ROS for physiologic cellular events such as capacitation and acrosome reaction would be abolished. This condition is then called "reductive stress" and is as dangerous for cells as oxidative stress.

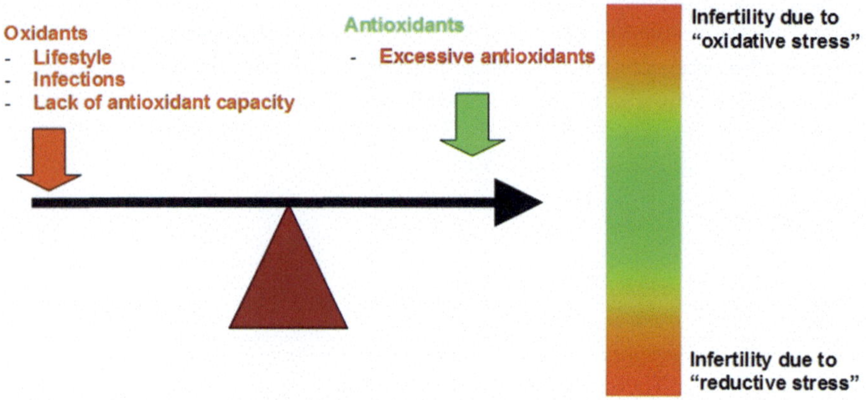

Fig. 11.3 Schematic representation of the balance between oxidation and reduction. Too many oxidants or too little antioxidants cause "oxidative stress," while a lack of oxidants or an excessive amount of antioxidants is causing "reductive stress"

11.4 Consequences of Oxidative Stress

Considering the high reactivity of ROS, the extraordinarily high amount of PUFAs, as well as the lack of sufficient antioxidative protection of spermatozoa, this has dire consequences for male germ cells if they are exposed to oxidative stress as spermatozoa are particularly susceptible to this stress. The chemical nature of PUFAs is to have numerous double bonds in the molecules which can easily be oxidized by excessive ROS levels present in the sperm cells' environment. These ROS can either originate from an extrinsic source (e.g., ROS from activated leukocytes in case the patient is suffering from an infection or inflammation) [58–61] or intrinsic ROS from apoptotic or damaged spermatozoa [62]. Extrinsic ROS derived from external sources like leukocytes or damaged spermatozoa preferably attack the plasma membrane lipids initiating a process called "lipid peroxidation" (LPO). Ultimately, this process decreases membrane fluidity of both plasma and organelle membranes and, as a result, damages membrane function, ion gradients, receptor-mediated signal transduction, etc. [63, 64]. As a result, the plasma membrane loses its function; hence, the male germ cell loses its functional ability and fertilization is impaired [65, 66]. While extrinsic ROS affect the plasma membrane and its functions, intrinsic ROS rather affect the sperm nuclear DNA integrity [62] and possibly mitochondrial membrane potential and mitochondrial DNA integrity [67–69].

11.4.1 Lipid Peroxidation

Lipid peroxidation is the oxidative degradation of lipids. This process has three phases, namely, the initiation, propagation, and termination phases. In the initiation phase, ROS attack carbon atoms adjacent to the double bonds in PUFAs. This reaction creates reactive methylene groups by abstraction of hydrogen atoms and transforms the lipid molecule into a lipid radical, which is stabilized by delocalization of the free electron in so-called resonance structures, which are energetically more stable than the initiating ROS. Lipid radicals, in turn, are unstable and react spontaneously with O_2 to form lipid peroxides.

These lipid peroxide radicals react with neighboring lipids in a so-called radical chain reaction, thus propagating the degradation process of lipids. In turn, these newly created lipid peroxides react with oxygen to form yet more lipid peroxides. Thus, in this way, numerous lipid molecules are damaged just by one initiating radical leading to the oxidization of almost 60% of the PUFAs present in the plasma membrane [70].

When one radical reacts with another radical, the two free electrons form a covalent bond resulting in a non-radical, thereby terminating the propagation of the radical chain reaction. This termination takes place when a sufficiently high concentration of lipid radicals is available. In addition to the described propagation and termination processes of lipid peroxidation, lipid molecules are also broken down to a number of stable carbonyl by-products such as malondialdehyde and 4-hydroxy-2-alkenals such as 4-hydroxy-nonenal. Malondialdehyde is highly mutagenic, and 4-hydroxy-nonenal is genotoxic [71], hence posing additional danger to spermatozoa, namely, cytotoxicity and DNA damage by forming DNA adducts [72], mainly pyrimido[1,2-a]purin-10(3H)-one [73], thereby indirectly causing DNA damage.

Semen samples from patients with high oxidative stress levels show significantly higher malondialdehyde levels compared to the controls and correlate negatively with the sperm count [74–76]. The thiobarbituric acid reactive substance as measured for the malondialdehyde concentration was negatively correlated with fertilization rates after IVF [77]. Antioxidants like vitamins C or E as well as ROS-scavenging enzymes such as superoxide dismutase or catalase reduce the risk of lipid peroxidation-induced cell damage. However, due to the genotoxicity and mutagenicity of the mentioned lipid peroxidation by-products and their ability to form DNA adducts, it is obvious that the cellular defense mechanisms are not 100% efficient [78], particularly in spermatozoa.

11.4.2 Nuclear and Mitochondrial DNA Damage

Apart from the above described damage to the plasma membrane initiated by ROS through lipid peroxidation and its consequences to motility and membrane-associated sperm functions, ROS can cause damage to nuclear (nDNA) [79–82] and mitochondrial DNA (mtDNA) [83, 84]. The association between nDNA damage and poor fertilization and pregnancy rates has repeatedly been demonstrated [80, 85, 86] and confirmed in a meta-analysis [87]. For intrauterine insemination and IVF, this connection appears to be without doubt [80, 88]. However, for intracytoplasmic sperm injection (ICSI), the effect of nDNA damage on fertilization and pregnancy is controversial [89, 90], and reasons for this are still unknown.

For mtDNA damage, St. John and co-workers [91] described a potential risk of abnormal transmission of mtDNA for patients undergoing assisted reproduction procedures. More recent findings suggest that ROS, mtDNA mutations, increased sperm mtDNA content as well as mtDNA depletion have to be considered major etiological factors in male infertility [68, 92, 93]. Unlike nDNA, mtDNA is highly sensitive to oxidative stress as it is not protected by histones or protamines, replicates very fast without proper proofreading, and has only a basic repair mechanism [94]. As a result, it was suggested that the mitochondrial genome is about 100 times more sensitive to assaults and mutations [95]. However, a more recent study by Lim et al. [96] indicates that the level of mtDNA damage in vivo is not higher than that of nDNA as the detected damage might be artifactual. On the other hand, high levels of mtDNA mutations strongly correlate with poor sperm motility [97]. mtDNA appears to show defects in oligoasthenozoospermic men that makes DNA unavailable for amplification. Only in motile sperm, mitochondria were functional to execute the electron transfer chain [83]. These results appear to be consistent with recent findings by Treulen et al. [98] indicating that damage to the mitochondrial outer membrane increases the production of ROS and thereby decreases sperm motility and velocity, but with only negligible effects on sperm DNA integrity. On the contrary, Bonanno et al. [99] reported that asthenozoospermic patients not only show elevated ROS levels but also a significantly increased number of mtDNA copies and decreased mtDNA integrity and mitochondrial membrane potential. The latter parameters were also closely associated with elevated ROS levels. Yet, nDNA fragmentation was only increased in 20% of the patients. If this patient group with increased nDNA damage represents an end point due to an extended or increased exposure of these spermatozoa to elevated levels of oxidative stress, still remains unclear.

11.5 Treatment of Oxidative Stress

In the light of the potential significant detrimental effects of oxidative stress on numerous medical conditions including male fertility, questions related to reducing oxidative stress point in two directions, namely, the causes of its generation and possible medical treatments. With regard to the causes of oxidative stress, a modern western lifestyle, with its relatively low intake of natural antioxidants such as vegetables or fruit as well as a relatively high exposure to exogenous sources of ROS including alcohol, cigarettes, or environmental pollutants, may be an important cause of oxidative stress [12, 14, 100, 101]. Male genital tract infections, varicocele [102], toxins [103, 104], or even cell phone radiation [105] represent other causes of oxidative stress. The prevalence of oxidative stress is estimated to be up to 35% in a nonselected group of men consulting for infertility, and up to 45% in patients with a history of urethral discharge have been reported [24, 25]. Many causes of oxidative stress are potentially correctable, either by avoiding the exposure to ROS-generating and causing agents, correcting the varicocele, or treating infection or inflammation. In practice, surgical or medical therapy (e.g., antibiotics or anti-inflammatories in the form of tables) seems to be easier for patients than changing the lifestyle, which would include the reduction/cessation of drinking, smoking, or the abandonment of other habits such as the use cell phones or eating low-vitamin processed or fast foods. Occupational exposure in certain professional groups such as long-distance drivers, welders or office workers (heat exposure), or workers in the chemical industry (environmental toxins) might also be at risk.

In order to compensate for the low of vitamin intake in the modern diet, many people are taking high dosages of antioxidants such as food supplements which contain ROS scavengers like vitamin C [106] and E [107]. In addition, numerous antioxidant herbal products containing polyphenols flavonoids are advertised to counteract oxidative stress [108–112]. However, such therapies, although beneficial in many cases, might have either no effect or even detrimental effects [113–118]. In addition, Aitken and co-workers [117] reported that not all polyphenols have beneficial effects. In fact, except for resveratrol, genistein, and 2,2,′4,4′-tetrahydroxy-diphenyl at concentrations below 100 μM, all other compounds investigated in the study caused loss of motility and mitochondrial membrane potential and stimulated ROS production with subsequent nDNA fragmentation. This is consistent with earlier findings of polyphenols inducing DNA damage and therefore might act as chemopreventives for cancer [119, 120]. This might be a result of the chemical nature of the compound in question as many biomolecules either donate electrons (antioxidant) or function as electron acceptor (antireductant) depending of the respective chemical conditions. While vitamin E is relatively bad electron acceptor, but good electron donor, resveratrol has better electron-accepting and poorer electron-donating properties. Compounds like vitamin A or β-carotene exhibit the latter properties even much more so [121]. Therefore, antioxidative therapies are debated [23, 122] as it seems that the effectiveness of an antioxidant therapy is dependent on the composition and concentration of the preparation.

11.5.1 The Antioxidant Paradox

The apparent contradictory results might be due to several reasons. First, one certainly has to differentiate between the different chemical natures of various antioxidants. Second, vitamins, such as vitamins C or E, are rather regarded as antioxidants, while polyphenols, besides having antioxidant capacity, also appear to have other effects. Moreover, a single antioxidant compound administered to a patient might be less effective than a combination of different antioxidants at specific concentrations. The third major problem is that scientists and clinicians still do not know what is the normal redox status in the human body is; no tests for this parameter are clinically performed. Due to this lack of knowledge with respect to the redox status, uncontrolled antioxidant treatment could have detrimental effects to the patient. Clinically, this might play a role as Henkel et al. observed spontaneous pregnancy in a couple who discontinued all antioxidant intake recommended by the fertility specialist and the additional over-the-counter antioxidants (Henkel et al., unpublished).

The phenomenon that antioxidants can have such paradoxical effects is called the "antioxidant paradox," a term which was coined by Halliwell [123], and postulates that the body's "total antioxidant capacity" seems unresponsive to high doses of dietary antioxidants and that manipulation of endogenous antioxidant levels (e.g., by supplying weak prooxidants) may be a more useful approach to treatment and prevention of diseases in which reactive oxygen species are important rather than the consumption of high doses of antioxidants. According to the principle, the human body needs an essential amount of antioxidants for normal cell function as cells are generally functioning in a reduced state. Conversely, a certain limited level of ROS in is also necessary for normal cell function. In the case of the male germ cell, ROS are essential to trigger capacitation, hyperactivation, and acrosome reaction [36–39]. Moreover, for the regulation of MAP kinases or normal function of several gene transcription factors [124, 125], a controlled amount of ROS is necessary. Even the induction of apoptosis, which is on the one hand caused by oxidative stress, is characterized by a shift toward a more oxidized status of the cell since caspases are sensitive to the redox status of the cell. Thus, this whole process is regulated by a fine balance between oxidation and reduction which is triggering or inhibiting the process [126, 127]. Therefore, an overdose of antioxidants can be detrimental and even cause cancer [123] or male infertility.

11.6 Reductive Stress

Since oxidative stress can derail cellular functions, the redox status must be finely balanced. In case of an overexposure of cells to antioxidants, this fine balance will be shifted from oxidation status into reduction status, a condition which has been termed "reductive stress" [128]. Accordingly, reductive stress is defined as an imbalance in the redox status with increased levels of reducing equivalents in form of redox couples such as GSH/GSSG or NADPH/NADP [129]. Reductive stress can cause cardiac injury, neurological diseases such as Alzheimer's disease [130, 131], and dysregulations of embryogenesis [132]. Thus, reductive stress is as dangerous for cells and organs as oxidative stress [133]. Paradoxically, the injury induced to cells under reductive stress conditions is of oxidative nature since high levels of antioxidants (reducing equivalents) promote excessive ROS production exceeding the ROS-scavenging capacity. This results in a mitochondrial spillover of hydrogen peroxide [134] and might also explain the observation of a spontaneous pregnancy in the couple who was asked to discontinue their excessive intake of antioxidants.

Henkel [135] and Chen et al. [136] pointed out the problem of a possible overtreatment of patients which may lead to male infertility due to reductive stress. Therefore, relevant standardized assays and proper cutoff values need to be established. These assays would have to include both sides of the redox scale, oxidation, and reduction, to establish what is "normal" in this context. One assay for which a seminal cutoff value was established by means of ROC curve analysis is the total antioxidant capacity [137]. Another, perhaps easier and cheaper, tests system might be measuring the oxidation-reduction potential with the MiOXSYS system [138]. A clinical evaluation of this method, however, is still outstanding.

11.7 Summary

Under aerobic conditions, cells metabolize oxygen in a stepwise reaction in the mitochondria to generate energy in the form of ATP. During this process, about 5% of the oxygen leaks in the form of highly reactive radicals from the mitochondrial electron transfer chain. Normally, these oxidants are neutralized by antioxidants. However, in the case of an imbalance toward elevated levels of reactive oxygen radicals, this can cause oxidative stress. In spermatozoa, the unique plasma membrane is rich in high amounts of polyunsaturated fatty acids. Oxidative stress causes damage of these membrane lipids by induction of lipid peroxidation. This process does not only lead to the loss of membrane function and functional capacity of the male germ cell but can also cause sperm nuclear DNA damage as the stable carbonyl by-products and 4-hydroxy-2-alkenals of lipid peroxidation are highly mutagenic and genotoxic. Therefore, it is important to minimize oxidative stress. This can either be achieved by elimination of conditions causing oxidative stress or by antioxidants. However, an oversupply of antioxidants in the body can cause the opposite condition of oxidative stress known as reductive stress, which is as dangerous for cells as oxidative stress as it can also be the cause of various diseases and infertility. The challenge is that up to now, the normal value for this fine balance between oxidation and reduction is unclear. Relevant tests still need to be developed and evaluated.

References

1. Zegers-Hochschild F, Adamson GD, de Mouzon J, Ishihara O, Mansour R, Nygren K, Sullivan E, van der Poel S. International Committee for Monitoring Assisted Reproductive Technology; World Health Organization. The International Committee for Monitoring Assisted Reproductive Technology (ICMART) and the World Health Organization (WHO) revised glossary on ART terminology, 2009. Hum Reprod. 2009;24:2683–7.
2. Boivin J, Bunting L, Collins JA, Nygren KG. International estimates of infertility prevalence and treatment-seeking: potential need and demand for infertility medical care. Hum Reprod. 2007;22:1506–12.
3. World Health Organization. Towards more objectivity in diagnosis and management of male infertility. Int J Androl. 1987;7. Suppl.:1–53.
4. de Kretser DM. Male infertility. Lancet. 1997;349:787–90.
5. World Health Organization. WHO Laboratory Manual for the Examination and Processing of Human Semen. Fifth edition, WHO Press; 2010.
6. Hull MG, Glazener CM, Kelly NJ, Conway DI, Foster PA, Hinton RA, Coulson C, Lambert PA, Watt EM, Desai KM. Population study of causes, treatment, and outcome of infertility. Br Med J (Clin Res Ed). 1985;291:1693–7.

7. Abid S, Maitra A, Meherji P, Patel Z, Kadam S, Shah J, Shah R, Kulkarni V, Baburao V, Gokral J. Clinical and laboratory evaluation of idiopathic male infertility in a secondary referral center in India. J Clin Lab Anal. 2008;22:29–38.
8. Nieschlag E, Behre HM. Andrology. Male reproductive health and dysfunction. 2nd ed. Berlin: Springer; 2000.
9. Tournaye HJ, Cohlen BJ. Management of male-factor infertility. Best Pract Res Clin Obstet Gynaecol. 2012;26:769–75.
10. Haidl G, Allam JP, Schuppe HC. Chronic epididymitis: impact on semen parameters and therapeutic options. Andrologia. 2008;40:92–6.
11. Howell SJ, Shalet SM. Testicular function following chemotherapy. Hum Reprod Update. 2001;7:363–9.
12. Bonde JP, Storgaard L. How work-place conditions, environmental toxicants and lifestyle affect male reproductive function. Int J Androl. 2002;25:262–8.
13. Smith R, Kaune H, Parodi D, Madariaga M, Rios R, Morales I, Castro A. Increased sperm DNA damage in patients with varicocele: relationship with seminal oxidative stress. Hum Reprod. 2006;21:986–93.
14. Wright C, Milne S, Leeson H. Sperm DNA damage caused by oxidative stress: modifiable clinical, lifestyle and nutritional factors in male infertility. Reprod BioMed Online. 2014;28:684–703.
15. Agarwal A, Makker K, Sharma R. Clinical relevance of oxidative stress in male factor infertility: an update. Am J Reprod Immunol. 2008;59:2–11.
16. Sies H. Oxidative stress: introductory remarks. In: Sies H, editor. Oxidative stress. London: Academic; 1985. p. 1–8.
17. Sies H. Biochemistry of oxidative stress. Angew Chem Int Ed Eng. 1986;25:1058–71.
18. Finkel T, Holbrook NJ. Oxidants, oxidative stress and the biology of ageing. Nature. 2000;408:239–47.
19. Gagnon C, Iwasaki A, De Lamirande E, Kovalski N. Reactive oxygen species and human spermatozoa. Ann N Y Acad Sci. 1991;637:436–44.
20. de Lamirande E, Gagnon C. Impact of reactive oxygen species on spermatozoa: a balancing act between beneficial and detrimental effects. Hum Reprod. 1995;10(Suppl 1):15–21.
21. Agarwal A, Gupta S, Sikka S. The role of free radicals and antioxidants in reproduction. Curr Opin Obstet Gynecol. 2006;18:325–32.
22. Aitken RJ. Sperm function tests and fertility. Int J Androl. 2006;29:69–75.
23. Tremellen K. Oxidative stress and male infertility—a clinical perspective. Hum Reprod Update. 2008;14:243–58.
24. Bayasgalan G, Naranbat D, Tsedmaa B, Tsogmaa B, Sukhee D, Amarjargal O, Lhagvasuren T, Radnaabazar J, Rowe PJ. Clinical patterns and major causes of infertility in Mongolia. J Obstet Gynaecol Res. 2004;30:386–93.
25. Henkel R, Maaß G, Jung A, Haidl G, Schill WB, Schuppe HC. Age-related changes in seminal polymorphonuclear elastase in men with asymptomatic inflammation of the genital tract. Asian J Androl. 2007;9:299–304.
26. Halliwell B. Oxidative stress and neurodegeneration: where are we now? J Neurochem. 2006;97:1634–58.
27. Halliwell B, Gutteridge J. Cellular responses to oxidative stress: adaptation, damage, repair, senescence and death. In: Halliwell B, Gutteridge J, editors. Free radicals in biology and medicine. New York: Oxford University Press; 2007. p. 187–267.
28. Rasmussen B, Fletcher IR, Brocks JJ, Kilburn MR. Reassessing the first appearance of eukaryotes and cyanobacteria. Nature. 2008;455:1101–4.
29. Hohmann-Marriott MF, Blankenship RE. Evolution of photosynthesis. Annu Rev Plant Biol. 2011;62:515–48.
30. Winslow RM, Monge CC. Hypoxia, polycythemia and chronic mountain sickness. Baltimore: The Johns Hopkins University Press; 1987.

31. Gnaiger E, Steinlechner-Maran R, Mendez G, Eberl T, Margreiter R. Control of mitochondrial and cellular respiration by oxygen. J Bioenerg Biomembr. 1995;27:583–96.
32. Naviaux RK. Oxidative shielding or oxidative stress? J Pharmacol Exp Ther. 2012;342:608–18.
33. Cavalier-Smith T. Cell evolution and earth history: stasis and revolution. Philos Trans R Soc Lond Ser B Biol Sci. 2006;361:969–1006.
34. Tang KH, Blankenship RE. Both forward and reverse TCA cycles operate in green sulfur bacteria. J Biol Chem. 2010;285:35848–54.
35. Cadenas E. Biochemistry of oxygen toxicity. Annu Rev Biochem. 1989;58:79–110.
36. de Lamirande E, Gagnon C. A positive role for the superoxide anion in triggering hyperactivation and capacitation of human spermatozoa. Int J Androl. 1993;16:21–5.
37. de Lamirande E, Gagnon C. Capacitation-associated production of superoxide anion by human spermatozoa. Free Radic Biol Med. 1995;18:487–95.
38. de Lamirande E, Jiang H, Zini A, Kodama H, Gagnon C. Reactive oxygen species and sperm physiology. Rev Reprod. 1997;2:48–54.
39. O'Flaherty CM, Beorlegui NB, Beconi MT. Reactive oxygen species requirements for bovine sperm capacitation and acrosome reaction. Theriogenology. 1999;52:289–301.
40. Storey BT. Mammalian sperm metabolism: oxygen and sugar, friend and foe. Int J Dev Biol. 2008;52:427–37.
41. Caldwell K, Blake ET, Sensabaugh GF. Sperm diaphorase: genetic polymorphism and isozyme pattern of sperm in infertile men. Science. 1976;191:1185–7.
42. Gavella M, Lipovac V. NADH-dependent oxidoreductase (diaphorase) activity and isozyme pattern of sperm in infertile men. Arch Androl. 1992;28:135–41.
43. Andreyev AY, Kushnareva YE, Starkov AA. Mitochondrial metabolism of reactive oxygen species. Biochemistry (Mosc). 2005;70:200–14.
44. Aitken RJ, Clarkson JS. Cellular basis of defective sperm function and its association with the genesis of reactive oxygen species by human spermatozoa. J Reprod Fertil. 1987;81:459–69.
45. Koppers AJ, De Iuliis GN, Finnie JM, McLaughlin EA, Aitken RJ. Significance of mitochondrial reactive oxygen species in the generation of oxidative stress in spermatozoa. J Clin Endocrinol Metab. 2008;93:3199–207.
46. Boveris A, Chance B. The mitochondrial generation of hydrogen peroxide. General properties and effect of hyperbaric oxygen. Biochem J. 1973;134:707–16.
47. Chance B, Sies H, Boveris H. Hydroperoxide metabolism in mammalian organs. Physiol Rev. 1979;59:527–605.
48. Raha S, Robinson BH. Mitochondria, oxygen free radicals, disease and ageing. Trends Biochem Sci. 2000;25:502–8.
49. Gomez E, Buckingham DW, Brindle J, Lanzafame F, Irvine DS, Aitken RJ. Development of an image analysis system to monitor the retention of residual cytoplasm by human spermatozoa: correlation with biochemical markers of the cytoplasmic space, oxidative stress, and sperm function. J Androl. 1996;17:276–87.
50. Aitken RJ, Fisher HM, Fulton N, Gomez E, Knox W, Lewis B, Irvine S. Reactive oxygen species generation by human spermatozoa is induced by exogenous NADPH and inhibited by the flavoprotein inhibitors diphenylene iodonium and quinacrine. Mol Reprod Dev. 1997;47:468–82.
51. Aziz N, Saleh RA, Sharma RK, Lewis-Jones I, Esfandiari N, Thomas AJ Jr, Agarwal A. Novel association between sperm reactive oxygen species production, sperm morphological defects, and the sperm deformity index. Fertil Steril. 2004;81:349–54.
52. Garrido N, Meseguer M, Simon C, Pellicer A, Remohi J. Pro-oxidative and anti-oxidative imbalance in human semen and its relation with male fertility. Asian J Androl. 2004;6:59–65.
53. Zini A, Al-Hathal N. Antioxidant therapy in male infertility: fact or fiction? Asian J Androl. 2011;13:374–81.
54. Sies H. Strategies of antioxidant defense. Eur J Biochem. 1993;215:213–9.
55. Parks JE, Lynch DV. Lipid composition and thermotropic phase behavior of boar, bull, stallion, and rooster sperm membranes. Cryobiology. 1992;29:255–66.

56. Zalata AA, Christophe AB, Depuydt CE, Schoonjans F, Comhaire FH. The fatty acid composition of phospholipids of spermatozoa from infertile patients. Mol Hum Reprod. 1998;4:111–8.
57. Sanocka D, Kurpisz M. Reactive oxygen species and sperm cells. Reprod Biol Endocrinol. 2004;2:12.
58. Villegas J, Schulz M, Vallejos V, Henkel R, Miska W, Sanchez R. Indirect immunofluorescence using monoclonal antibodies for the detection of leukocytospermia: comparison with peroxidase staining. Andrologia. 2002;34:69–73.
59. Fraczek M, Kurpisz M. Inflammatory mediators exert toxic effects of oxidative stress on human spermatozoa. J Androl. 2007;28:325–33.
60. Aitken RJ, Baker MA. Oxidative stress, spermatozoa and leukocytic infiltration: relationships forged by the opposing forces of microbial invasion and the search for perfection. J Reprod Immunol. 2013;100:11–9.
61. Agarwal A, Mulgund A, Alshahrani S, Assidi M, Abuzenadah AM, Sharma R, Sabanegh E. Reactive oxygen species and sperm DNA damage in infertile men presenting with low level leukocytospermia. Reprod Biol Endocrinol. 2014;12:126.
62. Henkel R, Kierspel E, Stalf T, Mehnert C, Menkveld R, Tinneberg HR, Schill WB, Kruger TF. Effect of reactive oxygen species produced by spermatozoa and leukocytes on sperm functions in non-leukocytospermic patients. Fertil Steril. 2005;83:635–42.
63. Sikka SC, Rajasekaran M, Hellstrom WJ. Role of oxidative stress and antioxidants in male infertility. J Androl. 1995;16:464–8.
64. Sikka SC. Relative impact of oxidative stress on male reproductive function. Curr Med Chem. 2001;8:851–62.
65. Carpino A, Siciliano L, Petroni MF, De Stefano C, Aquila S, Ando S, Petroni MF. Low seminal zinc bound to high molecular weight proteins in asthenozoospermic patients: evidence of increased sperm zinc content in oligoasthenozoospermic patients. Hum Reprod. 1998;13:111–4.
66. Veaute C, Andreoli MF, Racca A, Bailat A, Scalerandi MV, Bernal C, Malan Borel I. Effects of isomeric fatty acids on reproductive parameters in mice. Am J Reprod Immunol. 2007;58:487–96.
67. Wang X, Sharma RK, Gupta A, George V, Thomas AJ, Falcone T, Agarwal A. Alterations in mitochondria membrane potential and oxidative stress in infertile men: a prospective observational study. Fertil Steril. 2003;80(Suppl 2):844–50.
68. Venkatesh S, Deecaraman M, Kumar R, Shamsi MB, Dada R. Role of reactive oxygen species in the pathogenesis of mitochondrial DNA (mtDNA) mutations in male infertility. Indian J Med Res. 2009;129:127–37.
69. Sousa AP, Amaral A, Baptista M, Tavares R, Caballero Campo P, Caballero Peregrín P, Freitas A, Paiva A, Almeida-Santos T, Ramalho-Santos J. Not all sperm are equal: functional mitochondria characterize a subpopulation of human sperm with better fertilization potential. PLoS One. 2011;6:e18112.
70. Kothari S, Thompson A, Agarwal A, du Plessis S. Free radicals: their beneficial and detrimental effects on sperm function. Indian J Exp Biol. 2010;48:425–35.
71. Luczaj W, Skrzydlewska E. DNA damage caused by lipid peroxidation products. Cell Mol Biol Lett. 2003;8:391–413.
72. Esterbauer H. Cytotoxicity and genotoxicity of lipid-oxidation products. Am J Clin Nutr. 1993;57(5 Suppl):779S–86S.
73. Marnett LJ. Lipid peroxidation-DNA damage by malondialdehyde. Mutat Res. 1999;424:83–95.
74. Gomez E, Irvine DS, Aitken RJ. Evaluation of a spectrophotometric assay for the measurement of malondialdehyde and 4-hydroxyalkenals in human spermatozoa: relationships with semen quality and sperm function. Int J Androl. 1998;21:81–94.
75. Hsieh YY, Chang CC, Lin CS. Seminal malondialdehyde concentration but not glutathione peroxidase activity is negatively correlated with seminal concentration and motility. Int J Biol Sci. 2006;2:23–9.

76. Saraniya A, Koner BC, Doureradjou P, Selvaraj N, Shivagourou V. Altered malondialdehyde, protein carbonyl and sialic acid levels in seminal plasma of microscopically abnormal semen. Andrologia. 2008;40:56–7.
77. Zabludovsky N, Eltes F, Geva E, Berkovitz E, Amit A, Barak Y, Har-Even D, Bartoov B. Relationship between human sperm lipid peroxidation, comprehensive quality parameters and IVF outcome. Andrologia. 1999;31:91–8.
78. Burcham PC. Genotoxic lipid peroxidation products: their DNA damaging properties and role in formation of endogenous DNA adducts. Mutagenesis. 1998;13:287–305.
79. De Jonge C. The clinical value of sperm nuclear DNA assessment. Hum Fertil. 2002;5:51–3.
80. Henkel R, Hajimohammad M, Stalf T, Hoogendijk C, Mehnert C, Menkveld R, Gips H, Schill W-B, Kruger TF. Influence of deoxyribonucleic acid damage on fertilization and pregnancy. Fertil Steril. 2004;81:965–72.
81. Seli E, Gardner DK, Schoolcraft WB, Moffatt O, Sakkas D. Extent of nuclear DNA damage in ejaculated spermatozoa impacts on blastocyst development after in vitro fertilization. Fertil Steril. 2004;82:378–83.
82. Shamsi MB, Kumar R, Dada R. Evaluation of nuclear DNA damage in human spermatozoa in men opting for assisted reproduction. Indian J Med Res. 2008;127:115–23.
83. Carra E, Sangiorgi D, Gattuccio F, Rinaldi AM. Male infertility and mitochondrial DNA. Biochem Biophys Res Commun. 2004;322:333–9.
84. Wai T, Ao A, Zhang X, Cyr D, Dufort D, Shoubridge EA. The role of mitochondrial DNA copy number in mammalian fertility. Biol Reprod. 2010;83:52–62.
85. Lopes S, Jurisicova A, Sun JG, Casper RF. Reactive oxygen species: potential cause for DNA fragmentation in human spermatozoa. Hum Reprod. 1998;13:896–900.
86. Bungum M, Humaidan P, Axmon A, Spano M, Bungum L, Erenpreiss J, Giwercman A. Sperm DNA integrity assessment in prediction of assisted reproduction technology outcome. Hum Reprod. 2007;22:174–9.
87. Zini A, Boman JM, Belzile E, Ciampi A. Sperm DNA damage is associated with an increased risk of pregnancy loss after IVF and ICSI: systematic review and meta-analysis. Hum Reprod. 2008;23:2663–8.
88. Duran EH, Morshedi M, Taylor S, Oehninger S. Sperm DNA quality predicts intrauterine insemination outcome: a prospective cohort study. Hum Reprod. 2002;17:3122–8.
89. Speyer BE, Pizzey AR, Ranieri M, Joshi R, Delhanty JD, Serhal P. Fall in implantation rates following ICSI with sperm with high DNA fragmentation. Hum Reprod. 2010;7:1609–18.
90. Anifandis G, Bounartzi T, Messini CI, Dafopoulos K, Markandona R, Sotiriou S, Tzavella A, Messinis IE. Sperm DNA fragmentation measured by halosperm does not impact on embryo quality and ongoing pregnancy rates in IVF/ICSI treatments. Andrologia. 2015;47:295–302.
91. St John JC, Lloyd R, El Shourbagy S. The potential risks of abnormal transmission of mtDNA through assisted reproductive technologies. Reprod BioMed Online. 2004;8:34–44.
92. Kao SH, Chao HT, Liu HW, Liao TL, Wei YH. Sperm mitochondrial DNA depletion in men with asthenospermia. Fertil Steril. 2004;82:66–73.
93. Shamsi MB, Kumar R, Bhatt A, Bamezai RN, Kumar R, Gupta NP, Das TK, Dada R. Mitochondrial DNA mutations in etiopathogenesis of male infertility. Indian J Urol. 2008;24:150–4.
94. Croteau DL, Stierum RH, Bohr VA. Mitochondrial DNA repair pathways. Mutat Res. 1999;434:137–48.
95. Pesole G, Gissi C, De Chirico A, Saccone C. Nucleotide substitution rate of mammalian mitochondrial genomes. J Mol Evol. 1999;48:427–34.
96. Lim KS, Jeyaseelan K, Whiteman M, Jenner A, Halliwell B. Oxidative damage in mitochondrial DNA is not extensive. Ann N Y Acad Sci. 2005;1042:210–20.
97. Spiropoulos J, Turnbull DM, Chinnery PF. Can mitochondrial DNA mutations cause sperm dysfunction? Mol Hum Reprod. 2002;8:719–21.
98. Treulen F, Uribe P, Boguen R, Villegas JV. Mitochondrial outer membrane permeabilization increases reactive oxygen species production and decreases mean sperm velocity but is not associated with DNA fragmentation in human sperm. Mol Hum Reprod. 2015;30:767–76.

99. Bonanno O, Romeo G, Asero P, Pezzino FM, Castiglione R, Burrello N, Sidoti G, Frajese GV, Vicari E, D'Agata R. Sperm of patients with severe asthenozoospermia show biochemical, molecular, and genomic alterations. Reproduction. 2016;Sept 20. pii: REP-16–0342. [Epub ahead of print].
100. Homan GF, Davies M, Norman R. The impact of lifestyle factors on reproductive performance in the general population and those undergoing infertility treatment: a review. Hum Reprod Update. 2007;13:209–23.
101. Kumar S, Murarka S, Mishra VV, Gautam AK. Environmental & lifestyle factors in deterioration of male reproductive health. Indian J Med Res. 2014;140. Suppl:S29–35.
102. Will MA, Swain J, Fode M, Sonksen J, Christman GM, Ohl D. The great debate: varicocele treatment and impact on fertility. Fertil Steril. 2011;95:841–52.
103. Kovacic P, Jacintho JD. Reproductive toxins: pervasive theme of oxidative stress and electron transfer. Curr Med Chem. 2001;8:863–92.
104. Lavranos G, Balla M, Tzortzopoulou A, Syriou V, Angelopoulou R. Investigating ROS sources in male infertility: a common end for numerous pathways. Reprod Toxicol. 2012;34:298–307.
105. De Iuliis GN, Newey RJ, King BV, Aitken RJ. Mobile phone radiation induces reactive oxygen species production and DNA damage in human spermatozoa in vitro. PLoS One. 2009;4(7):e6446.
106. Niki E. Action of ascorbic acid as scavenger of active and stable oxygen radicals. Am J Clin Nutr. 1991;54:1119S–24S.
107. Chow CK. Vitamin E and oxidative stress. Free Radic Biol Med. 1991;11:215–32.
108. Moskaug JO, Carlsen H, Myhrstad MC, Blomhoff R. Polyphenols and glutathione synthesis regulation. Am J Clin Nutr. 2005;81(1 Suppl):277S–83S.
109. Bharti S, Misro MM, Rai U. Quercetin supplementation restores testicular function and augments germ cell survival in the estrogenized rats. Mol Cell Endocrinol. 2014;383:10–20.
110. Chen M, Hao J, Yang Q, Li G. Effects of icariin on reproductive functions in male rats. Molecules. 2014;19:9502–14.
111. Ly C, Yockell-Lelievre J, Ferraro ZM, Arnason JT, Ferrier J, Gruslin A. The effects of dietary polyphenols on reproductive health and early development. Hum Reprod Update. 2015;21:228–48.
112. Quek R, Henry CJ. Influence of polyphenols from lingonberry, cranberry, and red grape on in vitro digestibility of rice. Int J Food Sci Nutr. 2015;66:378–82.
113. Comhaire FH, Christophe AB, Zalata AA, Dhooge WS, Mahmoud AM, Depuydt CE. The effects of combined conventional treatment, oral antioxidants and essential fatty acids on sperm biology in subfertile men. Prostaglandins Leukot Essent Fat Acids. 2000;63:159–65.
114. Comhaire FH, El Garem Y, Mahmoud A, Eertmans F, Schoonjans F. Combined conventional/antioxidant "Astaxanthin" treatment for male infertility: a double blind, randomized trial. Asian J Androl. 2005;7:257–62.
115. Vicari E, Calogero AE. Effects of treatment with carnitines in infertile patients with prostato-vesiculo-epididymitis. Hum Reprod. 2001;16:2338–42.
116. Menezo YJ, Hazout A, Panteix G, Robert F, Rollet J, Cohen-Bacrie P, Chapuis F, Clement P, Benkhalifa M. Antioxidants to reduce sperm DNA fragmentation: an unexpected adverse effect. Reprod BioMed Online. 2007;14:418–21.
117. Aitken RJ, Muscio L, Whiting S, Connaughton HS, Fraser BA, Nixon B, Smith ND, De Iuliis GN. Analysis of the effects of polyphenols on human spermatozoa reveals unexpected impacts on mitochondrial membrane potential, oxidative stress and DNA integrity; implications for assisted reproductive technology. Biochem Pharmacol. 2016;121:78–96.
118. Silberstein T, Har-Vardi I, Harlev A, Friger M, Hamou B, Barac T, Levitas E, Saphier O. Antioxidants and polyphenols: concentrations and relation to male infertility and treatment success. Oxidative Med Cell Longev. 2016;2016:9140925. https://doi.org/10.1155/2016/9140925. Epub 2016 May 12

119. Ide H, Yu J, Lu Y, China T, Kumamoto T, Koseki T, Muto S, Horie S. Testosterone augments polyphenol-induced DNA damage response in prostate cancer cell line, LNCaP. Cancer Sci. 2011;102:468–71.
120. Amararathna M, Johnston MR, Rupasinghe HP. Plant polyphenols as chemopreventive agents for lung cancer. Int J Mol Sci. 2016;Aug 19;17(8). pii: E1352. doi: https://doi.org/10.3390/ijms17081352.
121. Johns JR, Platts JA. Theoretical insight into the antioxidant properties of melatonin and derivatives. Org Biomol Chem. 2014;12:7820–7.
122. Lanzafame FM, La Vignera S, Vicari E, Calogero AE. Oxidative stress and medical antioxidant treatment in male infertility. Reprod BioMed Online. 2009;19:638–59.
123. Halliwell B. The antioxidant paradox. Lancet. 2000;355:1179–80.
124. Sen CK. Redox signalling and the emerging therapeutic potential of thiol antioxidants. Biochem Pharmacol. 1998;55:1747–58.
125. Filomeni G, Rotilio G, Ciriolo MR. Disulfide relays and phosphorylative cascades: partners in redox-mediated signaling pathways. Cell Death Differ. 2005;12:1555–63.
126. Hampton MB, Orrenius S. Redox regulation of apoptotic cell death. Biofactors. 1998;8:1–5.
127. Hampton MB, Fadeel B, Orrenius S. Redox regulation of the caspases during apoptosis. Ann N Y Acad Sci. 1998;854:328–35.
128. Wendel A. Measurement of in vivo lipid peroxidation and toxicological significance. Free Radic Biol Med. 1987;3:355–8.
129. Christians ES, Benjamin IJ. Proteostasis and REDOX state in the heart. Am J Physiol Heart Circ Physiol. 2012;302:H24–37.
130. Brewer A, Banerjee Mustafi S, Murray TV, Namakkal Soorappan R, Benjamin I. Reductive stress linked to small HSPs, G6PD and NRF2 pathways in heart disease. Antioxid Redox Signal. 2013;18:1114–27.
131. Lloret A, Fuchsberger T, Giraldo E, Vina J. Reductive stress: a new concept in Alzheimer's disease. Curr Alzheimer Res. 2016;13:206–11.
132. Ufer C, Wang CC, Borchert A, Heydeck D, Kuhn H. Redox control in mammalian embryo development. Antioxid Redox Signal. 2010;13:833–75.
133. Castagné V, Lefèvre K, Natero R, Clarke PG, Bedker DA. An optimal redox status for the survival of axotomized ganglion cells in the developing retina. Neuroscience. 1999;93:313–20.
134. Murphy MP. How mitochondria produce reactive oxygen species. Biochem J. 2009;417:1–13.
135. Henkel R. Leukocytes and oxidative stress: dilemma for sperm function and male fertility. Asian J Androl. 2011;13:43–52.
136. Chen SJ, Allam JP, Duan YG, Haidl G. Influence of reactive oxygen species on human sperm functions and fertilizing capacity including therapeutical approaches. Arch Gynecol Obstet. 2013;288:191–9.
137. Roychoudhury S, Sharma R, Sikka S, Agarwal A. Diagnostic application of total antioxidant capacity in seminal plasma to assess oxidative stress in male factor infertility. J Assist Reprod Genet. 2016;33:627–35.
138. Agarwal A, Sharma R, Roychoudhury S, Du Plessis S, Sabanegh E. MiOXSYS: a novel method of measuring oxidation reduction potential in semen and seminal plasma. Fertil Steril. 2016;106:566–73.

Chapter 12
Apoptosis in Ejaculated Spermatozoa and in the Normal and Pathological Testes: Abortive Apoptosis and Sperm Chromatin Damage

Denny Sakkas and Hasan M. El-Fakahany

12.1 Introduction

The term "programmed cell death" was originally used to describe the coordinated series of events leading to cell demise during development. The term "apoptosis" refers to a morphologically distinct form of cell death that plays a major role during the normal development and homeostasis of multicellular organisms. This mode of cell death is a tightly regulated series of energy-dependent molecular and biochemical events orchestrated by a genetic program [1].

Apoptosis is either developmentally regulated (launched in response to specific stimuli, such as deprivation of survival factors, exposure to ionizing radiation and chemotherapeutic drugs, or activation by various death factors and their ligands) or induced in response to cell injury or stress. It is now widely accepted that apoptosis serves as a prominent force in sculpting body parts, deleting unneeded structures, maintaining tissue homeostasis, and as a defense mechanism to remove unwanted and potentially dangerous cells, such as self-reactive lymphocytes, virus-infected cells and tumor cells. Apoptosis has also been recognized in the pathogenesis of many diverse human diseases including cancer, acquired immune deficiency syndrome, neurodegenerative disorders, atherosclerosis, and cardiomyopathy. Maintaining the homeostatic relationship between apoptosis and cell proliferation is important for tissue development and degeneration. Decreased apoptosis may lead to neoplasia, whereas increased apoptosis may lead to a dystrophic condition [1].

D. Sakkas (✉)
Boston IVF, Waltham, MA, USA
e-mail: dsakkas@bostonivf.com

H.M. El-Fakahany
Department of Dermatology, STDs and Andrology, Al-Minya University, Al-Minya, Egypt

A. Zini, A. Agarwal (eds.), *A Clinician's Guide to Sperm DNA and Chromatin Damage*, https://doi.org/10.1007/978-3-319-71815-6_12

Table 12.1 Key events occurring during spermatogenesis when comparing apoptosis and necrosis

	APOPTOSIS ACTION	ROLE IN SPERMATOGENESIS	NECROSIS
STIMULATED BY	Tissue remodeling Maintenance of cell pool size Genomic Damage Metabolic derangement hypoxia Imbalance in signaling pathways	Cytoplasmic remodelling Maintains spermatogonia numbers Important in Spermatocytes	Metabolic stresses Absence of nutrients Changes in pH, temperature Hypoxia, anoxia
MORPHOLOGICAL CHANGES			
Affected cells	Individual Cells	Can impact overall sperm morphology	Groups of cells
Cell volume	Decreased		Increased
Chromatin	Condensed		Fragmented
Lysosomes	Unaffected		Abnormal
Mitochondria	Initially remain normal		Morphologically Aberrant
Inflammatory response	None		
Cell fate	Apoptotic bodies consumed by neighboring cells	Sertoli Cells can act as macrophages	Lysis
MOLECULAR CHANGES			
Gene activity	Required for program	Replacement of Histones by Protamine shuts down gene activity and also changes the ability for uniform DNA fragments to occur	Not needed
Chromosomal DNA	Cleaved at Specific sites leading to uniform sized DNA fragments		Random Cleavage

The impact of apoptosis on aspects of spermatogenesis is highlighted in the Role in Spermatogenesis column

12.1.1 Cellular Characteristics of Apoptosis Versus Necrosis

The process of apoptosis is associated with well-defined morphological and biochemical changes, including a reduction in cell volume, blebbing of the cell membrane, chromatin condensation and margination, and formation of apoptotic bodies (Table 12.1). In contrast to physiological cell death or apoptosis, necrosis is a passive process that does not require energy expenditure by the cell and occurs in response to a wide variety of noxious agents. Necrosis (Table 12.1) does not occur in a developmental context, usually affects a group of contiguous cells, and is characterized by swelling of the cell and its organelles (as a result of ion pump failure) and results ultimately in membrane rupture and cell lysis [1].

A unique biochemical event in apoptosis is the activation of calcium–magnesium-dependent endonuclease activity, which specifically cleaves cellular DNA between regularly spaced nucleosomal units. Such fragments are a characteristic DNA pattern, which is considered the hallmark of apoptosis. In necrosis, as opposed to apoptosis, the genomic DNA is degraded randomly by a host of cytosolic and lysosomal endonucleases, producing a continuous spectrum of sizes [2, 3].

Another important distinguishing feature of apoptosis is the rapid clearance of dead cells by "professional" phagocytes (such as macrophages) before they can lyse, spill their noxious contents, and cause an inflammatory reaction. This clearance mechanism is efficient and rapid. In contrast, during the pathological or accidental cell death that results from overwhelming cellular injury, cells swell and lyse, releasing noxious contents that often trigger an inflammatory response. An additional change associated with cells during the early phases of apoptosis is the alteration of plasma membrane phosphatidylserine asymmetry. In normal cells, the phosphatidylserine is located on the cytoplasmic side or on the inner leaflet of the plasma membrane. Early in apoptosis, phosphatidylserine is translocated from the inner to the outer surface of the plasma membrane and, consequently, is exposed to the external cellular environment. Surface exposure of phosphatidylserine occurs along with chromatin condensation that precedes the increase in membrane permeability and constitutes one of the principal targets of phagocyte recognition [4].

A disruption in the mitochondrial transmembrane potential occurring before nuclear changes has been observed in many cells undergoing apoptosis. This permeability transition involves the opening of a large channel in the inner membrane of the mitochondrion that leads to the release from mitochondria to the cytosol of apoptosis-inducing factors (AIF). In addition, permeability transition causes the mitochondrial generation of reactive oxygen species (ROS) and rapid expression of phosphatidylserine residues in the outer plasma membrane leaflet [5].

Moreover, during apoptosis, mitochondrial inner membrane proteins, such as cytochrome c, leak out into the cytosol. At least two other cytosolic proteins, apoptotic protease activating factors Apaf-1 and Apaf-3, have been identified that collaborate with cytochrome c (also known as Apaf-2) to induce proteolytic processing and CASPASE activation and, in turn, kill cells by apoptosis [3, 6].

These key differences between classic apoptosis and necrosis are confounded by the intricate changes occurring during spermatogenesis to the nuclear and cytoplasmic architecture (Table 12.1). For example, the replacement of histones by protamines: (i) creates a shutdown of gene activity during spermiogenesis hence inhibiting any active orchestrated contribution of apoptosis to this process and (ii) alters chromatin architecture so that the classic ordered fragmentation of nucleosomes seen in most cells cannot occur in sperm. For these reasons, we believe that although aspects of apoptosis are used to control spermatogenesis, it cannot be viewed as true apoptosis; hence some of the signals we associate with apoptosis become more complicated to understand.

12.1.1.1 Programmed Cell Death Cascade

Broadly, the programmed cell death cascade can be divided into at least three to four phases: signal activation, control, execution, and structural alterations. Multiple signaling pathways lead from death-triggering extrinsic signals to a central control and execution stage [1].

Three major pathways are involved in the process of caspase activation and apoptosis in mammalian cells. The intrinsic pathway for apoptosis involves the release of cytochrome c into the cytosol where it binds to Apaf1. Once activated by the cytochrome c, Apaf-1 then binds to procaspase 9 resulting in the activation of the initiator caspase 9 and the subsequent proteolytic activation of the executioner caspases 3, 6, and 7. The active executioners are then involved in the cleavage of a set of proteins, such as poly ADP ribose polymerase (PARP), and causes morphological changes to the cell and nucleus typical of apoptosis. A major player in the process is the B-cell lymphoma/leukemia 2 (BCL2, Bcl2) family of proteins [7] which act to regulate apoptosis through the interplay of the pro- and anti-apoptotic BCL family members. Members of the Bcl2 family of proteins play a major role in governing this mitochondria-dependent apoptotic pathway, with proteins such as Bax functioning as inducers and proteins such as Bcl2 as suppressors of cell death [3].

The extrinsic pathway for apoptosis involves ligation of a death receptor (e.g., Fas) to its ligand (e.g., Fas ligand (FasL). For the Fas pathway, binding of FasL to Fas activates Fas receptors, which recruit the Fas-associated death domain, which in turn binds to the initiator caspase 8 or 10 [8].

A third subcellular compartment, the endoplasmic reticulum has also shown to be involved in apoptotic execution. Crosstalk between these pathways does occur at numerous levels. In certain cells, caspase 8 through cleavage of Bid, a pro-apoptotic Bcl2 family member, can induce cytochrome c release from mitochondria in Fas-mediated death signaling. All these pathways converge on caspase 3 and other executioner caspases and nucleases that drive the terminal events of programmed cell death [8].

In this chapter, we will discuss apoptosis in relation to how and if it occurs in mature spermatozoa and how apoptosis functions in testes of men with normal spermatogenesis and different pathologies.

12.1.2 Apoptosis in Mature Spermatozoa

Numerous studies have now reported the presence of apoptotic protein markers on sperm membranes, including Fas [9], Bcl family proteins [10], and annexin V [11, 12]. As stated above the question of whether spermatozoa undergo apoptosis has perplexed a number of researchers. This question was raised in our initial study [9] of the presence of apoptotic proteins in ejaculated sperm, and we even coined the phrase abortive apoptosis [9] to convey a distinction from normal apoptosis. In addition, the finding that human spermatozoa can exhibit high levels of DNA fragmentation [13–20] has further pointed to apoptosis being a key mechanism in the control of spermatogenesis. Unfortunately, it has not been helped by the use of various DNA assessment techniques that have been confused with the diagnosis of apoptosis. The distinct mechanisms described above and in Table 12.1, including morphological and biochemical changes, reduction in cell volume, blebbing of the cell membrane, chromatin condensation, controlled DNA fragmentation and margination, and formation of apoptotic bodies, are not always evident in such a specialized cell like a mature spermatozoon.

The discovery of the internucleosomal fragmentation of genomic DNA to regular repeating oligonucleosomal fragments generated by Ca/Mg-dependent endonuclease is accepted as one of the best characterized biochemical markers of apoptosis (programmed cell death). In 1970, Williamson [21] described that cytoplasmic DNA isolated from mouse liver cells after culture was characterized by DNA fragments with a molecular weight consisting of multiples of 135 kDa. This finding was consistent with the hypothesis that these DNA fragments were a specific degradation product of nuclear DNA. In 1978, Zakharyan and Pogosyan presented a paper revealing that glucocorticoid-induced DNA degradation in rat lymphoid tissue, thymus, and spleen occurred in a specific pattern producing fragments of DNA that were electrophoretically similar to those observed after treatment of chromatin with micrococcal nuclease, which indicated that an internucleosomal cleavage pattern of DNA degradation occurred during apoptosis [22–24].

This classic ordered DNA fragmentation seen in apoptotic cells is not evident in human spermatozoa because of the differences in chromatin packaging imparted by protamines [13] (Table 12.1). There are however some hallmarks of apoptosis. For example, it has been shown that human sperm contains the proteins necessary for the autophagy process. Proteins related to the autophagy/mitophagy process (LC3, Atg5, Atg16, Beclin 1, p62, m-TOR, AMPKα 1/2, and PINK1) were all found present in human spermatozoa. Aparicio et al. [25] showed that autophagy-related proteins and upstream regulators were present and functional in human spermatozoa.

Overall, mature spermatozoa display several features of apoptotic cells; however, they also appear to be able to escape programmed cell death once transcription is shut down. Improving our understanding of this enigma is one area of research that requires further attention.

12.1.3 Testicular Germ Cell Apoptosis in Normal Spermatogenesis

In contrast to mature ejaculated spermatozoa, the role of apoptosis is quite clear in the testes. The testes of normal men produce more than 100 million spermatozoa daily; however up to 75% of the spermatogonia die in the process of programmed cell death before reaching maturity. Spermatogenesis is therefore a dynamic process, and both germ cell proliferation and differentiation need to be tightly regulated. This output depends on proliferative activity in the basal compartment of the seminiferous epithelium where the spermatogonial cells are found and differentiate toward the lumen where meiosis and spermatogenesis occur. During regular spermatogenesis, testicular germ cells therefore degenerate by an apoptotic process. In mammals, germ cell death is conspicuous during spermatogenesis and occurs spontaneously at various phases of germ cell development such that seminiferous epithelium yields fewer spermatozoa than might be anticipated from spermatogonial proliferations [26].

In normal newborns, apoptotic cells in the seminiferous cords were identified as being mostly spermatogonia, even though Sertoli cells were also detected. The extent of testicular cell proliferation during fetal and neonatal development determines the final adult testis size and potential for sperm output in the human with subsequent stabilization during the first years of prepuberty. Even though gonadotropins start to increase during the first month of life, it is remarkable that the peak of the activation of the hypothalamic–pituitary–gonadal (HPG) axis that takes place during the second and third months of life was not associated with a lower rate of apoptosis or with increase in testis weight. Hormonal or growth factors present in the feto-placental unit might influence testicular cell growth for a few weeks after birth. The newborn period is characterized by increased cell mass in the two compartments of the testis. This cell growth seems to be mainly mediated by decreased apoptosis. The main mechanism for modulation of cell number in the prepubertal testis is the regulation of apoptotic cell death relative to cell proliferation [27].

Similarly, apoptosis is the underlying mechanism of germ cell death during normal spermatogenesis in adult humans. Human testes exhibit a spontaneous occurrence of germ cell apoptosis involving all three classes of germ cells, including spermatogonia, spermatocytes, and spermatids. The incidence of spontaneous germ cell apoptosis in humans varies with ethnic background. For example, the incidence of spermatogonial and spermatid apoptosis was higher in Chinese men than in Caucasian men. The triggering factors for spontaneous germ cell apoptosis during normal spermatogenesis are not known, and it is uncertain why there are ethnic differences in the inherent susceptibility of germ cells to programmed cell death. However, it should be noted that, in testes, as in many other tissues, the contribution of spontaneous germ cell apoptosis has been grossly underestimated due to the rapid and efficient clearance of apoptotic cells by professional phagocytes (Sertoli cells) [1]. The Sertoli cells, lining the seminiferous epithelium, supervise spermatogenesis by providing structural and nutritional support to germ cells.

The survival of conjoined spermatogonial cell progenies depends in part on maintaining structural and functional relationships with both neighboring Sertoli cells and with the basal lamina of the seminiferous tubular wall. Spermatocytes are less dependent on the basal lamina relationship and more dependent on Sertoli cell support. When apoptosis signaling is activated, the CASPASEs initiate a cell disassembling procedure, generating apoptotic bodies leading to the final demise of entire spermatogonial and spermatocyte progenies [28].

During spermatogenesis, spermatogonia and round spermatids almost certainly die by apoptosis [29]. Peak germ cell loss has been observed during the stages of mitosis of type A spermatogonia, meiotic division of spermatocytes, and during spermiogenesis [30]. Apoptotic germ cells are either sloughed into the tubule lumen or phagocytosed by Sertoli cells. Spermatozoa also demonstrate changes consistent with apoptosis. The percentage of germ cells undergoing apoptosis in normal subjects is significantly lower than that seen in men with oligoasthenoteratozoospermia, Hodgkin's disease, and testicular cancer [31].

Five possible functional roles have been proposed in the literature for the presence of apoptosis during normal spermatogenesis:

- Maintenance of an optimal germ cell/Sertoli cell ratio. It has been established that each Sertoli cell can support only a finite number of germ cells throughout their development into spermatozoa. Therefore, supraoptimal numbers of spermatogonia may undergo apoptosis to maintain an optimal ratio [32].
- Elimination of abnormal germ cells. There may be a selective process in which abnormal germ cells, especially chromosomally abnormal germ cells, are eliminated from the population by apoptosis [26].
- The formation of the blood-testis barrier by tight junctions between Sertoli cells requires the elimination of excessive germ cells. Suppression of germ cell apoptosis by means of inactivating Bax, an apoptosis-inducing gene, prevents the formation of these tight junctions [33].
- Creation of a prepubertal apoptotic wave facilitates the eventual functional development of mature spermatogenesis. A massive wave of germ cell apoptosis normally takes place as mammalian species approach puberty. This wave serves as a regulator of the ratio between germinal cells in various stages and Sertoli cells. There is evidence that preventing this wave of apoptosis by expression of apoptosis inhibitory proteins, such as BclxL or Bcl2, results in highly abnormal adult spermatogenesis accompanied by sterility [34].
- Selective removal of unneeded portions of sperm cytoplasm. Apoptosis contributes during spermatogenesis in the process of removing abnormal sperm. For example, spermatids display many of the histological and molecular fingerprints of apoptosis. Maturing spermatids form darkly staining basophilic bodies and express multiple CASPASEs within these "residual bodies." In addition, these bodies contain proteins linked to the regulation of cell death such as Fas and p53. The cytoplasm of maturing spermatids is collected and removed by residual bodies. This is probably done by neighboring Sertoli cells, which recognize and phagocytose them as they are shed. All of this has led to the idea that developing spermatozoa use the apoptotic machinery to selectively dissipate unneeded portions of their cytoplasm. In this view, apoptotic factors are somehow segregated to the cytoplasm—away from the nucleus—and this segregation permits the emerging sperm to utilize the apoptotic machinery without dying [35].

12.1.4 Regulators of Testicular Apoptosis

Apoptotic cell death seems to be strictly regulated by extrinsic and intrinsic factors and can be triggered by a wide variety of stimuli. Examples of extrinsic stimuli potentially important in testicular apoptosis are irradiation, trauma, viral infection, toxin exposure, and the withdrawal of hormonal support. It has been widely assumed that certain hormones, growth factors, or cytokines are necessary for cell survival and cell cycle progression and that their absence leads to apoptosis of their target cells. Moreover, genetic control plays a prominent role in apoptosis through molecular regulatory factors, which act as intrinsic mediators [36].

12.2 Intrinsic Regulators

12.2.1 Genes Regulating Germ Cell Apoptosis

Disruption of a number of genes results in infertility through accelerated germ cell apoptosis in mice. These findings give a first glimpse of the mechanisms involved in the regulation of germ cell apoptosis and may help in defining important genetic principles that may apply to genes important for human fertility. Male mice deficient in Bax were infertile and displayed accumulation of premeiotic germ cells with complete loss of advanced spermatids. In addition, mice misexpressing Bcl2 in spermatogonia displayed an accumulation of spermatogonia before puberty but, during adulthood, exhibited loss of germ cells in the majority of the tubules [37].

12.2.1.1 Fas-FasL

The cell surface receptor, Fas, is a transmembrane glycoprotein that belongs to the tumor necrosis factor/nerve growth factor family. The Fas-FasL interaction triggers the death of cells expressing Fas. Expression of Fas and FasL is not only detected on the Sertoli cells but also in germ cells and Leydig cells [38].

In testis, the Fas system has been implicated in maintaining immune privilege. According to this hypothesis, FasL-expressing Sertoli cells eliminate Fas-positive activated T cells, providing general protection against rejection in the testicular environment. Moreover, if Sertoli cells are injured, they increase the expression of FasL to eliminate Fas-positive germ cells, which cannot be supported adequately. These findings and the response of FasL and Fas, expressed by Sertoli cells and germ cells, respectively, to environmental conditions by initiating germ cell death implicate the Sertoli cell in the paracrine control of germ cell output during spermatogenesis by a Fas-mediated pathway [39].

Although Fas may contribute to germ cell homeostasis, it is not essential. Mice with complete lack of Fas are fertile without any overt defects in germ cell apoptosis [40]. It may still play a key role in coordinating the number of sperm in human. Recently, Wang et al. [41] investigated whether single nucleotide polymorphisms (SNP) in the promoter regions of two Fas pathway genes can influence their transcriptional activities and result in abnormal cell apoptosis, thus leading to impairment of spermatogenesis. They showed that frequencies of FASLG -844CC, CT, and TT genotypes among infertile men were significantly different from those among controls ($P = 0.024$). Men with FASLG -844TT genotype had an increased risk of idiopathic azoospermia or severe oligozoospermia compared with those with

CC and CT genotype (odds ratio 2.72, 95% confidence interval 1.25–5.93). The results suggest that FASLG -844C/T SNP may be a genetic predisposing factor of idiopathic azoospermia or severe oligozoospermia.

12.2.1.2 Bcl2 Family

Bcl2 is the first identified member of a growing family of genes that regulates cell death in either a positive or a negative fashion. The Bcl2 family of proteins, which contains both pro-apoptotic (Bax, Bak, Bclxs, Bad) and anti-apoptotic (Bcl2, Bcl-xL, Mcl, A1) proteins, constitutes a critical, intracellular checkpoint within a common cell death pathway that determines the susceptibility of a cell to apoptosis. It is generally believed that the ratio of pro-apoptotic to anti-apoptotic Bcl2 family proteins is the critical determinant of cell fate, with an excess of Bcl2 resulting in cell survival but an excess of Bax resulting in cell death. Although these molecules compete, it has not been established firmly yet whether anti-apoptotic or pro-apoptotic members are dominant in determining the key survival-promoting decision point. Paradoxically, a given family member may perform either function, depending on the cell systems used [8].

Bcl2 protects cells from apoptosis by its capacity to reduce production of ROS. Other members of the Bcl2 family, including Bax, Bak, and Bad, can block the ability of Bcl2 to inhibit apoptosis and subsequently to promote cell death. Bax, for example, functions to increase the sensitivity of cells to apoptotic stimuli [42]. Disruption of Bax, an apoptosis-inducing gene, prevented the process of apoptosis in the testis and resulted in an accumulation of immature germ cells (mainly spermatocytes) in the tubules [33].

The impact of the Bcl pathway may differ in varying male infertility pheno types as Stronati et al. [43] have shown that when exposed to environmental pollutants, certain chemicals might alter sperm DNA integrity and BclxL levels in European adult males. Finally, it is also known that normal testicular function is dependent upon hormones acting through endocrine and paracrine pathways both in vivo and in vitro. Sertoli cells provide factors and it has been shown that their removal induces germ cell apoptosis. One classic example is the proteins of the Bcl-2 family. These key apoptotic proteins in particular provide one signaling pathway which appears to be essential for male germ cell homeostasis controlled hormonally [44].

12.2.1.3 p53

The p53 family of transcription factors, including p53, p63, and p73, are critical for many physiological processes, including female fertility, but little is known about their functions in spermatogenesis. p53 suppresses oncogenic transformation by promoting apoptosis. p53 is found in high concentration in the testis and plays a significant role in temperature-induced germ cell apoptosis. This cell cycle regulator also seems to be required for radiation-induced apoptosis of spermatogonia, as evidenced by de novo induction of p53 expression in spermatogonia and degenerating giant cells in the testis following irradiation [36].

p53-induced testicular apoptosis involves:

1. Activation of redox-related genes also known as p53-induced genes
2. Generation of ROS
3. Oxidative degradation of mitochondrial components permitting the release of apoptosis-inducing factors, including AIF, cytochrome c, Apaf1, and Apaf3, into the cytosol to activate the CASPASEs [45]

In mouse models, it has also been reported that deficiency of the TAp73 isoform, but not p53 or DeltaNp73, results in male infertility because of severe impairment of spermatogenesis [46]. These results indicate that abnormal regulation of p53 family members could impact human male infertility.

12.2.1.4 CASPASEs

CASPASEs are cysteine proteases that promote apoptosis in mammals. Evidence for the role of CASPASEs in cell death is based on findings that their inhibition can prevent apoptosis, whereas their overexpression and activation cause apoptosis. CASPASEs mediate apoptosis by cleaving selected intracellular proteins, including poly (ADP-ribose)polymerase (PARP), lamin, and actin, and cause morphological changes to the cell and nuclei [47, 48].

In vitro, apoptosis of human male germ cells can be prevented by CASPASE inhibition [49]. On the other hand, CASPASE activity could not be detected in human adult germ cells obtained from men with normal spermatogenesis and cultured in vitro under conditions that led to massive DNA fragmentation, suggesting the implication of an alternative, CASPASE-independent mechanism [50, 51]. In contrast, Kim et al. [52] have shown that the expression of FasL is upregulated in the testes of patients with SCO and MA, which suggests that it may be associated with apoptotic elimination or altered maturation of Fas-expressing germ cells through the activation of caspase 3.

12.2.1.5 c-Myc

c-Myc is a nuclear phosphoprotein, encoded by a proto-oncogene, c-Myc. It plays a key role in the control of cell proliferation by acting as a transcription factor. Overexpression of the c-Myc gene in transgenic rats induces germ cell apoptosis at the meiotic prophase of primary spermatocytes. Depletion of sperm and seminiferous tubule atrophy causing sterility have been observed in the male transgenic rats [53].

12.2.1.6 Cyclic Adenosine Monophosphate Responsive Element Modulator (CREM)

The transcriptional activator, cyclic adenosine monophosphate (cAMP)-responsive element modulator (CREM), which is highly expressed in postmeiotic cells, may be responsible for the activation of haploid germ cell-specific genes involved in the structuring of the spermatozoa. CREM is responsive to the cAMP signal pathway and is required for expression of postmeiotic germ cell-specific genes. Mice that are CREM-deficient are phenotypically normal but have a maturation arrest at the early spermatid stage associated with a marked increase in apoptosis [54].

CREM is expressed in nuclei of round spermatids but not in elongated spermatids. CREM may be important for spermatid development and as a stage-specific regulator of human spermatogenesis. Absence of CREM may play a causative role in testicular failure associated with various types of human male infertility [55].

12.2.1.7 c-kit

c-kit has been identified as a germ cell apoptosis-preventing gene. Blockade or loss of the c-kit receptor results in the inability of mature spermatozoa to undergo the acrosome reaction. Decreased expression of the c-kit receptor and its ligand, stem cell factor, may alter the balance between cell proliferation/differentiation and cell death, resulting in increased apoptosis in the testes [56].

In mice, c-kit is involved in the migration of primordial germ cells and is expressed early in spermatogenesis. It is expressed in type A, intermediate, and type B spermatogonia, and its ligand is expressed in Sertoli cells [57].

12.2.2 Genetic Regulators of DNA Repair

DNA damage is one of the most potent triggers of apoptosis. DNA damage (e.g., chromosomal abnormalities, failure of DNA repair or genetic recombination, ionizing radiation, chemotherapy) leads to the elimination of damaged cells scattered within the epithelium via apoptosis [58].

PARP is a chromatin-associated enzyme with a presumptive role in DNA repair during replication and recovery from strand breaks caused by genotoxic agents. It is particularly active in the testis, where its expression varies according to the stage of germ cell differentiation. The degradation of PARP is also one of the classic indicators of apoptosis [59].

12.3 Extrinsic Regulation (Hormonal Regulation)

Withdrawal of gonadotropins or testosterone can markedly accelerate germ cell apoptosis. In rodents, spermatogenesis and apoptosis have been shown to be hormonally dependent. As in other hormonally sensitive reproductive organs, such as the prostate, endometrium, and ovary, the withdrawal of hormonal stimulation results in the selective degeneration of specific cell types [36].

Assessing the relationship between hormonal deprivation and the induction of germ cell apoptosis in adult rats following the withdrawal of testosterone demonstrated a significant rise in testicular cells with a low DNA content in combination with a decrease in haploid cells after testosterone deprivation [60].

Glucocorticoids act at the level of the pituitary and testis to suppress testosterone secretion and as a result may generate testicular apoptosis [61, 62]. Also, administration of exogenous glucocorticoid resulted in testicular germ cell apoptosis in rats [61, 62]. Severe stress may provoke the release of endogenous glucocorticoids in men, resulting in decreased serum testosterone and possibly triggering apoptosis [63].

There is an increase in DNA fragmentation in seminiferous tubules after hypophysectomy [64], further supporting the concept that androgen deprivation increases programmed cell death in the seminiferous epithelium. GnRH antagonist-induced germ cell apoptosis is most prominent among meiotic spermatocytes. Administration of a GnRH antagonist resulted in morphologic signs of germ cell degeneration in spermatocytes and spermatids [1].

Gonadotropin-dependent germ cell apoptosis seems to be age-related. A marked increase in apoptotic DNA fragmentation was seen in aging rats treated with a potent GnRH antagonist to suppress circulating levels of FSH, LH, and testosterone. Testicular apoptosis may, therefore, be enhanced in the aging male, given the decline in free testosterone levels that occur with advancing age [65].

12.3.1 Testicular Germ Cell Apoptosis During Testicular Dysfunction Conditions

12.3.1.1 Aging

With aging, both potential daily sperm production and Leydig cell function decline. As for spermatogenesis, histopathological examination reveals that there is a significant decline in the number of Sertoli cells per seminiferous tubule and the number of spermatids and primary spermatocytes per Sertoli cell [66].

Germ cell loss associated with aging occurs by apoptosis, probably because of a combination of a primary testicular defect and secondary hypothalamic pituitary dysfunction. Reproductive aging in the rat is characterized by decreased Leydig cell steroidogenesis associated with seminiferous tubule dysfunction. Accelerated germ cell apoptosis involving spermatogonia, spermatocytes, and spermatids is greater in the testes of aging rats than in the testes of younger animals [67].

We have previously explored the relationship between men's age and DNA damage repair proteins related to apoptosis in human testicular germ cells [68]. Statistically significant differences in DNA damage repair-associated proteins (PARP1, PAR, XRCC1, and APE1) and apoptosis markers (caspase 9, active caspase 3, and cleaved PARP1) were observed in testicular samples from older men. These differences were most marked in spermatocytes. It is clearly apparent that there is an age-related increase in human testicular germ cell DNA break repair and apoptosis with age.

Diminished spermatogonial proliferation was also found concomitant with low spermatogonial apoptosis. The decline of spermatogonial apoptosis might reflect a compensatory role of apoptosis in spermatogonia for the diminished proliferation that occurred during aging. Accelerated apoptosis of primary spermatocytes was detected in the testis of elderly men. It was speculated that apoptosis of primary spermatocytes might be the most relevant cause of impaired spermatogenesis in the aged testis. Sertoli cells might already have digested many apoptotic spermatids at the time of the detection of DNA fragmentation, because those cells are phagocytosed in the early phase of the apoptotic process in the rat testis [69].

The aspect of declining sperm quality in aged men has further implications with a number of studies now showing that there is a paternal age-related decline in fertility, a higher rate of certain neurodegenerative pathologies in offspring fathered by aged men, and possible transgenerational effects related to the paternal lineage [70–75].

12.3.1.2 Varicocele

Several varicocele-associated factors, including heat stress, androgen deprivation, and exposure to toxic elements, may induce pathways, which result in apoptosis [76]. Our own studies have shown that that there is an increase in human testicular germ cell DNA repair and apoptosis in infertile varicocele patients and that their profile resembles that of premature aging [77].

Apoptosis in the Ejaculate of Men with Varicocele

Varicocele induces apoptosis, which is initiated in the testicular tissue and is then expressed in the semen. Up to 10% of sperm cells in the ejaculate of men with a varicocele were apoptotic, as compared with 0.1% in fertile controls [78]. Saleh et al. [79] showed that infertile men with varicoceles had significantly greater DNA damage in spermatozoa than had normal men. Bertolla et al. [80] also evaluated DNA fragmentation in adolescents with clinically diagnosed varicoceles and determined that these boys had a higher percentage of cells with DNA fragmentation than did adolescents with no varicocele.

The expression of Fas protein was upregulated in semen samples obtained from patients with varicocele when compared to a control group, whereas little or no changes in FasL expression were detected in both groups. The relationship between varicoceles and apoptosis was explored by monitoring the concentrations of the soluble form of Fas (s-Fas) in seminal plasma, to characterize the Fas-signaling system with regard to hypospermatogenesis as a result of varicocele. By screening the seminal plasma of oligospermic men with varicoceles, oligospermic men with no varicocele, and normal controls, for the levels of s-Fas and the s-Fas ligand, s-Fas ligand was not detected in any of the cases, whereas s-Fas levels were specifically lower only in cases of varicocele [81, 82].

These reduced s-Fas levels were reversed by varicocelectomy. However, although higher temperatures may inhibit s-Fas production in patients with varicocele, the reason for this decrease in s-Fas levels remains unknown [81, 82].

In contrast, Chen et al. [83] identified no relationship between semen quality and apoptosis in fresh semen samples obtained from 30 patients with varicocele and 15 fertile controls. Although the varicocele patients had a significantly higher apoptotic index (AI) than fertile controls, semen quality and sperm motion characteristics were not significantly different between the two groups.

Seminal ROS may result in sperm DNA damage in patients with varicoceles. At the molecular level, ROS affect DNA directly and alter the levels of intracellular Ca+2, which is known to be one of the most effective means of inducing apoptosis. Morphological alterations in testicular tissues have been reported as "stress patterns" in patients with varicoceles. This stress pattern is reminiscent of, although not identical to, the cytomorphological changes in apoptosis [76].

High levels of seminal ROS and reduced total antioxidant capacity were detected in both fertile and infertile men with a clinical diagnosis of varicocele. Therefore, it was hypothesized that spermatozoal dysfunction in association with varicoceles may be related, at least in part, to elevated levels of sperm DNA damage induced by the high levels of ROS which are common in such patients [84].

Interestingly in a recent study, Agarwal and colleagues [85] identified and analyzed proteins of interest in infertile men with unilateral varicocele by searching for differentially expressed proteins (DEP) compared to fertile men. They identified 29 proteins of interest involved in spermatogenesis and other fundamental reproductive events such as sperm maturation, acquisition of sperm motility, hyperactivation, capacitation, acrosome reaction, and fertilization. Proteins expressed uniquely in the unilateral varicocele group were cysteine-rich secretory protein 2 precursor (CRISP2) and arginase-2 (ARG2). They concluded that expressions of these proteins of interest are altered and possibly functionally compromised in infertile men with unilateral varicocele.

Apoptosis in the Testicular Tissue in Men with Varicocele

Simsek et al. [86] evaluated the presence of apoptosis in testicular tissue, using the TUNEL assay. Apoptosis was very rare in the testicular tissues of the control group compared to the varicocele group. The mean percentage of apoptotic cells per total germ cell was 2% in the control and 14.7% in the varicocele group. Hassan et al. [87] showed that testicular apoptosis is increased in varicocele-associated men either fertile or infertile. They found that the occurrence of apoptotic changes comprised all types of germ cells but did not affect Sertoli cells. Mean tubular apoptotic indices of fertile or infertile men with varicocele were significantly higher than controls (mean of 4.55 and 6.29% versus 2.71; $P < 0.05$). Mean Leydig cells apoptotic indices of infertile men with varicocele were also significantly higher than those of fertile men without varicocele as well as controls.

Benoff et al. [88] also reported that there were far more apoptotic nuclei, as assessed by TUNEL labeling in testis biopsy sections, in the seminiferous tubules of men with varicocele than in normal controls and that the percentage of apoptotic nuclei was noticeably higher in some men with varicoceles.

Although Bcl2 was not expressed in the germ cells in infertile patients with varicocele, these cells expressed low levels of Bax, with no significant differences to the specimens from fertile men. In the testes from infertile patients with varicoceles stained for Caspase 3, significantly fewer germ cells were detected than those in the testes of normal controls. It was suggested that apoptosis might be suppressed as the result of reduced expression of caspase 3 and that the mitochondrial pathway involving Bcl2 and Bax may not be involved in apoptotic regulation in germ cells [89].

12.3.1.3 Failure of Spermiogenesis

The causes of complete spermiogenesis failure are not completely known. These include the withdrawal of some developmentally important ligands, such as testosterone [90] or vitamin A [91]; mutations of the receptors with which these ligands and their metabolites can act, such as the retinoic acid receptor A [92] or the retinoid X receptor B [93]; alterations of molecules involved in signal transduction pathways, downstream of receptors, such as CREM protein [54]; or mutations of components of cell DNA repair enzyme systems [94]. Such conditions are often associated with germ cell apoptosis [95].

Reduced expression of CREM was also detected in patients with predominant round spermatid maturation arrest in comparison with men with normal spermatogenesis or with mixed testicular atrophy [55], and increased apoptosis of testicular cells has been demonstrated in patients with abnormal spermatogenesis [96]. It can thus be postulated that the low efficacy of round spermatid sperm injection in cases of complete spermiogenesis failure is due to the activation of apoptosis-promoting mechanisms similar to those operating in the experimental models of spermiogenesis arrest [97].

Apoptosis is involved in the removal of arrested germ cells from the testis of patients with spermatogenic disorders. The degree of spermatocyte and spermatid DNA fragmentation in the group of patients with incomplete spermiogenesis failure appears higher as compared to men with normal sperm production [1].

In addition to DNA fragmentation, apoptotic cells also undergo a rearrangement of plasma membrane lipids, leading to translocation of phosphatidylserine from the inner side of the plasma membrane to the outer layer, probably as a result of disintegration of plasma membrane cytoskeleton that, in healthy cells, stabilizes membrane structure by connecting plasma membrane components to the cellular interior. It was suggested that this plasma membrane modification may serve to mark apoptotic cells for subsequent recognition and removal by the phagocytotic machinery [98].

Tesarik et al. [99], using double labeling with TUNEL and annexin V, concluded that patients with complete spermiogenesis failure (round spermatids is the latest stage detected histologically in the testicular biopsy in azoospermic patients) had significantly higher frequencies of primary spermatocytes and round spermatids carrying the apoptosis-specific DNA damage in comparison with patients with incomplete spermiogenesis failure (elongated spermatids is the latest stage detected histologically in the testicular biopsy in azoospermic patients). Apoptosis-related phosphatidylserine externalization occurs rarely until the advanced stages of spermiogenesis. Since externalized phosphatidylserine is expected to be involved in the recognition of apoptotic cells by phagocytes, apoptotic spermatocytes and round spermatids may not be removed easily by phagocytosis. The high frequency of DNA damage in round spermatids from patients with complete spermiogenesis failure explains the low success rates of spermatid conception in these cases. They also recommended that the evaluation of apoptosis could help to predict success rates of spermatid conception.

CASPASE activation and DNA fragmentation are frequent phenomena in germ cells from men with non-obstructive azoospermia, especially in cases of meiotic and postmeiotic maturation arrest. The incidence of CASPASE activation and DNA fragmentation is somewhat lower in samples from patients with hypospermatogenesis, in which some germ cells achieve the late elongated spermatid stage [50].

12.3.1.4 Obstructive Azoospermia

The mechanism inducing apoptosis after obstruction remains unknown. Since the obstruction of the vas deferens would also induce an increase of pressure in the seminal tract, it may cause apoptosis. Increased pressure occurring prior to testicular development might have a more adverse effect than that occurring in adulthood. The difference in apoptotic change between prepubertal and adult cases might thus relate to the susceptibility to pressure. However, these pressure increases also seem to be reduced by epididymal development [100].

Flickinger et al. [101] reported that obstruction of the seminal tract in immature rats caused epididymal granulomas, which might in turn have caused fairly high pressure to the seminal tract. In case of prepubertal obstruction when epididymis is not well developed, the increased pressure may directly affect the testis to cause increased germ cell apoptosis.

Patients with congenital absence of the vas deferens who generally have good spermatogenesis are somewhat different from acquired obstructions. They have lifelong history of seminal tract obstruction; however, the increase or the fluctuation of the pressure may not occur. This could be supported by the report that the vasectomized men showed significantly greater seminiferous tubular wall thickness than the patients who had congenital absence of the vas deferens [102].

12.4 Conclusion

The importance of understanding how apoptosis functions in both the normal and abnormal testes is paramount. It is becoming clear that subtle abnormalities in a sperm can become a significant factor in defining the progress of not only pregnancy but also of fetal and childhood development [72, 74, 103]. Improving our understanding of apoptosis and the factors that control it in the testes may allow us to better define male infertility and also treat it in a way that can limit any adverse paternal effects from spermatozoa that escape apoptosis.

References

1. Sinha HA, Swerdloff RS. Hormonal and genetic control of germ cell apoptosis in the testis. Rev Reprod. 1999;4(1):38–47.
2. Tilly JL. Apoptosis and ovarian function. Rev Reprod. 1996;1(3):162–72.
3. Reed JC. Mechanisms of apoptosis. Am J Pathol. 2000;157(5):1415–30.
4. Kroemer G, Petit P, Zamzami N, Vayssiere JL, Mignotte B. The biochemistry of programmed cell death. FASEB J. 1995;9(13):1277–87.
5. Kroemer G, Zamzami N, Susin SA. Mitochondrial control of apoptosis. Immunol Today. 1997;18(1):44–51.
6. Reed JC. Double identity for proteins of the Bcl-2 family. Nature. 1997;387(6635):773–6.
7. Youle RJ, Strasser A. The BCL-2 protein family: opposing activities that mediate cell death. Nat Rev Mol Cell Biol. 2008;9(1):47–59.
8. Sinha Hikim AP, Lue Y, Diaz-Romero M, Yen PH, Wang C, Swerdloff RS. Deciphering the pathways of germ cell apoptosis in the testis. J Steroid Biochem Mol Biol. 2003;85(2–5):175–82.
9. Sakkas D, Mariethoz E, St John JC. Abnormal sperm parameters in humans are indicative of an abortive apoptotic mechanism linked to the Fas-mediated pathway. Exp Cell Res. 1999;251(2):350–5.
10. Cayli S, Sakkas D, Vigue L, Demir R, Huszar G. Cellular maturity and apoptosis in human sperm: creatine kinase, caspase-3 and Bcl-XL levels in mature and diminished maturity sperm. Mol Hum Reprod. 2004;10(5):365–72.
11. Barroso G, Morshedi M, Oehninger S. Analysis of DNA fragmentation, plasma membrane translocation of phosphatidylserine and oxidative stress in human spermatozoa. Hum Reprod. 2000;15(6):1338–44.
12. Grunewald S, Paasch U, Glander HJ. Enrichment of non-apoptotic human spermatozoa after cryopreservation by immunomagnetic cell sorting. Cell Tissue Bank. 2001;2(3):127–33.
13. Bianchi PG, Manicardi GC, Bizzaro D, Bianchi U, Sakkas D. Effect of deoxyribonucleic acid protamination on fluorochrome staining and in situ nick-translation of murine and human mature spermatozoa. Biol Reprod. 1993;49(5):1083–8.
14. Manicardi GC, Bianchi PG, Pantano S, Azzoni P, Bizzaro D, Bianchi U, et al. Presence of endogenous nicks in DNA of ejaculated human spermatozoa and its relationship to chromomycin A3 accessibility. Biol Reprod. 1995;52(4):864–7.

15. Sakkas D, Moffatt O, Manicardi GC, Mariethoz E, Tarozzi N, Bizzaro D. Nature of DNA damage in ejaculated human spermatozoa and the possible involvement of apoptosis. Biol Reprod. 2002;66(4):1061–7.
16. Bungum M, Bungum L, Giwercman A. Sperm chromatin structure assay (SCSA): a tool in diagnosis and treatment of infertility. Asian J Androl. 2011;13(1):69–75.
17. Erenpreiss J, Spano M, Erenpreisa J, Bungum M, Giwercman A. Sperm chromatin structure and male fertility: biological and clinical aspects. Asian J Androl. 2006;8(1):11–29.
18. Evenson DP, Larson KL, Jost LK. Sperm chromatin structure assay: its clinical use for detecting sperm DNA fragmentation in male infertility and comparisons with other techniques. J Androl. 2002;23(1):25–43.
19. Lewis SE, Agbaje I, Alvarez J. Sperm DNA tests as useful adjuncts to semen analysis. Syst Biol Reprod Med. 2008;54(3):111–25.
20. Seli E, Sakkas D. Spermatozoal nuclear determinants of reproductive outcome: implications for ART. Hum Reprod Update. 2005;11(4):337–49.
21. Williamson R. Properties of rapidly labelled deoxyribonucleic acid fragments isolated from the cytoplasm of primary cultures of embryonic mouse liver cells. J Mol Biol. 1970;51(1):157–68.
22. Kerr JF, Wyllie AH, Currie AR. Apoptosis: a basic biological phenomenon with wide-ranging implications in tissue kinetics. Br J Cancer. 1972;26(4):239–57.
23. Wyllie AH, Kerr JF, Currie AR. Cell death: the significance of apoptosis. Int Rev Cytol. 1980;68(2):251–306.
24. Wyllie AH. Glucocorticoid-induced thymocyte apoptosis is associated with endogenous endonuclease activation. Nature. 1980;284(5756):555–6.
25. Aparicio IM, Espino J, Bejarano I, Gallardo-Soler A, Campo ML, Salido GM, et al. Autophagy-related proteins are functionally active in human spermatozoa and may be involved in the regulation of cell survival and motility. Sci Rep. 2016;6:33647.
26. Sharpe RM. Regulation of spermatogenesis. In: Knobil E, Neill JD, editors. The physiology of reproduction. New York: Raven Press; 2006. p. 1363–434.
27. Berensztein EB, Sciara MI, Rivarola MA, Belgorosky A. Apoptosis and proliferation of human testicular somatic and germ cells during prepuberty: high rate of testicular growth in newborns mediated by decreased apoptosis. J Clin Endocrinol Metab. 2002;87(11):5113–8.
28. Tres LL, Kierszenbaum AL. Cell death patterns of the rat spermatogonial cell progeny induced by sertoli cell geometric changes and Fas (CD95) agonist. Dev Dyn. 1999;214(4):361–71.
29. Henriksen K, Hakovirta H, Parvinen M. In-situ quantification of stage-specific apoptosis in the rat seminiferous epithelium: effects of short-term experimental cryptorchidism. Int J Androl. 1995;18:256–62.
30. de Rooij DG. Proliferation and differentiation of spermatogonial stem cells. Reproduction. 2001;121(3):347–54.
31. Gandini L, Lombardo F, Paoli D, Caponecchia L, Familiari G, Verlengia C, et al. Study of apoptotic DNA fragmentation in human spermatozoa. Hum Reprod. 2000;15(4):830–9.
32. Orth JM, Gunsalus GL, Lamperti AA. Evidence from Sertoli cell-depleted rats indicates that spermatid number in adults depends on numbers of Sertoli cells produced during perinatal development. Endocrinology. 1988;122(3):787–94.
33. Knudson CM, Tung KS, Tourtellotte WG, Brown GA, Korsmeyer SJ. Bax-deficient mice with lymphoid hyperplasia and male germ cell death. Science. 1995;270(5233):96–9.
34. Rodriguez I, Ody C, Araki K, Garcia I, Vassalli P. An early and massive wave of germinal cell apoptosis is required for the development of functional spermatogenesis. EMBO J. 1997;16(9):2262–70.
35. Blanco-Rodriguez J, Martinez-Garcia C. Apoptosis is physiologically restricted to a specialized cytoplasmic compartment in rat spermatids. Biol Reprod. 1999;61(6):1541–7.
36. Kim ED, Barqawi AZ, Seo JT, Meacham RB. Apoptosis: its importance in spermatogenic dysfunction. Urol Clin N Am. 2002;29(4):755–65. vii
37. Furuchi T, Masuko K, Nishimune Y, Obinata M, Matsui Y. Inhibition of testicular germ cell apoptosis and differentiation in mice misexpressing Bcl-2 in spermatogonia. Development. 1996;122(6):1703–9.

38. Sugihara A, Saiki S, Tsuji M, Tsujimura T, Nakata Y, Kubota A, et al. Expression of Fas and Fas ligand in the testes and testicular germ cell tumors: an immunohistochemical study. Anticancer Res. 1997;17(5B):3861–5.
39. Lee J, Richburg JH, Shipp EB, Meistrich ML, Boekelheide K. The Fas system, a regulator of testicular germ cell apoptosis, is differentially up-regulated in Sertoli cell versus germ cell injury of the testis. Endocrinology. 1999;140(2):852–8.
40. Adachi M, Suematsu S, Kondo T, Ogasawara J, Tanaka T, Yoshida N, et al. Targeted mutation in the Fas gene causes hyperplasia in peripheral lymphoid organs and liver. Nat Genet. 1995;11(3):294–300.
41. Wang W, Lu N, Xia Y, Gu A, Wu B, Liang J, et al. FAS and FASLG polymorphisms and susceptibility to idiopathic azoospermia or severe oligozoospermia. Reprod BioMed Online. 2009;18(1):141–7.
42. Kane DJ, Sarafian TA, Anton R, Hahn H, Gralla EB, Valentine JS, et al. Bcl-2 inhibition of neural death: decreased generation of reactive oxygen species. Science. 1993;262(5137):1274–7.
43. Stronati A, Manicardi GC, Cecati M, Bordicchia M, Ferrante L, Spano M, et al. Relationships between sperm DNA fragmentation, sperm apoptotic markers and serum levels of CB-153 and p,p′-DDE in European and Inuit populations. Reproduction. 2006;132(6):949–58.
44. Sofikitis N, Giotitsas N, Tsounapi P, Baltogiannis D, Giannakis D, Pardalidis N. Hormonal regulation of spermatogenesis and spermiogenesis. J Steroid Biochem Mol Biol. 2008;109(3–5):323–30.
45. Polyak K, Xia Y, Zweier JL, Kinzler KW, Vogelstein B. A model for p53-induced apoptosis. Nature. 1997;389(6648):300–5.
46. Inoue S, Tomasini R, Rufini A, Elia AJ, Agostini M, Amelio I, et al. TAp73 is required for spermatogenesis and the maintenance of male fertility. Proc Natl Acad Sci U S A. 2014;111(5):1843–8.
47. Salvesen GS, Dixit VM. Caspase activation: the induced-proximity model. Proc Natl Acad Sci U S A. 1999;96(20):10964–7.
48. Salvesen GS, Dixit VM. Caspases: intracellular signaling by proteolysis. Cell. 1997;91(4):443–6.
49. Pentikainen V, Erkkila K, Dunkel L. Fas regulates germ cell apoptosis in the human testis in vitro. Am J Phys. 1999;276(2 Pt 1):310–6.
50. Tesarik J, Ubaldi F, Rienzi L, Martinez F, Iacobelli M, Mendoza C, et al. Caspase-dependent and -independent DNA fragmentation in Sertoli and germ cells from men with primary testicular failure: relationship with histological diagnosis. Hum Reprod. 2004;19(2):254–61.
51. Tesarik J, Martinez F, Rienzi L, Iacobelli M, Ubaldi F, Mendoza C, et al. In-vitro effects of FSH and testosterone withdrawal on caspase activation and DNA fragmentation in different cell types of human seminiferous epithelium. Hum Reprod. 2002;17(7):1811–9.
52. Kim SK, Yoon YD, Park YS, Seo JT, Kim JH. Involvement of the Fas-Fas ligand system and active caspase-3 in abnormal apoptosis in human testes with maturation arrest and Sertoli cell-only syndrome. Fertil Steril. 2007;87(3):547–53.
53. Kodaira K, Takahashi R, Hirabayashi M, Suzuki T, Obinata M, Ueda M. Overexpression of c-myc induces apoptosis at the prophase of meiosis of rat primary spermatocytes. Mol Reprod Dev. 1996;45(4):403–10.
54. Nantel F, Monaco L, Foulkes NS, Masquilier D, LeMeur M, Henriksen K, et al. Spermiogenesis deficiency and germ-cell apoptosis in CREM-mutant mice. Nature. 1996;380(6570):159–62.
55. Weinbauer GF, Behr R, Bergmann M, Nieschlag E. Testicular cAMP responsive element modulator (CREM) protein is expressed in round spermatids but is absent or reduced in men with round spermatid maturation arrest. Mol Hum Reprod. 1998;4(1):9–15.
56. Sandlow JI, Feng HL, Zheng LJ, Sandra A. Migration and ultrastructural localization of the c-kit receptor protein in spermatogenic cells and spermatozoa of the mouse. J Urol. 1999;161(5):1676–80.
57. Feng HL, Sandlow JI, Sparks AE, Sandra A, Zheng LJ. Decreased expression of the c-kit receptor is associated with increased apoptosis in subfertile human testes. Fertil Steril. 1999;71(1):85–9.

58. Blanco-Rodriguez J. A matter of death and life: the significance of germ cell death during spermatogenesis. Int J Androl. 1998;21(5):236–48.
59. Tramontano F, Malanga M, Farina B, Jones R, Quesada P. Heat stress reduces poly(ADPR) polymerase expression in rat testis. Mol Hum Reprod. 2000;6(7):575–81.
60. Henriksen K, Hakovirta H, Parvinen M. Testosterone inhibits and induces apoptosis in rat seminiferous tubules in a stage-specific manner: in situ quantification in squash preparations after administration of ethane dimethane sulfonate. Endocrinology. 1995;136(8):3285–91.
61. Yazawa H, Sasagawa I, Nakada T. Apoptosis of testicular germ cells induced by exogenous glucocorticoid in rats. Hum Reprod. 2000;15(9):1917–20.
62. Yazawa H, Sasagawa I, Suzuki Y, Nakada T. Glucocorticoid hormone can suppress apoptosis of rat testicular germ cells induced by testicular ischemia. Fertil Steril. 2001;75(5):980–5.
63. Sasagawa I, Yazawa H, Suzuki Y, Nakada T. Stress and testicular germ cell apoptosis. Arch Androl. 2001;47(3):211–6.
64. Tapanainen JS, Tilly JL, Vihko KK, Hsueh AJ. Hormonal control of apoptotic cell death in the testis: gonadotropins and androgens as testicular cell survival factors. Mol Endocrinol. 1993;7(5):643–50.
65. Billig H, Furuta I, Rivier C, Tapanainen J, Parvinen M, Hsueh AJ. Apoptosis in testis germ cells: developmental changes in gonadotropin dependence and localization to selective tubule stages. Endocrinology. 1995;136(1):5–12.
66. Johnson L. Spermatogenesis and aging in the human. J Androl. 1986;7(6):331–54.
67. Wang C, Sinha Hikim AP, Lue YH, Leung A, Baravarian S, Swerdloff RS. Reproductive aging in the Brown Norway rat is characterized by accelerated germ cell apoptosis and is not altered by luteinizing hormone replacement. J Androl. 1999;20(4):509–18.
68. El-Domyati M, Al-Din A, Barakat M, El-Fakahany H, Xu J, Sakkas D. DNA repair and apoptosis in testicular germ cells of ageing fertile males: the role of the poly(ADP-ribosyl)ation pathway. Fertil Steril. 2009;91(5):2221–9.
69. Kimura M, Itoh N, Takagi S, Sasao T, Takahashi A, Masumori N, et al. Balance of apoptosis and proliferation of germ cells related to spermatogenesis in aged men. J Androl. 2003;24(2):185–91.
70. Aitken RJ, Koopman P, Lewis SE. Seeds of concern. Nature. 2004;432(7013):48–52.
71. Fisch H. Older men are having children, but the reality of a male biological clock makes this trend worrisome. Geriatrics. 2009;64(1):14–7.
72. Humm KC, Sakkas D. Role of increased male age in IVF and egg donation: is sperm DNA fragmentation responsible? Fertil Steril. 2013;99(1):30–6.
73. Jenkins TG, Carrell DT. The paternal epigenome and embryogenesis: poising mechanisms for development. Asian J Androl. 2011;13(1):76–80.
74. Zini A, Boman JM, Belzile E, Ciampi A. Sperm DNA damage is associated with an increased risk of pregnancy loss after IVF and ICSI: systematic review and meta-analysis. Hum Reprod. 2008;23(12):2663–8.
75. Northstone K, Golding J, Davey SG, Miller LL, Pembrey M. Prepubertal start of father's smoking and increased body fat in his sons: further characterisation of paternal transgenerational responses. Eur J Hum Genet. 2014;22(12):1382–6.
76. Ku JH, Shim HB, Kim SW, Paick JS. The role of apoptosis in the pathogenesis of varicocele. BJU Int. 2005;96(7):1092–6.
77. El-Domyati MM, Al-Din AB, Barakat MT, El-Fakahany HM, Honig S, Xu J, et al. The expression and distribution of deoxyribonucleic acid repair and apoptosis markers in testicular germ cells of infertile varicocele patients resembles that of old fertile men. Fertil Steril. 2010;93(3):795–801.
78. Baccetti B, Collodel G, Piomboni P. Apoptosis in human ejaculated sperm cells (notulae seminologicae 9). J Submicrosc Cytol Pathol. 1996;28(4):587–96.
79. Saleh RA, Agarwal A, Sharma RK, Said TM, Sikka SC, Thomas AJ Jr. Evaluation of nuclear DNA damage in spermatozoa from infertile men with varicocele. Fertil Steril. 2003;80(6):1431–6.

80. Bertolla RP, Cedenho AP, Hassun Filho PA, Lima SB, Ortiz V, Srougi M. Sperm nuclear DNA fragmentation in adolescents with varicocele. Fertil Steril. 2006;85(3):625–8.
81. Fujisawa M, Hiramine C, Tanaka H, Okada H, Arakawa S, Kamidono S. Decrease in apoptosis of germ cells in the testes of infertile men with varicocele. World J Urol. 1999;17(5):296–300.
82. Fujisawa M, Ishikawa T. Soluble forms of Fas and Fas ligand concentrations in the seminal plasma of infertile men with varicocele. J Urol. 2003;170(6 Pt 1):2363–5.
83. Chen CH, Lee SS, Chen DC, Chien HH, Chen IC, Chu YN, et al. Apoptosis and kinematics of ejaculated spermatozoa in patients with varicocele. J Androl. 2004;25(3):348–53.
84. Hendin BN, Kolettis PN, Sharma RK, Thomas AJ Jr, Agarwal A. Varicocele is associated with elevated spermatozoal reactive oxygen species production and diminished seminal plasma antioxidant capacity. J Urol. 1999;161(6):1831–4.
85. Agarwal A, Sharma R, Durairajanayagam D, Ayaz A, Cui Z, Willard B, et al. Major protein alterations in spermatozoa from infertile men with unilateral varicocele. Reprod Biol Endocrinol. 2015;13:8.
86. Simsek F, Turkeri L, Cevik I, Bircan K, Akdas A. Role of apoptosis in testicular tissue damage caused by varicocele. Arch Esp Urol. 1998;51(9):947–50.
87. Hassan A, El-Nashar EM, Mostafa T. Programmed cell death in varicocele-bearing testes. Andrologia. 2009;41(1):39–45.
88. Benoff SH, Millan C, Hurley IR, Napolitano B, Marmar JL. Bilateral increased apoptosis and bilateral accumulation of cadmium in infertile men with left varicocele. Hum Reprod. 2004;19(3):616–27.
89. Tanaka H, Fujisawa M, Tanaka H, Okada H, Kamidono S. Apoptosis-related proteins in the testes of infertile men with varicocele. BJU Int. 2002;89(9):905–9.
90. O'Donnell L, McLachlan RI, Wreford NG, de Kretser DM, Robertson DM. Testosterone withdrawal promotes stage-specific detachment of round spermatids from the rat seminiferous epithelium. Biol Reprod. 1996;55(4):895–901.
91. Troen G, Eskild W, Fromm SH, De Luca LM, Ong DE, Wardlaw SA, et al. Vitamin A-sensitive tissues in transgenic mice expressing high levels of human cellular retinol-binding protein type I are not altered phenotypically. J Nutr. 1999;129(9):1621–7.
92. Akmal KM, Dufour JM, Kim KH. Retinoic acid receptor alpha gene expression in the rat testis: potential role during the prophase of meiosis and in the transition from round to elongating spermatids. Biol Reprod. 1997;56(2):549–56.
93. Kastner P, Mark M, Leid M, Gansmuller A, Chin W, Grondona JM, et al. Abnormal spermatogenesis in RXR beta mutant mice. Genes Dev. 1996;10(1):80–92.
94. Roest HP, van Klaveren J, de Wit J, van Gurp CG, Koken MH, Vermey M, et al. Inactivation of the HR6B ubiquitin-conjugating DNA repair enzyme in mice causes male sterility associated with chromatin modification. Cell. 1996;86(5):799–810.
95. Sassone-Corsi P. Transcriptional checkpoints determining the fate of male germ cells. Cell. 1997;88(2):163–6.
96. Lin WW, Lamb DJ, Wheeler TM, Lipshultz LI, Kim ED. In situ end-labeling of human testicular tissue demonstrates increased apoptosis in conditions of abnormal spermatogenesis. Fertil Steril. 1997;68(6):1065–9.
97. Amer M, Soliman E, El-Sadek M, Mendoza C, Tesarik J. Is complete spermiogenesis failure a good indication for spermatid conception? Lancet. 1997;350(9071):116.
98. van Engeland M, Kuijpers HJ, Ramaekers FC, Reutelingsperger CP, Schutte B. Plasma membrane alterations and cytoskeletal changes in apoptosis. Exp Cell Res. 1997;235(2):421–30.
99. Tesarik J, Greco E, Cohen-Bacrie P, Mendoza C. Germ cell apoptosis in men with complete and incomplete spermiogenesis failure. Mol Hum Reprod. 1998;4(8):757–62.
100. Inaba Y, Fujisawa M, Okada H, Arakawa S, Kamidono S. The apoptotic changes of testicular germ cells in the obstructive azoospermia models of prepubertal and adult rats. J Urol. 1998;160(2):540–4.

101. Flickinger CJ, Herr JC, Baran ML, Howards SS. Testicular development and the formation of spermatic granulomas of the epididymis after obstruction of the vas deferens in immature rats. J Urol. 1995;154(4):1539–44.
102. Hirsch IH, Choi H. Quantitative testicular biopsy in congenital and acquired genital obstruction. J Urol. 1990;143(2):311–2.
103. Aitken RJ, De Iuliis GN, McLachlan RI. Biological and clinical significance of DNA damage in the male germ line. Int J Androl. 2009;32(1):46–56.

Chapter 13
Defective DNA Repair in Spermiogenesis

Tiphanie Cavé, Olivier Simard, Marie-Chantal Grégoire, and Guylain Boissonneault

13.1 Introduction

DNA repair offers essential protection from endogenous or exogenous genotoxic sources. Faulty repair has been shown to increase de novo mutations, translocations, or persistent DNA damage, leading to apoptosis or cancer.

DNA damage in mature sperm may have important consequences as it may be transmitted to the next generation. Andrologists are now aware of the many potential origins of DNA alterations during spermatogenesis given the multiple steps involved in this differentiation program. Over the past 10 years, our research has focused on the postmeiotic events of spermatogenesis (spermiogenesis) given the genetic threat potentially associated with the major chromatin-remodeling steps in spermatids. The eviction of most of the histones and their replacement by protamines lead to a six- to tenfold compaction of the chromatin, providing greater mechanical and chemical stability to the genome. However, the specific steps of nuclear protein exchange offer a window of opportunity for genetic alterations [1–3]. Most strikingly, we and others have established that the transition is characterized by a transient surge in DNA strand breaks including a significant proportion of double-strand breaks (DSBs) that become repaired once differentiation proceeds to the final steps [4]. Although evidence suggests that DSBs are seemingly conserved from *Drosophila* to humans [5–9], the function of the endogenous breaks remains unknown. One leading hypothesis is that DNA breaks would relieve the massive increase in free DNA supercoiling created by the nucleosome withdrawal. Regardless of whether these DSBs arise enzymatically or as a result of high torsional stress, effective and global DNA repair must be operating so as to minimize residual breaks in the mature gamete. Potential inducers of DSBs in

T. Cavé • O. Simard • M.-C. Grégoire • G. Boissonneault (✉)
Department of Biochemistry, Université de Sherbrooke, Sherbrooke, QC, Canada
e-mail: tiphanie.cave@usherbrooke.ca; olivier.simard@usherbrooke.ca; marie-chantal.gregoire@usherbrooke.ca; guylain.boissonneault@usherbrooke.ca

A. Zini, A. Agarwal (eds.), *A Clinician's Guide to Sperm DNA and Chromatin Damage*, https://doi.org/10.1007/978-3-319-71815-6_13

spermatids, haploid DNA repair mechanisms, and genetic consequences of faulty repair are briefly discussed in this chapter. This may prove to represent a major component of the well-known male bias for transmission of de novo mutations [10].

13.2 Topoisomerases and Elimination of Torsional Stress

As outlined above, torsional stress from the accumulation of negative supercoiling must be eliminated during chromatin remodeling, allowing for efficient DNA compaction by protamines [11]. Evidence of transient DSBs in spermatids were obtained by pulsed-field gel electrophoresis (PFGE), comet assays, TUNEL determination of DSBs, and in situ DNA end labeling ([4] and Grégoire et al. personal communication). It is worth noting that because mechanical DNA breaks do not generate 3′OH DNA ends (Grégoire et al. personal communication), the surge of 3′OH end labeling, specifically detected by the latter two techniques, provides strong evidence that enzymes must also be involved in the process. Studies from our group showed that topoisomerase IIβ is present in elongating spermatids in mice during chromatin remodeling [12, 13], and the use of type II topoisomerase inhibitors led to a significant decrease in DSB [4]. In addition, topoisomerase I, topoisomerase IIα[alpha], topoisomerase IIIα, and Sp011 have also been detected by immunofluorescence, whereas type I and type II topoisomerase activities have been detected in vitro by plasmid relaxation using nuclear extract from sonication-resistant spermatids (SRS) (unpublished data). Type II topoisomerase proceeds through the induction of a DSB to decrease the linking number in steps of two, thereby reducing supercoiling [13]. Evidence of impaired topoisomerase ligation activity in elongating spermatids was provided by immunofluorescence detection of TDP1 [13] and TDP2 in nuclei (unpublished data). Both proteins are found at stalled topoisomerase in order to remove the covalently bound protein on DNA and recruit the DSBs DNA repair machinery. The deposition of transition proteins and protamines may in part be responsible to hinder the topoisomerase catalytic cycle and to trigger TDP1 and TDP2 signaling. However, confirmation of the role of topoisomerase in the transient DNA DSBs must await deletion of topoisomerase in spermatids by conditional knockout in mice.

13.3 Nonhomologous End Joining

The sharp but transient increase in endogenous DSBs implies that an efficient DNA repair mechanism is operating in spermatids in order to prevent accumulation of unrepaired DNA DSBs in the mature sperm. A rough estimate based on preliminary data from PFGE analysis suggests an induction of around 45,000 transient DSBs in elongating spermatids compared to round spermatids (Grégoire et al. unpublished).

This may be considered important relative to somatic cells [14] although an undetermined fraction of the detected surge in DSBs may arise from intermediates of the topoisomerase II catalytic cycle released by proteolytic treatment during DNA extraction. A significant number of DSBs, however, are still observed following extensive treatment by an efficient topoisomerase II inhibitor (HU-331) in short-term culture of seminiferous tubules (unpublished data) and leading to the complete loss of 3′OH labeling. The persistent DSBs suggest that they must arise from mechanical breaks. Persistence of DSBs in mature sperm is likely to impact fertility if the level exceeds a given threshold or impacts the genetic program of the developing embryo [15]. Spermatids are haploid cells and so cannot rely on a sister chromatids for reliable templated DNA repair [10]. Under haploid conditions, only nonhomologous end joining (NHEJ) is operating to repair DSB as homologous recombination (HR) is unlikely to proceed. However, NHEJ is error-prone and has been shown to create small insertions or deletions at break sites [16, 17]. Mutational insertions and deletions can be especially deleterious, if, for instance, they create a frame shift in coding sequences, hence generating alternative proteins.

Evidence for NHEJ as a prominent DNA repair mechanism in spermatids includes detection of key proteins involved in this pathway, using immunoblots or immunofluorescence [5], as well as in vitro inhibition of NHEJ in SRS nuclear extracts using ligase IV inhibitors such as SCR7 (unpublished data). Pioneer in vitro studies using testicular extracts also demonstrated NHEJ activity from cloning and sequencing of the repair template [18].

NHEJ deserves some attention to better appreciate how functional alteration of key components of the repair pathways may impact DNA integrity in spermatids. Two general NHEJ repair mechanisms are now emerging: the canonical NHEJ (C-NHEJ, which is also called classical NHEJ) and the alternative end joining (Alt-EJ, also referred to as Alt-NHEJ or A-NHEJ). The C-NHEJ is the primary repair pathway, while Alt-EJ is considered a backup pathway [14, 17, 19–23] (Fig. 13.1). During C-NHEJ repair, DNA overhangs are simply ligated together avoiding search for complementary sequence, thus resulting in small insertions and deletions, generally of one or few nucleotides [17] (Fig. 13.1a). However, in some instances, the resulting modifications may involve structural changes such as chromosomal translocation or chromosomal aberrations [24, 25]. Although the Alt-EJ detailed mechanism is still unclear, a consensus is shown in Fig. 13.1b. Larger insertions or deletions are expected from this mechanism [17, 22, 26].

As recently shown, both small or larger paternally transmitted insertions and deletions may be implicated in diseases with a genetic component such as autism spectrum disorder (ASD) [27]. Because DSB repair in spermatids must depend solely on NHEJ-related pathways and given that NHEJ activity declines with age [28–30], the impact of such a functional decline is expected to be worse in spermatids than for somatic cells. We suspect that it may be in part responsible for the observed age dependence of male-transmitted de novo mutations and the higher propensity for transmission of neurological disorders [31–35].

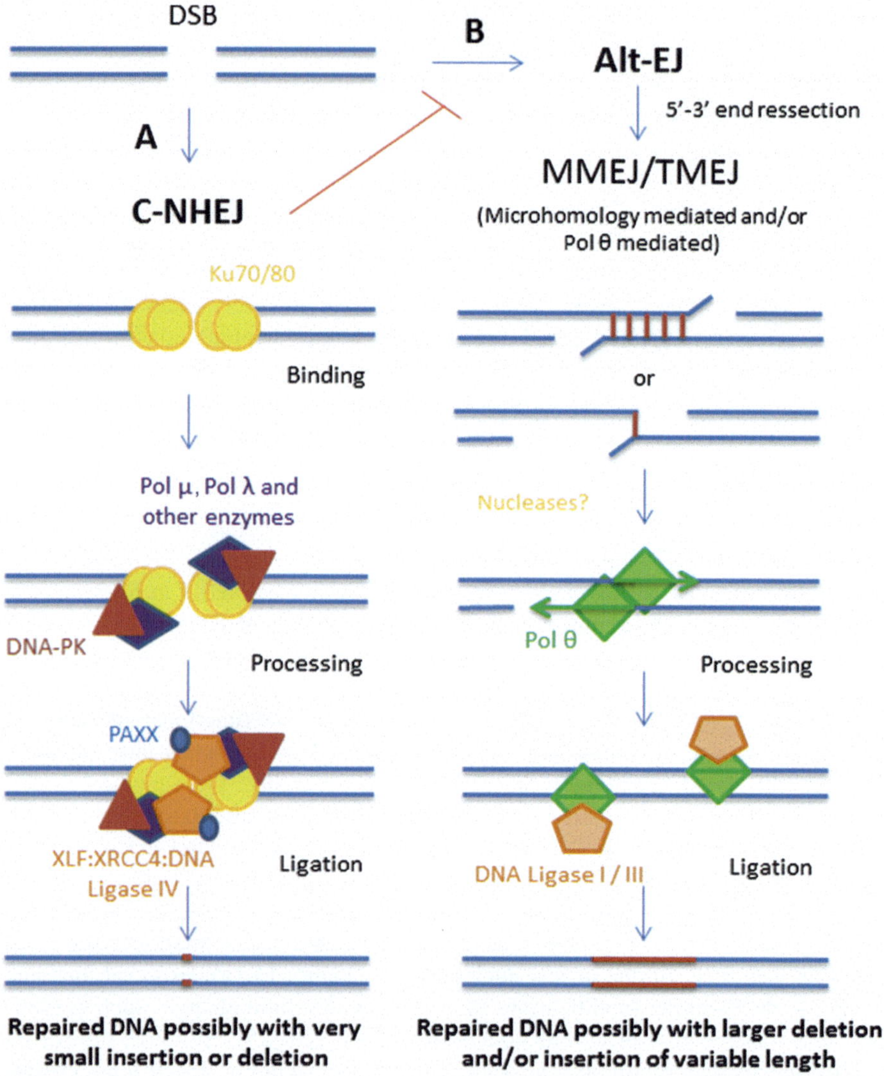

Fig. 13.1 NHEJ repair pathways. (**a**) During C-NHEJ repair, the Ku70–80 heterodimer detects and binds the broken ends of the DSB. DNA-dependent protein kinase catalytic subunit (DNA-PKcs) is recruited and specifically binds the Ku70–80 heterodimer. In the case of minor DNA damage, the ligation is then possible with minimal processing involving the core complex XLF:XRCC4:DNA ligase IV and PAXX. However, in the case of more severe damages, polymerases (Pol μ and Pol λ) and additional enzymes are required at the break site in order to process the DNA ends. (**b**) The Alt-EJ pathway is an alternative to C-NHEJ and is available when C-NHEJ cannot operate. Two Alt-EJ sub-pathways become available depending on the DNA sequence to be processed. One is mediated by Pol θ (TMEJ), and one can be directed by microhomology (MMEJ). Both DNA ligases I and III are required in the Alt-EJ pathway. Although C-NHEJ repair is more efficient than Alt-EJ, both are error-prone and may lead to insertions or deletions (See references [14, 17, 19–23] for further details)

13.4 Defective Mismatch Repair and Trinucleotide Repeat Instability

The mismatch repair (MMR) is used for the repair of base-base mismatches, insertions, and deletions that occur during DNA replication and recombination. MMR is also involved in suppression of homologous recombination and also has a role in DNA damage response in eukaryotic cells [36]. Inactivation of the MMR leads to an increase in spontaneous mutations and predisposes to the development of tumors and cancers [36, 37]. MMR is therefore generally recognized as a repair mechanism promoting genome stability.

Trinucleotide repeats (TNRs) such as CAG, CTG, or CGG are involved in several neurological disorders, such as Huntington disease, spinocerebellar ataxias, and more [38]. In these diseases, symptoms are observed once a critical number of repeats are reached in the corresponding gene. In the case where TNRs are localized within coding regions such as Huntington disease, an inverse correlation between the number of repeats and the age at onset of symptoms has been observed. TNRs are dynamic and have been shown to either extend or contract, mostly when a hairpin structure is adopted by the repeat during various cellular processes [38]. In such a situation, MMR recognizes the hairpin but displays defective repair activity, which leads to TNR length variation [39].

TNR extensions and contractions also occur during gametogenesis, which directly affects the number of repeats transmitted to the offspring. When an extension occurs, this results in the anticipation of the disease whereby an increased number of repeats is being transmitted to the offspring, resulting in an earlier age at onset of the symptoms. Using a mouse model for Huntington's disease, we showed that CAG repeats can be extended toward the end of the chromatin-remodeling steps in spermatid [40]. This extension was previously shown to be dependent on MMR activity [41]. Hence, the genetic instability in spermatids is also reflected by TNR extension within neurodevelopmental genes. The potential for spermiogenesis to create both de novo insertion/deletion and TNR variations that impact neurodevelopment emphasizes the need to further study this chromatin transition when searching the etiology of these genetic diseases.

13.5 Other Sources of DNA Damage in Spermatids

We briefly outline other important sources of DNA damage in spermatids for which the repair mechanisms have not yet been characterized.

13.6 Reactive Oxygen Species

Reactive oxygen species (ROS) can be considered an additional endogenous [42] or exogenous [43] factor capable of inducing DNA damages in the form of strand breakage in spermatids. However, it is yet unclear whether the observed surge in DSBs is associated with a timely increase in ROS. A proper balance of ROS is apparently needed in order to promote proper sperm maturation [44], but an excess in oxidative stress may induce cellular damage [45–47]. Hence, not only the integrity of DNA but also the sperm chromatin state can be impacted by ROS. Interestingly, studies have shown a negative correlation between the efficiency of sperm chromatin protamination and the degree of oxidative DNA damage [48]. Base excision repair (BER) and nucleotide excision repair (NER) have a leading role in repair of various DNA lesions [49–51], including oxidative damages [52]. Whether BER or NER is operating in spermatids has yet to be determined.

13.6.1 Chemotherapy

Chemotherapy or radiation therapy induces a wide range of DNA damage in the male reproductive system [53–57] and often leads to infertility because replicating cells at premeiotic stages are exquisitely sensitive to genotoxic drugs [55–57]. The chromatin-remodeling steps in spermatids have also been shown to be sensitive to chemotherapy [58, 59]. Although the underlying mechanisms are yet to be identified, one can speculate that the transient DSB and active repair process are especially vulnerable to such genotoxic insults. Further discussion regarding the impact of chemotherapy on spermatogenesis can be found in Chap. 15.

13.7 Conclusions and Future Direction

Further studies may lead to the identification of genetic conditions that can alter DNA repair processes during spermiogenesis. Mutations leading to defective DNA repair in spermatids have so far not been identified, but the impact of genetic alteration in the DNA damage response has been confirmed at other stages of spermatogenesis. For instance, deletion of Ku70 gene prevents the synthesis of the associated protein (which is central to C-NHEJ) and established that this protein is critical for DNA repair during meiosis [60]. BRD7 gene knockout mice displayed alteration of p53 activity which is a key factor for proper regulation of several testis genes involved in DNA repair [61]. Although p53 is known to participate in most DNA repair processes including HR, BER, NER, and MMR, it has been also recently linked to NHEJ [62]. Given the extent of DNA DSBs in elongating spermatids, any impairment in DNA repair could trigger programmed cell death. Apoptosis of germ cells is a normal process allowing for the elimination of cells unable to process a threshold level of DNA damage. "Abortive apoptosis" has therefore been proposed as a source of persistent DNA damage in spermatids and spermatozoa since in this case normal elimination of cells with a high level of DNA damage does not proceed normally [63, 64].

In summary, spermiogenesis may prove to represent a very vulnerable chromatin structure transition and a significant source of genetic instability potentially leading to de novo genetic disorders in the offspring.

References

1. Rathke C, Baarends WM, Awe S, Renkawitz-Pohl R. Chromatin dynamics during spermiogenesis. Biochim Biophys Acta BBA Gene Regul Mech. 2014;1839(3):155–68.
2. Hermo L, Pelletier R-M, Cyr DG, Smith CE. Surfing the wave, cycle, life history, and genes/proteins expressed by testicular germ cells. Part 1: background to spermatogenesis, spermatogonia, and spermatocytes. Pelletier R-M, editor. Microsc Res Tech. 2010;73(4):241–78.
3. Pradeepa MM, Rao MRS. Chromatin remodeling during mammalian spermatogenesis: role of testis specific histone variants and transition proteins. Soc Reprod Fertil Suppl. 2007;63:1–10.
4. Laberge R-M, Boissonneault G. On the nature and origin of DNA strand breaks in elongating spermatids. Biol Reprod. 2005;73(2):289–96.
5. Cabrero J, Palomino-Morales RJ, Camacho JPM. The DNA-repair Ku70 protein is located in the nucleus and tail of elongating spermatids in grasshoppers. Chromosom Res. 2007;15(8):1093–100.
6. Rathke C, Baarends WM, Jayaramaiah-Raja S, Bartkuhn M, Renkawitz R, Renkawitz-Pohl R. Transition from a nucleosome-based to a protamine-based chromatin configuration during spermiogenesis in Drosophila. J Cell Sci. 2007;120(9):1689–700.
7. Roca J, Mezquita C. DNA topoisomerase II activity in nonreplicating, transcriptionally inactive, chicken late spermatids. EMBO J. 1989;8(6):1855–60.
8. Morse-Gaudio M, Risley MS. Topoisomerase II expression and VM-26 induction of DNA breaks during spermatogenesis in Xenopus laevis. J Cell Sci. 1994;107(Pt 10):2887–98.
9. Marcon L, Transient DNA. Strand breaks during mouse and human spermiogenesis: new insights in stage specificity and link to chromatin remodeling. Biol Reprod. 2003;70(4):910–8.
10. Gregoire M-C, Massonneau J, Simard O, Gouraud A, Brazeau M-A, Arguin M, et al. Male-driven de novo mutations in haploid germ cells. Mol Hum Reprod. 2013;19(8):495–9.
11. Gouraud A, Brazeau M-A, Grégoire M-C, Simard O, Massonneau J, Arguin M, et al. "Breaking news" from spermatids. Basic Clin Androl. 2013;23(1):11.
12. Leduc F, Nkoma GB, Boissonneault G. Spermiogenesis and DNA repair: a possible etiology of human infertility and genetic disorders. Syst Biol Reprod Med. 2008;54(1):3–10.
13. Leduc F, Maquennehan V, Nkoma GB, Boissonneault G. DNA damage response during chromatin remodeling in elongating spermatids of mice. Biol Reprod. 2008;78(2):324–32.
14. Lieber MR. The mechanism of double-strand DNA break repair by the nonhomologous DNA end-joining pathway. Annu Rev Biochem. 2010;79(1):181–211.
15. Evenson DP, Larson KL, Jost LK. Sperm chromatin structure assay: its clinical use for detecting sperm DNA fragmentation in male infertility and comparisons with other techniques. J Androl. 2002;23(1):25–43.
16. Budman J, Chu G. Processing of DNA for nonhomologous end-joining by cell-free extract. EMBO J. 2005;24(4):849–60.
17. Rodgers K, McVey M. Error-prone repair of DNA double-strand breaks: ERROR-PRONE REPAIR OF DNA DSBs. J Cell Physiol. 2016;231(1):15–24.

18. Raghavan SC, Raman MJ. Nonhomologous end joining of complementary and noncomplementary DNA termini in mouse testicular extracts. DNA Repair. 2004;3(10):1297–310.
19. Lieber MR, Ma Y, Pannicke U, Schwarz K. Mechanism and regulation of human nonhomologous DNA end-joining. Nat Rev Mol Cell Biol. 2003;4(9):712–20.
20. Black S, Kashkina E, Kent T, Pomerantz R. DNA polymerase θ: a unique multifunctional end-joining machine. Genes. 2016;7(9):67.
21. Yang K, Guo R, Xu D. Non-homologous end joining: advances and frontiers. Acta Biochim Biophys Sin. 2016;48(7):632–40.
22. Iliakis G, Murmann T, Soni A. Alternative end-joining repair pathways are the ultimate backup for abrogated classical non-homologous end-joining and homologous recombination repair: implications for the formation of chromosome translocations. Mutat Res Toxicol Environ Mutagen. 2015;793:166–75.
23. Liang L, Deng L, Nguyen SC, Zhao X, Maulion CD, Shao C, et al. Human DNA ligases I and III, but not ligase IV, are required for microhomology-mediated end joining of DNA double-strand breaks. Nucleic Acids Res. 2008;36(10):3297–310.
24. Agarwal S, Tafel AA, Kanaar R. DNA double-strand break repair and chromosome translocations. DNA Repair. 2006;5(9–10):1075–81.
25. Byler M, Lebel R. Risks of reproducing with a genetic disorder. Semin Reprod Med. 2013;31(4):258–66.
26. Wyatt DW, Feng W, Conlin MP, Yousefzadeh MJ, Roberts SA, Mieczkowski P, et al. Essential roles for polymerase θ-mediated end joining in the repair of chromosome breaks. Mol Cell. 2016;63(4):662–73.
27. Dong S, Walker MF, Carriero NJ, DiCola M, Willsey AJ, Ye AY, et al. De novo insertions and deletions of predominantly paternal origin are associated with autism Spectrum disorder. Cell Rep. 2014;9(1):16–23.
28. Seluanov A, Mittelman D, Pereira-Smith OM, Wilson JH, Gorbunova V. DNA end joining becomes less efficient and more error-prone during cellular senescence. Proc Natl Acad Sci. 2004;101(20):7624–9.
29. Vyjayanti VN, Rao KS. DNA double strand break repair in brain: reduced NHEJ activity in aging rat neurons. Neurosci Lett. 2006;393(1):18–22.
30. Vaidya A, Mao Z, Tian X, Spencer B, Seluanov A, Gorbunova V. Knock-in reporter mice demonstrate that DNA repair by non-homologous end joining declines with age. Hasty P, editor. PLoS Genet. 2014;10(7):e1004511.
31. Kong A, Frigge ML, Masson G, Besenbacher S, Sulem P, Magnusson G, et al. Rate of de novo mutations and the importance of father's age to disease risk. Nature. 2012;488(7412):471–5.
32. Whelan EC, Nwala AC, Osgood C, Olariu S. Selective mutation accumulation: a computational model of the paternal age effect. Bioinformatics. 2016;32:3790–3797.
33. Reichenberg A, Gross R, Weiser M, Bresnahan M, Silverman J, Harlap S, et al. Advancing paternal age and autism. Arch Gen Psychiatry. 2006;63(9):1026.
34. Sipos A. Paternal age and schizophrenia: a population based cohort study. BMJ. 2004;329(7474):1070. 0
35. Vestergaard M, Mork A, Madsen KM, Olsen J. Paternal age and epilepsy in the offspring. Eur J Epidemiol. 2005;20(12):1003–5.
36. Li G-M. Mechanisms and functions of DNA mismatch repair. Cell Res. 2008;18(1):85–98.
37. Modrich P. Mechanisms in eukaryotic mismatch repair. J Biol Chem. 2006;281(41):30305–9.
38. Pearson CE, Edamura KN, Cleary JD. Repeat instability: mechanisms of dynamic mutations. Nat Rev Genet. 2005;6(10):729–42.
39. Owen BAL, Yang Z, Lai M, Gajek M, Badger JD, Hayes JJ, et al. (CAG)n-hairpin DNA binds to Msh2–Msh3 and changes properties of mismatch recognition. Nat Struct Mol Biol. 2005;12(8):663–70.
40. Simard O, Grégoire M-C, Arguin M, Brazeau M-A, Leduc F, Marois I, et al. Instability of trinucleotidic repeats during chromatin remodeling in spermatids. Hum Mutat. 2014;35(11):1280–1284.
41. Kovtun IV, McMurray CT. Trinucleotide expansion in haploid germ cells by gap repair. Nat Genet. 2001;27(4):407–11.

42. Twigg J, Fulton N, Gomez E, Irvine DS, Aitken RJ. Analysis of the impact of intracellular reactive oxygen species generation on the structural and functional integrity of human spermatozoa: lipid peroxidation, DNA fragmentation and effectiveness of antioxidants. Hum Reprod. 1998;13(6):1429–36.
43. Harlev A, Agarwal A, Gunes SO, Shetty A, du Plessis SS. Smoking and male infertility: an evidence-based review. World J Mens Health. 2015;33(3):143.
44. Guerriero G, Trocchia S, Abdel-Gawad FK, Ciarcia G. Roles of reactive oxygen species in the spermatogenesis regulation. Front Endocrinol. 2014. 5:56. [Internet]. [cited 2016 Sep 29]. Available from: http://journal.frontiersin.org/article/10.3389/fend0.2014.00056/abstract.
45. Jena NR. DNA damage by reactive species: mechanisms, mutation and repair. J Biosci. 2012;37(3):503–17.
46. Li Z, Yang J, Huang H. Oxidative stress induces H2AX phosphorylation in human spermatozoa. FEBS Lett. 2006;580(26):6161–8.
47. Agarwal A, Said TM. Oxidative stress, DNA damage and apoptosis in male infertility: a clinical approach. BJU Int. 2005;95(4):503–7.
48. De Iuliis GN, Thomson LK, Mitchell LA, Finnie JM, Koppers AJ, Hedges A, et al. DNA damage in human spermatozoa is highly correlated with the efficiency of chromatin remodeling and the formation of 8-hydroxy-2′-deoxyguanosine, a marker of oxidative stress. Biol Reprod. 2009;81(3):517–24.
49. Gillet LCJ, Schärer OD. Molecular mechanisms of mammalian global genome nucleotide excision repair. Chem Rev. 2006;106(2):253–76.
50. Krokan HE, Bjoras M. Base excision repair. Cold Spring Harb Perspect Biol. 2013;5(4):a012583.
51. Robertson AB, Klungland A, Rognes T, Leiros I. DNA repair in mammalian cells: base excision repair: the long and short of it. Cell Mol Life Sci. 2009;66(6):981–93.
52. Melis JPM, van Steeg H, Luijten M. Oxidative DNA damage and nucleotide excision repair. Antioxid Redox Signal. 2013;18(18):2409–19.
53. Howell SJ. Spermatogenesis after cancer treatment: damage and recovery. J Natl Cancer Inst Monogr. 2005;2005(34):12–7.
54. van Loon AAWM, Sonneveld E, Hoogerbrugge J, van der Schans GP, Grootegoed JA, Lohman PHM, et al. Induction and repair of DNA single-strand breaks and DNA base damage at different cellular stages of spermatogenesis of the hamster upon in vitro exposure to ionizing radiation. Mutat Res Repair. 1993;294(2):139–48.
55. Muslimović A, Nyström S, Gao Y, Hammarsten O. Numerical analysis of etoposide induced DNA breaks. Sullivan BA, editor. PLoS One. 2009;4(6):e5859.
56. Cheung-Ong K, Giaever G, Nislow C. DNA-damaging agents in cancer chemotherapy: serendipity and chemical biology. Chem Biol. 2013;20(5):648–59.
57. Klapacz J, Pottenger LH, Engelward BP, Heinen CD, Johnson GE, Clewell RA, et al. Contributions of DNA repair and damage response pathways to the non-linear genotoxic responses of alkylating agents. Mutat Res Mutat Res. 2016;767:77–91.
58. Codrington AM, Hales BF, Robaire B. Spermiogenic germ cell phase-specific DNA damage following cyclophosphamide exposure. J Androl. 2004;25(3):354–62.
59. Aguilar-Mahecha A. Chronic cyclophosphamide treatment alters the expression of stress response genes in rat male germ cells. Biol Reprod. 2002;66(4):1024–32.
60. Ahmed EA, Sfeir A, Takai H, Scherthan H. Ku70 and non-homologous end joining protect testicular cells from DNA damage. J Cell Sci. 2013;126(14):3095–104.
61. Wang H, Zhao R, Guo C, Jiang S, Yang J, Xu Y, et al. Knockout of BRD7 results in impaired spermatogenesis and male infertility. Sci Rep. 2016;6:21776.
62. Gatz SA, Wiesmüller L. p53 in recombination and repair. Cell Death Differ. 2006;13(6):1003–16.
63. Sakkas D, Mariethoz E, Manicardi G, Bizzaro D, Bianchi PG, Bianchi U. Origin of DNA damage in ejaculated human spermatozoa. Rev Reprod. 1999;4(1):31–7.
64. Sakkas D, Seli E, Bizzaro D, Tarozzi N, Manicardi GC. Abnormal spermatozoa in the ejaculate: abortive apoptosis and faulty nuclear remodelling during spermatogenesis. Reprod BioMed Online. 2003;7(4):428–32.

Chapter 14
Defective Spermatogenesis and Sperm DNA Damage

Rakesh Sharma and Ashok Agarwal

14.1 Neurological Pathways

Spermatogenesis is initiated through hormonal controls in the hypothalamus (Fig. 14.1). The hypothalamus secretes gonadotropin-releasing hormone (GnRH), triggering the release of luteinizing hormone (LH) and follicle-stimulating hormone (FSH) from the adenohypophysis or anterior lobe of the pituitary. LH assists with steroidogenesis by stimulating the Leydig cells which are located in the testicular interstitium, while FSH stimulates the Sertoli cells to aid with the proliferative and developmental stages of spermatogenesis. In addition to LH and FSH, the adenohypophysis also secretes adrenocorticotropic hormone, prolactin, growth hormone, and thyroid-stimulating hormone—all of these hormones play an important role throughout spermatogenesis. The primary hormones are responsible for initiating spermatogenesis inside the testes, which is the central organ of the reproductive axis. GnRH stimulations are regulated through three types of rhythmicity: (1) seasonal, peak GnRH production occurring during the spring; (2) circadian, daily regulator with the highest output during the early morning; and (3) pulsatile, highest output occurring on average every 90–120 min.

R. Sharma
American Center for Reproductive Medicine, Cleveland Clinic, Cleveland, OH, USA

A. Agarwal (✉)
American Center for Reproductive Medicine, Glickman Urological & Kidney Institute, Cleveland Clinic, Cleveland, OH, USA
e-mail: Agarwaa@ccf.org

A. Zini, A. Agarwal (eds.), *A Clinician's Guide to Sperm DNA and Chromatin Damage*, https://doi.org/10.1007/978-3-319-71815-6_14

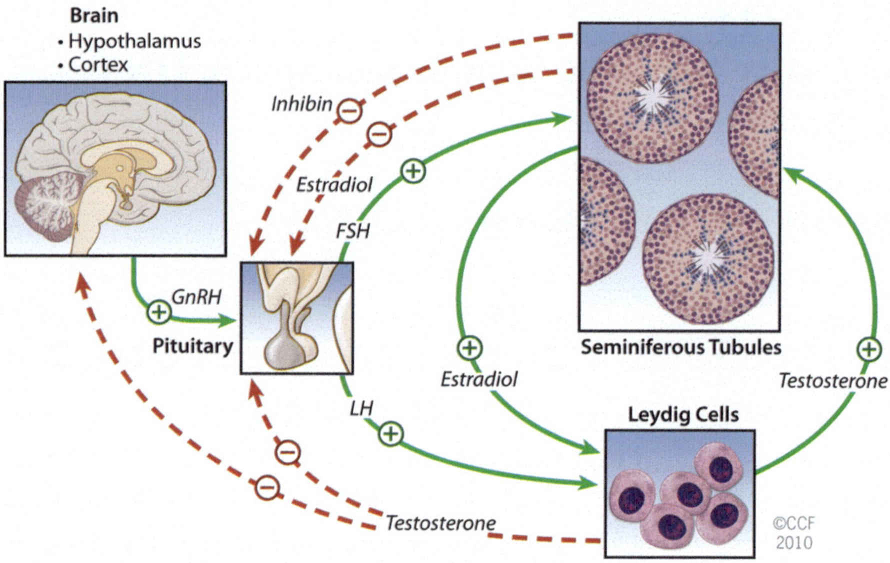

Fig. 14.1 Schematic representation of the hypothalamic pituitary axis and the hormonal feedback system (Reprinted with permission, Cleveland Clinic Center for Medical Art & Photography © 2010. All Rights Reserved)

14.1.1 Steroid Hormone Interaction and Neurological Axis

Androgens are an integral part of spermatogenesis. Dihydrotestosterone is formed by metabolizing testosterone with 5α-reductase. Both testosterone and dihydrotestosterone regulate various genes and the various developmental stages during gestation [1]. Estrogen, on the other hand, as commonly regarded "female" hormone, is also necessary for proper spermatogenesis [2, 3]. During Sertoli cell differentiation, estrogen levels drop to a minimum, and during the pre-pubescent years, estrogen shuts off androgen production by the Leydig cells. When puberty begins, estrogen levels fall to enable androgen production by Leydig cells and initiate spermatogenesis. Thyroid hormones play a key role in spermatogenesis involving Sertoli cell proliferation and development. All of these hormones interact with one another in the testicular axis in both the interstitial region and the Sertoli cells to enable spermatogenesis. In addition to hormones, growth factors secreted directly by the Sertoli cells also play an important role in regulating spermatogenesis. Specifically, transforming growth factor (alpha and beta), insulin-like growth factor, and β-fibroblast growth factor facilitates germ cell migration during embryonic development, proliferation, and regulation of meiosis and cellular differentiation.

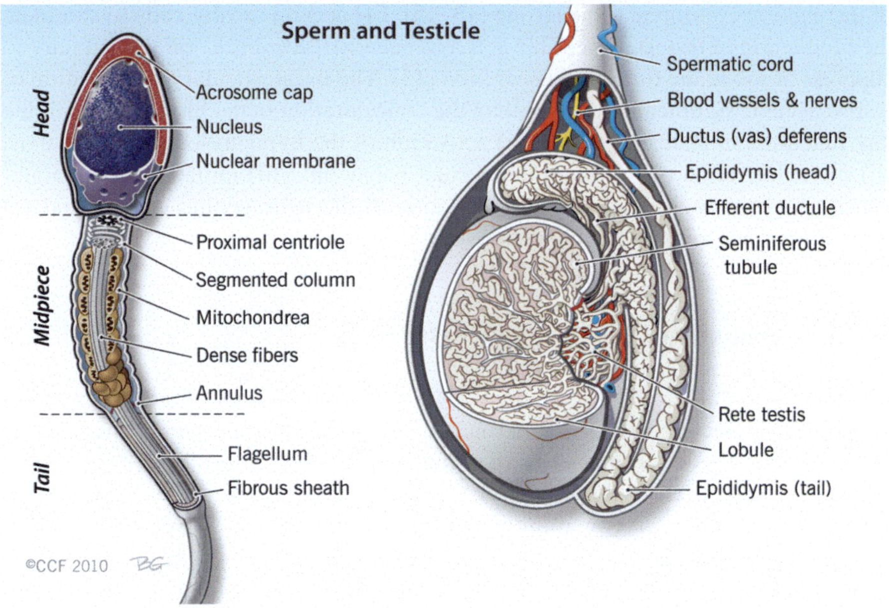

Fig. 14.2 The human testis and the epididymis. The testis shows the tunica vaginalis and tunica albuginea, seminiferous tubule septa, rete testis and the overlying head, body, and tail of the epididymis. To the left is a diagrammatic representation of a fully mature spermatozoon (Reprinted with permission, Cleveland Clinic Center for Medical Art & Photography © 2010. All Rights Reserved)

14.2 Organization of the Testis

The testes are ellipsoid in shape, measuring of 4.5–5.1 cm in length [4, 5], 2.5 × 4 cm in width [6], and have a volume of 15–25 mL [7]. They are engulfed by a strong connective tissues capsule (tunica albuginea) [6] and are the only organs in the human that are located outside the body. The reason for the extracorporal localization of the testes is that Sertoli cells are temperature-sensitive. Therefore, spermatogenesis occurs at temperatures that are optimally 2–4° lower than body temperature [8]. The testis is loosely connected along its posterior border to the epididymis, which gives rise to the vas deferens at its lower pole [9]. The testis has two main functions: produce hormones, in particular testosterone, and produce male gamete—the spermatozoa (Fig. 14.2).

14.2.1 Supporting Cells

14.2.1.1 Leydig Cells

The Leydig cells are irregularly shaped cells that have granular cytoplasm present individually or more often in groups within the connective tissue. They contribute to about 5–2% of the testicular volume [10–12]. Leydig cells are the prime source of the male sex hormone testosterone [13–15]. LH acts on Leydig cells to stimulate the production of testosterone. This acts as a negative "feedback" on the pituitary to suppress or modulate further LH secretion [15]. The intratesticular concentration of testosterone is significantly higher than the concentration in the blood. Some of the key functions of testosterone are: (i) activation of the hypophyseal-testicular axis, (ii) masculinization of the brain and sexual behaviors, (iii) initiation and maintenance of spermatogenesis, (iv) differentiation of the male genital organs, and (v) acquisition of secondary sex characteristics.

14.2.1.2 Seminiferous Tubules and Sertoli Cells

Most of the volume of the testis is made up of seminiferous tubules, which are packed in connective tissue within the confines of the fibrous septa. The testis is incompletely divided into a series of about 370 lobules or fibrous septae consisting of the seminiferous tubules and the intertubular tissue. The seminiferous tubules are a series of convoluted tubules within the testes. Spermatogenesis takes place in these tubules, scattered into many different proliferating and developing pockets (Fig. 14.3). The seminiferous tubules are looped or blind-ended and separated by groups of Leydig cells, blood vessels, lymphatics, and nerves. Each seminiferous tubule is about 180 μm in diameter. The height of the germinal epithelium measures 80 μm, and the thickness of the peritubular tissue is about 8 μm [16].

Seminiferous tubules consist of three layers of peritubular tissue: (1) the outer adventitial layer of fibrocytes that originate from primitive connective tissue from the interstitium, (2) the middle layer composed of myoid cells that are distributed next to the connective tissue lamellae, and (3) the peritubular layer, a thick, inner lamella that mainly consists of collagen. The seminiferous tubule space is divided into basal (basement membrane) and adluminal (lumen) compartments by strong intercellular junctional complexes called "tight junctions." The seminiferous tubules are lined with highly specialized Sertoli cells that rest on the tubular basement membrane and extend into the lumen with a complex ramification of cytoplasm. They encourage Sertoli cell proliferation and development during the gestational period. Both ends of the seminiferous tubules open into the spaces of the rete testis [17]. The fluid secreted by the seminiferous tubules is collected in the rete testis and delivered into the excurrent ductal system of the epididymis.

Approximately 40% of the seminiferous tubules consist of Sertoli cells, and roughly 40% of the Sertoli cells are occupied with elongated spermatids [18, 19]. Sertoli cells have larger nuclei than most cells, ranging from 250 to 850 cm^3 [19]. Each Sertoli cell makes contact with five other Sertoli cells and about 40–50 germ cells in various stages of development and differentiation. The Sertoli cells provide structural, functional, and metabolic support to germ cells. Functionally and endocrinologically competent Sertoli cells are necessary for optimal spermatogenesis. During spermatogenesis, the earlier germinal cells rest toward the epithelium region of the seminiferous tubules in order to develop and mature, while the more devel-

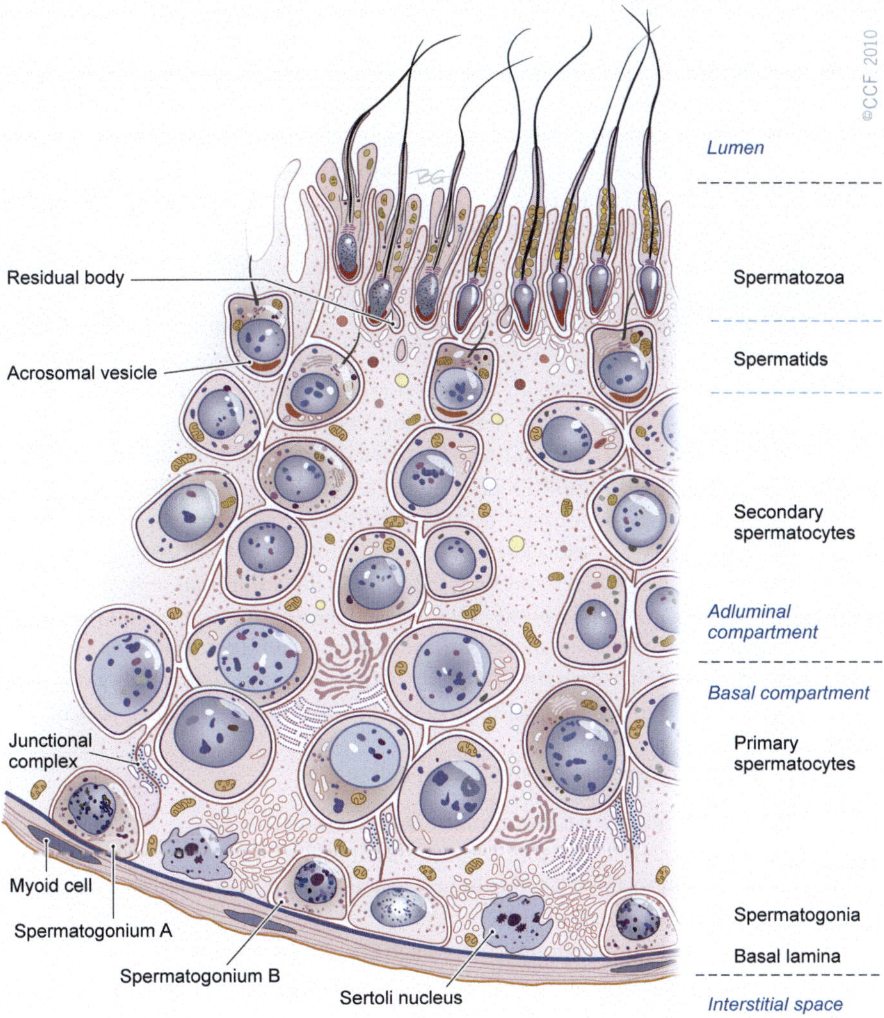

Fig. 14.3 Section of the germinal epithelium in the seminiferous tubule. Sertoli cells divide the germinal epithelium in a basal and adluminal compartment, via the Sertoli cell. Spermatozoa are released into the lumen (Reprinted with permission, Cleveland Clinic Center for Medical Art & Photography © 2010. All Rights Reserved)

oped germinal cells move toward the lumen of the seminiferous tubules in order to exit the seminiferous tubule system and continue with the final phases of spermatogenesis.

Sertoli cells function as "nurse" cells for spermatogenesis, nourishing germ cells as they develop and participating in germ cell phagocytosis. Multiple sites of communication exist between Sertoli cells and developing germ cells for the maintenance of spermatogenesis within an appropriate hormonal milieu. FSH binds to the high-affinity FSH receptors found on Sertoli cells, signaling the secretion of androgen-binding protein (ABP). ABP allows androgens such as testosterone and dihydrotestosterone to bind and increase their concentrations to initiate and/or continue the process of spermatogenesis. Sertoli cells also release anti-Müllerian hormone that allows for the embryonic development of the male by reducing the growth of the Müllerian ducts [20, 21], which in females develop into the fallopian tubes. Sertoli cells also secrete inhibin, a key macromolecule hormone that is participating in pituitary FSH regulation by providing negative feedback.

Considering that spermatozoa are only produced as from puberty, the male germ cells are not recognized by the immune system which develops during the first year of life. Therefore, spermatozoa must be protected from immunological attack. The structure providing this essential protection and forming a special microenvironment for spermatogenesis to occur in an immunologically privileged site is the blood-testis barrier. It is formed by neighboring Sertoli cells that are connected via so-called tight junctions. The blood-testis barrier divides the seminiferous tubules into two regions: a basal region located near the seminiferous epithelium and an adluminal region that is positioned toward the lumen region of the seminiferous tubules. The basal region is the spermatogenic site for the development of the diploid spermatogonia and primary spermatocyte, while the adluminal region serves as a developmental site for the haploid cells, secondary spermatocytes, and spermatids. The blood-testis barrier has three different levels: (1) tight junctions between Sertoli cells, which help separate premeiotic spermatogonia from the rest of the germ cells, (2) the endothelial cells in both the capillaries, and (3) peritubular myoid cells.

Some of the main functions of the Sertoli cell are:

1. Maintenance of integrity of seminiferous epithelium
2. Compartmentalization of seminiferous epithelium
3. Secretion of fluid to form tubular lumen to transport sperm within the duct
4. Participation in spermiation
5. Phagocytosis and elimination of cytoplasm
6. Delivery of nutrients to germ cells
7. Steroidogenesis and steroid metabolism
8. Movement of cells within the epithelium
9. Secretion of inhibin and androgen-binding protein
10. Regulation of spermatogenic cycle
11. Providing a target for LH, FSH, and testosterone receptors present on Sertoli cells

14.3 Spermatogenesis

The process of differentiation of a simple diploid spermatogonium into a spermatid is known as spermatogenesis [17]. It is a complex, temporal event whereby primitive, totipotent stem cells divide to either renew themselves or produce daughter

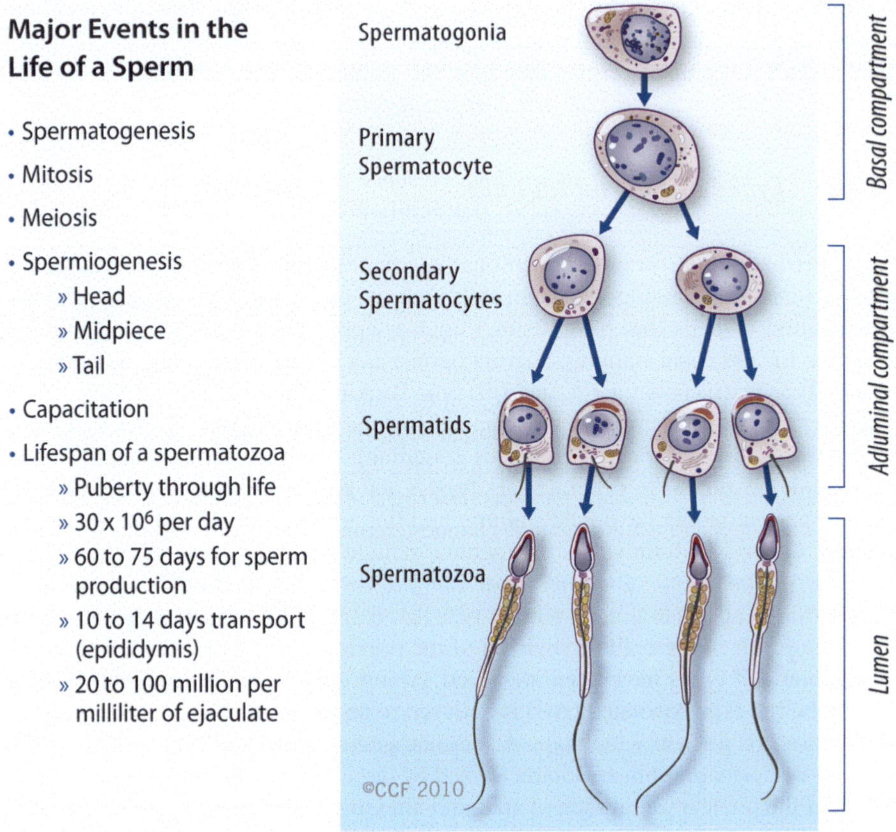

Fig. 14.4 A diagrammatic representation of major events in the life of a sperm involving spermatogenesis, spermiogenesis, and spermiation during which the developing germ cells undergo mitotic and meiotic division to reduce the chromosome content (Reprinted with permission, Cleveland Clinic Center for Medical Art & Photography © 2010. All Rights Reserved)

cells that are transformed into a specialized testicular spermatozoon (Fig. 14.4). It involves both mitotic and meiotic divisions and extensive cellular remodeling. Spermatogenesis can be divided into three phases: (i) proliferation and differentiation of spermatogonia, (ii) meiosis, and (iii) spermiogenesis, a complex process that transforms round spermatids after meiosis into a complex structure called the spermatozoon. In humans, the process of spermatogenesis starts at puberty and continues throughout the entire life span of the individual. Once the gonocytes have differentiated into fetal spermatogonia, an active process of mitotic replication begins very early in the embryonic development.

Within the seminiferous tubule, germ cells are arranged in a highly ordered sequence from the basement membrane to the lumen. Spermatogonia lie directly on the basement membrane, followed by primary spermatocytes, secondary spermatocytes, and spermatids, as they progress toward the tubule lumen. The tight junction barrier supports spermatogonia and early spermatocytes within the basal compartment and all subsequent germ cells within the adluminal compartment.

14.3.1 *Types of Spermatogonia*

Fetal spermatogonia become transitional spermatogonia and later spermatogonia type Ad (dark). Spermatogonial stem cells undergo proliferative events and produce a population of cells that have distinct nuclear appearance that can be seen with hematoxylin and eosin staining. Spermatogonia can be categorized into three types: (i) dark type A, (ii) pale type A, and (iii) type B spermatogonia (Fig. 14.5).

Dark type A spermatogonia are stem cells of the seminiferous tubules that have an intensely stained dark ovoid nucleus containing fine granular chromatin. These cells divide by mitosis to generate dark type A and pale type A spermatogonia. Pale type A spermatogonia have pale staining and fine granular chromatin in the ovoid nucleus. Other proliferative spermatogonia include Apaired (Apr), resulting from dividing Aisolated and subsequently dividing to form Aaligned (Aal). Further differentiation of spermatogonia includes type A1, A2, A3, A4, intermediate, and type B, each a result of the cellular division of the previous type. In humans, four spermatogonial cell types have been identified: Along, Adark, Apale, and type B [22–24]. In the rat, type Aisolated (Ais) is believed to be the stem cell [25, 26], whereas in humans, it is unclear which type A spermatogonia is the stem cell.

Type B spermatogonia are characterized by large clumps of condensed chromatin under the nuclear membrane of an ovoid nucleus. These cells divide mitotically to produce primary spermatocytes (preloptotene, leptotene, zygotene, and pachytene), secondary spermatocytes, and spermatids (Sa, Sb, Sc, Sd1, and Sd2) [23] (Fig. 14.6). Spermatogonia do not separate completely after meiosis but remain joined by intercellular bridges, which persist throughout all stages of spermatogenesis. This facilitates biochemical interactions and synchronizes germ cell maturation [27].

14.3.2 *Spermatocytogenesis*

Spermatocytogenesis consists of the meiotic phase in which primary spermatocytes undergo meiosis I and meiosis II to give rise to haploid spermatids. This takes place in the basal compartment. Primary spermatocytes enter the first meiotic division to form secondary spermatocytes. The prophase of the first meiotic division is very long. Primary spermatocytes have the longest life span. Secondary spermatocytes undergo the second meiotic division to produce spermatids. Secondary spermatocytes are short lived (1.1—1.7 days).

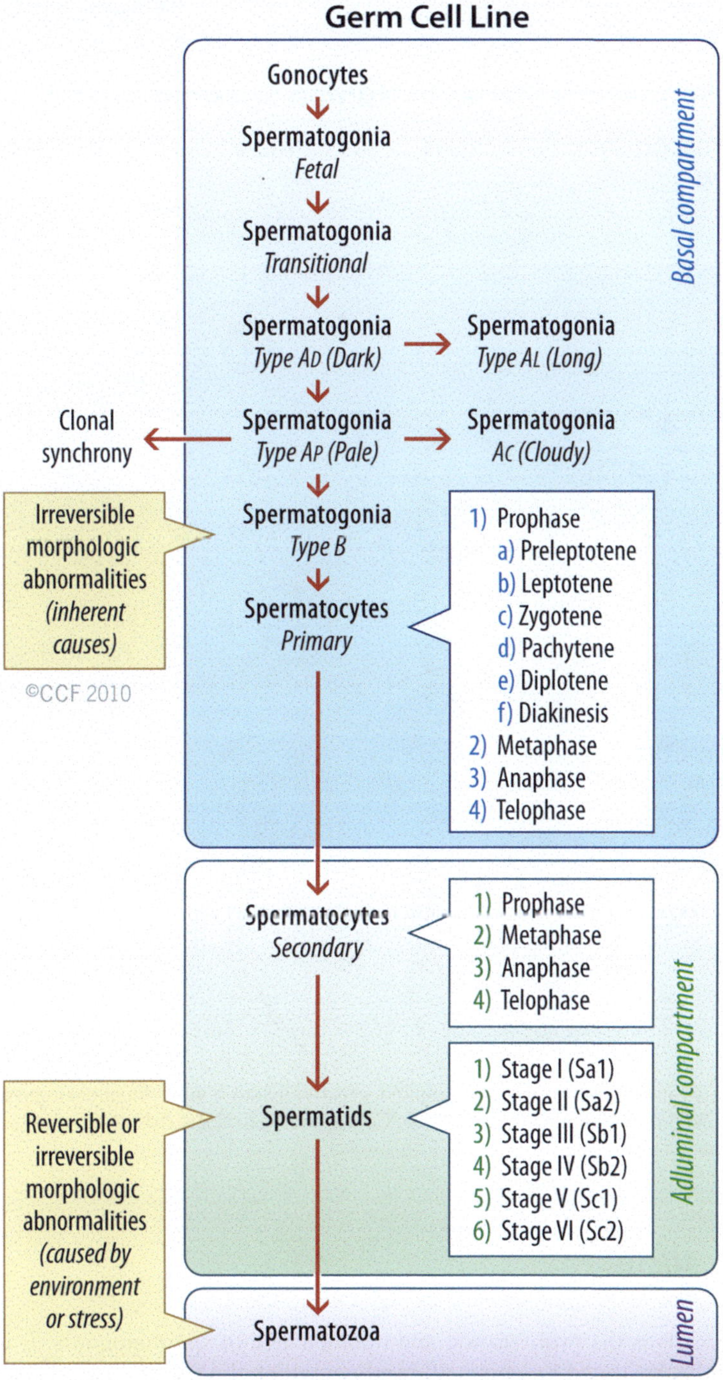

Fig. 14.5 Schematic representation of the development of a diploid undifferentiated germ cell into a fully functional haploid spermatozoon along the basal to the adluminal compartment and final release into the lumen. Different steps in the development of primary, secondary, and spermatid stages are also shown and the irreversible and reversible morphological abnormalities that may occur during various stages of spermatogenesis (Reprinted with permission, Cleveland Clinic Center for Medical Art & Photography © 2010. All Rights Reserved)

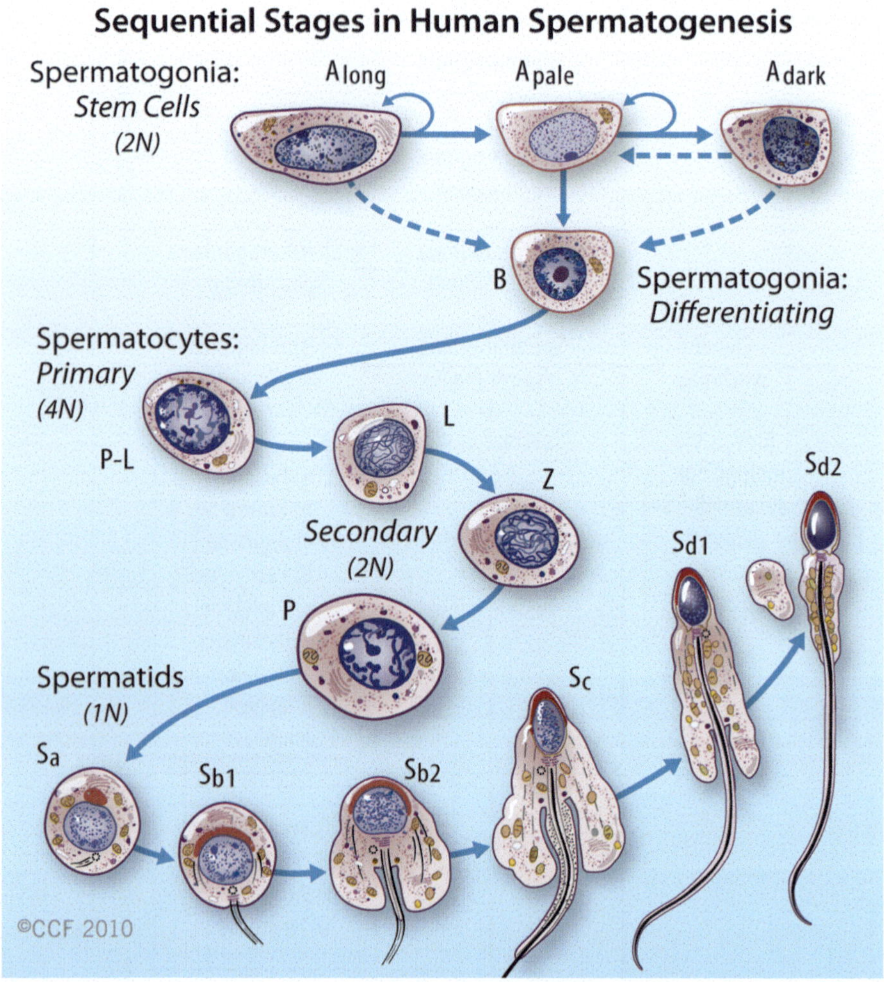

Fig. 14.6 Differentiation of a human diploid germ cell into a fully functional spermatozoon (Reprinted with permission, Cleveland Clinic Center for Medical Art & Photography © 2010. All Rights Reserved)

14.3.3 Mitosis

Mitosis involves the proliferation and maintenance of spermatogonia. It is a precise, well-orchestrated sequence of events in which the genetic material (chromosomes) is duplicated, with breakdown of the nuclear envelope and formation of two daughter cells as a result of equal division of the chromosomes and cytoplasm [28]. DNA is organized into loop domains on which specific regulatory proteins interact [29–33]. The mitotic phase involves spermatogonia (types A and B) and primary spermatocytes (spermatocytes I). Primary spermatocytes are produced by developing germ cells interconnected by intracellular bridges through a series of mitotic divisions. Once the baseline number of spermatogonia is established after puberty, the mitotic component proceeds to provide precursor cells and initiate the process of differentiation and maturation. Chromosomes are most vulnerable during mitosis, and all DNA repair processes are shut down to prevent fusion of telomeres [34].

14.3.4 Meiosis

The meiotic phase involves primary spermatocytes until spermatids are formed, and during this process, chromosome pairing, crossover, and genetic exchange take place until a new genome is determined. Meiosis consists of two successive divisions to yield four haploid spermatids from one diploid primary spermatocyte. After the first meiotic division (reduction division), each daughter cell contains one partner of the homologous chromosome pair, and they are called secondary spermatocytes (2n).

Meiosis is characterized by prophase, metaphase, anaphase, and telophase. The process starts when type B spermatogonia lose contact with the basement membrane and form preleptotene primary spermatocytes. During the leptotene stage of prophase, the chromosomes are arranged as long filaments. During the zygotene stage, the homologous chromosomes called tetrads are arranged linearly by a process known as synapsis and form synaptonemal complexes. Crossing over takes place during this phase, and chromosomes shorten in the pachytene stage. The homologous chromosomes condense and separate from sites of crossing over during diakinesis. This random sorting is important to maintaining genetic diversity in sperm. At the end of prophase, the nuclear envelope breaks down, and in metaphase, chromosomes are arranged in the equatorial plate. At anaphase, each chromosome consists of two chromatids migrating to opposite poles. In telophase, cell division occurs with the formation of secondary spermatocytes having half the number of chromosomes. Thus, each primary spermatocyte can theoretically yield four spermatids, although fewer actually result, as the complexity of meiosis is associated with a loss of some germ cells. The primary spermatocytes are the largest germ cells of the germinal epithelium.

The prophase of the second meiotic division is very short, and in this phase, the DNA content is reduced to half as the two chromatids of each chromosome separate and move to the opposite poles. At the end of telophase, the spermatids do not separate completely but remain interconnected by fine bridges for synchronous development. These spermatids are haploid with (22, X) or (22, Y) chromosome and undergo complete differentiation/morphogenesis known as spermiogenesis.

14.3.5 Spermiogenesis

Spermiogenesis is the process of differentiation of the spermatids into a spermatozoon with fully compacted chromatin. During this process, morphological changes occur once the process of meiosis is completed. In humans, six different stages have been described in the process of spermatid maturation; these are termed as Sa-1 and Sa-2, Sb-1 and Sb-2, and Sc-1 and Sc-2 (Fig. 14.6). Each stage can be identified by the morphological characteristics. During the Sa-1 stage, both the Golgi complex and mitochondria are well developed and differentiated. In addition, the acrosomal vesicle appears, the chromatoid body develops in one pole of the cell opposite from the acrosomal vesicle, and the proximal centriole and the axial filament appear. During the Sb-1 and Sb-2 stages, acrosome formation is completed, the intermediate piece is formed, and the tail develops. This process is completed during the Sc stages. During the postmeiotic phase, progressive condensation of the nucleus occurs with inactivation of the genome. Testicular histones are replaced by transitional proteins and, finally, by protamines, specific alkaline proteins that allow arrangement of the DNA in arrays instead of supercoiled solenoids. In addition, protamines are stabilized by disulfide bonds which essentially provide for nuclear stability in the male germ cell. During spermiogenesis, the developing male germ cells are extremely sensitive to oxidative stress. Spermatids have limited capacity for renewing glutathione and DNA repair and are therefore dependent on the antioxidant protection conferred by the Sertoli cells [35].

14.3.6 Spermiation

A mature spermatid frees itself from the Sertoli cell and enters the lumen of the tubule as a spermatozoon in a process called spermiation. Spermatids that originate from the same spermatogonia remain connected by bridges to facilitate the transport of cytoplasmic products. Sertoli cells actively participate in spermiation, which may also involve the actual movement of the cell as the spermatid advances toward the lumen of the seminiferous tubules [19]. The mature spermatids close their intracellular bridges, disconnect their contact with the germinal epithelium, and become free cells called spermatozoa. Portions of the cytoplasm in the Sertoli cell known as the cytoplasmic droplet are completely eliminated, or, at times, they may be retained in the immature spermatozoon during the process of spermiation [36].

14.3.7 The Cycle or Wave of Seminiferous Epithelium

A cycle of spermatogenesis involves the division of primitive spermatogonial stem cells into subsequent germ cell types through the process of meiosis. Type A spermatogonial divisions occur at a shorter time interval than the entire process of spermatogenesis. Therefore, at any given time, several cycles of spermatogenesis coexist within the germinal epithelium. Spermatogenesis is not a random but well-orchestrated series of well-defined events in the seminiferous epithelium. Germ cells are localized in spatial units referred as stages. Each stage is recognized by development of the acrosome: meiotic divisions and shape of the nucleus and release of the sperm into lumen of the seminiferous tubule. A stage is designated by Roman numerals. Each cell type of the stage is morphologically integrated with the others in its development process. Each stage has a defined morphological entity of spermatid development called a step, which is designated by an Arabic number. Several steps occur together to form a stage, and several stages are necessary to form a mature sperm from immature stem cells [37, 38]. In rodent spermatogenesis, only one stage can be found in a cross section of seminiferous tubule.

Within any given cross section of the seminiferous tubule, there are four to five layers of germ cells. Cells in each layer comprise a generation or a cohort of cells that develop as a synchronous group. Each group has a similar appearance and function. Stages I–III have four generations comprising type A spermatogonia, two primary spermatocytes, and an immature spermatid. Stages IV–VIII have five generations: type A spermatogonia, one generation of primary spermatocyte, one generation of secondary spermatocytes, and one generation of spermatids. Thus, a position in the tubule that is occupied by cells comprising stage I will become stage II, followed by stage III, until the cycle repeats. The cycle of spermatogenesis can be identified for each species, but the duration of the cycle varies for each species [23].

The stages of spermatogenesis are sequentially arranged along the length of the tubule in such a way that it results in a "wave of spermatogenesis." Although it appears that the spatial organization is lacking or is poor in the human seminiferous tubule, these stages are tightly organized in an intricate helicine pattern [39]. In addition to the steps being organized spatially within the seminiferous tubule, the stages are organized in time. Spermatozoa are released only in certain cross sections along the length of the seminiferous tubule. In the rat, all stages are involved in spermatogenesis, but spermatozoa are released only in stage VIII. In humans, this wave appears to be a spiral cellular arrangement as they progress down the tubule. This spatial arrangement probably exists to ensure that sperm production is a continuous and not a pulsatile process. The spermatocyte takes 25.3 days to mature. Spermiogenesis occurs in 21.6 days, and the duration of the cycle is 16 days. The progression from spermatogonia to spermatozoa or spermatogenesis is 74 days or four and a half cycles of the seminiferous cycle.

14.4 Chromatin Remodeling/Alterations During Sperm Differentiation

Mammalian sperm chromatin is unique in that it is highly organized, condensed, and compacted. This feature protects the paternal genome during transport through the male and the female reproductive tracts and helps ensure that it is delivered to the ova in good condition. Mammalian sperm DNA is the most tightly compacted eukaryotic DNA [40]. This feature is in sharp contrast to the DNA structure in somatic cell nuclei. Somatic cell nuclear DNA is wrapped around an octamer of histones and packaged into a solenoid structure [41]. This type of packaging adds histones, which increase the chromatin volume. The sperm nucleus does not have this type of packaging, and the volume is highly compacted. Chromatin changes occur in the testis during meiosis in which copies of the genome are partitioned into haploid spermatid cells and during spermiogenesis in which spermatids elongate to form sperm with fully compacted chromatin. These events are largely controlled by posttranslational events for transcription. Translation greatly subsides as DNA becomes compacted, and the cytoplasm is jettisoned during spermiogenesis [42, 43]. After meiosis, sperm DNA experiences extreme chromosome compaction during spermiogenesis.

Chromatin modeling is accompanied by changes in the nuclear shape, conversion of negatively supercoiled nucleosomal DNA into a non-supercoiled state [44], induction of transient DNA breaks [45], and chromatin condensation. It is mediated by drastic changes at the most fundamental level of DNA packaging where a nucleosomal architecture shifts to a toroidal structure [46]. This change is implemented by sperm nuclear basic proteins (SNBs) that include variants of histone subunits, transition proteins, and protamine proteins [47, 48]. Chromatin proteins do not act exclusively to compact sperm DNA. This transition occurs in a stepwise manner, replacing somatic histones with testis-expressed histone variants, transition proteins, and finally protamines [49]. Histone localization and posttranslational modification of histones encode epigenetic information that may regulate transcription important for sperm development [50]. They may also serve to mark the heterochromatin state of specific regions of the genome that may be important after fertilization, when somatic histones are incorporated back into paternal chromatin or during subsequent zygotic development [51]. Male infertility can result from deficits of SNBs [52–54].

14.4.1 Histone and Basic Nuclear Protein Transitions in Spermatogenesis

In the course of spermatogenesis, histones are replaced in developing sperm by testis-specific histone variants that are important for fertility [55]. The cells depend on posttranslational modifications to implement subsequent stages of sperm formation, maturation, and activation as de Novo transcription in postmeiotic sperm is largely silenced [43]. During this whole process, sperm chromatin undergoes a series of modifications in which histones are lost and replaced with transition proteins and subsequently with protamines [56–58]. Approximately 15% of the histones are retained in human sperm chromatin, subsequently making chromatin less tightly compacted [59, 60]. Chromatin remodeling is facilitated by the coordinated loosening of the chromatin by histone hyperacetylation and by the DNA topoisomerase II (topo II), which produce temporary nicks in the sperm DNA to relieve torsional stress that results from supercoiling [45, 61–63]. However, if these nicks are not repaired, DNA-fragmented sperm may be present in the ejaculate [64].

14.4.2 Role of Transition Proteins

The histone-to-protamine transition is important in the formation of spermatozoa [65]. This occurs in two steps in mammals: replacement of histones by transition nuclear proteins (TPs)—TP1 and TP2—and replacement of TPs by protamines (protamine 1 and protamine 2). TPs are required for normal chromatin condensation, for reducing the number of DNA breaks, and for preventing the formation of secondary defects in spermatozoa and the eventual loss of genomic integrity and sterility.

The transition proteins are localized exclusively to the nuclei of elongating and condensing spermatids [66] and were first detected in steps 10–11 spermatids [67, 68] (Figs. 14.7 and 14.8). Maximum levels of these TPs are acquired during steps 12–13, when they constitute about 90% of the chromatin basic protein, with TP1 being about 2.5 times of those of the TP2 levels [53]. After the early stages of step 15, both proteins are no longer detected in the nucleus [67, 68]. Defective protamine 2 processing is correlated with infertility in humans [69] and mouse mutants [53, 54] and could be due solely to the secondary cytoplasmic effects on sperm development resulting in a reduced ability to penetrate the egg.

14.4.3 Protamines as Checkpoints of Spermatogenesis

Sperm from infertile men show an altered P1/P2 ratio and/or no detectable P2 in mature sperm. Protamine abnormalities in sperm from fertile men are extremely rare [69–73].

Protamines are approximately half the size of histones [74]. They are highly basic sperm-specific nuclear proteins that are characterized by an arginine-rich core and cysteine residues [75, 76]. Protamines confer a higher order of DNA packaging in sperm than that found in somatic cells. All of these levels of compaction and organization help protect sperm chromatin during transport through the male and female reproductive tract. This also ensures delivery of the paternal genome in a form that allows developing embryo to accurately express genetic information [60, 77–79].

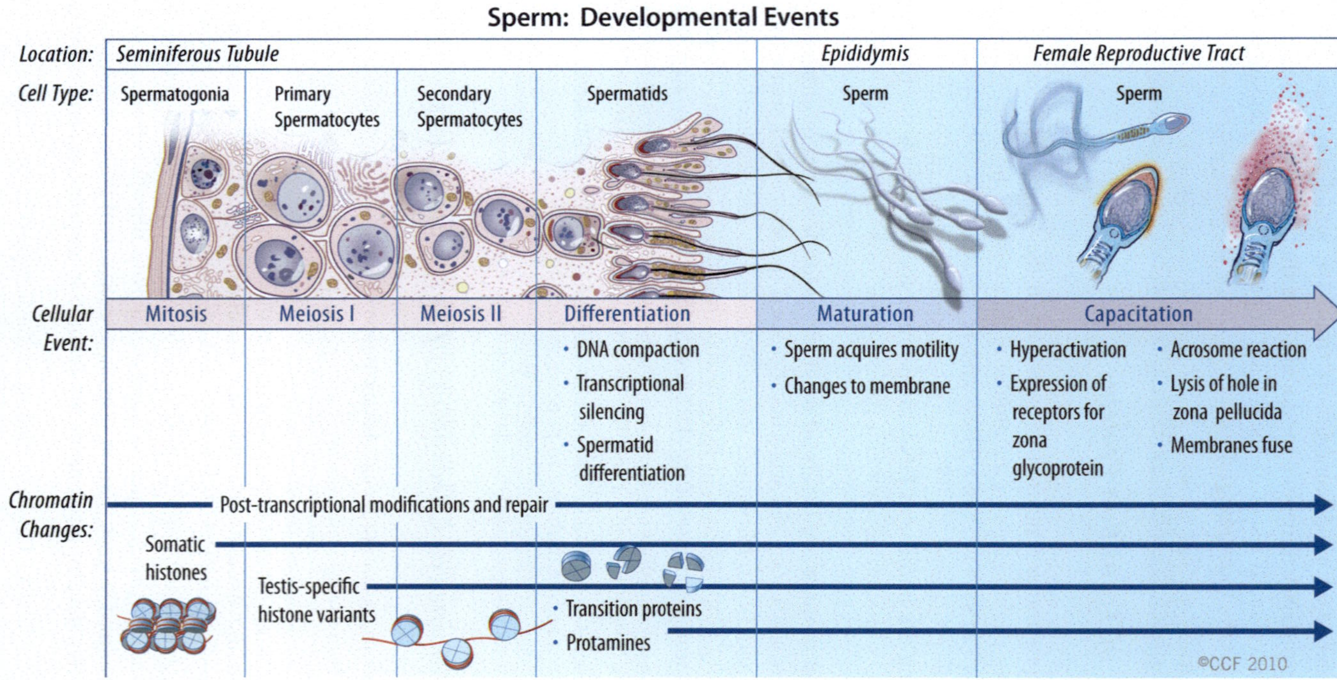

Fig. 14.7 Diagrammatic representation of the series of cellular and chromatin changes during the development of the germ cell into a spermatozoon and its subsequent release and storage into the epididymis and its journey into the female reproductive tract (Reprinted with permission, Cleveland Clinic Center for Medical Art & Photography © 2010. All Rights Reserved)

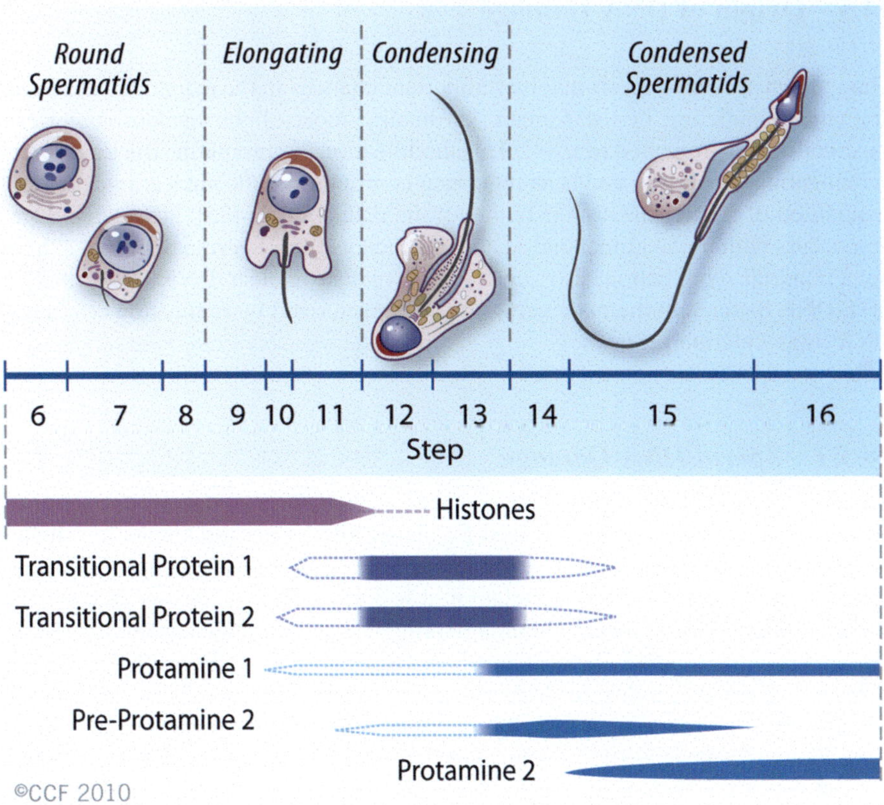

Fig. 14.8 Diagrammatic representation of the steps where the histones are replaced with the transition proteins and protamines in the round spermatid progresses into a condensed spermatid just before it is released into the lumen (Reprinted with permission, Cleveland Clinic Center for Medical Art & Photography © 2010. All Rights Reserved)

14.4.4 DNA Methylation During Spermatogenesis

Nucleohistones are present in human and rat sperm and are absent in mouse sperm. About 15% of the histones are retained in the mature human spermatozoa [60]. There are widespread differences in methylation of specific sequences during oogenesis and spermatogenesis. DNA methylation may be involved in genomic imprinting in mammals and is one of the major epigenetic marks established during spermatogenesis [80]. Mature sperm shows a unique DNA methylation profile, one that is different from that of somatic cells [81]. The level of DNA methylation does not correlate with fertilization but with pregnancy rate after IVF [82].

14.5 Origin of DNA Damage

Mammalian spermiogenesis involves important changes in the cytoarchitecture and dramatic remodeling of the somatic chromatin; most of the nucleosomal DNA supercoiling is eliminated [83, 84]. This modification in chromatin structure occurs in elongating spermatids and is an important contributor to the nuclear integrity and acquisition of full fertilization potential of the male gamete [85]. DNA fragmentation occurs both in the mitochondria and the nucleus [86]. Spermatozoa that exhibit mitochondrial dysfunction also show a high rate of nuclear DNA fragmentation [87]. DNA damage in the male germ line is characterized by replication errors and DNA fragmentation [88].

14.5.1 Sperm DNA Damage

Sperm DNA damage is characterized by abasic sites, base modifications, single-strand and double-strand breaks, and DNA protein cross-links. Although DNA fragmentation does not constitute a mutation, it is a promutagenic change that has the potential to generate mutations in the offspring if the repair mechanisms are defective or inadequate. DNA damage involves (1) post-meiotically initiated abortive apoptosis when the ability to drive this process to completion is in decline, (2) unresolved strand breaks created during spermiogenesis to relieve torsional stress associated with chromatin remodeling, and (3) oxidative stress as a result of reactive oxygen species. Three major mechanisms for the creation of DNA damage in the male germ line have been proposed: chromatin remodeling by topoisomerase, oxidative stress, and abortive apoptosis.

DNA damage could arise due to a combination of all three mechanisms. Furthermore, a two-step hypothesis has been proposed [85, 89]. Defects in the chromatin remodeling process result in the production of spermatozoa that are characterized by reduction in the efficiency of protamination, abnormal protamine 1 to protamine 2 ratio, and relatively high nucleohistone content [79, 90, 91]. These defects in chromatin modeling create a state of vulnerability whereby spermatozoa become increasingly susceptible to oxidative damage. In the second step of this DNA cascade, reactive oxygen species attack chromatin. Sperm chromatin compaction is believed to play an important role in protecting the male genome from insult. This specific chromatin structure of the sperm essential for proper fertility is, in part, due to the proteins that are bound to the DNA, including histones, protamines, and components of the nuclear matrix [92, 93]. The cascade of events leading to DNA damage involves an error in chromatin remodeling during spermiogenesis. This leads to generation of spermatozoa with poorly protaminated nuclear DNA that is increasingly susceptible to oxidative attack [89].

14.5.2 Sperm Apoptosis

Spermatogenesis is accompanied by germ cell apoptosis in the seminiferous epithelium, a process which normally occurs throughout the life span. In addition, germ cell loss can be triggered by a variety of factors such as exposure to toxicants, alterations in the hormonal support, heat, radiation, or chemotherapeutic exposure [94–97]. Apoptosis of germ cells is necessary to maintain the optimal germ cell to Sertoli cell ratio and eliminate abnormal germ cells, especially during puberty. Approximately 75% of the spermatogonia are eliminated by programmed cell death before they can attain maturity [98, 99]. Spermatozoa do exhibit some of the hallmarks of apoptosis including caspase activation and phosphatidylserine exposure on the surface of the cell [100]. Sertoli cells can support only a limited number of germ cells in the testis. Therefore, apoptosis normally occurs to prevent the overproduction of germ cells and to selectively remove injured germ cells [101]. Clonal expansion of the germ cells in the testis occurs at very high levels, and thus, apoptosis is necessary to limit the size of the germ cell population to one which the Sertoli cell is able to support [102]. Men with poor seminal parameters often display a large percentage of Fas-expressing sperm in their ejaculate [79]. Some of these sperm with DNA damage and Fas expression may have undergone "abortive apoptosis" in which they started but subsequently escaped the apoptotic pathway [103]. Reactive oxygen and nitrogen species can trigger the intrinsic apoptotic pathways. The extrinsic apoptosis is mediated by activation of Fas protein receptors. These receptors are activated by binding of Fas ligand.

The combination of both intrinsic and extrinsic pathway results in a lethal cell response and activation of caspase-9, which in turn will activate executioner caspases resulting in the fragmentation of the cell [104, 105]. Fas receptors are present in less than 10% of ejaculated spermatozoa from healthy spermatozoa and more than 50% of ejaculated spermatozoa from infertile men with oligozoospermia [106]. Sperm apoptosis can be recognized by both early and late stage markers—the early sign of phagocytosis is the translocation of the phosphatidyl serine residues from the inner to the outer plasma membrane of the spermatozoa. It is also an indication that abortive apoptosis is occurring in men with abnormal semen parameters [79]. DNA fragmentation is the late stage marker of apoptosis.

14.5.3 Oxidative Stress in the Testis

Sertoli cells provide nutritional support to the differentiating germ cells in the testis. They protect the differentiating germ cells from oxidative stress as these cells pass through meiosis and emerge as haploid cells known as round spermatids. At this stage of development, these cells are transcriptionally silent. Even in the absence of any regulated gene transcription, they are able to undergo cellular transformation into a fully differentiated, highly specialized cell—the spermatozoon. This is accomplished thorough a highly orchestrated differential translation of preexisting mRNA species through a process called spermiogenesis. Cells are sensitive to oxidative stress during spermiogenesis. Throughout this phase, they are highly dependent on the nurturing Sertoli cells, which possess antioxidants such as superoxide dismutase, glutathione reductase, transferase, and peroxidase [35]. Isolated spermatozoa have a limited capacity for DNA repair [107] and do not transcribe novel RNA [108].

14.5.4 Spermiogenesis and Etiology of DNA Damage

Spermiogenesis, the process by which haploid round spermatids differentiate into spermatozoa, is a key event in the etiology of DNA damage in the male germ line. During this process, the chromatin undergoes extensive remodeling, which enables the entire haploid genome to be compacted into a sperm head measuring $5 \times 2.5\ \mu$. This occurs as physiological DNA strand breaks are introduced by topoisomerase to relieve the torsional stresses involved in DNA packaging during sperm differentiation. These strand breaks are corrected by a complex process involving H2Ax expression, formation of poly(ADP-ribose) by nuclear poly(ADP-ribose) polymerases (PARP), and topoisomerase [109]. If the process of spermiogenesis is disrupted for any reason, restoration of the cleavage sites is impaired, and defective spermatozoa with unresolved physiological strand breaks are released from the germinal epithelium. Transition proteins play a key role in maintaining DNA integrity during spermiogenesis as they move into the sperm nucleus between the removal of histones and the entry of protamines. Functional deletion of these proteins results in the production of spermatozoa with poor fertilizing ability, poor chromatin compaction, and high levels of DNA fragmentation [65]. DNA damage in human spermatozoa is associated with the disruption and poor chromatin remodeling during spermiogenesis [91, 110].

The efficiency of spermatogenesis is reflected by conventional semen characteristics such as sperm count and morphology and the correlation with DNA damage [111, 112]. Poor protamination results in spermatozoa that possess nucleohistone-rich regions of chromatin that is vulnerable to oxidative attack [85]. Oxidative stress is a major determinant of the quality of spermiogenesis, and disruption will lead to the production of spermatozoa vulnerable to oxidative stress, 8-OHdG formation, and, ultimately, DNA fragmentation as a consequence of apoptosis [108, 113, 114].

14.5.5 Efficiency of Spermatogenesis

The efficiency of spermatogenesis varies between different species; it appears to be relatively constant in man. The time needed for spermatogonia to differentiate into mature spermatozoa is estimated to be 70 ± 4 days [115]. In comparison to animals, the spermatogenetic efficiency in man is poor, and the daily rate of spermatozoa production is about 3–4 million per gram of testicular tissue [116]. Although a much higher sperm count than the 15 million/mL described by WHO manual [117] should be expected in the ejaculate, this is not the case. This is largely because most developed cells (>75%) are eliminated as a result of apoptosis. In the remaining cells, more than half are abnormal. Therefore, only about 12% of the spermatogenetic potential is available for reproduction [118]. Furthermore, daily sperm production in men also declines with age, a process which is associated with the loss of Sertoli cells, an increase in germ cell degeneration during prophase of meiosis, or the loss of primary spermatocytes along with a reduction in the number of Leydig cells, non-Leydig interstitial cells, and myoid cells.

14.6 Post-Spermiation Events

The process of spermiation and the journey of a sperm through the excurrent duct of the testis to a site where it can be included in the ejaculate take an additional 10–14 days. The nucleus progressively elongates as its chromatin condenses; the head is characterized by a flattened and pointed paddle shape, which is specific to each species, and involves the Golgi phase where the centrioles migrate from the cytoplasm to the base of the nucleus; and the proximal centriole becomes the implantation apparatus to anchor flagellum to the nucleus and the distal centriole becomes the axoneme. In the cap phase, the acrosome forms a distinct cap over the nucleus covering about 30% to 50% of the nuclear surface [119]. The acrosome contains the hydrolytic enzymes necessary for fertilization. The manchette is formed, and the spermatids are embedded in Sertoli cells. During the maturation phase, mitochondria migrate toward the segment of the growing tail to form the mitochondrial sheath and outer dense fibers. A fibrous sheath is formed to complete the assembly of the tail. Most of the spermatid cytoplasm is discarded as a residual body, and the spermatid moves toward the lumen of the seminiferous tubule. Once elongation of the spermatid is complete, Sertoli cell cytoplasm retracts around the developing sperm, all unnecessary cytoplasm is stripped, and spermatozoa are finally released it into the tubule lumen. The mature spermatozoon is an elaborate, highly specialized cell produced in large numbers—about 300 per g of testis per second.

14.7 DNA Repair Mechanisms

About 105 DNA lesions/cells are produced daily in the mammalian genome as a result of cellular metabolism and replication errors [120]. There are five repair mechanisms in place irrespective of the cause of DNA damage to compensate for the DNA damage and maintain genomic integrity in the spermatozoa: (1) nucleotide excision repair, (2) base excision repair, (3) mismatch repair, (4) double-strand break repair, and (5) post-replication repair.

14.7.1 Nucleotide Excision Repair

Nucleotide excision repair or NER mechanism acts upon lesions caused by oxidative stress damage, mismatched bases, or DNA intra-strand cross-links causing distortion of the helical DNA structure [121, 122]. Global genome NER (GG-NER) and transcription-coupled NER (TC-NER) are the two pathways responsible for the underlying mechanism of NER. GG-NER is responsible for DNA damage, and TC-NER is responsible for detecting lesions in the coding strand of actively transcribed genes.

14.7.2 Base Excision Repair

Base pair excision repair (BER) is responsible for removal of non-helix-distorting base lesions; these excisions are increased by deamination or oxidation [122, 123]. 8-Oxo-2′-deoxyguanosine is the most significant and a well-characterized lesion. Abasic sites are generated in spermatozoa when 8-OHdg is cut by 8-oxoguanine glycosylase I (OGG1) [124]. Since the apyrimidinic endonuclease is absent in spermatozoa, the apyrimidinic sites created by OGG1 in DNA-damaged spermatozoa are repaired in the S-phase of the first mitotic division in the zygote [124, 125].

14.7.3 Mismatch Repair Mechanism

Mismatches are caused by inefficient proofreading by DNA polymerase [126]. The common mismatches are the base-base mismatches such as G-T or A-C and insertion-deletion loops. Mismatch repair mechanism increases the DNA replication fidelity by 100-fold and suppresses genomic instability [125]. Four important proteins involved in MMR are also involved in male infertility, namely, MLH1, MLH2, MSH4, and RAD51. Meiotic arrest is seen at the pachytene stage as a result of deficiency or absence of these genes [127].

14.7.4 DNA Double-Strand Repair

Double strand DNA breaks can occur as a result of a variety of factors such as failed DNA replication and repair, recombination, ionizing radiation, and chemotherapeutic agents and reactive oxygen species. If these double strands are not repaired, these can result in translocations, DNA fusions, and cell death. Nonhomologous end-joining repair (NHEJR) mechanisms help in repairing the DNA double-strand breaks [122].

14.7.5 Homologous Recombination

Homologous recombination repair mechanism operates mainly during the interphase and G2 phase where the double-strand DNA breaks are protected from exonuclease activity by the binding of Rad51 protein to the strand. DNA double-strand breaks activate both ataxia-telangiectasia mutated (ATM) and MRE11-RAD50-NBS1 complex and generate 3′-ssDNA [128, 129]. Gonadal atrophy and azoospermia are seen in men with ATM as a result of failure of primary spermatocytes at the leptotene-zygotene transition. Meiotic recombinations are blocked by mutations of MRE11 [127].

14.7.6 Nonhomologous End Joining

Ku70 and Ku 8–0 heterodimer recognize and bind to the double-stranded breaks in DNA and recruit DNA-dependent protein kinase [127]. This results in recruitment of MRE11 complex, which induces the removal of non-ligatable termini. Deficiency in the nonhomologous end joining predisposes to cancer and immune deficiency syndrome [122, 130].

In addition, there are proteins associated with DNA repair and infertility such as the retinoblastoma gene (RB1) which results in hypermethylation of O6-methylguanine-DNA methyltransferases (MGMT) when inactivated resulting in silencing and reduction of MGMT. Knockout mice studies have demonstrated that retinoblastoma is essential for proper terminal differentiation of Sertoli cells.

Ubiquitin-protease pathway (UPP) is involved in the DNA repair, protein folding, and translocation, and apoptosis and maximum mammalian UPP activity are seen in the testis. UPP is involved in different stages of spermatogenesis such as meiosis and acrosome biogenesis. Sperm malfunction and increased risk of infertility are seen as a result of abnormal or deficient UPP [131]. Fanconi anemia (FA) genes are essential for DNA inter-strand cross-link repair. Of the 16 FA pathway proteins, eight are essential for inter-strand cross-link repair and involved in monoubiquitination FANCD2 and FANCI [127, 132]. In addition to homologous recombinational repair of double-strand breaks, FANCN mutant male mice exhibited reduced fertility as a result of defective meiosis and increased apoptosis in germ cells [133].

14.8 Regulation of Spermatogenesis

Both intrinsic and extrinsic regulation influence spermatogenic process.

14.8.1 Intrinsic Regulation

Testosterone, neurotransmitters (neuroendocrine substances), and growth factors are secreted by Leydig cells to neighboring Leydig cells, blood vessels, the lamina propria of the seminiferous tubules, and Sertoli cells [12, 118, 134]. In this sense, Leydig cells help maintain the nutrition of the Sertoli cells, and the cells of the peritubular tissue influence the contractility of myofibroblasts and regulate the peristaltic movements of seminiferous tubules and transportation of the spermatozoa. Leydig cells also help regulate blood flow in the intertubular microvasculature [6]. Sertoli cells, in turn, deliver different growth factors, and various germ cells participate in the development and regulation of germ cells. These factors represent an independent intratesticular regulation of spermatogenesis.

14.8.2 Extrinsic Influences

The hypothalamus and hypophysis control local regulation of spermatogenesis by pulsatile secretion of GnRH and release of LH. Leydig cells produce testosterone, which influences spermatogenesis and provides feedback to the hypophysis that regulates the secretory activity of Leydig cells. FSH action on the Sertoli cells is necessary for maturation of the germ cells. Both FSH and LH are necessary for complete spermatogenesis. Testicular function is determined by interaction between the endocrine and paracrine mechanisms [135, 136]. Sertoli cells secrete inhibin, which functions in the feedback mechanism directed to the hypophysis. Thus, both growth and differentiation of testicular germ cells involve a series of complex interactions between somatic and germinal elements [135, 137, 138].

14.8.3 Immune Status of the Testis

Mature spermatozoa, late pachytene spermatocytes, and spermatids express unique antigens that are not formed until puberty, and therefore, immune tolerance is not developed. Considering that the blood-testis barrier develops as these autoantigens develop, the testis is regarded an immune-privileged site, i.e., transplanted foreign tissue can survive for a period of time without immunological rejection. Yet, an immune surveillance is present in the testis and the epididymis, which shows an active immunoregulation to prevent autoimmune disease [139, 140].

14.8.4 Disturbances of Spermatogenesis

Disturbances in both proliferation and differentiation of the male germ cells and the intratesticular and extratesticular mechanisms regulating spermatogenesis can occur as a result of environmental influences or as a result of diseases that directly or indirectly affect spermatogenesis [141, 142]. In addition, nutrition, therapeutic drugs, hormones and their metabolites, increased scrotal temperature, toxic substances, and radiation can reduce or completely inhibit spermatogenesis. Thus, all these series of changes are necessary to transform the stem cells into fully mature, functional spermatozoa equipped to fertilize an egg (Fig. 14.7).

14.9 Sperm Transport in the Epididymis, Storage, and Capacitation

The epididymis is an androgen-dependent organ with both absorptive and secretory functions that lies along the dorsolateral border of each testis. It comprises the vasa efferentia, which emanates from the rete testis and the epididymal ducts and is divided into three functionally distinct regions: the head, body, and tail, otherwise known as the caput epididymis, corpus epididymis, and cauda epididymis, respectively. Its primary function is post-testicular maturation and storage of spermatozoa during their passage from the testis to the vas deferens. Much of the testicular fluid that transports spermatozoa from the seminiferous tubules is reabsorbed in the caput, thereby increasing the concentration of the spermatozoa by 10- to 100-fold. As the newly developed spermatozoa pass through these regions of the epididymis, many changes occur including alterations in net surface charge, membrane protein composition, immunoreactivity, phospholipid and fatty acid content, and adenylate cyclase activity.

14.9.1 Epididymal Sperm Storage

As many as half of the spermatozoa released from the testis die and disintegrate within the epididymis and are reabsorbed by the epididymal epithelium. The remaining mature spermatozoa are stored in the cauda epididymis providing a capacity for repetitive fertile ejaculations. This storage capacity decreases distally, and the spermatozoa in the vas deferens may only be motile for a few days. After prolonged sexual activity, caudal spermatozoa first lose their fertilizing ability, followed by their motility and then their vitality; they ultimately disintegrate. Older, senescent spermatozoa must be eliminated from the male tract at regular intervals. Otherwise, their relative contribution to the next ejaculate(s) increases, reducing semen quality, even though such ejaculates do have a high sperm concentration. The vas deferens is not a physiological site of sperm storage and contains only about 2% of the total spermatozoa in the male tract. Sperms transit through the fine tubules of the epididymis in approximately 10–15 days in humans.

Sperm mature outside the testis but have very limited motility or none at all and are incapable of fertilizing an egg while still being within the testis. Both epididymal maturation and capacitation are necessary before fertilization. Capacitation is the final step required for fertilization and involves the elimination of the so-called de-capacitation factors that are added on the sperm plasma membranes during testicular development and epididymal maturation. This function may be an evolutionary consequence of the development of a storage system for inactive sperm in the caudal epididymis. Preservation of optimal sperm function during this period of storage requires adequate testosterone levels in the circulation.

14.9.2 Capacitation and Acrosome Reaction

Capacitation is a series of cellular or physiological changes that spermatozoa must undergo in order to fertilize an egg [143, 144]. It is characterized by the ability to undergo the acrosome reaction, bind to the zona pellucida, and acquire hypermotility. During capacitation, the seminal plasma factors that coat the surface of the sperm are removed, and the surface charge is modified along with the sperm membrane, sterols, lipids, and glycoproteins and the outer acrosomal membrane lying immediately under it. Levels of intracellular free calcium also increase [145].

The acrosome reaction enables sperm to penetrate the zona pellucida and also spurs the fusogenic state in the plasmalemma overlying the nonreactive equatorial segment, which is needed for interaction with the oolemma. The changes termed as "acrosome reaction" prepare the sperm to fuse with the egg membrane and involve the removal of cholesterol from the surface membrane in preparation for the acrosome reaction [146, 147]. In addition, d-mannose-binding lectins are also involved in the binding of human sperm to the zona pellucida [148, 149]. Thus, all these series of changes are necessary to transform the stem cells into fully mature, functional spermatozoa equipped to fertilize an egg (Fig. 14.7).

14.10 Conclusion

The testis is an immune-privileged site in the adluminal compartment that is set up in the blood-testis barrier and provides a microenvironment for spermatogenesis to occur. The seminiferous tubules are the site of sperm production. The process of differentiation of a spermatogonium into a spermatid is known as spermatogenesis. It involves both mitotic and meiotic proliferation as well as extensive cell remodeling. In humans, the process of spermatogenesis starts at puberty and continues throughout life. Spermatogenesis produces genetic material necessary for the replication of the species. Meiosis assures genetic diversity. Along the length of the seminiferous tubule, there are only certain cross sections where spermatozoa are released. Sperm production is a continuous and not a pulsatile process. Spermatozoa are highly specialized cells that do not grow or divide. The spermatogenic process is maintained by different intrinsic and extrinsic influences. Proper expression of genes is a prerequisite for regulation of mitosis, meiosis, apoptosis, and maintenance of genomic integrity, which is important for reproduction and survival of the species. Oxidative stress together with apoptosis specifically during spermiogenesis is the key event in the etiology of DNA damage resulting in defective spermatogenesis. Aberrations in recombination, defective chromatin packaging, abortive apoptosis, and oxidative stress are all involved in the etiology of DNA damage in the germ line. Controlling of oxidative stress experienced by the germ cells during differentiation and maturation is important. Spermatozoa have to undergo a series of changes such as capacitation and acrosome reaction before they can fertilize.

References

1. Wilson JD. Syndromes of androgen resistance. Biol Reprod. 1992;46:168–73.
2. Lubahn DB, Moyer JS, Golding TS, Couse JF, Korach KS, Smithies O. Alteration of reproductive function but not prenatal sexual development after insertional disruption of the mouse estrogen receptor gene. Proc Natl Acad Sci U S A. 1993;90:11162–6.
3. Smith EP, Boyd J, Frank GR, Takahashi H, Cohen RM, Specker B, Williams TC, Lubahn DB, Korach KS. Estrogen resistance caused by a mutation in the estrogen-receptor gene in a man. N Engl J Med. 1994;331:1056–61.
4. Tishler PV. Diameter of testicles. N Engl J Med. 1971;285:1489.
5. Winter JS, Faiman C. Pituitary-gonadal relations in male children and adolescents. Pediatr Res. 1972;6:126–35.
6. Middendorff R, Müller D, Mewe M, Mukhopadhyay AK, Holstein AF, Davidoff MS. The tunica albuginea of the human testis is characterized by complex contraction and relaxation activities regulated by cyclic GMP. J Clin Endocrinol Metab. 2002;87:3486–99.
7. Prader A. Testicular size: assessment and clinical importance. Triangle; Sandoz J Med Sci. 1966;7:240–3.
8. Agger P. Scrotal and testicular temperature: its relation to sperm count before and after operation for varicocele. Fertil Steril. 1971;22:286–97.
9. de Kretser DM, Temple-Smith PD, Kerr JB. Anatomical and functional aspects of the male reproductive organs. In: Bandhauer K, Fricks JB, editors. Handbook of urology, vol. XVI. Berlin: Springer-Verlag; 1982. p. 1–131.
10. Christensen AK. Leydig cells. In: Hamilton DW, Greep RO, editors. Handbook of physiology. Baltimore: Williams and Wilkins; 1975. p. 57–94.
11. Kaler LW, Neaves WB. Attrition of the human Leydig cell population with advancing age. Anat Rec. 1978;192:513–8.
12. de Kretser DM, Kerr JB. The cytology of the testis. In: Knobill E, Neil JD, editors. The physiology of reproduction. New York: Raven Press; 1994. p. 1177–290.
13. Payne AH, Wong KL, Vega MM. Differential effects of single and repeated administrations of gonadotropins on luteinizing hormone receptors and testosterone synthesis in two populations of Leydig cells. J Biol Chem. 1980;255:7118–22.
14. Glover TD, Barratt CLR, Tyler JJP, Hennessey JF. Human male fertility. London: Academic; 1980. p. 247.
15. Ewing LL, Keeney DS. Leydig cells: structure and function. In: Desjardins C, Ewin LL, editors. Cell and molecular biology of the testis. New York: Oxford University Press; 1993.
16. Davidoff MS, Breucker H, Holstein AF, Seidel K. Cellular architecture of the lamina propria of human tubules. Cell Tissue Res. 1990;262:253–61.
17. Roosen-Runge EC, Holstein A. The human rete testis. Cell Tissue Res. 1978;189:409–33.
18. de França LR, Ghosh S, Ye SJ, Russell LD. Surface and surface-to-volume relationships of the Sertoli cell during the cycle of the seminiferous epithelium in the rat. Biol Reprod. 1993;49:1215–28.

19. Russell LD, Griswold MD. In: Russell LD, Griswold MD, editors. The Sertoli cell. Clearwater: Cache Press; 1993.
20. Behringer RR. The Müllerian inhibitor and mammalian sexual development. Philos Trans R Soc Lond: Ser B Biol Sci. 1995;350:285–8.
21. Josso N, di Clemente N, Gouédard L. Anti-Müllerian hormone and its receptors. Mol Cell Endocrinol. 2001;179:25–32.
22. Clermont Y. The cycle of the seminiferous epithelium in man. Am J Anat. 1963;112:35–51.
23. Clermont Y. Kinetics of spermatogenesis in mammals: seminiferous epithelium cycle and spermatogonial renewal. Physiol Rev. 1972;52:198–236.
24. Schulze C. Morphological characteristics of the spermatogonial stem cells in man. Cell Tissue Res. 1974;198:191–9.
25. Clermont Y, Bustos-Obregon E. Re-examination of spermatogonial renewal in the rat by means of seminiferous tubules mounted "in toto". Am J Anat. 1968;122:237–47.
26. Huckins C. The spermatogonial stem cell population in adult rats. I. Their morphology, proliferation and maturation. Anat Rec. 1971;169:533–57.
27. Dym M, Fawcett DW. Further observations on the numbers of spermatogonia, spermatocytes, and spermatids connected by intercellular bridges in the mammalian testis. Biol Reprod. 1971;4:195–215.
28. Berezney R, Coffey DS. Nuclear matrix. Isolation and characterization of a framework structure from rat liver nuclei. J Cell Biol. 1977;73:616–37.
29. Mirkovitch J, Mirault ME, Laemmli UK. Organization of the higher-order chromatin loop: specific DNA attachment sites on nuclear scaffold. Cell. 1984;39:223–32.
30. Gasse S. Studies on scaffold attachment sites and their relation to genome function. Int Rev Cytol. 1989;119:57.
31. Adachi Y, Kas E, Laemmli UK. Preferential cooperative binding of DNA topoisomerase II to scaffold-associated regions. EMBO J. 1989;13:3997.
32. Izaurralde E, Kas E, Laemmli UK. Highly preferential nucleation of histone H1 assembly on scaffold-associated regions. J Mol Biol. 1989;210:573–85.
33. Dickinson LA, Joh T, Kohwi Y, Kohwi-Shigematsu T. A tissue-specific MAR/SAR DNA-binding protein with unusual binding site recognition. Cell. 1992;70:631–45.
34. Orthwein A, Fradet-Turcotte A, Noordermeer SM, Canny MD, Brun CM, Strecker J, Escribano-Diaz C, Durocher D. Mitosis inhibits DNA double-strand break repair to guard against telomere fusions. Science. 2015;344:189–93.
35. Bauché F, Fouchard MH, Jégou B. Antioxidant system in rat testicular cells. FEBS Lett. 1994;349:392–6.
36. Breucker H, Schäfer E, Holstein AF. Morphogenesis and fate of the residual body in human spermiogenesis. Cell Tissue Res. 1985;240:303–9.
37. Leblond CP, Clermont Y. Definition of the stages of the cycle of the seminiferous epithelium in the rat. Ann N Y Acad Sci. 1952;55:548–73.
38. Clermont Y, Perey B. The stages of the cycle of the seminiferous epithelium of the rat: practical definitions in PA-Schiff-hematoxylin and hematoxylin-eosin stained sections. Rev Can Biol. 1957;16:451–62.
39. Schulze W, Rehder U. Organization and morphogenesis of the human seminiferous epithelium. Cell Tissue Res. 1984;237:395–407.
40. Ward WS, Coffey DS. DNA packaging and organization in mammalian spermatozoa: comparison with somatic cells. Biol Reprod. 1991;44:569–74.
41. McGhee JD, Felsenfeld G, Eisenberg H. Nucleosome structure and conformational changes. Biophys J. 1980;32:261–70.
42. Sassone-Corsi P. Unique chromatin remodeling and transcriptional regulation in spermatogenesis. Science. 2002;296:2176–8.
43. Dadoune JP, Siffroi JP, Alfonsi MF. Transcription in haploid male germ cells. Int Rev Cytol. 2004;237:1–56.

44. Ward WS, Partin AW, Coffey DS. DNA loop domains in mammalian spermatozoa. Chromosoma. 1989;98:153–9.
45. McPherson S, Longo FJ. Chromatin structure-function alterations during mammalian spermatogenesis: DNA nicking and repair in elongating spermatids. Eur J Histochem. 1993;37:109–28.
46. Allen MJ, Lee C, Lee JD 4th, Pogany GC, Balooch M, Siekhaus WJ, Balhorn R. Atomic force microscopy of mammalian sperm chromatin. Chromosoma. 1993;102:623–30.
47. Lewis JD, Abbott DW, Ausió J. A haploid affair: core histone transitions during spermatogenesis. Biochem Cell Biol. 2003a;81:131–40.
48. Lewis JD, Song Y, de Jong ME, Bagha SM, Ausió J. A walk though vertebrate and invertebrate protamines. Chromosoma. 2003b;111:473–82.
49. Braun RE. Packaging paternal chromosomes with protamine. Nat Genet. 2001;28:10–2.
50. Wu TF, Chu DS. Sperm chromatin: fertile grounds for proteomic discovery of clinical tools. Mol Cell Proteomics. 2008;7:1876–86.
51. Ooi SL, Henikoff S. Germline histone dynamics and epigenetics. Curr Opin Cell Biol. 2007;19:257–65.
52. Cho C, Willis WD, Goulding EH, Jung-Ha H, Choi YC, Hecht NB, Eddy EM. Haploinsufficiency of protamine-1 or -2 causes infertility in mice. Nat Genet. 2001;28:82–6.
53. Yu YE, Zhang Y, Unni E, Shirley CR, Deng JM, Russell LD, Weil MM, Behringer RR, Meistrich ML. Abnormal spermatogenesis and reduced fertility in transition nuclear protein 1-deficient mice. Proc Natl Acad Sci U S A. 2000;97:4683–8.
54. Zhao M, Shirley CR, Yu YE, Mohapatra B, Zhang Y, Unni E, Deng JM, Arango NA, Terry NH, Weil MM, Russell LD, Behringer RR, Meistrich ML. Targeted disruption of the transition protein 2 gene affects sperm chromatin structure and reduces fertility in mice. Mol Cell Biol. 2001;21:7243–55.
55. Churikov D, Zalenskaya IA, Zalensky AO. Male germline-specific histones in mouse and man. Cytogenet Genome Res. 2004;105:203–14.
56. Dadoune JP. The nuclear status of human sperm cells. Micron. 1995;26:323–45.
57. Lee CH, Cho YH. Aspects of mammalian spermatogenesis: electrophoretical analysis of protamines in mammalian species. Mol Cells. 1999;9:556–9.
58. Kierszenbaum AL. Transition nuclear proteins during spermiogenesis: unrepaired DNA breaks not allowed. Mol Reprod Dev. 2001;58:357–8.
59. Bench GS, Friz AM, Corzett MH, Morse DH, Balhorn R. DNA and total protamine masses in individual sperm from fertile mammalian subjects. Cytometry. 1996;23:263–71.
60. Gatewood JM, Cook GR, Balhorn R, Bradbury EM, Schmid CW. Sequence-specific packaging of DNA in human sperm chromatin. Science. 1987;236:962–4.
61. McPherson SM, Longo FJ. Nicking of rat spermatid and spermatozoa DNA: possible involvement of DNA topoisomerase II. Dev Biol. 1993a;158:122–30.
62. Marcon L, Boissonneault G. Transient DNA strand breaks during mouse and human spermiogenesis new insights in stage specificity and link to chromatin remodeling. Biol Reprod. 2004;70:910–8.
63. Laberge RM, Boissonneault G. On the nature and origin of DNA strand breaks in elongating spermatids. Biol Reprod. 2005;73:289–96.
64. Muratori M, Marchiani S, Maggi M, Forti G, Baldi E. Origin and biological significance of DNA fragmentation in human spermatozoa. Front Biosci. 2006;11:1491–9.
65. Zhao M, Shirley CR, Mounsey S, Meistrich ML. Nucleoprotein transitions during spermiogenesis in mice with transition nuclear protein Tnp1 and Tnp2 mutations. Biol Reprod. 2004;71:1016–25.
66. Meistrich ML. Calculation of the incidence of infertility in human populations from sperm measures using the two-distribution model. Prog Clin Biol Res. 1989;302:275–85.
67. Heidaran MA, Showman RM, Kistler WS. A cytochemical study of the transcriptional and translational regulation of nuclear transition protein 1 (TP1), a major chromosomal protein of mammalian spermatids. J Cell Biol. 1988;106:1427–33.

68. Alfonso PJ, Kistler WS. Immunohistochemical localization of spermatid nuclear transition protein 2 in the testes of rats and mice. Biol Reprod. 1993;48:522–9.
69. de Yebra L, Ballescá JL, Vanrell JA, Corzett M, Balhorn R, Oliva R. Detection of P2 precursors in the sperm cells of infertile patients who have reduced protamine P2 levels. Fertil Steril. 1998;69:755–9.
70. Oliva R. Protamines and male infertility. Hum Reprod Update. 2006;12:417–35.
71. Chevaillier P, Mauro N, Feneux D, Jouannet P, David G. Anomalous protein complement of sperm nuclei in some infertile men. Lancet. 1987;2:806–7.
72. Balhorn R, Reed S, Tanphaichitr N. Aberrant protamine 1/protamine 2 ratios in sperm of infertile human males. Experientia. 1988;44:52–5.
73. Aoki VW, Moskovtsev SI, Willis J, Liu L, Mullen JB, Carrell DT. DNA integrity is compromised in protamine-deficient human sperm. J Androl. 2005;26:741–8.
74. Fuentes-Mascorro G, Serrano H, Rosado A. Sperm chromatin. Arch Androl. 2000;45:215–25.
75. Dixon GH, Aiken JM, Jankowski JM, McKenzie D, Moir R, States JC. Organization and evolution of protamine gene of salmoind fishes. In: Reeck GR, Goodwin GH, Puigdomenech P, editors. Chromosomal proteins and gene expression. New York: Plenum Publishing Corp; 1986.
76. Krawetz SA, Dixon GH. Sequence similarities of the protamine genes: implications for regulation and evolution. J Mol Evol. 1988;27:291–7.
77. Brewer L, Corzett M, Balhorn R. Condensation of DNA by spermatid basic nuclear proteins. J Biol Chem. 2002;277:38895–900.
78. Balhorn R, Cosman M, Thornton K, Krishnan VV, Corzett M, Bench G, Kramer C, Lee J, Hud NV, Allen MJ, et al. In: Gagnon C, editor. The male gamete: from basic science to clinical applications. Vienna: Cache River Press; 1999.
79. Sakkas D, Mariethoz E, Manicardi G, et al. Origin of DNA damage in ejaculated human spermatozoa. Rev Reprod. 1999;4:31–7.
80. Trasler JM. Epigenetics in spermatogenesis. Mol Cell Endocrinol. 2009;306:33–6.
81. Oakes CC, La Salle S, Smiraglia DJ, Robaire B, Trasler JM. Developmental acquisition of genome-wide DNA methylation occurs prior to meiosis in male germ cells. Dev Biol. 2007;307:368–79.
82. Benchaib M, Braun V, Lornage J, et al. Sperm DNA fragmentation decreases the pregnancy rate in an assisted reproductive technique. Hum Reprod. 2003;18:1023–8.
83. Risley MS, Einheber S, Bumcrot DA. Changes in DNA topology during spermatogenesis. Chromosoma. 1986;94:217–27.
84. Ward WS. The structure of the sleeping genome: implications of sperm DNA organization for somatic cells. J Cell Biochem. 1994;55:77–82.
85. Aitken RJ, De Iuliis GN. On the possible origins of DNA damage in human spermatozoa. Mol Hum Reprod. 2010;16:3–13.
86. Cummins JM. Fertilization and elimination of the paternal mitochondrial genome. Hum Reprod. 2000;15:92–101.
87. Donnelly ET, O'Connell M, McClure N, Lewis SE. Differences in nuclear DNA fragmentation and mitochondrial integrity of semen and prepared human spermatozoa. Hum Reprod. 2000;15:1552–61.
88. Crow JF. The high spontaneous mutation rate: is it a health risk? ProcNat Acad Sci USA. 1997;94:8380–6.
89. Aitken RJ, De Iuliis GN, McLachlan RI. Biological and clinical significance of DNA damage in the male germ line. Int J Androl. 2009;32:46–56.
90. Carrell DT, Emery BR, Hammoud S. The aetiology of sperm protamine abnormalities and their potential impact on the sperm epigenome. Int J Androl. 2008;31:537–45.
91. De Iuliis GN, Thomson LK, Mitchell LA, Finnie JM, Koppers AJ, Hedges A, Nixon B, Aitken RJ. DNA damage in human spermatozoa is highly correlated with the efficiency of chromatin remodeling and the formation of 8-hydroxy-2′-deoxyguanosine, a marker of oxidative stress. Biol Reprod. 2009;81:517–24.

92. Kramer JA, Krawetz SA. Nuclear matrix interactions within the sperm genome. J Biol Chem. 1996;271:11619–22.
93. Ward WS, Kimura Y, Yanagimachi R. An intact sperm nuclear matrix may be necessary for the mouse paternal genome to participate in embryonic development. Biol Reprod. 1999;60:702–6.
94. Casanueva FF, Villanueva L, Dieguez C, Diaz Y, Cabranes JA, Szoke B, Scanlon MF, Schally AV, Fernandez-Cruz A. Free fatty acids block growth hormone (GH) releasing hormone-stimulated GH secretion in man directly at the pituitary. J Clin Endocrinol Metab. 1987;65:634–42.
95. Nieschlag E, Leifke E. Empirical therapies for idiopathic infertility. In: Nieschlag E, Behre HM, editors. Andrology: male reproductive health and dysfunction, vol. 12. Heidelberg: Springer; 1997. p. 313–9.
96. Ferlin A, Speltra E, Patassini C, Pati MA, Garolla A, Caretta N, Foresta C. Heat shock protein and heat shock factor expression in sperm: relation to oligozoospermia and varicocele. J Urol. 2010;183:1248–52.
97. Rendtorff R, Hohmann C, Reinmuth S, Müller A, Dittrich R, Beyer M, Wickmann L, Keil T, Henze G, Staudt BA. Hormone and sperm analyses after chemo- and radiotherapy in childhood and adolescence. Klin Padiatr. 2010;222:145–9.
98. Print CG, Loveland KL. Germ cell suicide: new insights into apoptosis during spermatogenesis. Bioassays. 2000;22:423–30.
99. Martincic DS, Virant Klun I, Zorn B, Vrtovec HM. Germ cell apoptosis in the human testis. Pflugers Arch. 2001;442:59–60.
100. Weng SL, Taylor SL, Morshedi M, Schuffner A, Duran EH, Beebe S, Oehninger S. Caspase activity and apoptotic markers in ejaculated human sperm. Mol Hum Reprod. 2002;8:984–91.
101. Sinha Hikim AP, Swerdloff RS. Hormonal and genetic control of germ cell apoptosis in the testis. Rev Reprod. 1999;4:38–47.
102. Rodriguez I, Ody C, Araki K, Garcia I, Vassalli P. An early and massive wave of germinal cell apoptosis is required for the development of functional spermatogenesis. EMBO J. 1997;16:2262–70.
103. Sakkas D, Seli E, Bizzaro D, Tarozzi N, Manicardi GC. Abnormal spermatozoa in the ejaculate: abortive apoptosis and faulty nuclear remodelling during spermatogenesis. Reprod Biomed Online. 2003;7:428–32.
104. Epstein J. Male genital system and urinary tract infection. In: Robbins Basic Pathology, editors. Kumar V, Abbas AK, Aster JC. Ninth Edition, Elsevier Saunders, PA; 2012. p. 651–680.
105. Martin SJ, Reutelingsperger CP, McGahon AJ, Rader JA, Van Schie RC, Laface DM, Green DR. Early redistribution of plasma membrane phosphatidylserine is a general feature of apoptosis regardless of the initiating stimulus: inhibition by overexpression of Bcl-2 and Abl. J Exp Med. 1995;182:1545–56.
106. Sakkas D, Mariethoz E, St John JC. Abnormal sperm parameters in humans are indicative of an abortive apoptotic mechanism linked to the Fas-mediated pathway. Exp Cell Res. 1999b;251:350–5.
107. Fraga CG, Motchnik PA, Wyrobek AJ, Rempel DM, Ames BN. Smoking and low antioxidant levels increase oxidative damage to sperm DNA. Mutat Res. 1996;351:199–203.
108. Grunewald S, Paasch U, Glander HJ, Anderegg U. Mature human spermatozoa do not transcribe novel RNA. Andrologia. 2005;37:69–71.
109. Meyer-Ficca ML, Lonchar J, Credidio C, Ihara M, Li Y, Wang ZQ, Meyer RG. Disruption of poly(ADP-ribose) homeostasis affects spermiogenesis and sperm chromatin integrity in mice. Biol Reprod. 2009;81:46–55.
110. Bianchi PG, Manicardi GC, Bizzaro D, Bianchi U, Sakkas D. Effect of deoxyribonucleic acid protamination on fluorochrome staining and in situ nick-translation of murine and human mature spermatozoa. Biol Reprod. 1993;49:1083–8.
111. Irvine DS, Twigg JP, Gordon EL, Fulton N, Milne PA, Aitken RJ. DNA integrity in human spermatozoa: relationships with semen quality. J Androl. 2000;21:33–44.

112. Aitken RJ, Gordon E, Harkiss D, Twigg JP, Milne P, Jennings Z, Irvine DS. Relative impact of oxidative stress on the functional competence and genomic integrity of human spermatozoa. Biol Reprod. 1998;59:1037–46.
113. Piña-Guzmán B, Solís-Heredia MJ, Rojas-García AE, Urióstegui-Acosta M, Quintanilla-Vega B. Genetic damage caused by methyl-parathion in mouse spermatozoa is related to oxidative stress. Toxicol Appl Pharmacol. 2006;216:216–24.
114. Zubkova EV, Robaire B. Effects of ageing on spermatozoal chromatin and its sensitivity to in vivo and in vitro oxidative challenge in the Brown Norway rat. Hum Reprod. 2006;11:2901–10.
115. Heller C, Clermont Y. Kinetics of the germinal epithelium in man. Recent Prog Horm Res. 1964;20:545–75.
116. Sculze W, Salzbrunn A. Spatial and quantitative aspects of spermatogenetic tissue in primates. In: Neischlag E, Habenicht U, editors. Spermatogenesis-fertilization-contraception. Berlin: Springer, New York; 1992. p. 267–83.
117. World Health Organization. WHO laboratory manual for the examination and processing of human semen. 5th ed. Geneva: WHO Press; 2010.
118. Sharpe RM. Regulation of spermatogenesis. In: Knobill E, Neil JD, editors. The physiology of reproduction. New York: Raven Press; 1994. p. 1363–434.
119. De Kretser DM. Ultrastructural features of human spermiogenesis. Z Zellforsch Mikrosk Anat. 1969;98:477–505.
120. Hoeijmakers JH. DNA damage, aging, and cancer. N Engl J Med. 2009;361:1475–85.
121. Gillet LC, Scharer OD. Molecular mechanisms of mammalian global genome nucleotide excision repair. Chem Rev. 2006;106:253–76.
122. Lyama T, Wilson DM. DNA repair mechanisms in dividing and non-dividing cells. DNA Repair (Amst). 2013;12:620–36.
123. Boiteux S, Radicella JP. Base excision repair of 8-hydroxyguanine protects DNA from endogenous oxidative stress. Biochimie. 1999;81:59–67.
124. Aitken RJ, Smith TB, Jobling MS, Baker MA, De Iuliis GN. Oxidative stress and male reproductive health. Asian J Androl. 2014;16:31–8.
125. Shimura T, Inoue M, Taga M, Shiraishi K, Uematsu N, Takei N, Yuan ZM, Shinohara T, Niwa O. p53-dependent S-phase damage checkpoint and pronuclear cross talk in mouse zygotes with X-irradiated sperm. Mol Cell Biol. 2002;22:2220–8.
126. Champe PC, Harvey RA, Ferrier DR. DNA structure and replication. In: Lippincott's illustrated reviews: biochemistry. 3rd ed. London: Lippincott Williams & Wilkins; 2005. p. 393–412.
127. Gordon FKE, Lamb DJ. DNA repair genes and genomic instability in severe male factor infertility. In: Carrell DT, editor. The genetics of male infertility. New York: Humana Press; 2006.
128. You Z, Bailis JM. DNA damage and decisions: CtIP coordinates DNA repair and cell cycle checkpoints. Trends Cell Biol. 2010;20:402–9.
129. Stracker TH, Petrini JH. The MRE11 complex: starting from the ends. Nat Rev Mol Cell Biol. 2011;12:90–103.
130. Kohl KP, Sekelsky J. Meiotic and mitotic recombination in meiosis. Genetics. 2013;194:327–34.
131. Hou CC, Yang WX. New insights to the ubiquitin-proteasome pathway (UPP) mechanism during spermatogenesis. Mol Biol Rep. 2013;40:3213–30.
132. Koczorowska AM, Bialkowska A, Kluzek K, Zdzienicka MZ. The role of the Fanconi anemia pathway in DNA repair and maintenance of genome stability. Postepy Hig Med Dosw. 2014;68:459–72.
133. Simhadri S, Peterson S, Patel D, Huo Y, Cai H, Bowman-Colin C, Miller S, Ludwig T, Ganesan S, Bhaumik M, Bunting S, Jasin M, Xia B. Male fertility defect associated with disrupted BRCA1-PALB2 interaction in mice. J Biol Chem. 2014;289:24617–29.
134. Jegou B. The Sertoli cell. Bailliere Clin Endocrinol Metab. 1992;6:273–311.

135. Bellve AR, Zheng W. Growth factors as autocrine and paracrine modulators of male gonadal functions. J Reprod Fertil. 1989;85:771–93.
136. Skinner MK. Cell-cell interactions in the testis. Endocr Rev. 1991;12:45–77.
137. Sharpe T. Intratesticular control of steroidogenesis. Clin Endocrinol. 1990;33:787–807.
138. Sharpe RM. Monitoring of spermatogenesis in man-measurement of Sertoli cell- or germ cell-secreted proteins in semen or blood. Int J Androl. 1992;15:201–10.
139. Mahi-Brown CA, Yule TD, Tung KS. Evidence for active immunological regulation in prevention of testicular autoimmune disease independent of the blood-testis barrier. Am J Reprod Immunol Microbiol. 1988;16:165–70.
140. Barratt CL, Bolton AE, Cooke ID. Functional significance of white blood cells in the male and female reproductive tract. Hum Reprod. 1990;5:639–48.
141. Holstein AF, Schulze W, Breucker H. Histopathology of human testicular and epididymal tissue. In: Hargreave TB, editor. Male infertility. London: Springer; 1994. p. 105–48.
142. Nieschlag E, Behre H. Andrology. Male reproductive health and dysfunction. Berlin: Springer; 2001.
143. Eddy EM, O'Brien DA. The spermatozoon. In: Knobill EO, NO'Nneill JD, editors. The physiology of reproduction. New York: Raven Press; 1994.
144. Yanagamachi R. Mammalian Fertilization. In: Knobill E, O'Brien NJ, editors. The physiology of reproduction. New York: Raven Press; 1994.
145. Thomas P, Meizel S. Phosphatidylinositol 4,5-bisphosphate hydrolysis in human sperm stimulated with follicular fluid or progesterone is dependent upon Ca2+ influx. Biochem J. 1989;264:539–46.
146. Parks JE, Ehrenwalt E. Cholesterol efflux from mammalian sperm and its potential role in capacitation. In: Bavister BD, Cummins J, Raldon E, editors. Fertilization in mammals. Norwell: Serono Symposia; 1990.
147. Ravnik SE, Zarutskie PW, Muller CH. Purification and characterization of a human follicular fluid lipid transfer protein that stimulates human sperm capacitation. Biol Reprod. 1992;47:1126–33.
148. Benoff S, Cooper GW, Hurley I, Mandel FS, Rosenfeld DL. Antisperm antibody binding to human sperm inhibits capacitation induced changes in the levels of plasma membrane sterols. Am J Reprod Immunol. 1993;30:113–30.
149. Benoff S, Hurley I, Cooper GW, Mandel FS, Hershlag A, Scholl GM, et al. Fertilization potential in vitro is correlated with head-specific mannose-ligand receptor expression, acrosome status and membrane cholesterol content. Hum Reprod. 1993;8:2155–66.

Chapter 15
Sperm Chromatin and Lifestyle Factors

Sarah K. Fatool and Avi Harlev

15.1 Introduction

DNA fragmentation refers to an accumulation of multiple double-stranded DNA breaks that are not repairable by nuclear proteins. Sperm have limited repair mechanisms and, thus, are more susceptible to oxidative stress, which may lead to DNA fragmentation [1, 2]. In addition, sperm DNA fragmentation can occur during spermatogenesis, and in fact, excessive DNA fragmentation is an indicator of apoptosis.

Men with a high percentage of sperm DNA fragmentation are more likely to be infertile and have abnormal offspring [3]. The loss of sperm DNA integrity affects practically every stage of conception and embryo development [3].

Furthermore, DNA fragmentation is a predictor of infertility in couples with unknown fertility status [4]. After establishing the significant difference in sperm DNA fragmentation in couples with successful IVF treatment to those who failed (33.8 ± 3.6% vs. 68.5 ± 2.3%, $p < 0.001$), Simon et al. [5] reported that men with DNA fragmentation of over 25% are more likely to fail IVF treatment with a sensitivity of 63.6% and a specificity of 93.3%) [5]. Moreover, such ability of sperm DNA fragmentation in predicting infertility was found to be consistent regardless of the DNA fragmentation assay used: DFI, SCSA, TUNEL, or comet [3].

Sperm DNA fragmentation begets inferior embryos. In a sample of couples undergoing IVF, men with high sperm DNA fragmentation produced embryos of lower quality [5]. In mice models, embryos fertilized with DNA-fragmented sperm

S.K. Fatool
Faculty of Health Sciences, Medical School for International Health,
Ben-Gurion University of the Negev, Be'er Sheva, Israel

Soroka University Medical Center, Ben-Gurion University of the Negev, Be'er Sheva, Israel
e-mail: sarahkrl8@gmail.com

A. Harlev (✉)
Soroka University Medical Center, Ben-Gurion University of the Negev, Be'er Sheva, Israel
e-mail: harlev@bgu.ac.il

A. Zini, A. Agarwal (eds.), *A Clinician's Guide to Sperm DNA and Chromatin Damage*, https://doi.org/10.1007/978-3-319-71815-6_15

using intracytoplasmic sperm injection (ICSI) grew slower than those embryos fertilized with normal sperm [6]. If implantation did occur, the mouse fetus would often not survive to term [6]. Such findings mirror the observations seen in fertility [7] and IVF clinics [8]. In mice models, when ICSI is performed using sperm with high DNA fragmentation, the offspring had a shorter lifespan, organomegaly, and solid tumors, while the female offspring showed increased anxiety, deficit in short-term special memory, and age-dependent hypolocomotion ($p < 0.5$) [6]. Therefore, distinguishing factors that damage sperm DNA may help to improve reproductive outcomes.

The objectives of this chapter are to identify lifestyle factors that affect sperm DNA integrity, investigate mechanism(s) for such damage, explore alleviating factors, and propose future investigations. Although there are many different lifestyle factors that are involved, the most relevant topics have been selected for discussion, including obesity, nutrition, smoking, alcohol consumption, and radiation.

15.2 Mechanisms of DNA Fragmentation

Impaired spermatogenesis, abortive apoptosis, and oxidative stress are the three primary mechanisms of sperm DNA damage. Spermatogenesis is a dynamic process involving both intracellular development and extracellular signaling, and this process can easily awry if the proper conditions are not maintained. Protamine distribution is an example of the impact of intracellular development on fertility. During spermatogenesis, DNA packaging proteins change from histones to lysine-rich transition proteins, and then replaced by protamines [9]. Protamines are cross-linked with disulfide bonds to maintain DNA stability [10]. Protamine 1 (P1) and protamine 2 (P2) are equally distributed in the sperm DNA, and deficiency of P2 is found to be associated with male infertility [11].

Apoptosis is physiological cell death that plays a major role in regulating sperm development [12]. Fas, a ubiquitously expressed apoptosis initiator, requires Fas ligand (FasL) to begin the apoptotic cascade, and FasL is only expressed in selective cell populations [13]. Sertoli cells express FasL [14] and can reduce spermatozoa population to 25% [15] of its potential in order to prevent abnormal sperm from developing and to keep the sperm population at capacity. After initiation of the apoptotic cascade, the increase in endonuclease activity induces double-stranded DNA breaks. Many sperm that have DNA fragmentation, however, do not have apoptotic signaling molecules and display signs of immaturity [12]. Sakkas et al. proposed that while these sperm are "earmarked" for apoptosis, a malfunction in the Fas/FasL signaling caused the sperm to abort the process [12]. Such "escape" or abortive apoptosis seems to play a role in sperm DNA fragmentation in smoking [16], alcohol [17–19], and radiation exposures [20].

Oxidative stress in semen primarily originates from leukocytes and, in lesser amount, from the mitochondria and dead sperm. Within the sperm, mitochondria house the electron transport chain (ETC), and the containment of these electrons are important for the redox balance. When electrons leak from Complex I and III in the ETC, intrinsic reactive oxygen species (ROS) are generated [21]. Outside of the sperm cells, the presence of leukocytes is the main contributor to ROS, in part from the production of bactericidal hydrogen peroxide [22]. Oxidative stress from the neighboring dead sperm cells also contributes to the oxidative stress in the ejaculate [23]. Oxidative stress caused by leukocytes and dead sperm, however, was reported to be correlated more with loss of sperm mobility and less with DNA fragmentation [22]. ROS generated from the mitochondria or intrinsic ROS, on the other hand, was found to be present in sperm with higher DNA damage [22].

The ejaculate contains several antioxidant compounds that can reduce ROS levels [24], but sperm have limited capacity to deal with intrinsic oxidative stress and the resulting DNA damage. Sperm that are subjected to large amounts of oxidative stress can lose their mobility [2] and ability to fuse with the oocyte for successful fertilization [2] and may also result in sperm DNA damage. As mentioned before, sperm DNA fragmentation is correlated with infertility [4], impaired early embryo development [5], pregnancy loss [6–8], and poor long-term health outcomes of the offspring [3, 6]. Many modifiable lifestyle factors, such as smoking [25] and toxin exposure [26], and non-modifiable factors, such as age [2], are involved in causing oxidative stress.

While presented separately, defective spermatogenesis, abortive apoptosis, and oxidative stress are intertwined. Some studies have suggested that abortive apoptosis could be caused by oxidative stress [27], while other evidence demonstrates the opposite [28]. Apoptosis is initiated in sperm undergoing defective spermatogenesis. This chapter will address mechanism in more detail in each section.

Obesity rate continues to rise in the United States and globally [29]. The negative effects of obesity on cardiovascular, endocrine, and overall health has led to the hypothesis that there may be a link between obesity and male sub- and infertility. Molecular studies substantiate their suspicions; obesity has been found to increase seminal oxidative stress [30]. In fact, some researchers have proposed a connection between the high rates of obesity in young men [31] and the global decline in sperm quality [32]. After adjusting for marital status, obese men were found to father less children than their normal weight counterparts [33]. Additionally, a Norwegian study found that couples with overweight or obese male partners were more likely to be infertile even when adjusting for female BMI, male and female ages, smoking, and coital frequency (OR 1.36; CI 95% = 1.13–1.63) [34].

Many studies show a clear correlation between obese and overweight men and increased sperm DNA fragmentation [35, 36]. In a recent meta-analysis, Campbell et al. [32] asserted that obese men have a statistically significant increase of sperm with DNA fragmentation compared to their normal weight peers. However, other studies have asserted the opposite conclusion. Bandel et al. [37] pooled several study populations and found that normal weight men had higher DNA fragmentation index (DFI) measurements than overweight men, and there was no correlation between BMI and DNA fragmentation after adjusting for cofounders. The study population primarily consisted of Swedish nationals, and since the effects of oxidative stress has been linked to a complex interaction of exposure and genetics in other lifestyle factors such as smoking, Bandel et al.'s conclusion may only apply to Swedes. Rybar et al. [38] conducted a similar study and also found no association between obesity and DNA fragmentation. However, the obese group was only 16 participants and did not examine morbid obesity as a separate group. So, does obesity cause an increase in sperm DNA fragmentation?

An experiment conducted by Duale et al. [35] on mice models may help to clear up the confusion. DNA fragmentation was studied in three different mice models of obesity: high-fat-diet-induced obesity, leptin-deficient obesity, and leptin-induced obesity on a high-fat diet. In both models, the average sperm DNA fragmentation was higher than the lean controls, as was the variability. Some mice within the experimental group had normal chromatin structure, and others had measurements that indicated infertility [38]. Some obese mice were able to compensate or prevent DNA damage while their genetically similar littermates had a dramatic increase in sperm DNA fragmentation. Finally, sperm DNA damage was nonsignificant ($p < 0.05$) between dietary groups, indicating that a high-fat diet is a possible cofounder. Keeping in mind the importance of cofounders and genetics, more studies are needed to establish a firm connection between obesity and sperm DNA damage if one exists.

If obesity is associated with sperm DNA fragmentation, identifying the mechanism involved is important to mitigate the effects, and several mechanisms have been proposed. Obesity has been established as a low-inflammation state. Tunc et al. [30] identified that an increased BMI was correlated with increased testicular oxidative stress possibly due to seminal macrophages [30]. Obese men also have increased estrogen and decreased testosterone [30], and such hormone imbalance may affect spermatogenesis. Obesity is correlated with scrotal hyperthermia, a known cause of poor sperm quality, and increased fat around the genital region may be the mechanism involved [39]. Other researchers have proposed that cofounders, such as diet and metabolic syndrome [40], and not obesity itself may be responsible for the change in sperm parameters. Hakonsen et al. [41] studied the effect of weight loss on sperm parameters in obese adults. While many sperm parameters improved after weight loss, DFI did not [41]. However, animal models have shown that antioxidants, diet, and exercise may reverse or prevent DNA damage resulting from a high-fat diet [42, 43].

More studies are required in order to further explore the effect of obesity on sperm DNA integrity. During these investigations, researchers should also keep in mind the heterogeneity of the obese population. A patient who has been obese since childhood would possibly have more exposure to oxidative stress than another patient with adult-onset obesity. Fat percentage may be a better indicator than BMI. Morbid obesity should be analyzed separately from obesity in future studies. Finally, if hyperthermia is the mechanism, fat distribution may be the most important variable. Future work should strive to find why obesity affects some men's sperm DNA and not others.

15.3 Nutrition

Diet is another possible factor contributing to sperm DNA damage as nutrition deficiency or overabundance may affect the balance between ROS and antioxidants. Instead of focusing on the effect of specific food groups of sperm DNA fragmentation, Jurewicz et al. [44] examined diet holistically to account for food interactions. Jurewicz et al. [44] surveyed 336 infertile men with respect to their diet. Diets were categorized into a "prudent diet" (fish, chicken fruit, cruciferous vegetables, tomatoes, leafy green vegetables, legumes, and whole grains), a Western diet (red and processed meat, butter, high-fat dairy, refined grains, pizza, snacks, high-energy drinks, mayonnaise, and sweets), and a mixed diet. It was found that men with a prudent diet had a significantly lower DFI (15.20%) than men on mixed (16.04%) or Western (17.98%) diets ($p < 0.05$) [44]. These findings suggest that a Western diet may be responsible for declining sperm quality in Western civilizations. Vujkovic et al. [45] conducted a similar study in subfertile men and found that men who made more health-conscious food choices (diet high in fish, chicken, vegetables, and whole grains) had lower percentage of sperm DNA fragmentation ($p = 0.05$). When stratified by food group, fruits, vegetables, and nuts were significantly associated with lower sperm DNA fragmentation ($p < 0.05$). These studies suggest that a diet with a high amount of fruits, vegetables, and nuts may prevent sperm DNA fragmentation, and a traditional Western diet may increase sperm DNA fragmentation.

While consumption of fruits, vegetables, and nuts seem to be a protective factor for sperm DNA fragmentation, would a diet that consists of only these food groups—vegetarians and vegans—lower the sperm DNA fragmentation? A population study was conducted on lifelong vegans, lacto-ovo-vegetarians, and nonvegetarians, and no difference in chromatin integrity was found between the three groups. Furthermore, vegan and vegetarian diet had a negative impact on other sperm variables [46].

The Western diet has been proven to be damaging to sperm DNA integrity in animal models as well. When compared to those who are fed a normal diet, rats on a high-fat diet have an increase of lipid peroxidation (increase of 30%; $p < 0.05$) [47] and DNA damage ($p < 0.05$) [50]. Two alleviating or protective factors have been identified. Yan et al. [48] found that metformin reduced the number of spermatozoa with DNA damage in rats on a high-fat diet ($p < 0.05$). In fact, metformin reduced DNA damage so much that there was no significant difference between the normal diet group and the metformin group [48]. Another alleviating factor found was change in diet and increased exercise. Palmer et al. [43] investigated rats on a high-fat diet that were put on a diet improvement regimen, exercise program, or both. In all cases with such lifestyle intervention, the sperm DNA damage reduced to that of the lean controls ($p < 0.01$) [43].

Besides diet choice, antioxidant supplementation may prove beneficial in ameliorating sperm DNA damage keeping in mind that the primary mechanism involved in sperm DNA damage is redox imbalance. Dattilo et al. [42] administered an antioxidant cocktail to the male partners of infertile couples who have failed at least two assisted reproduction technology (ART) attempts and had a DFI or SDI greater than 20%. The antioxidant treatment consisted of B vitamins, zinc, opuntia fig extract, N-acetyl-cysteine, and vitamin E, taken one to two times a day for 2–12 months. In addition to half of the men found to have decreased levels in both the SDI and DFI, 20% of the couples achieved a spontaneous pregnancy. The final live birth rate was 39% in the overall study group and 57% in the couples with improved SDI and DFI measurements ($p < 0.001$) [42].

Overall, diet appears to have an impact on sperm DNA fragmentation. A "generally healthy" diet consisting of chicken fish, fruits, vegetables, and nuts is associated with lower rates of sperm DNA fragmentation, while a high-fat and Western diet is associated with more oxidative stress and subsequently DNA damage. Lifestyle modifications including diet change and exercise as well as medication such as metformin are the potential solutions to alleviate the sperm DNA damage caused by high-fat diet. Antioxidant supplements may also be potentially useful for infertile couples with a high DFI.

15.4 Smoking

In addition to the numerous detrimental effects cigarette smoking has on the cardiovascular and pulmonary systems, the carcinogenic and genotoxic nature of its substance causes cancer in multiple systems including the testes. In spite of numerous campaigns held to end smoking by the World Health Organization (WHO), over 1.1 billion smokers still burden the health care system globally [49]. Furthermore, the rates of smokers are on the rising trend in Eastern Mediterranean and African countries [49], so immigrants from these countries should also be thoroughly questioned about their smoking habits and secondhand smoke exposure. As smoking is more prevalent in males [49], it has become a major issue in men's health. In a large meta-analysis done by Sharma et al. [50], smoking was found to be associated with reduced sperm count, motility, and morphology; however, the link between sperm DNA damage and smoking was less clear.

Compounds in cigarette are directly and indirectly mutagenic. In vitro experiments in human sperm have shown that cigarette smoke causes sperm DNA fragmentation in a dose-dependent manner [51]. Nicotine, cadmium, and lead have all been found to be associated with sperm DNA damage. When sperm from healthy volunteers were incubated in nicotine levels similar to those found in smoker's seminal fluid, sperm DNA fragmentation significantly increased ($p < 0.05$) [52]. Higher levels of cadmium and lead have been found in men with fertility disorders [53]. In mice, cadmium was associated with increased sperm DNA fragmentation [54]. Cadmium also downregulates 8-oxoguanine DNA glycosylase [55], which is involved in repairing DNA oxidative damage, perpetuating the fragmentation. Finally, lead increases DFI rate in vitro in both fertile and infertile men [56].

Smoking reduces the activity of catalase. Catalase, an antioxidant, reduces hydrogen peroxide to water, thereby protecting the sperm cells from oxidative damage. Peltola et al. [26] studied the effects of smoking on this antioxidative enzyme using a rat model. After a single smoking session, catalase activity was found to be reduced in rat testes for 12 h to 5 days [26].

Smoking reduces the expression of Chk1. After analyzing semen from infertile men in North China, Cui et al. [57] found not only in vitro sperm DNA fragmentation rate associated with smoking regardless of the exposure to smoking (30% vs. 70%; $p < 0.05$) but also found reduced levels of mRNA of Chk1 ($p < 0.05$). Chk1, a checkpoint protein that promotes the survival and repair of sperm with DNA damage, is usually associated with loss of DNA integrity; however, Chk1 mRNA levels were inversely related to sperm DNA fragmentation in smokers. The reduction of Chk1 with smoking indicates that this habit not only increases the existing sperm DNA fragmentation but also prevents DNA repair and encourages apoptosis [57].

Smoking also induces apoptosis. Men with infertility and idiopathic oligoasthenoteratozoospermia showed a positive correlation between the number of cigarettes per day and apoptotic markers such as s-Fas and caspase-3 ($r = 0.907$ and $r = 0.867$, respectively; $p < 0.001$ in both) [16]. The percentage of DNA fragmentation was also highly associated with s-Fas and caspase-3 ($r = 0.908$ and $r = 0.919$, respectively; $p < 0.001$ in both) [16]. One possible explanation is that these abnormal sperm are undergoing "abortive apoptosis" where the normal apoptotic mechanism causes double-stranded DNA breaks but not complete death of the sperm [58].

While in vitro studies and studies of certain populations indicate that cigarette toxins have a negative effect on sperm DNA and chromatin, the effects of smoking on sperm DNA in the general population remain somewhat controversial [25]. Several studies prove that smoking is significantly associated with decreased DNA integrity in men who are seeking treatment for infertility [57, 59, 60], while other studies show there was no significant association [61, 62]. Part of the challenge of these studies is that it is difficult to determine the dose-response smoking has on SDF. A high number of pack years tends to come with increasing age, and SDF also increases with age [63]. Hence, this could be one of the cofounder that could explain the contradicting conclusions drawn by the studies.

Some men are more genetically susceptible to oxidative stress and more sensitive to the toxins in cigarette smoking. As seen in Table 15.1, polymorphisms in several genes that reduce oxidative stress and are involved in detoxification of the tobacco toxins are linked to idiopathic infertility [25, 64–67]. One of the genes, OGG1, is involved in such process, and a homozygotic polymorphism in this gene is linked to increased oxidative DNA damage in sperm and increased risk of infertility [67]. Taken together, these studies show a complex relationship between exposure and genetics. Moreover, genetic polymorphism may determine the primary mechanism of the sperm DNA damage in smokers.

Nongenetic factors may also play a role in determining the severity of DNA damage caused by cigarette smoke. Anifandis et al. [68] analyzed semen samples that were gathered for fertility evaluation and found that smoking and alcohol consumption were significantly associated with SDF, and the combination of these two lifestyle habits enhanced the damage. Another susceptible population is patients diagnosed with varicocele. Patients with this pathology are more likely to have

Table 15.1 Effects of various polymorphisms on infertility in smoking men and other populations

Gene polymorphism	Function of gene	Polymorphism	Effect of polymorphism
Cytochrome P450 1A1	Metabolizes xenobiotics, drugs, oxidative toxins, and polyunsaturated fatty acids	3801T>C	Increases risk of male infertility in smokers*
N-acetyltransferase	Metabolizes xenobiotics, arylamines, aromatic amines, and hydrazines	590G>A	Increases risk of male infertility in smokers,* alcohol abusers,* and low fruit and vegetable consumers*
Glutathione S-transfer genes	Responsible for detoxification of xenobiotics and redox reaction	GSTM1+/ GSTT1 del; GSTP1 105IV/ GSTT1+	Increases the risk of male infertility in smokers*
8-Oxoguanine DNA glycosylase 1	Repairs oxidative DNA damage	Ser326Cys	Increases the risk of infertility in male smokers*

*$p < 0.05$ [64–67]

higher DNA fragmentation than those without. Varicocele results in venous stasis in the testes, allowing toxins from cigarette smoke, such as cadmium, to accumulate, and it also causes a decrease in the amount of antioxidants [69]. In a population of men with varicoceles, Fariello et al. [70] evaluated moderate smoking and heavy smoking groups for sperm DNA fragmentation using comet assay, comparing them to a control group. A significant dose-dependent relationship between smoking and sperm DNA fragmentation was observed in men with varicocele, especially in the moderate smoking and high DNA fragmentation groups ($p = 0.033$ and $p < 0.0001$, respectively) [70].

There is strong molecular evidence on smoking causing sperm DNA damage, even though specific population-based investigations have conflicting findings. Perhaps the most convincing evidence lies in the group of patients with specific polymorphisms in checkpoint and DNA repair genes. Nongenetic factors, such as varicocele, may also increase the effects of smoking on sperm DNA.

15.5 Alcohol

Alcohol is one of the most widely abused substances globally. More than half of the men in the United States reported using alcohol in the past 30 days, and almost 25% of men binge drink five times a month [71]. The effects of alcohol on the reproductive system include gynecomastia, erectile dysfunction, loss of libido, disturbance in sex hormones [72, 73], and testicular atrophy [74]. Chronic alcohol exposure was found to cause vast histological changes in mice including the following: germative cell loss, lipid droplet accumulation, irregular diameter of seminiferous tubules, and dilated interstitial blood vessels [74].

Alcohol damages chromatin integrity and increases DNA fragmentation in mouse [17], rat [18, 75], and human sperm [68, 76]. Robbins et al. [76] found an association between alcohol consumption and the following sperm chromosome abnormalities: aneuploidy, diploidy, and duplication. Diabetic patients and smokers are at increased risk of sperm DNA fragmentation from alcohol consumption. Pourentezari et al. [77] found that while diabetes and alcohol individually increased sperm DNA fragmentation in mice ($p < 0.001$), the two factors seemed to have a cumulative effect ($p < 0.05$). Finally, as mentioned before, patients who consume alcohol and smoke are at increased risk of DNA fragmentation [68]. However, while smoking has multiple different proposed mechanisms for sperm DNA damage, ethanol seems to have a clear primary mechanism.

Evidence suggests that apoptosis is the primary mechanism of sperm DNA damage in chronic ethanol users [17, 19]. Eid et al. [19] studied histological changes in the sperm and testes in rats after chronic exposure to ethanol. Significantly higher number of apoptotic germinal cells, depletion of germinal epithelium, and apoptotic seminiferous tubules were seen in the experimental group ($p < 0.01$). Germinal cells intensely stained with Fas and caspase-3 in the ethanol group. While FasL was observed on the basal side of the Sertoli cells in the control group, it translocated to the spermatogonia side in the ethanol-exposed group. Caspase-3, caspase-8, and caspase-9 were all higher in the testicular homogenate in ethanol-treated group ($p < 0.5$, $p < 0.5$, and $p < 0.9$, respectively). Zhu et al. [18] observed that rats with chronic alcohol exposure had higher testicular p53 levels, which is a major regulator of apoptosis.

While it is evident that alcohol causes apoptosis, what initiates the cascade? Talebi et al. [75] suggested that apoptosis is in part due to DNA denaturation, suggesting that ethanol is genotoxic. Other studies suggest that apoptosis is due to low testosterone levels in alcohol users [73]. An alternative hypothesis is oxidative stress. While several articles showed link between alcohol and oxidative stress in general [78], the link between alcohol intake and ROS damages in the testes has not been thoroughly examined [75]. Alcohol alters the redox balance, especially in the liver, by changing the NAD+/NADH ratio, damaging mitochondria, inducing mild hypoxia, and affecting antioxidant enzymes [78]. Two studies linked redox imbalance to ethanol consumption in prepubescent [79] and adult rats [80], while antioxidants were found to alleviate the redox imbalance [80]. However, without a clear link between oxidative stress and sperm DNA fragmentation (SDF) from alcohol exposure or a clear link between antioxidant use and increased fertility in a chronic alcoholic, these findings are purely esoteric.

Finally, another possible mechanism of action is impaired spermatogenesis [17]. Koh et al. [81] identified a reduction in a proliferative marker in ethanol-exposed rats. However, spermatogenesis is a dynamic process requiring a specific environment and signals, making it difficult to observe the real-time effects of ethanol exposure.

Chronic alcohol users are at higher risk for loss of sperm DNA integrity most likely due to an increased rate of apoptosis. Future research should determine the role of oxidative stress and impaired spermatogenesis in SDF due to alcohol exposure. Supplemental antioxidants may play a role in reversing SDF in chronic alcoholics if oxidative stress is truly the main mechanism involved in this process.

15.6 Irradiation

Radiation clearly affects fertility [82], and one well-established associated mechanism is radiation-induced sperm DNA damage [83, 84]. The mechanism of DNA damage on sperm depends on the type and length of exposure. This chapter will examine only a few sources of irradiation: hospital occupational exposure, X-ray radiation, radiotherapy, and cell phones.

The carcinogenic and mutagenic effects of chronic exposure to ionizing radiation are well established, and sperm DNA are not spared. A cross-sectional study conducted by Kumar et al. [85] identified a connection between sperm DNA fragmentation and ionizing radiation exposure in a hospital setting ($p < 0.05$). However, there was no association with aneuploidy [85].

High doses of radiation exposure in healthcare are harmful to male fertility, and the two types of radiation that will be examined in this chapter are X-rays and radiotherapy treatment. X-rays are a common medical tool used for routine diagnosis of cardiovascular, pulmonary, gastrointestinal, and orthopedic conditions. Haines et al. [83] found an increase in sperm DNA fragmentation 45 days after mice were exposed to a single dose of X-ray radiation. Interestingly, the authors found that even though spermatogonia have DNA repair proteins that mature spermatozoa do not, damaged spermatogonia were allowed to mature with existing DNA damage instead of inducing the apoptotic mechanism [83]. Also, using a mouse model, Cordelli et al. [20] discovered that spermatogonia responded to the immediate and direct X-ray damage by an initial attempt of DNA repair. As the damaged spermatogonia mature, the double-stranded breaks and apoptotic markers increased as well [20]. Taken together, these studies suggest that X-rays cause direct and immediate DNA fragmentation in spermatogonia and a delayed apoptotic double-stranded breaks.

Radiotherapy is used for localized cancers such as testicular cancer. In the United States, testicular cancer has an estimated 5-year survival rate of 80% for all stages [86] leaving hundreds of young survivors with questions about their quality of life and fertility potential. Paoli et al. [87] found that while DFI increased 3 months after initiating radiotherapy ($p < 0.001$), the increase was not affected by the patients' age or the histotypes of the cancer ($p > 0.05$ in all cases). Of note, the DFI normalized in 3–5 years after radiotherapy, but it took 5 years for normalization in the chemotherapy group [87]. As with most exposures, polymorphisms may influence the extent of damage that radiotherapy causes. Zhu et al. identified that hMSH5 P29S could augment DNA damage induced by testicular radiotherapy in patients with testicular germ cell tumor [88]. Melatonin may be a protective factor for radiotherapy. Preliminary results in mice suggest that pretreatment of melatonin may prevent DNA strand breaks by the reduction of apoptotic signaling [89]. However, the clinical implications of preventing apoptosis in a cancerous tissue may be counterproductive.

The final source of radiation that will be examined in this section is the cell phone. Seldom does the industrialized world males have a cell phone further than an arm reach away, in spite of the numerous studies that link cell phone use with sperm DNA fragmentation [84, 90, 91]. In a retrospective population study, Radwan et al. [90] found that cell phone use for more than 10 years was associated with a higher degree if sperm DNA fragmentation ($p < 0.04$). Moreover, in vitro studies conducted on sperm from healthy males confirm these epidemiological findings. Gorpinchenko et al. [92] treated semen from men with normozoospermia for 5 h with cell phone exposure and compared it to sperm that was not exposed. Sperm in the experimental group had significantly higher DNA fragmentation than the control group (8.8% vs. 4.2%, $p < 0.05$) [92].

While cell phone exposure may increase sperm DNA damage in men without any previous fertility issues [90], it probably has a higher impact in men with existing fertility issues [91].

Zalata et al. [91] exposed semen samples of men with normozoospermia, asthenozoospermia, asthenoteratozoospermia, and oligoasthenoteratozoospermia to radiation similar to a cell phone 10 cm away for 60 min and measured the sperm DNA fragmentation. In all groups, the exposed group significantly increased in DNA damage. The oligoasthenoteratozoospermic group showed the most significant increase (40.0% vs. 80%, $p < 0.001$) [91], while the normozoospermic group showed the slightest increase (11.5% vs. 30.8%, $p < 0.01$) [91], indicating that men with existing fertility issues are more sensitive to the radiation from cell phone use. Cell phone use also affects other sperm parameters. For example, Zilberlicht et al. [93] found that there was a statistically significant decrease in sperm concentration in men talking on the phone for more than 1 h a day ($p = 0.04$) and talking while charging the cell phone ($p = 0.02$).

Cell phones generate small amounts of radiation via radiofrequency electromagnetic field (RF-EMF). De Iuliis et al. [84] found that RF-EMF increases the ROS generation in the mitochondria, increasing intracellular oxidative stress and DNA damage [84]. De Iuliis et al. were also able to link oxidative stress resulting from RF-EMR to both oxidative DNA damage (formation of 8-hydroxy-2′-deoxyguanosine) and fragmentation ($r^2 = 0.727$ and $r^2 = 0.861$, respectively) [84]. One possible explanation for the ROS release from mitochondria is that RF-EMF also damages mitochondrial DNA, resulting in dysfunction mitochondrial proteins, inadequate electron sequestration, and ROS generation from redox imbalance [94]. Future work on cell phone radiation should focus on how to reduce exposure.

Radiation from occupational exposure, X-ray radiation, radiotherapy, and cell phone radiation have all been linked to increased sperm DNA fragmentation. Although the exact mechanism for the damage seems to be different for each exposure, a study comparing these mechanisms is yet to be done. Further investigation is needed to solidify the exact mechanism and identify the alleviating factors for sperm DNA damage.

15.7 Conclusion

As sperm DNA fragmentation is a relatively new sperm parameter in fertility, researchers are rapidly discovering lifestyle factors that correlate with increased sperm DNA damage. While obesity has yet to be definitively correlated with high sperm DNA fragmentation [37], a high-fat diet is positively associated, and a health-conscious diet is negatively associated [44, 45]. Moreover, since damage from a high-fat diet can be alleviated by diet and exercise in rat models [43, 48], the cause of obesity, such as diet and sedentary lifestyle, is more likely a risk factor than obesity itself. Studies on rat models show that sperm DNA damage from a high-fat diet may also be alleviated by metformin [48]. Vegans and vegetarians were no different than nonvegetarians in terms of sperm DNA damage [46].

Smoking is only a risk factor for high sperm DNA fragmentation in the following populations: genetically susceptible males [64–67], alcoholics [68], and men with varicocele [70]. Alcohol consumption increases DNA fragmentation [68, 76], especially in those who also smoke [68]. Unfortunately, alleviating factors for sperm DNA damage due to smoking and chronic alcoholism have yet to be determined.

Radiation exposure in the form of X-rays, radiotherapy, and cell phones are risk factors for loss of sperm DNA integrity. Radiotherapy temporarily increases the sperm DNA damage but then normalized in 3–5 years [89]. Melatonin pretreatment was identified as a protective factor for radiotherapy-induced sperm DNA damage in mice [89]. Cell phone use increases sperm DNA fragmentation, especially in men who have existing fertility issues such as asthenozoospermia [91]. Future research of these and other factors should focus on the interplay between genetics and lifestyle.

This chapter only covered a few major lifestyle factors that can affect sperm DNA integrity (Table 15.2), but many more have yet to be studied. Unfortunately, industrial advancement has created many of these risk factors. For example, though

Table 15.2 Summary of lifestyle factors in this chapter

Lifestyle	Correlation with SDF	Future work
Obesity	Controversial	Identify cofounders such as high-fat diet and metabolic syndrome
High-fat diet	Positive correlation with SDF	Determine the effects of different fat sources (e.g., vegetable fat vs. animal fat)
Health-conscious diet	Negative correlation with SDF	Continue to identify specific foods that prevent SDF
Vegan/vegetarian diet vs. meat-inclusive diet	No significant difference	Conduct more studies needed to confirm there is no significant difference
Smoking	Controversial for general population; genetic susceptibility in some men	Continue to identify genetically susceptible populations and possible alleviating factors
Alcohol consumption	Positive correlation	Identify possible cofounders and determine if there is genetic susceptibility
X-rays	Positive correlation	Develop protective or alleviating factors
Radiotherapy	Positive correlation	Develop protective or alleviating factors
Cell phone use	Positive correlation	Develop protective or alleviating factors

SDF sperm DNA fragmentation

previously a rarity, a high-fat diet is normal in an increasing number of countries feeding the recent obesity epidemic. Moreover, cell phones are almost ubiquitously available in developed nations. While increased food availability and improved communications have advanced society in some aspects, continuous research is needed to keep up with the effects of the evolving global environment on male health.

References

1. Aitken RJ, De Iuliis GN, Finnie JM, Hedges A, McLachlan RI. Analysis of the relationships between oxidative stress, DNA damage and sperm vitality in a patient population: development of diagnostic criteria. Hum Reprod. 2010;25(10):2415–26.
2. Aitken RJ, Smith TB, Jobling MS, Baker MA, De Iuliis GN. Oxidative stress and male reproductive health. Asian J Androl. 2014;16(1):31–8.
3. Lewis SE, John Aitken R, Conner SJ, et al. The impact of sperm DNA damage in assisted conception and beyond: recent advances in diagnosis and treatment. Reprod Biomed Online. 2013;27(4):325–37.
4. Spanò M, Bonde JP, Hjøllund HI, Kolstad HA, Cordelli E, Leter G. Sperm chromatin damage impairs human fertility. The Danish first pregnancy planner study team. Fertil Steril. 2000;73(1):43–50.
5. Simon L, Lutton D, McManus J, Lewis SE. Sperm DNA damage measured by the alkaline comet assay as an independent predictor of male infertility and in vitro fertilization success. Fertil Steril. 2011;95(2):652–7.
6. Fernández-Gonzalez R, Moreira PN, Pérez-Crespo M, et al. Long-term effects of mouse intracytoplasmic sperm injection with DNA-fragmented sperm on health and behavior of adult offspring. Biol Reprod. 2008;78(4):761–72.
7. Evenson DP, Jost LK, Marshall D, et al. Utility of the sperm chromatin structure assay as a diagnostic and prognostic tool in the human fertility clinic. Hum Reprod. 1999;14(4):1039–49.
8. Zini A, Boman JM, Belzile E, Ciampi A. Sperm DNA damage is associated with an increased risk of pregnancy loss after IVF and ICSI: systematic review and meta-analysis. Hum Reprod. 2008;23(12):2663–8.
9. Steger K. Transcriptional and translational regulation of gene expression in haploid spermatids. Anat Embryol (Berl). 1999;199(6):471–87.
10. Jager S. Sperm nuclear stability and male infertility. Arch Androl. 1990;25(3):253–9.
11. Balhorn R, Reed S, Tanphaichitr N. Aberrant protamine 1/protamine 2 ratios in sperm of infertile human males. Experientia. 1988;44(1):52–5.
12. Sakkas D, Seli E, Manicardi GC, Nijs M, Ombelet W, Bizzaro D. The presence of abnormal spermatozoa in the ejaculate: did apoptosis fail? Hum Fertil (Camb). 2004;7(2):99–103.
13. Nagata S. Apoptosis by death factor. Cell. 1997;88(3):355–65.
14. Francavilla S, D'Abrizio P, Rucci N, et al. Fas and Fas ligand expression in fetal and adult human testis with normal or deranged spermatogenesis. J Clin Endocrinol Metab. 2000;85(8):2692–700.
15. Huckins C. The morphology and kinetics of spermatogonial degeneration in normal adult rats: an analysis using a simplified classification of the germinal epithelium. Anat Rec. 1978;190(4):905–26.
16. El-Melegy NT, Ali ME. Apoptotic markers in semen of infertile men: association with cigarette smoking. Int Braz J Urol. 2011;37(4):495–506.
17. Rahimipour M, Talebi AR, Anvari M, Sarcheshmeh AA, Omidi M. Effects of different doses of ethanol on sperm parameters, chromatin structure and apoptosis in adult mice. Eur J Obstet Gynecol Reprod Biol. 2013;170(2):423–8.

18. Zhu Q, Meisinger J, Emanuele NV, Emanuele MA, LaPaglia N, Van Thiel DH. Ethanol exposure enhances apoptosis within the testes. Alcohol Clin Exp Res. 2000;24(10):1550–6.
19. Eid NA, Shibata MA, Ito Y, Kusakabe K, Hammad H, Otsuki Y. Involvement of Fas system and active caspases in apoptotic signalling in testicular germ cells of ethanol-treated rats. Int J Androl. 2002;25(3):159–67.
20. Cordelli E, Eleuteri P, Grollino MG, et al. Direct and delayed X-ray-induced DNA damage in male mouse germ cells. Environ Mol Mutagen. 2012;53(6):429–39.
21. Koppers AJ, De Iuliis GN, Finnie JM, McLaughlin EA, Aitken RJ. Significance of mitochondrial reactive oxygen species in the generation of oxidative stress in spermatozoa. J Clin Endocrinol Metab. 2008;93(8):3199–207.
22. Henkel R, Kierspel E, Stalf T, et al. Effect of reactive oxygen species produced by spermatozoa and leukocytes on sperm functions in non-leukocytospermic patients. Fertil Steril. 2005;83(3):635–42.
23. Shannon P, Curson B. Site of aromatic L-amino acid oxidase in dead bovine spermatozoa and determination of between-bull differences in the percentage of dead spermatozoa by oxidase activity. J Reprod Fertil. 1982;64(2):469–73.
24. Opuwari CS, Henkel RR. An update on oxidative damage to spermatozoa and oocytes. Biomed Res Int. 2016;2016:9540142.
25. Harlev A, Agarwal A, Gunes SO, Shetty A, du Plessis SS. Smoking and male infertility: an evidence-based review. World J Mens Health. 2015;33(3):143–60.
26. Peltola V, Mäntylä E, Huhtaniemi I, Ahotupa M. Lipid peroxidation and antioxidant enzyme activities in the rat testis after cigarette smoke inhalation or administration of polychlorinated biphenyls or polychlorinated naphthalenes. J Androl. 1994;15(4):353–61.
27. Aitken RJ, Koppers AJ. Apoptosis and DNA damage in human spermatozoa. Asian J Androl. 2011;13(1):36–42.
28. Muratori M, Tamburrino L, Marchiani S, et al. Investigation on the origin of sperm DNA fragmentation: role of apoptosis, immaturity and oxidative stress. Mol Med. 2015;21:109–22.
29. Finucane MM, Stevens GA, Cowan MJ, et al. National, regional, and global trends in body-mass index since 1980: systematic analysis of health examination surveys and epidemiological studies with 960 country-years and 9·1 million participants. Lancet. 2011;377(9765):557–67.
30. Tunc O, Bakos HW, Tremellen K. Impact of body mass index on seminal oxidative stress. Andrologia. 2011;43(2):121–8.
31. Ogden CL, Carroll MD, Kit BK, Flegal KM. Prevalence of childhood and adult obesity in the United States, 2011–2012. JAMA. 2014;311(8):806–14.
32. Campbell JM, Lane M, Owens JA, Bakos HW. Paternal obesity negatively affects male fertility and assisted reproduction outcomes: a systematic review and meta-analysis. Reprod Biomed Online. 2015;31(5):593–604.
33. Jokela M, Elovainio M, Kivimäki M. Lower fertility associated with obesity and underweight: the US National Longitudinal Survey of youth. Am J Clin Nutr. 2008;88(4):886–93.
34. Nguyen RH, Wilcox AJ, Skjaerven R, Baird DD. Men's body mass index and infertility. Hum Reprod. 2007;22(9):2488–93.
35. Duale N, Steffensen IL, Andersen J, Brevik A, Brunborg G, Lindeman B. Impaired sperm chromatin integrity in obese mice. Andrology. 2014;2(2):234–43.
36. Kort HI, Massey JB, Elsner CW, et al. Impact of body mass index values on sperm quantity and quality. J Androl. 2006;27(3):450–2.
37. Bandel I, Bungum M, Richtoff J, et al. No association between body mass index and sperm DNA integrity. Hum Reprod. 2015;30(7):1704–13.
38. Rybar R, Kopecka V, Prinosilova P, Markova P, Rubes J. Male obesity and age in relationship to semen parameters and sperm chromatin integrity. Andrologia. 2011;43(4):286–91.
39. Sharpe RM. Environmental/lifestyle effects on spermatogenesis. Philos Trans R Soc Lond Ser B Biol Sci. 2010;365(1546):1697–712.
40. Kasturi SS, Tannir J, Brannigan RE. The metabolic syndrome and male infertility. J Androl. 2008;29(3):251–9.

41. Håkonsen LB, Thulstrup AM, Aggerholm AS, et al. Does weight loss improve semen quality and reproductive hormones? Results from a cohort of severely obese men. Reprod Health. 2011;8:24.
42. Dattilo M, Cornet D, Amar E, Cohen M, Menezo Y. The importance of the one carbon cycle nutritional support in human male fertility: a preliminary clinical report. Reprod Biol Endocrinol. 2014;12:71.
43. Palmer NO, Bakos HW, Owens JA, Setchell BP, Lane M. Diet and exercise in an obese mouse fed a high-fat diet improve metabolic health and reverse perturbed sperm function. Am J Physiol Endocrinol Metab. 2012;302(7):E768–80.
44. Jurewicz J, Radwan M, Sobala W, Radwan P, Bochenek M, Hanke W. Dietary patterns and their relationship with semen quality. Am J Mens Health. 2016. pii: 1557988315627139.
45. Vujkovic M, de Vries JH, Dohle GR, et al. Associations between dietary patterns and semen quality in men undergoing IVF/ICSI treatment. Hum Reprod. 2009;24(6):1304–12.
46. Orzylowska EM, Jacobson JD, Bareh GM, Ko EY, Corselli JU, Chan PJ. Food intake diet and sperm characteristics in a blue zone: a Loma Linda study. Eur J Obstet Gynecol Reprod Biol. 2016;203:112–5.
47. Ferramosca A, Conte A, Moscatelli N, Zara V. A high-fat diet negatively affects rat sperm mitochondrial respiration. Andrology. 2016;4(3):520–5.
48. Yan WJ, Mu Y, Yu N, et al. Protective effects of metformin on reproductive function in obese male rats induced by high-fat diet. J Assist Reprod Genet. 2015;32(7):1097–104.
49. Organization WH. Prevalence of tobacco smoking. Global health observatory data: tobacco control. 2016. http://www.who.int/gho/tobacco/use/en/. Accessed 13 Sept 2016.
50. Sharma R, Harlev A, Agarwal A, Esteves SC. Cigarette smoking and semen quality: a new meta-analysis examining the effect of the 2010 World Health Organization Laboratory methods for the examination of human semen. Eur Urol. 2016;70:635–45.
51. Calogero A, Polosa R, Perdichizzi A, et al. Cigarette smoke extract immobilizes human spermatozoa and induces sperm apoptosis. Reprod Biomed Online. 2009;19(4):564–71.
52. Condorelli RA, La Vignera S, Giacone F, et al. In vitro effects of nicotine on sperm motility and bio-functional flow cytometry sperm parameters. Int J Immunopathol Pharmacol. 2013;26(3):739–46.
53. Wdowiak A, Bakalczuk G, Bakalczuk S. Evaluation of effect of selected trace elements on dynamics of sperm DNA fragmentation. Postepy Hig Med Dosw (Online). 2015;69:1405–10.
54. Oliveira H, Spanò M, Santos C. Pereira MeL. Adverse effects of cadmium exposure on mouse sperm. Reprod Toxicol. 2009;28(4):550–5.
55. Youn CK, Kim SH, Lee DY, et al. Cadmium down-regulates human OGG1 through suppression of Sp1 activity. J Biol Chem. 2005;280(26):25185–95.
56. Gomes M, Gonçalves A, Rocha E, et al. Effect of in vitro exposure to lead chloride on semen quality and sperm DNA fragmentation. Zygote. 2015;23(3):384–93.
57. Cui X, Jing X, Wu X, Wang Z, Li Q. Potential effect of smoking on semen quality through DNA damage and the downregulation of Chk1 in sperm. Mol Med Rep. 2016;14(1):753–61.
58. Sakkas D, Mariethoz E, St John JC. Abnormal sperm parameters in humans are indicative of an abortive apoptotic mechanism linked to the Fas-mediated pathway. Exp Cell Res. 1999;251(2):350–5.
59. Antoniassi MP, Intasqui Lopes P, Camargo M, et al. Analysis of the sperm functional aspects and seminal plasma proteomic profile from male smokers. BJU Int. 2016;118:814–22.
60. Mitra A, Chakraborty B, Mukhopadhay D, et al. Effect of smoking on semen quality, FSH, testosterone level, and CAG repeat length in androgen receptor gene of infertile men in an Indian city. Syst Biol Reprod Med. 2012;58(5):255–62.
61. Bounartzi T, Dafopoulos K, Anifandis G, et al. Pregnancy prediction by free sperm DNA and sperm DNA fragmentation in semen specimens of IVF/ICSI-ET patients. Hum Fertil (Camb). 2016;19(1):56–62.
62. Bojar I, Witczak M, Wdowiak A. Biological and environmental conditionings for a sperm DNA fragmentation. Ann Agric Environ Med. 2013;20(4):865–8.

63. Johnson SL, Dunleavy J, Gemmell NJ, Nakagawa S. Consistent age-dependent declines in human semen quality: a systematic review and meta-analysis. Ageing Res Rev. 2015;19:22–33.
64. Yarosh SL, Kokhtenko EV, Starodubova NI, Churnosov MI, Polonikov AV. Smoking status modifies the relation between CYP1A1*2C gene polymorphism and idiopathic male infertility: the importance of gene-environment interaction analysis for genetic studies of the disease. Reprod Sci. 2013;20(11):1302–7.
65. Yarosh SL, Kokhtenko EV, Churnosov MI, Solodilova MA, Polonikov AV. Joint effect of glutathione S-transferase genotypes and cigarette smoking on idiopathic male infertility. Andrologia. 2015;47(9):980–6.
66. Yarosh SL, Kokhtenko EV, Churnosov MI, Ataman AV, Solodilova MA, Polonikov AV. Synergism between the N-acetyltransferase 2 gene and oxidant exposure increases the risk of idiopathic male infertility. Reprod Biomed Online. 2014;29(3):362–9.
67. Ji G, Yan L, Liu W, Qu J, Gu A. OGG1 Ser326Cys polymorphism interacts with cigarette smoking to increase oxidative DNA damage in human sperm and the risk of male infertility. Toxicol Lett. 2013;218(2):144–9.
68. Anifandis G, Bounartzi T, Messini CI, Dafopoulos K, Sotiriou S, Messinis IE. The impact of cigarette smoking and alcohol consumption on sperm parameters and sperm DNA fragmentation (SDF) measured by Halosperm(®). Arch Gynecol Obstet. 2014;290(4):777–82.
69. Smith R, Kaune H, Parodi D, et al. Increased sperm DNA damage in patients with varicocele: relationship with seminal oxidative stress. Hum Reprod. 2006;21(4):986–93.
70. Fariello RM, Pariz JR, Spaine DM, et al. Effect of smoking on the functional aspects of sperm and seminal plasma protein profiles in patients with varicocele. Hum Reprod. 2012;27(11):3140–9.
71. CDC. Fact sheets – excessive alcohol use and risks to men's health. 2016. http://www.cdc.gov/alcohol/fact-sheets/mens-health.htm.
72. Boyden TW, Pamenter RW. Effects of ethanol on the male hypothalamic-pituitary-gonadal axis. Endocr Rev. 1983;4(4):389–95.
73. Tadic SD, Elm MS, Subbotin VM, Eagon PK. Hypogonadism precedes liver feminization in chronic alcohol-fed male rats. Hepatology. 2000;31(5):1135–40.
74. Martinez M, Macera S, de Assis GF, et al. Structural evaluation of the effects of chronic ethanol ingestion on the testis of Calomys callosus. Tissue Cell. 2009;41(3):199–205.
75. Talebi AR, Sarcheshmeh AA, Khalili MA, Tabibnejad N. Effects of ethanol consumption on chromatin condensation and DNA integrity of epididymal spermatozoa in rat. Alcohol. 2011;45(4):403–9.
76. Robbins WA, Vine MF, Truong KY, Everson RB. Use of fluorescence in situ hybridization (FISH) to assess effects of smoking, caffeine, and alcohol on aneuploidy load in sperm of healthy men. Environ Mol Mutagen. 1997;30(2):175–83.
77. Pourentezari M, Talebi AR, Mangoli E, Anvari M, Rahimipour M. Additional deleterious effects of alcohol consumption on sperm parameters and DNA integrity in diabetic mice. Andrologia. 2016;48(5):564–9.
78. Wu D, Cederbaum AI. Alcohol, oxidative stress, and free radical damage. Alcohol Res Health. 2003;27(4):277–84.
79. Emanuele NV, LaPagli N, Steiner J, Colantoni A, Van Thiel DH, Emanuele MA. Peripubertal paternal EtOH exposure. Endocrine. 2001;14(2):213–9.
80. Amanvermez R, Demir S, Tunçel OK, Alvur M, Agar E. Alcohol-induced oxidative stress and reduction in oxidation by ascorbate/L-cys/L-met in the testis, ovary, kidney, and lung of rat. Adv Ther. 2005;22(6):548–58.
81. Koh PO, Kim MO. Ethanol exposure decreases cell proliferation and increases apoptosis in rat testes. J Vet Med Sci. 2006;68(10):1013–7.
82. Ash P. The influence of radiation on fertility in man. Br J Radiol. 1980;53(628):271–8.
83. Haines GA, Hendry JH, Daniel CP, Morris ID. Increased levels of comet-detected spermatozoa DNA damage following in vivo isotopic- or X-irradiation of spermatogonia. Mutat Res. 2001;495(1–2):21–32.

84. De Iuliis GN, Newey RJ, King BV, Aitken RJ. Mobile phone radiation induces reactive oxygen species production and DNA damage in human spermatozoa in vitro. PLoS One. 2009;4(7):e6446.
85. Kumar D, Salian SR, Kalthur G, et al. Semen abnormalities, sperm DNA damage and global hypermethylation in health workers occupationally exposed to ionizing radiation. PLoS One. 2013;8(7):e69927.
86. Kopp HG, Kuczyk M, Classen J, et al. Advances in the treatment of testicular cancer. Drugs. 2006;66(5):641–59.
87. Paoli D, Gallo M, Rizzo F, et al. Testicular cancer and sperm DNA damage: short- and long-term effects of antineoplastic treatment. Andrology. 2015;3(1):122–8.
88. Zhu Y, Gao G, Xia L, et al. The polymorphic hMSH5 C85T allele augments radiotherapy-induced spermatogenic impairment. Andrology. 2016;4(5):873–9.
89. Khan S, Adhikari JS, Rizvi MA, Chaudhury NK. Radioprotective potential of melatonin against ^{60}Co γ-ray-induced testicular injury in male C57BL/6 mice. J Biomed Sci. 2015;22:61.
90. Radwan M, Jurewicz J, Merecz-Kot D, et al. Sperm DNA damage-the effect of stress and everyday life factors. Int J Impot Res. 2016;28(4):148–54.
91. Zalata A, El-Samanoudy AZ, Shaalan D, El-Baiomy Y, Mostafa T. In vitro effect of cell phone radiation on motility, DNA fragmentation and clusterin gene expression in human sperm. Int J Fertil Steril. 2015;9(1):129–36.
92. Gorpinchenko I, Nikitin O, Banyra O, Shulyak A. The influence of direct mobile phone radiation on sperm quality. Cent Eur J Urol. 2014;67(1):65–71.
93. Zilberlicht A, Wiener-Megnazi Z, Sheinfeld Y, Grach B, Lahav-Baratz S, Dirnfeld M. Habits of cell phone usage and sperm quality – does it warrant attention? Reprod Biomed Online. 2015;31(3):421–6.
94. Aitken RJ, Bennetts LE, Sawyer D, Wiklendt AM, King BV. Impact of radio frequency electromagnetic radiation on DNA integrity in the male germline. Int J Androl. 2005;28(3):171–9.

Chapter 16
Cancer and Sperm DNA Damage

Peter T.K. Chan and Bernard Robaire

16.1 Introduction

Recent epidemiological studies indicate that there is a worldwide rise in the incidence of many cancers that affect boys and young men [1–3]. Simultaneously, with the advances in medical technology for early detection of cancer and the improvement in the efficacy of cancer therapies, the survival rates of many of these cancer patients have improved dramatically in the past decades. Many young cancer survivors have not started or completed forming a family. Thus, the impact of cancer and cancer therapies on male reproductive health and the options for fertility preservation are important issues in survivorship for young cancer patients.

16.2 Epidemiology of Cancer in Boys and Young Men

Common cancers in men that receive most attention in the public media include lung, colon, prostate, skin, and liver cancers. These cancers, however, tend to affect men who have passed the reproductive age. For boys and young men, the most common cancers include testicular cancer, lymphoma, leukemia, sarcoma, and brain cancers. The incidence of childhood cancer worldwide has been steadily increasing over the past 50 years [1–3]. With an estimated cumulative incidence of 1720 per million, equivalent to a risk of 1 in 581, childhood cancer is indeed one of the

P.T.K. Chan
Department of Surgery (Urology), McGill University and the McGill Univeristy Health Centre, Montreal, QC, Canada

B. Robaire (✉)
Departments of Pharmacology & Therapeutics and of Obstetrics & Gynecology, McGill University, 3655 Promenade Sir William Osler, Montreal, QC, Canada
e-mail: bernard.robaire@mcgill.ca

A. Zini, A. Agarwal (eds.), *A Clinician's Guide to Sperm DNA and Chromatin Damage*, https://doi.org/10.1007/978-3-319-71815-6_16

leading causes of death among children younger than 15 years of age [4, 5]. According to the recent data from the American Cancer Society [4], 10,380 children in the United States under the age of 15 will be diagnosed with cancer in 2016. Interestingly, boys were affected 1.2 times more frequently than girls [6].

Thanks to tremendous strides in cancer management, including early detection strategies and advances in various treatment modalities such as surgeries, radiation, and combination chemotherapy regimens, the survival rates of many childhood cancers have increased dramatically over the past 40 years [7, 8]. In particular, testicular cancer, which is the most commonly diagnosed solitary cancer in young men between the ages of 18 and 35 years [9], has a 5-year survival rate of over 90%, even in cases with metastasis. Approximately half of childhood cancers are hematologic malignancies (leukemia and lymphoma) with an anticipated long-term survival greater than 75%. Improvements in prognosis and survival rates have also been observed for many other childhood malignancies, including Wilms' tumor, malignant bone tumors, and rhabdomyosarcomas. The latest statistics indicate that the relative 5-year survival rate for all childhood cancers combined is approximately 84% [3]. It is estimated that in North America approximately 1 in 900 of the population aged 20–45 years is a childhood cancer survivor [10]. In Canada, this translates to approximately 10,000 people who are survivors of childhood cancer and are expected to have 70 years or more of life after successful treatment [11].

16.3 Fertility After Cancer Therapy: Patients' Perspectives

While many of these young cancer survivors can expect a good quality of life, they may also face a series of undesired consequences related to their cancer and cancer therapies. Impairment in reproductive health is a well-known complication of cancer therapy; it occurs in a significant proportion of cancer survivors due to the inhibition of spermatogenesis (spermatotoxicity) of cancer treatments such as chemotherapy and radiation therapy. Many young cancer survivors have not initiated or completed forming a family. Interestingly, surveys indicated that almost 80% of childless cancer survivors report the desire to have children and believe that their experience of surviving cancer will make them better parents [12–14]. In a recent study, adolescents prioritized fertility as a top goal after good health [15].

For the majority of cancer survivors who desire to have children but have poor sperm quantity and quality, assisted reproductive technologies (ART), including in vitro fertilization (IVF) and intracytoplasmic sperm injection (ICSI), are sought to help them to father their own children [16]. While ART is becoming more popular and available, and our knowledge and experience in its efficacy and safety have expanded tremendously in recent years, some studies reported an association of ART with significant health risks to the offspring, including an increased risk of congenital malformations, genetic anomalies, low birth weight, and multiple pregnancies [17–21]. Health-care professionals counseling cancer patients and survivors must be prepared to provide them with precise and up-to-date options on post-cancer fertility.

16.4 Reproductive Health Before Cancer Treatment

It should be pointed out that the reproductive health of many cancer patients may be suboptimal even before receiving specific cancer therapies, as revealed by studies on the sperm density and morphology of pre-chemotherapy sperm banked samples and on case-control studies of their natural fecundity [22–25]. The reason for the impaired fertility status may, in part, be due to the decline in the physical state (poor nutrition, fever, cachexia, pain, etc.) of the patients due to cancer. The psychosocial stress attributed to the cancer diagnosis may play a role in the well-being of the subject. Prolonged periods of sexual abstinence may also contribute to the poor sperm quality before chemotherapy. In testicular cancer, poor sperm profile may be explained by the fact that there is only one remaining contralateral noncancerous testis to produce sperm. Indeed, some studies have shown that the contralateral noncancerous testis may have compromised reproductive function due to a higher risk of coexisting intraepithelial germ cell tumors and abnormal spermatogenesis, both quantitatively and qualitatively [24, 26].

Using a complementary panel of molecular genetic assays, including the AO/SCSA, TUNEL, and comet assays to determine sperm DNA damage and mBBr-SH labeling and the CMA3 assay to assess chromatin packaging, we have recently reported that, prior to chemotherapy, 37% of men with testis cancer and 81% of men with Hodgkin lymphoma demonstrate abnormal sperm chromatin structure despite having normal sperm density and motility [25]. Although several studies have supported our findings [27–32], other investigators [33, 34] have failed to confirm all our observations, but Smith et al. [34] did observe a higher level of sperm DNA fragmentation rate in non-Hodgkin lymphoma patients. Taken together, these studies suggest that with subsequent cytotoxic cancer therapy, sperms from cancer patients are at risk for further genetic damage.

16.5 Cancer Management Strategies

Generally, cancer management involves three major modalities, namely, surgery, radiation, and chemotherapy. The choice of treatment depends on the nature and stage of the cancer and the comorbidity of the subject. Not uncommonly, a combination of these modalities in various orders may be required to achieve optimal cancer control.

Complications of each modality also vary. Mechanisms of how each treatment modality may potentially compromise male reproductive health are discussed in this section.

16.5.1 Impact of Surgical Management for Cancer on Male Reproductive Status

The purpose of surgical resection of tumor is to remove the tumor with adequate surgical margins to aim for cure or to debulk the volume of tumor to facilitate the effect of adjuvant therapy with radiation or chemotherapy and thus control the cancer. A common surgical management for testicular cancer in young males is radical orchiectomy. Removal of one testis may affect the total spermatogenic activity in an individual.

Indeed, men with testicular cancer are at risk of having decreased spermatogenic activity in the contralateral testis. Other surgical managements for cancers in young males may result in damage to the autonomic nervous system required for semen emission.

Pelvic and lower intestine surgeries, retroperitoneal lymph node dissection for advanced testicular cancer, or any procedures involving the spine and other parts of the central nervous system may result in postoperative anejaculation. Despite the fact that spermatogenic function is generally not affected in these patients, they are at risk of having impaired fertility due to the absence of semen emission. Although it is well established in several animal models, including the monkey, that compensatory hypertrophy of the remaining testis occurs in the adult when one testis is removed prior to puberty [35–37], in human subjects, clinical studies indicate that this occurs only to a limited extent [38–40] and is insufficient to compensate for the loss of one testis.

With regard to the sperm chromatin integrity, a study using Swedish tumor registry data from 1970 to 2002 [41] reported that sperm DNA fragmentation index increased significantly in men aged 18–45 who were previously treated for childhood cancer (brain tumors, lymphomas, leukemia, Wilms' tumor, testicular cancer, and other malignancies) before 18 years of age with surgery only without radiation or chemotherapy. Their findings implied that childhood cancer patients have underlying genomic instability or defects in DNA repair mechanisms, as reported by other investigators [42].

16.5.2 Radiation Therapy

Germ cells and somatic cells in testes are prone to damage postradiation. The usual clinical dosage of radiation therapy for cancer ranges from 0.2 to 70 Gy, depending on the nature, stage, and anatomical location of the tumor. A cumulative dosage of 2.5–6 Gy directly to the testes may permanently damage germ cells, leading to prolonged or permanent azoospermia [43]. Even for radiation therapy outside the pelvic areas (e.g., para-aortic lymph nodes) with gonadal shielding to reduce the extent of gonadal toxicity, the scattering effects of radiation may still contribute to impaired fertility postirradiation. Such damage to sperm production may be further attributed to damage to cells in the somatic compartment of the testis. Using spermatogonial stem cell (SCC) transplantation in rat, Zhang et al. [44] demonstrated that transplantation of SCCs from irradiated animals into testes of irradiated nude mice (which had normal differentiation of their own spermatogonia) permitted differentiation of the donor spermatogonia to spermatozoa. Conversely, transplantation of SCCs from untreated prepubertal rats into irradiated rat testes showed that the donor spermatogonia were able to colonize along the seminiferous tubules but could not differentiate. Their findings suggest that the defect caused by radiation in the rat testes that hinder spermatogonial differentiation is due to damage to the somatic compartment [44].

Clinically, radiation therapy appeared to have a negative impact on sperm chromatin integrity for men treated with childhood cancers [41, 45] or prostate cancer as adult [46]. Fluorescence in situ hybridization (FISH) further demonstrated an increase in the incidence of sperm aneuploidy on chromosomes 18, X, and Y in men treated with radiotherapy for testicular seminoma [47]. Taken together, current evidence supports the presence of a significant risk of impairment of the male reproductive status after radiotherapy for cancer. In order to allow clinicians to properly counsel these patients, further longitudinal studies are required to evaluate the trajectory of sperm chromatin changes over time post therapy and to evaluate the health risks of offspring.

16.5.3 Chemotherapy

Chemotherapy is generally indicated in advanced and metastatic cancer, although its use in certain cancers, such as germ cell tumors at an early, localized stage, may help to lower the risks of subsequent metastasis. In addition to malignant cells, any rapidly dividing cells, including germ cells at various phases of spermatogenesis, are targets of chemotherapy. Gonadotoxicity of chemotherapy to an individual depends on at least three factors: (1) the nature of the malignancy, which dictates the type of chemotherapeutic agents to be used; (2) the stage of the disease, which dictates the duration and dosages of chemotherapy; and (3) the host factors, such as the baseline reproductive health of the individual. The impact of chemotherapy on male reproductive health is discussed in the next section.

16.5.3.1 Impact of Chemotherapy on Male Reproductive Health: Animal Studies

Using rodents (rats and mice) as models, a large body of evidence has emerged demonstrating that treatment with chemotherapeutic agents usually has dramatic effects on the production of male germ cells [48, 49]. Depending on the mechanism by which such agents act on the different phases of spermatogenesis (spermatogonial mitotic cell division, meiosis, or spermiogenesis), consequences can range from complete elimination of germ cells from the testis, resulting in Sertoli-cell-only syndrome, to no apparent histological effects on spermatogenesis but functional effects on germ cells (their motility, fertilizing ability, or capacity to produce normal viable offspring). Over the past 20 years, studies on male-mediated adverse effects of chemotherapeutic drugs, such as cyclophosphamide (CPA), bleomycin, etoposide, cisplatin, or procarbazine, on fertility and progeny outcome have clearly established some of the underlying molecular mechanisms that result in loss of fertility and altered progeny outcome [50–53].

Using CPA or the combination of drugs used for treating testicular cancer (bleomycin, etoposide, and cisplatin, BEP) as model drugs and the rat as the model animal, it has been demonstrated that paternal exposures result in adverse reproductive outcomes that range from increased preimplantation and postimplantation loss or early postnatal death to growth retardation and congenital malformation; significantly, some of these outcomes are transmitted to subsequent generations [54, 55]. It is particularly noteworthy that the action of such drugs on germ cells not only affects the number of germ cells that the testis can produce but also alters markers of chromatin structure (comet, acridine orange, TUNEL, mBBr, and CMA3 assays, nuclear proteome) in spermatozoa [56, 57]. It is clear from animal studies that spermatozoa that have damaged chromatin as a result of paternal drug treatment are capable of fertilizing oocytes [54, 58–60]. These studies have also revealed that the effects of paternal exposure on progeny can be wide ranging. While treatment with BEP caused a decrease in both sperm production and sperm motility, no apparent effects were observed on progeny at the end of gestation, yet postnatal death rates were dramatically increased [58]. By contrast, chronic CPA treatment had minimal effects on sperm number and motility, yet a wide range of effects were observed in progeny, ranging from abnormalities at birth to learning deficits as adults and in subsequent generations as well as abnormal reproductive capacity [51, 54, 61].

The effects of such chemotherapeutic treatments cannot only result in DNA breaks and cross-links but can also cause epigenetic modifications; these include an alteration in DNA methylation profile [62] and changes in sperm nuclear proteins [63, 64]. Remarkably, proteins implicated in the translational control and post-translational processing of protamine 1 are also significantly elevated 9 weeks post-BEP treatment, suggesting that histone eviction may dictate the DNA availability for protamine binding [65]. Males mated to control females 9 weeks after BEP treatment have reduced litter sizes; moreover, the profile of gene expression in the developing testes of their pups is altered [65]. Liu et al. [66] recently reported that exposure of male germ cells to a BEP induces telomere shortening in all stages of rat spermatogenesis. Thus altering epigenetic marks or nuclear proteins in mature spermatozoa impacts on male fecundity, potentially threatening normal progeny development; this raises concerns regarding transgenerational risks of chemotherapy exposure.

16.5.3.2 Clinical Studies

The assessment of the consequences on progeny outcome of exposure of men to chemotherapeutic drugs presents remarkable challenges. Chemotherapy often results in transient or permanent azoospermia or oligozoospermia in cancer patients [67]. Large epidemiological studies, discussed above, have revealed that there is clearly an effect on fertility and time to pregnancy [14]. In addition, the standard semen parameters (sperm number, motility, and morphology) as established by the World Health Organization (WHO) [68] are not sufficiently reliable predictors of male fertility [25, 69–71].

Consequently, the focus has shifted in recent years to assessing the nature and quality of chromatin in spermatozoa. In recent comprehensive reviews, Barratt et al. [72] and Zini et al. [73] have outlined our current clinical understanding and uncertainties related to the many assays used to ascertain sperm chromatin quality. Aneuploidy, an abnormal number of chromosomes, is one of the more striking consequences of anticancer drugs on sperm chromatin quality. Using multicolor fluorescent in situ hybridization to detect sperm aneuploidy for chromosomes 13, 21, X, and Y in testicular cancer and Hodgkin lymphoma patients before and up to 24 months after the initiation of chemotherapy, Tempest et al. [74] found that at 6 months, all cancer patients showed significantly increased frequencies of XY disomy and nullisomy for chromosomes 13 and 21. Although frequencies of aneuploidy generally declined over time after termination of treatment, increased aneuploidy frequencies persisted in some chromosomes for up to 24 months.

Using a series of assays that provide complementary information on sperm chromatin structure, e.g., extent of single- and double-strand breaks, degree of protamination, and cross-linking of sulfhydryl bonds, O'Flaherty et al. [25] have shown that, prior to initiation of chemotherapy, sperm chromatin integrity was poorer in cancer patients than in a control population. After treatment with chemotherapeutics, not only was there the expected decline in sperm production and chromatin quality but also, up to 2 years later, a reduction in spermatozoal chromatin integrity in over 40% of the patients who had a return of spermatogenesis [75, 76]. Subsequent multicenter prospective longitudinal studies of Hodgkin and non-Hodgkin lymphomas [32] and testicular germ cell tumors [31] supported these findings.

The negative impact of antineoplastic agents appears to extend beyond the genome in humans as well as it does in animals. It has recently been reported that temozolomide, an oral alkylating agent used for treatment of advanced astrocytoma and melanoma, affected sperm quantity and quality (increased aneuploidy rate) as well as epigenome integrity [77]. One of the mechanisms of action of temozolomide is alkylation/methylation of DNA at the O-6 position of guanine residues resulting in DNA mismatch repair and subsequent double-strand breaks and apoptosis. Epigenetic analysis of human sperm following treatment with temozolomide demonstrated hypomethylation at the DMR (differentially methylated region) locus of the H19 (a gene with CpG-rich regions important for human tumor growth) [77].

This locus is paternally imprinted and hypermethylated in normospermic men. Alteration of spermatozoal DNA methylation profiles has a known association with clinical male infertility with oligozoospermia [78]. Hypomethylation of normally hypermethylated paternally imprinted loci is associated with neoplasia and other metabolic and growth defects such as Beckwith-Wiedemann syndrome and disorders in neurodevelopment, cognition, and behavior. Further studies are thus required to evaluate if such an imprinting error is corrected after fertilization and the potential extent of transgenerational risks to children.

Based on the limited studies to date, it is clear that the presence of several cancers in young men results, to varying degrees, in sperm chromatin with reduced integrity. Furthermore, treatment of cancer may cause transient partial or complete loss of spermatozoa. Under some conditions, it is clear that the germ cells that eventually return to repopulate the seminiferous epithelium are still damaged, while under others, they appear to be normal. Whether spermatogonial stem cells (SCC) are able to repair all the damages caused by radiation or chemotherapy or not remains to be established.

16.6 Male Fertility Preservation and Restoration Strategies

Fertility preservation has become recognized as part of the important global care of cancer patients at the time of cancer diagnosis. This has come about because of the potential long-term negative impact of cytotoxic cancer therapies on male reproductive health and the expressed desire of many young cancer survivors to have children.

Continuing research efforts are being made to contribute to the development of multidisciplinary counseling strategies to best advise cancer patients and survivors regarding their potential risks for adverse pregnancy and progeny outcomes.

16.6.1 Sperm Cryopreservation

Sperm cryopreservation or sperm “banking” is currently the only available strategy to preserve male fertility. Ideally, sperm samples should be collected before any cytotoxic cancer therapies, through ejaculation by masturbation after 2–4 days of sexual abstinence. Then, sperm samples should be analyzed, frozen, and stored in aliquots in liquid nitrogen for future use. With the advances in and increased access to ART, such as IVF/ICSI, a very low number of living spermatozoa are required to achieve fertilization; therefore, even sperm samples that are far from meeting the semen parameters set by the WHO may still be used to achieve fertilization. Sperm cryopreservation does have its limitations as a fertility preservation strategy. First, only subjects beyond the state of physical maturity of adolescence, when “spermarche” begins within the testes, can have spermatozoa in the semen for cryopreservation.

One study of 62 attempts by adolescents to bank sperm before cancer therapy resulted in totally normal semen in only 4 subjects [79]. Semen procurement by masturbation may not always be feasible among adolescents, even for those who have spermatogenesis. In fact, for cultural and religious reasons, the act of masturbation may be viewed as inappropriate by parents of young adolescent cancer patients [80]. Alternative methods to obtain mature sperms in adolescents using high-frequency penile vibratory stimulus, electroejaculation, or surgical testicular sperm extraction will require sedation/anesthesia and are deemed too invasive for youngsters. Thus, sperm banking is not universally practiced in pediatric oncology centers, and few adolescent-friendly facilities exist.

For preadolescent boys with cancer, there is currently no accepted and proven option for fertility preservation. Early investigators held the view that being prepubertal during anticancer therapy conferred protection against gonadal damage. However, a study evaluating 12 men who survived childhood malignancy revealed that although puberty had progressed apparently normally in all 12, 8 patients were azoospermic, and only 1 had normal semen analysis 2–16.5 years post-chemotherapy [81]. In addition, following treatment of Hodgkin lymphoma in childhood, severe germ cell damage was observed in the majority of patients, even 17 years after chemotherapy [76, 82]. Evidently, there is no gonadal protection in the prepubertal male against chemotherapy-induced damage [83, 84]. In fact, some investigators believe that prepubertal testes are more vulnerable to the cytotoxic effects of chemotherapy than adult testes [85].

16.6.2 Pharmacological Strategies

The hypothesis that blocking the hypothalamic-pituitary-gonadal axis prior to the initiation of chemotherapy preserves the nondividing germ cells or SSC population was first proposed by Glode et al. [86]. Hormonal manipulation, including the use of exogenous GnRH (gonadotropin-releasing hormone) analogs and steroids (testosterone) to suppress gonadotropin release, has been investigated as a potential fertility preservation strategy. Since cytotoxic treatment acts mainly on rapidly dividing cells, germ cells have been postulated to be less susceptible to cytotoxic effects if hormone treatments are used to render the testes quiescent. This technique has been successful in some rodents (rats but not mice) [87, 88]; in addition, in rats the extent of the damage of chemotherapeutic agents has been shown to extend beyond the germ cells to the somatic cells surrounding them [89]. There is no evidence of a similar spermatogonial block in monkeys [90]. Thus far, clinical trials have not shown any benefit of this method [83, 91]. Furthermore, this approach would be ineffective for prepubertal children as the proliferation of germ cells in prepubertal primates appears to be gonadotropin independent [92]. Clearly, there is an urgent need for novel strategies that are effective and minimally invasive for fertility preservation in young male cancer patients.

16.6.3 Fertility Restoration with Germ Cell Transplantation

Stem cells of the male germ line, termed SSCs, exist in the testis prior to birth. Harvesting either SSCs or tissue blocks from testes for cryopreservation before anti-cancer therapies offers the hope for prepubertal boys with cancer to preserve fertility and form their family in the future [93]. After the patient is cured and is at an appropriate state of maturity, preserved SSCs, or SSCs derived from frozen tissue blocks, could be autotransplanted back to the seminiferous tubules to regenerate complete spermatogenesis. Cryopreservation of the testis tissue from prepubertal boys has revealed that germ cells can be preserved [94]. An important feature of this strategy is that instead of just preserving fertility, it aims to "restore" fertility. This fertility restoration scheme, based on germ cell or tissue transplantation, has been established with mice and other species [89, 93–101] and is currently under investigation to extend its application to humans.

To date, several groups have reported different cell culture systems designed to maintain and expand human SSCs [102–108]. Further, xenotransplantation of cultured human SSCs to immunodeficient mice—a well-acknowledged and only available assay for functionality of human SSCs—demonstrated their migration to the niche at the basal membrane of the seminiferous tubules, indicating their SSC capabilities [102]. Initiation of human spermatogenesis in the host mice has yet to be achieved; nonetheless, the steady progress in the development of male fertility restoration strategy with SCCs in the past two decades gives hopes to breakthroughs that will affect clinical practice.

The advances of the SCC cell culture system open an opportunity to combine with the exciting germ line genomic editing technology to potentially improve clinical outcomes. Several recent reports demonstrated the feasibility of genetic and epigenetic editing in SSC transplantation [109–112]. The use of CRISPR-Cas9 system has been shown in human to successfully repair mutations in hemoglobin beta gene in β-thalassemia [113] and dystrophin gene in Duchenne muscular dystrophy patient-induced pluripotent stem cells [114]. Another report describes successful repair of the cystic fibrosis transmembrane conductor receptor locus in cultured intestinal stem cells from patients with cystic fibrosis [115]. Potentially, identified cancer-inducing genes can be corrected in SCCs harvested in cancer patient during fertility preservation to reduce or eliminate the risk of transmission of cancer to offspring.

While significant progress has been made in this fertility restoration regime in the recent years, several hurdles must be overcome prior to realizing its clinical application. In addition to using a minimally invasive surgical approach to harvest SCCs (particularly when dealing with preadolescent boys) from the testes and proper isolation of the SCC population for cryopreservation, culture, clonal expansion, and subsequent transplantation for spermatogenesis reintroduction, the risk of contamination with lingering cancer cells, as in the case of hematological cancers (e.g., leukemia) or metastatic cancers, must be reduced to zero. Several groups have reported mixed results in the elimination of cancer cells when harvesting SCCs

[116–118]. Additionally, the costs, risks, success rate, and efficacy along with the potential well-being of the offspring produced with the complex interplay of various biotechnologies must be considered through rigorous ethical reflection and societal debate, particularly when genomic or epigenomic editing of the SCCs aimed at correcting adverse mutations may soon be a reality.

16.7 Health of Offspring of Male Cancer Survivors

Whereas the nature, mechanisms, and extents of gamete damage from cytotoxic anticancer therapies are important research questions, for cancer survivors, one of the most important clinical questions is the health risks to their offspring after cancer. Several recent studies reported a nonsignificant risk of adverse offspring health outcomes from cancer survivors. Two studies from retrospective cohort analyses of the Childhood Cancer Survivor Study reported no increase in the risk of stillbirth, neonatal death [119], and congenital anomalies [120] among survivors of childhood cancers who had undergone radiation and chemotherapy. A Danish case-cohort study also reported no increased risks of genetic disease from cancer survivors exposed to childhood/adolescent alkylating chemotherapies or radiation [121]. Using data collected from 1953 to 2004 from registries (e.g., national cancer, population birth, and hospital discharge registries) on close to 7000 offspring of cancer survivors with congenital anomalies and over 35,000 offspring of these survivors' siblings, another recent study demonstrated no significant increase in offspring anomaly rates from cancer survivors, regardless of the age when the cancer was diagnosed. However, the researchers did note a significantly higher risk of congenital anomalies in the offspring of survivors with cancer diagnosed in earlier period (1955–1964, prevalence ratio 2.77, 95% CI 1.26–6.11) [122].

While messages from these new studies may be reassuring, a few important points must be noted. First, other earlier and contemporary series observed either increased [123–125] or no increased risks [14, 126–129] of congenital malformations in the offspring of cancer survivors. The inconsistency of the results may be in part related to the differences in sample size and power, definitions of outcomes, study designs, and selection bias. Further, it should be noted that most of these data focus on outcomes of offspring from natural conceptions rather than with assisted reproduction—which many male cancer survivors may need with fresh or cryopreserved sperm. Indeed Stahl et al. [125] reported a significantly higher risk of birth abnormalities in offspring of men with a history of cancer (relative risk 1.17, 95% CI = 1.02–1.31) with both natural conception and assisted reproduction. Perhaps most importantly, these data do not address adequately other important reproductive outcomes such as time required to achieve pregnancy, risks of lower number of offspring, or rate of miscarriage, particularly early (<20 weeks) miscarriage; these are some of the endpoints that might be predicted to be affected based on the animal studies described above.

Taken together, cytotoxic cancer therapies not only will have negative impact on the quantitative and qualitative changes in conventional semen parameters and sperm DNA quality leading potentially to adverse reproductive outcomes: clinical infertility, increased use of assisted reproduction, and potential adverse offspring outcomes. Even for male cancer survivors who managed to achieve live births naturally or via assisted reproduction, the potential risks of adverse outcomes including congenital malformation, genetic diseases, and low birth weight cannot be completely eliminated. Further large-scale prospective longitudinal studies of cancer survivor cohorts and multicenter cancer registry follow-up studies will shed lights on the actual reproductive risks to allow formulation of proper counseling to these young cancer survivors. Meanwhile, precancer treatment fertility preservation counseling is the key to minimize the potential risks of adverse outcomes in the reproductive status of these patients.

16.8 Clinical Perspectives on Male Fertility Preservation and Fertility Outcomes

Understanding that currently sperm banking through cryopreservation prior to cancer therapy is the only feasible option of male fertility preservation, important questions remain to be answered. These include:

- What are the key components of an effective strategy to increase the willingness of these young men with newly diagnosed cancer to bank sperm?
- What are the assisted reproductive outcomes on the usage of these banked sperm?

Young men with newly diagnosed cancer who require cytotoxic therapy experience simultaneously complex psychosocial stress [130]. We have previously evaluated important factors that influence the sperm banking decision of cancer patients [131]. These factors include health-care providers' role in discussing fertility preservation, importance of fatherhood, current fatherhood status, partner's/parent's influence, attitudes toward survival, complexity of sperm banking, cultural factors, sexual orientation, and cost. The negative impact of cost of sperm banking is further highlighted in our recent report [132] demonstrating that in the absence of fees for sperm banking and subsequent storage, young cancer patients are willing to come for significantly more sperm banking sessions to preserve their fertility prior to cancer treatment, despite the fact that they are under significant level of stress and time constraint to begin treatment. The result is that a great quantity of sperm would be available for their future use, potentially leading to a higher chance of procreation success.

For male cancer survivors who fail to achieve pregnancy either naturally or with assisted reproduction using their fresh ejaculated sperm, if available, the use of their cryopreserved sperm is the only option for them to father genetic children. With the reduction in sperm quantity, motility, morphology, and chromatin quality from cryo-damage, the majority of these patients will require ICSI as a choice of assisted reproductive technology when using their banked sperm. Little is known on the reproductive outcomes on their usage of cryopreserved sperm. We recently reported that, while the usage rate of cryopreserved sperm is significantly lower among cancer survivors compared to noncancer patients (e.g., for infertility treatment) (11% vs 31%), the live birth rate of ICSI in cancer survivors was comparable to that of noncancer patients (62% vs 40%) [133]. As noted earlier, some cancer patients may have impaired sperm DNA integrity even prior to anticancer therapy at the time of fertility preservation. Thus, for some cancer survivors, despite successful fertility preservation, subsequent use of the cryopreserved sperm with conventional ICSI may not necessarily lead to live birth due to impaired sperm DNA quality. Advanced sperm selection strategies such as ultra-morphological selection, electrophoresis selection, hyaluronan-binding selection, and magnetic-activated cell sorting may be used in selected cases to improve the assisted reproductive outcomes, as we previously reported [134].

16.9 Looking to the Future

While the risks of impaired fertility after cancer therapy have long been recognized, the biological mechanisms and the nature and extent of sperm damage at the molecular level have only been revealed recently. The importance of fertility after cancer is gradually being accepted as an essential survivorship issue for young cancer survivors.

The establishment of effective fertility preservation protocols and counseling strategies represents an ongoing effort of researchers and clinicians.

A multidisciplinary approach, including input from oncologists, urologists, reproductive biologists, social workers, ethicists, geneticists, and embryologists, is the essence of successful development and implementation of any fertility management plan for young cancer survivors. Many questions remain to be answered: What is the potential of further recovery of sperm quality in long-term post chemotherapy? How long should a patient wait post chemotherapy before he can safely use his fresh sperm for procreation? What is the nature and extent of risk of adverse reproductive outcomes using sperm with impaired sperm chromatin post chemotherapy? What are the transgenerational risks, particularly in the context of using assisted reproduction? To what extent would such risks be reduced by using sperm cryopreserved prior to chemotherapy for procreation? What sperm biological markers and what assays provide the best clinical prediction of the risks of adverse reproductive outcomes when using sperm with impaired chromatin quality? Further research to address these and other related questions is clearly needed to help health-care professionals and health policy makers to enhance the quality of counseling and to establish practice guidelines on the subject of fertility after cancer.

References

1. Burns KC, Boudreau C, Panepinto JA. Attitudes regarding fertility preservation in female adolescent cancer patients. J Pediatr Hematol Oncol. 2006;28:350–4.
2. Richiardi L, Bellocco R, Adami HO, Torrang A, Barlow L, Hakulinen T, et al. Testicular cancer incidence in eight northern European countries: secular and recent trends. Cancer Epidemiol Biomark Prev. 2004;13:2157–66.
3. American Cancer Society. http://www.cancer.org/acs/groups/content/@research/documents/document/acspc-047079.pdf. 2016. Accessed 6 Sep 2016.
4. American Cancer Society. http://www.cancer.org/cancer/cancerinchildren/detailedguide/cancer-in-children-key-statistics. 2016. Accessed 6 Sept 2016.
5. Stiller CA. Epidemiology and genetics of childhood cancer. Oncogene. 2004;23:6429–44.
6. Stiller CA, Allen MB, Eatock EM. Childhood cancer in Britain: the national registry of childhood tumours and incidence rates 1978–1987. Eur J Cancer. 1995;31A:2028–34.
7. Waring AB, Wallace WH. Subfertility following treatment for childhood cancer. Hosp Med. 2000;61:550–7.
8. National Cancer Institute. Surveillance epidemiology and end results program of the National Cancer Institute research: fact sheet. http://SEER.Cancer.gov. 2009. Accessed 2 Jan 2009.
9. Garner MJ, Turner MC, Ghadirian P, Krewski D. Epidemiology of testicular cancer: an overview. Int J Cancer. 2005;116:331–9.
10. Bhatia S. Cancer survivorship-pediatric issues. Hematology Am Soc Hematol Educ Program. 2005:507–15.
11. Meadows AT. Pediatric cancer survivorship: research and clinical care. J Clin Oncol. 2006;24:5160–5.
12. Schover LR, Brey K, Lichtin A, Lipshultz LI, Jeha S. Oncologists' attitudes and practices regarding banking sperm before cancer treatment. J Clin Oncol. 2002;20:1890–7.
13. Schover LR, Rybicki LA, Martin BA, Bringelsen KA. Having children after cancer. A pilot survey of survivors' attitudes and experiences. Cancer. 1999;86:697–709.
14. Green DM, Lange JM, Peabody EM, Grigorieva NN, Peterson SM, Kalapurakal JA, et al. Pregnancy outcome after treatment for Wilms tumor: a report from the national Wilms tumor long-term follow-up study. J Clin Oncol. 2010;28:2824–30.
15. Klosky JL, Simmons JL, Russell KM, Foster RH, Sabbatini GM, Canavera KE, et al. Fertility as a priority among at-risk adolescent males newly diagnosed with cancer and their parents. Support Care Cancer. 2015;23:333–41.
16. Chan PT, Palermo GD, Veeck LL, Rosenwaks Z, Schlegel PN. Testicular sperm extraction combined with intracytoplasmic sperm injection in the treatment of men with persistent azoospermia postchemotherapy. Cancer. 2001;92:1632–7.
17. Hansen M, Bower C, Milne E, de Klerk N, Kurinczuk JJ. Assisted reproductive technologies and the risk of birth defects–a systematic review. Hum Reprod. 2005;20:328–38.
18. Schieve LA, Cohen B, Nannini A, Ferre C, Reynolds MA, Zhang Z, Massachusetts Consortium for Assisted Reproductive Technology Epidemiologic Research (MCARTER), et al. A population-based study of maternal and perinatal outcomes associated with assisted reproductive technology in Massachusetts. Matern Child Health J. 2007;11:517–25.
19. Schieve LA, Meikle SF, Ferre C, Peterson HB, Jeng G, Wilcox LS. Low and very low birth weight in infants conceived with use of assisted reproductive technology. N Engl J Med. 2002;346:731–7.
20. Steel AJ, Sutcliffe A. Long-term health implications for children conceived by IVF/ICSI. Hum Fertil (Camb). 2009;12:21–7.
21. Qin J, Sheng X, Wang H, Liang D, Tan H, Xia J. Assisted reproductive technology and risk of congenital malformations: a meta-analysis based on cohort studies. Arch Gynecol Obstet. 2015;292:777–98.
22. Meirow D, Schenker JG. Cancer and male infertility. Hum Reprod. 1995;10:2017–22.

23. Meseguer M, Molina N, Garcia-Velasco JA, Remohi J, Pellicer A, Garrido N. Sperm cryopreservation in oncological patients: a 14-year follow-up study. Fertil Steril. 2006;85:640–5.
24. Baker JA, Buck GM, Vena JE, Moysich KB. Fertility patterns prior to testicular cancer diagnosis. Cancer Causes Control. 2005;16:295–9.
25. O'Flaherty C, Vaisheva F, Hales BF, Chan P, Robaire B. Characterization of sperm chromatin quality in testicular cancer and Hodgkin's lymphoma patients prior to chemotherapy. Hum Reprod. 2008;23:1044–52.
26. Dieckmann KP, Linke J, Pichlmeier U, Kulejewski M, German Testicular Cancer Study Group. Spermatogenesis in the contralateral testis of patients with testicular germ cell cancer: histological evaluation of testicular biopsies and a comparison with healthy males. BJU Int. 2007;99:1079–85.
27. O'Donovan M. An evaluation of chromatin condensation and DNA integrity in the spermatozoa of men with cancer before and after therapy. Andrologia. 2005;37:83–90.
28. Meseguer M, Santiso R, Garrido N, Fernandez JL. The effect of cancer on sperm DNA fragmentation as measured by the sperm chromatin dispersion test. Fertil Steril. 2008;90:225–7.
29. Ståhl O, Eberhard J, Cavallin-Ståhl E, Jepson K, Friberg B, Tingsmark C, et al. Sperm DNA integrity in cancer patients: the effect of disease and treatment. Int J Androl. 2009;32:695–703.
30. Rives N, Perdrix A, Hennebicq S, Saïas-Magnan J, Melin MC, Berthaut I, et al. The semen quality of 1158 men with testicular cancer at the time of cryopreservation: results of the French National CECOS Network. J Androl. 2012;33:1394–401.
31. Bujan L, Walschaerts M, Moinard N, Hennebicq S, Saias J, Brugnon F, et al. Impact of chemotherapy and radiotherapy for testicular germ cell tumors on spermatogenesis and sperm DNA: a multicenter prospective study from the CECOS network. Fertil Steril. 2013;100:673–80.
32. Bujan L, Walschaerts M, Brugnon F, Daudin M, Berthaut I, Auger J, et al. Impact of lymphoma treatments on spermatogenesis and sperm deoxyribonucleic acid: a multicenter prospective study from the CECOS network. Fertil Steril. 2014;102:667–74.
33. Ribeiro TM, Bertolla RP, Spaine DM, Fraietta R, Ortiz V, Cedenho AP. Sperm nuclear apoptotic DNA fragmentation in men with testicular cancer. Fertil Steril. 2008;90:1782–6.
34. Smit M, van Casteren NJ, Wildhagen MF, Romijn JC, Dohle GR. Sperm DNA integrity in cancer patients before and after cytotoxic treatment. Hum Reprod. 2010;25:1877–83.
35. Cunningham GR, Tindall DJ, Huckins C, Means AR. Mechanisms for the testicular hypertrophy which follows hemicastration. Endocrinology. 1978;102:16–23.
36. Medhamurthy R, Aravindan GR, Moudgal NR. Hemiorchidectomy leads to dramatic and immediate alterations in pituitary follicle-stimulating hormone secretion and the functional activity of the remaining testis in the adult male bonnet monkey (Macaca radiata). Biol Reprod. 1993;49:743–9.
37. Tsutsui T, Kurita A, Kirihara N, Hori T, Kawakami E. Testicular compensatory hypertrophy related to hemicastration in prepubertal dogs. J Vet Med Sci. 2004;66:1021–5.
38. Laron Z, Dickerman Z, Ritterman I, Kaufman H. Follow-up of boys with unilateral compensatory testicular hypertrophy. Fertil Steril. 1980;33:297–301.
39. Lin WW, Kim ED, Quesada ET, Lipshultz LI, Coburn M. Unilateral testicular injury from external trauma: evaluation of semen quality and endocrine parameters. J Urol. 1998;159:841–3.
40. Grinspon RP, Habib C, Bedecarrás P, Gottlieb S, Rey RA. Compensatory function of the remaining testis is dissociated in boys and adolescents with monorchidism. Eur J Endocrinol. 2016;174:399–407.
41. Romerius P, Ståhl O, Moëll C, Relander T, Cavallin-Ståhl E, Gustafsson H, et al. Sperm DNA integrity in men treated for childhood cancer. Clin Cancer Res. 2010;16:3843–50.
42. Papaefthymiou MA, Giaginis CT, Theocharis SE. DNA repair alterations in common pediatric malignancies. Med Sci Monit. 2008;14:RA8–15.
43. Clifton DK, Bremner WJ. The effect of testicular x-irradiation on spermatogenesis in man. A comparison with the mouse. J Androl. 1983;4:387–92.

44. Zhang Z, Shao S, Meistrich ML. The radiation-induced block in spermatogonial differentiation is due to damage to the somatic environment, not the germ cells. J Cell Physiol. 2007;211:149–58.
45. Spermon JR, Ramos L, Wetzels AM, Sweep CG, Braat DD, Kiemeney LA, et al. Sperm integrity pre- and post-chemotherapy in men with testicular germ cell cancer. Hum Reprod. 2006;21:1781–6.
46. Singh DK, Hersey K, Perlis N, Crook J, Jarvi K, Fleshner N. The effect of radiation on semen quality and fertility in men treated with brachytherapy for early stage prostate cancer. J Urol. 2012;187:987–9.
47. Le W, Huang S, Gui Y, Luo H, Wu D, Feng H, et al. Assessment of numerical chromosomal abnormalities of the sperms before and after radiotherapy in seminoma patient. Int J Clin Exp Med. 2014;7:703–8.
48. Robaire B, Hales BF, editors. Advances in male-mediated reproductive toxicology. New York: Kluwer Academic/Plenum; 2003.
49. Anderson D, Brinkworth MH, editors. Male mediated developmental toxicity. London: Royal Society of Chemistry; 2006.
50. Hales BF, Barton TS, Robaire B. Impact of paternal exposure to chemotherapy on offspring in the rat. J Natl Cancer Inst Monogr. 2005;34:28–31.
51. Hales BF, Crosman K, Robaire B. Increased postimplantation loss and malformations among the F2 progeny of male rats chronically treated with cyclophosphamide. Teratology. 1992;45:671–8.
52. Anderson D. Male-mediated developmental toxicity. Toxicol Appl Pharmacol. 2005;207(2 Suppl):506–13.
53. Meistrich ML. Male gonadal toxicity. Pediatr Blood Cancer. 2009;53:261–6.
54. Trasler JM, Hales BF, Robaire B. Paternal cyclophosphamide treatment of rats causes fetal loss and malformations without affecting male fertility. Nature. 1985;316:144–6.
55. Harrouk W, Codrington A, Vinson R, Robaire B, Hales BF. Paternal exposure to cyclophosphamide induces DNA damage and alters the expression of DNA repair genes in the rat preimplantation embryo. Mutat Res. 2000;461:229–41.
56. Codrington AM, Hales BF, Robaire B. Chronic cyclophosphamide exposure alters the profile of rat sperm nuclear matrix proteins. Biol Reprod. 2007;77:303–11.
57. Delbes G, Hales BF, Robaire B. Toxicants and human sperm chromatin integrity. Mol Hum Reprod. 2010;16:14–22.
58. Bieber AM, Marcon L, Hales BF, Robaire B. Effects of chemotherapeutic agents for testicular cancer on the male rat reproductive system, spermatozoa, and fertility. J Androl. 2006;27:189–200.
59. Menezo Y, Dale B, Cohen M. DNA damage and repair in human oocytes and embryos: a review. Zygote. 2010;21:1–9.
60. Sakkas D, Alvarez JG. Sperm DNA fragmentation: mechanisms of origin, impact on reproductive outcome, and analysis. Fertil Steril. 2010;93:1027–36.
61. Auroux M, Dulioust E, Selva J, Rince P. Cyclophosphamide in the F0 male rat: physical and behavioral changes in three successive adult generations. Mutat Res. 1990;229:189–200.
62. Chan D, Delbès G, Landry M, Robaire B, Trasler JM. Epigenetic alterations in sperm DNA associated with testicular cancer treatment. Toxicol Sci. 2012;125:532–43.
63. Maselli J, Hales BF, Chan P, Robaire B. Exposure to bleomycin, etoposide, and cis-platinum alters rat sperm chromatin integrity and sperm head protein profile. Biol Reprod. 2012;86(166):1–10.
64. Bagheri-Sereshki N, Hales BF, Robaire B. The effects of chemotherapeutic agents, bleomycin, etoposide, and cisplatin, on chromatin remodeling in male rat germ cells. Biol Reprod. 2016;94:81.
65. Maselli J, Hales BF, Robaire B. The effects of chemotherapy with bleomycin, etoposide, and cis-platinum (BEP) on rat sperm chromatin remodeling, fecundity and testicular gene expression in the progeny. Biol Reprod. 2013;89:85.

66. LiuM,MaselliJ,HalesBF,RobaireB.Theeffectsofchemotherapywithbleomycin,etoposideandcis-platinumontelomeresinratmalegermcells. Andrology. 2015;3:1104–12.
67. Gandini L, Sgro P, Lombardo F, Paoli D, Culasso F, Toselli L, et al. Effect of chemo- or radiotherapy on sperm parameters of testicular cancer patients. Hum Reprod. 2006;21:2882–9.
68. World Health Organization. WHO laboratory manual for examination and processing of human semen. 5th ed. Cambridge: University Press Cambridge; 2010.
69. Spano M, Bonde JP, Hjollund HI, Kolstad HA, Cordelli E, Leter G. Sperm chromatin damage impairs human fertility. The Danish First Pregnancy Planner Study Team. Fertil Steril. 2000;73:43–50.
70. Virro MR, Larson-Cook KL, Evenson DP. Sperm chromatin structure assay (SCSA) parameters are related to fertilization, blastocyst development, and ongoing pregnancy in in vitro fertilization and intracytoplasmic sperm injection cycles. Fertil Steril. 2004;81:1289–95.
71. Payne JF, Raburn DJ, Couchman GM, Price TM, Jamison MG, Walmer DK. Redefining the relationship between sperm deoxyribonucleic acid fragmentation as measured by the sperm chromatin structure assay and outcomes of assisted reproductive techniques. Fertil Steril. 2005;84:356–64.
72. Barratt CL, Aitken RJ, Bjorndahl L, Carrell DT, de Boer P, Kvist U, et al. Sperm DNA: organization, protection and vulnerability: from basic science to clinical applications-a position report. Hum Reprod. 2010;25:824–38.
73. Zini A, Albert O, Robaire B. Assessing sperm chromatin and DNA damage: clinical importance and development of standards. Andrology. 2014;2:322–5.
74. Tempest HG, Ko E, Chan P, Robaire B, Rademaker A, Martin RH. Sperm aneuploidy frequencies analysed before and after chemotherapy in testicular cancer and Hodgkin's lymphoma patients. Hum Reprod. 2008;23:251–8.
75. O'Flaherty C, Hales BF, Chan P, Robaire B. Impact of chemotherapeutics and advanced testicular cancer or Hodgkin lymphoma on sperm deoxyribonucleic acid integrity. Fertil Steril. 2010;94:1374–9.
76. Heikens J, Behrendt H, Adriaanse R, Berghout A. Irreversible gonadal damage in male survivors of pediatric Hodgkin's disease. Cancer. 1996;78:2020–4.
77. Bruno C, Dudkiewicz-Sibony C, Berthaut I, Weil E, Brunet L, Fortier C, et al. Survey of 243 ART patients having made a final disposition decision about their surplus cryopreserved embryos: the crucial role of symbolic embryo representation. Hum Reprod. 2016;31:1508–14.
78. Cui X, Jing X, Wu X, Yan M, Li Q, Shen Y, et al. DNA methylation in spermatogenesis and male infertility. Exp Ther Med. 2016;12:1973–9.
79. Postovsky S, Lightman A, Aminpour D, Elhasid R, Peretz M, Arush MW. Sperm cryopreservation in adolescents with newly diagnosed cancer. Med Pediatr Oncol. 2003;40:355–9.
80. Rosoff PM, Katsur ML. Preserving fertility in young cancer patients: a medical, ethical and legal challenge. J Philos Sci Law. 2003;3. http://www6.miami.edu/ethics/jpsl/archives/papers/preservingFert.html. Accessed 4 Sept 2010.
81. Mustieles C, Munoz A, Alonso M, Ros P, Yturriaga R, Maldonado S, et al. Male gonadal function after chemotherapy in survivors of childhood malignancy. Med Pediatr Oncol. 1995;24:347–51.
82. Shafford EA, Kingston JE, Malpas JS, Plowman PN, Pritchard J, Savage MO, et al. Testicular function following the treatment of Hodgkin's disease in childhood. Br J Cancer. 1993;68:1199–204.
83. Thomson AB, Anderson RA, Irvine DS, Kelnar CJ, Sharpe RM, Wallace WH. Investigation of suppression of the hypothalamic-pituitary-gonadal axis to restore spermatogenesis in azoospermic men treated for childhood cancer. Hum Reprod. 2002;17:1715–23.
84. van Casteren NJ, van der Linden GH, Hakvoort-Cammel FG, Hahlen K, Dohle GR, van den Heuvel-Eibrink MM. Effect of childhood cancer treatment on fertility markers in adult male long-term survivors. Pediatr Blood Cancer. 2009;52:108–12.
85. Revel A, Revel-Vilk S. Pediatric fertility preservation: is it time to offer testicular tissue cryopreservation? Mol Cell Endocrinol. 2008;282:143–9.

86. Glode LM, Robinson J, Gould SF. Protection from cyclophosphamide-induced testicular damage with an analogue of gonadotropin-releasing hormone. Lancet. 1981;1:1132–4.
87. Kurdoglu B, Wilson G, Parchuri N, Ye WS, Meistrich ML. Protection from radiation-induced damage to spermatogenesis by hormone treatment. Radiat Res. 1994;139:97–102.
88. Meistrich ML, Shetty G. Hormonal suppression for fertility preservation in males and females. Reproduction. 2008;136:691–701.
89. Zhang X, Ebata KT, Nagano MC. Genetic analysis of the clonal origin of regenerating mouse spermatogenesis following transplantation. Biol Reprod. 2003;69:1872–8.
90. Boekelheide K, Schoenfeld H, Hall SJ, Weng CCY, Shetty G, Leith J, et al. Gonadotropin-releasing hormone antagonist (cetrorelix) therapy fails to protect nonhuman primates (Macaca arctoides) from radiation- induced spermatogenic failure. J Androl. 2009;26:222–34.
91. Waxman JH, Ahmed R, Smith D, Wrigley PF, Gregory W, Shalet S, et al. Failure to preserve fertility in patients with Hodgkin's disease. Cancer Chemother Pharmacol. 1987;19:159–62.
92. Kelnar CJ, McKinnell C, Walker M, Morris KD, Wallace WH, Saunders PT, et al. Testicular changes during infantile "quiescence" in the marmoset and their gonadotrophin dependence: a model for investigating susceptibility of the prepubertal human testis to cancer therapy? Hum Reprod. 2002;17:1367–78.
93. Nagano MC. A surgical strategy using spermatogonial stem cells for restoring male fertility. In: Tulandi T, Gosden RG, editors. Preservation of fertility. London: Taylor & Francis; 2004. p. 125–40.
94. Keros V, Hultenby K, Borgstrom B, Fridstrom M, Jahnukainen K, Hovatta O. Methods of cryopreservation of testicular tissue with viable spermatogonia in pre-pubertal boys undergoing gonadotoxic cancer treatment. Hum Reprod. 2007;22:1384–95.
95. Oatley JM, Brinster RL. Regulation of spermatogonial stem cell self-renewal in mammals. Annu Rev Cell Dev Biol. 2008;24:263–86.
96. Nagano MC. Homing efficiency and proliferation kinetics of male germ line stem cells following transplantation in mice. Biol Reprod. 2003;69:701–7.
97. Ebata KT, Yeh JR, Zhang X, Nagano MC. The application of biomarkers of spermatogonial stem cells for restoring male fertility. Dis Markers. 2008;24:267–76.
98. Ebata KT, Zhang X, Nagano MC. Expression patterns of cell-surface molecules on male germ line stem cells during postnatal mouse development. Mol Reprod Dev. 2005;72:171–81.
99. Ebata KT, Zhang X, Nagano MC. Male germ line stem cells have an altered potential to proliferate and differentiate during postnatal development in mice. Biol Reprod. 2007;76:841–7.
100. Yeh JR, Zhang X, Nagano MC. Establishment of a short-term in vitro assay for mouse spermatogonial stem cells. Biol Reprod. 2007;77:897–904.
101. Schlatt S, Ehmcke J, Jahnukainen K. Testicular stem cells for fertility preservation: preclinical studies on male germ cell transplantation and testicular grafting. Pediatr Blood Cancer. 2009;53:274–80.
102. Nagano M, Patrizio P, Brinster RL. Long-term survival of human spermatogonial stem cells in mouse testes. Fertil Steril. 2002;78:1225–33.
103. Sadri-Ardekani H, Mizrak SC, van Daalen SK, Korver CM, Roepers-Gajadien HL, Koruji M, et al. Propagation of human spermatogonial stem cells in vitro. J Am Med Assoc. 2009;302:2127–34.
104. Sadri-Ardekani H, Akhondi MA, van der Veen F, Repping S, van Pelt AM. In vitro propagation of human prepubertal spermatogonial stem cells. JAMA. 2011;305:2416–8.
105. Lim J, Sung S, Kim H, Song S, Hong J, Yoon T, et al. Long-term proliferation and characterization of human spermatogonial stem cells obtained from obstructive and non-obstructive azoospermia under exogenous feeder-free culture conditions. Cell Prolif. 2010;43:405–17.
106. Kossack N, Terwort N, Wistuba J, Ehmcke J, Schlatt S, Scholer H, et al. A combined approach facilitates the reliable detection of human spermatogonia in vitro. Hum Reprod. 2013;28:3012–25.
107. Akhondi M, Mohazzab A, Jeddi-Tehrani M, Sadeghi M, Eidi A, Khodadadi A, et al. Propagation of human germ stem cells in long-term culture. Iran J Reprod Med. 2013;11:551–8.

108. Guo Y, Liu L, Sun M, Hai Y, Li Z, He Z. Expansion and long-term culture of human spermatogonial stem cells via the activation of SMAD3 and AKT pathways. Exp Biol Med (Maywood). 2015;240:1112–22.
109. Fanslow DA, Wirt SE, Barker JC, Connelly JP, Porteus MH, Dann CT. Genome editing in mouse spermatogonial stem/progenitor cells using engineered nucleases. PLoS One. 2014;9:e112652.
110. Wu Y, Zhou H, Fan X, Zhang Y, Zhang M, Wang Y, et al. Correction of a genetic disease by CRISPR-Cas9-mediated gene editing in mouse spermatogonial stem cells. Cell Res. 2015;25:67–79.
111. Chapman KM, Medrano GA, Jaichander P, Chaudhary J, Waits AE, Nobrega MA, et al. Targeted germline modifications in rats using CRISPR/Cas9 and spermatogonial stem cells. Cell Rep. 2015;10:1828–35.
112. Sato T, Sakuma T, Yokonishi T, Katagiri K, Kamimura S, Ogonuki N, et al. Genome editing in mouse spermatogonial stem cell lines using TALEN and double-nicking CRISPR/Cas9. Stem Cell Rep. 2015;5:75–82.
113. Xie F, Ye L, Chang JC, Beyer AI, Wang J, Muench MO, et al. Seamless gene correction of beta-thalassemia mutations in patient-specific iPSCs using CRISPR/Cas9 and piggyBac. Genome Res. 2014;24:1526–33.
114. Li HL, Fujimoto N, Sasakawa N, Shirai S, Ohkame T, Sakuma T, et al. Precise correction of the dystrophin gene in Duchenne muscular dystrophy patient induced pluripotent stem cells by TALEN and CRISPR-Cas9. Stem Cell Rep. 2015;4:143–54.
115. Schwank G, Koo BK, Sasselli V, Dekkers JF, Heo I, Demircan T, et al. Functional repair of CFTR by CRISPR/Cas9 in intestinal stem cell organoids of cystic fibrosis patients. Cell Stem Cell. 2013;13:653–8.
116. Geens M, Van de Velde H, De Block G, Goossens E, Van Steirteghem A, Tournaye H. The efficiency of magnetic-activated cell sorting and fluorescence-activated cell sorting in the decontamination of testicular cell suspensions in cancer patients. Hum Reprod. 2007;22:733–42.
117. Hermann BP, Sukhwani M, Salati J, Sheng Y, Chu T, Orwig KE. Separating spermatogonia from cancer cells in contaminated prepubertal primate testis cell suspensions. Hum Reprod. 2011;26:3222–31.
118. Sadri-Ardekani H, Homburg CH, van Capel TM, van den Berg H, van der Veen F, van der Schoot CE, et al. Eliminating acute lymphoblastic leukemia cells from human testicular cell cultures: a pilot study. Fertil Steril. 2014;101:1072–8. e1071
119. Signorello LB, Mulvihill JJ, Green DM, Munro HM, Stovall M, Weathers RE, et al. Stillbirth and neonatal death in relation to radiation exposure before conception: a retrospective cohort study. Lancet. 2010;376:624–30.
120. Signorello LB, Mulvihill JJ, Green DM, Munro HM, Stovall M, Weathers RE, et al. Congenital anomalies in the children of cancer survivors: a report from the childhood cancer survivor study. J Clin Oncol. 2012;30:239–45.
121. Winther JF, Olsen JH, Wu H, Shyr Y, Mulvihill JJ, Stovall M, et al. Genetic disease in the children of Danish survivors of childhood and adolescent cancer. J Clin Oncol. 2012;30:27–33.
122. Seppänen VI, Artama MS, Malila NK, Pitkäniemi JM, Rantanen ME, Ritvanen AK, et al. Risk for congenital anomalies in offspring of childhood, adolescent and young adult cancer survivors. Int J Cancer. 2016;139:1721–30.
123. Magelssen H, Melve KK, Skjaerven R, Fosså SD. Parenthood probability and pregnancy outcome in patients with a cancer diagnosis during adolescence and young adulthood. Hum Reprod. 2008;23:178–86.
124. Chow EJ, Kamineni A, Daling JR, Fraser A, Wiggins CL, Mineau GP, et al. Reproductive outcomes in male childhood cancer survivors: a linked cancer-birth registry analysis. Arch Pediatr Adolesc Med. 2009;163:887–94.
125. Ståhl O, Boyd HA, Giwercman A, Lindholm M, Jensen A, Kjær SK, et al. Risk of birth abnormalities in the offspring of men with a history of cancer: a cohort study using Danish and Swedish national registries. J Natl Cancer Inst. 2011;103:398–406.

126. Mueller BA, Chow EJ, Kamineni A, Daling JR, Fraser A, Wiggins CL, et al. Pregnancy outcomes in female childhood and adolescent cancer survivors: a linked cancer-birth registry analysis. Arch Pediatr Adolesc Med. 2009;163:879–86.
127. Nagarajan R, Robison LL. Pregnancy outcomes in survivors of childhood cancer. J Natl Cancer Inst Monogr. 2005;34:72–6.
128. Byrne J, Rasmussen SA, Steinhorn SC, Connelly RR, Myers MH, Lynch CF, et al. Genetic disease in offspring of long-term survivors of childhood and adolescent cancer. Am J Hum Genet. 1998;62:45–52.
129. Winther JF, Boice JD Jr, Frederiksen K, Bautz A, Mulvihill JJ, Stovall M, et al. Radiotherapy for childhood cancer and risk for congenital malformations in offspring: a population based cohort study. Clin Genet. 2009;75:50–6.
130. Rosberger Z, Carter J, Achille M, Bultz BD, Chan P. Communicating about infertility risks. In: Kissane DW, Bultz BD, Butow PM, Finlay IG, editors. Handbook of communication in oncology and palliative care. New York: Oxford University Press; 2010. p. 399–408.
131. Achille MA, Rosberger Z, Robitaille R, Lebel S, Gouin JP, Bultz BD, et al. Facilitators and obstacles to sperm banking in young men receiving gonadotoxic chemotherapy for cancer: the perspective of survivors and health care professionals. Hum Reprod. 2006;21:3206–16.
132. Herrero MB, García A, Buckett W, Tulandi T, Chan P. Quebec public funding facilitates fertility preservation to male cancer patients. Curr Oncol. 2016;23:20–5.
133. Garcia A, Herrero MB, Holzer H, Tulandi T, Chan P. Assisted reproductive outcomes of male cancer survivors. J Cancer Surviv. 2015;9:208–14.
134. Herrero MB, Delbes G, Chung JT, Son WY, Holzer H, Buckett W, et al. Case report: the use of annexin V coupled with magnetic activated cell sorting in cryopreserved spermatozoa from a male cancer survivor: healthy twin newborns after two previous ICSI failures. J Assist Reprod Genet. 2013;30:1415–9.

Chapter 17
Sperm Chromatin and Environmental Factors

Aleksander Giwercman and Marcello Spanó

17.1 Introduction

During the past 25 years, the possible time-related deterioration in the function of male reproductive organs has been a matter of debate [1]. In the 1990s alarming reports on declining sperm counts as well as on increasing incidence of congenital malformations of male genital organs—cryptorchidism and hypospadias—have been published, although the validity of these data is still a matter of discussion [2–4]. On the other hand, there is no doubt that testicular cancer has become significantly more common over the past four to five decades [5]. The rapid rise in the incidence of testicular cancer points towards a negative impact of environment- or lifestyle-related factors on male reproductive function. The deleterious effect of the environment and/or lifestyle on semen parameters might have a negative impact on the integrity of the sperm DNA. Such effect might not only have an impact on the fertility potential of the subject but also introduce genetic aberrations which might be transmitted to the next generation [6].

This chapter will focus on the available evidence regarding environment- and lifestyle-induced changes in the sperm DNA and the biological and clinical implications of such effect.

A. Giwercman (✉)
Lund University, Malmö, Sweden
e-mail: aleksander.giwercman@med.lu.se

M. Spanó (Deceased)
Laboratory of Biosafety and Risk Assessment, Division of Technologies and Methodologies for Health Protection, ENEA (Italian National Agency for New Technologies, Energy and Sustainable Economic Development), Rome, Italy

A. Zini, A. Agarwal (eds.), *A Clinician's Guide to Sperm DNA and Chromatin Damage*, https://doi.org/10.1007/978-3-319-71815-6_17

17.2 How Can Environment/Lifestyle Affect Sperm Chromatin?

Apart from numerical and structural chromosomal changes, environmental exposure may, in principle, affect sperm DNA by introducing DNA fragmentation (or DNA strand breaks) and/or epigenetic changes in the genome of the male gamete.

Meiotic crossing-over is associated with the genetically programmed introduction of DNA double-strand breaks (DSBs) by specific nucleases of SP011 family [7]. These DNA DSBs should be ligated until the end of meiosis I. Defective repair may interrupt spermatogenesis or lead to persistent sperm DNA fragmentation in ejaculated spermatozoa. Stage-specific occurrence of transient DNA strand breaks during spermiogenesis has been observed [8–10]. Both single-strand breaks (SSBs) and DSBs have been found in round and elongating spermatids. DNA breaks are necessary for transient relief of torsional stress, favouring casting off of the nucleosome histone cores and aiding their replacement with transitional proteins and protamines during maturation of elongating spermatids [9–11]. Thus, chromatin packaging necessitates endogenous nuclease activity to both create and ligate breaks, in order to reassemble DNA around the new protamine core. Chromatin packaging is completed and DNA integrity restored during epididymal transit [12]. Although there is little evidence that spermatid maturation-associated DNA breaks are fully ligated, biologically this must be the case [13]. Ligation of DNA breaks is necessary not only to preserve the integrity of the primary DNA structure but also for reassembly of the important unit of genome expression—the DNA loop domain.

Enzymatic activity involved in the creation of DNA breaks in spermatids has only been proven (by decatenating activity and specific inhibition) for topoisomerase II (Topo II) generating and ligating DSBs [9, 14]. Remodelling of chromatin by histone H4 hyperacetylation weakens the ionic interactions between the DNA and histone cores and is needed for Topo II activity to be introduced in spermatids [14]. Interestingly, Topo II activity seems to be androgen dependent [15], and, since many of the environmental toxicants act as endocrine disrupters, they may, in principle, have an impact on sperm DNA integrity.

Although deficiencies in recombination during spermiogenesis may be a cause of sperm DNA strand breaks, it has been proposed that the most important mechanism behind DNA damage in spermatozoa is a two-step process including (1) development of increased vulnerability to free radical attack and (2) oxidative stress mediated by variety of reactive oxygen species (ROS) [16].

A major factor leading to increased ROS vulnerability of the male gamete relates to the state of protamination of sperm chromatin. The exchange of histones with protamines occurs during the spermiogenesis, and insufficient protamination implies defective compaction of the DNA and subsequently an increased risk of damage following oxidative attack. Whereas it has been shown that drugs, as those used in cancer treatment, can negatively affect sperm chromatin [17], it remains to be investigated whether the protamination process can be negatively affected by environmental chemicals.

For several reasons spermatozoa are sensitive to the negative effects of oxidative stress. They have an abundance of substrates susceptible to free radical attack, including high amount of polyunsaturated fats in their plasma membrane. Their antioxidant defensive capacity is low because most of the cytoplasm is removed during the process of spermiogenesis. This leads to reduction of cytoplasmic antioxidants such as catalase and superoxide dismutase. Furthermore, the cells, by themselves, create ROS due to electron leakage from their mitochondria [18]. The most important activator of such ROS generation is the induction of apoptosis in response to senescence or other adverse circumstances, including exposure to toxic chemicals [19].

It has been shown that some men possess abnormal spermatozoa generating a particularly high level of ROS. Abnormal spermatozoa with excessive cellular content of polyunsaturated fatty acids, a phenomenon which may be related to impact of lifestyle or environmental factors on the male reproductive system, were observed.

Another external source of ROS having a negative impact on sperm DNA is leukocytes. However, since the male gametes come into contact with infiltrating leukocytes is at the moment of ejaculation, it is believed that this source of free radicals is of less importance for the level of sperm DNA damage in ejaculated spermatozoa due to the high antioxidant capacity of the seminal plasma. On the other hand, when seminal plasma was removed, as a part of preparation for assisted reproduction, ROS produced by the leukocytes may negatively affect the spermatozoa negatively, impacting on their motility and DNA integrity.

Furthermore, smoking and poor diet may add to reduction of the antioxidant protection of the spermatozoa and, thereby, lead to oxidative DNA damage [20, 21], whereas environmental toxicants were shown to increase the level of oxidative stress [22].

Another type of potentially environmentally induced sperm chromatin alterations are epigenetic changes in the genome. Epigenetics refers to changes in gene expression caused by mechanisms other than changes in the underlying DNA sequence. Examples of epigenetics include gene methylation or demethylation leading to their inactivation or deactivation, respectively [23].

17.3 Epidemiological Indications of Environmentally Induced Changes in Sperm DNA

Genetic or epigenetic changes in the sperm genome introduced by environment- and/or lifestyle-related factors may have a serious impact on the reproductive function of an individual. Thus, such alterations may not only lead to impaired male fertility but, once established, may be paternally passed to the subsequent generations [24, 25].

Although there is no direct evidence of sperm DNA alterations induced by environment/lifestyle and then subsequently passed to the offspring, there are some examples which can be considered as indirect evidence of existence of such mechanisms. The Y chromosome has been argued to be particularly vulnerable to DNA damage because it cannot correct double-stranded DNA deletions by homologous recombination [6].

Paternal smoking, reported to introduce sperm DNA damage [26], has been reported to lead to an increased risk of childhood cancer in offspring [27–29] although others could not find the association [30]. Another possible consequence of sperm DNA damage might be microdeletions in the Y chromosome, which will lead to infertility in the male offspring [31].

It has been suggested, although the data seem somewhat contradictory, that increasing paternal age is associated to a higher frequency of aneuploidies, point mutations, sperm DNA breaks, loss of apoptosis, genetic imprinting and other chromosomal abnormalities and has been considered as the major cause of new mutations in human populations [32]. Apart from age, paternal occupation has been linked to certain birth defects or diseases in the offspring which supposedly would act through genetic or epigenetic mechanisms [33]. Epigenetic abnormalities have been associated to imprinting diseases, for which a paternal role has been reported [34], and have been suggested to be increased in babies following conception by assisted reproduction.

A yet unresolved question being of great importance for evaluation of the risk of transmission of sperm DNA changes to the offspring is the ability of the fertilised oocyte to repair such changes. However, animal experiments might indicate that (1) sensitivity of induction of transmissible genetic damage is germ cell-stage dependent, the male postmeiotic cells being the most sensitive, (2) cytogenetic abnormalities at first metaphase after fertilisation are critical intermediates between paternal exposure and abnormal reproductive outcomes, and (3) the amount of sperm DNA damage that is converted into chromosomal aberrations in the zygote and that directly affects the risk for abnormal reproductive outcomes is regulated by maternal susceptibility factors [35]. The zygote has machinery necessary for the repair of sperm DNA damage, but the mechanism of action is not fully clarified. It is supposed that such repair should, preferably, take place prior to the first mitotic division and any inadequacies in the repair and replication process may have major adverse consequences for the embryo and also for the health of the offspring [19].

17.4 Sperm Chromatin and Environment

A significant number of studies have addressed the issue of association between certain environment-related exposures and sperm DNA integrity. Generally, the results are somewhat conflicting. This may be to some degree due to use of different methods for assessment of DNA damage, large variation in sample size, as well as variation in recruitment of study subjects, including men from general population, infertility patients, or occupationally exposed men. Below, these results, in relation to the most extensively studied exposures, will be summarised. An overview of studies related to this topic is given in Tables 17.1, 17.2, 17.3, and 17.4.

Table 17.1 List of studies dealing with impact of cigarette smoking on sperm DNA integrity

Smoking as main exposure or confounding factor	Assay used	No participants	Effect	Reference
Main exposure	8-OHdG	60	↑	[36]
Confounding factor	TUNEL	113	↑	[38]
Main exposure	SCSA	25	=	[105]
Main exposure	SCSA	277	=	[106]
Main exposure	TUNEL	70	↑	[39]
Main exposure	SCSA	70	↑	[39]
Main exposure	TUNEL	97	=	[107]
Main exposure	SCSA	65	=	[46]
Confounding factor	COMET (alkaline)	71	=	[54]
Confounding factor	8-OHdG	225	=	[45]
Main exposure	COMET (alkaline)	40	=	[108]
Main exposure	COMET (neutral)	257	=	[41]
Confounding factor	SCSA	176	=	[62]
Main exposure	TUNEL	108	↑	[40]
Confounding factor	COMET (neutral)	379	=	[43]
Main exposure	OxyDNA assay	55	=	[42]
Confounding factor	SCSA	279	=	[109]
Confounding factor	SCSA	225	=	[110]
Main exposure	TUNEL and 8-OHdG	116	↑	[111]
Main exposure (mother)	SCSA	265	=	[47]
Main exposure (mother and/or father)	SCSA	295	=	[48]

= No effect found

↑ Exposure-related increase in percentage of spermatozoa with DNA damage (Adapted from M Spanó, unpublished data)

17.4.1 Tobacco and Other Lifestyle Factors

The impact of cigarette smoking on sperm DNA integrity has been extensively studied. Some studies have shown increased level of sperm DNA damage in smoking men. Thus, Shen et al. [36] reported on positive correlation between 8-OHdG amount—considered as the best marker of oxidative sperm DNA damage [37]—and blood cotinine levels. The same was true for three studies based on use of TUNEL [38–40] and one using SCSA [39]. All these reports were based on relatively small sample sizes, none of them with a sample size more than 60.

On the other hand, a number of reports could not confirm the association between tobacco smoking and sperm DNA damage [41–45]. This list includes studies based on use of COMET, TUNEL, SCSA, as well as 8-oxodG analyses. Interestingly, Saleh et al. [46] reported higher levels of ROS but not sperm DNA strand breaks in smokers as compared to non-smokers. Similarly, Viloria et al. [42] found lower

Table 17.2 List of studies dealing with impact of environmental/occupational (except pesticide and PCB) exposure on sperm DNA integrity

Exposure	Assay used	No participants	Effect	Reference
Air pollution	SCSA	266	↑	[58]
Air pollution	SCSA	36	↑	[59]
Air pollution	SCSA and CMA	228	=	[60]
Air pollution	TUNEL	68	↑	[61]
Styrene (mandelic acid urinary concentration)	SCSA	44	↑	[52]
Styrene (mandelic acid urinary concentration)	COMET (alkaline)	73	↑	[54]
Styrene (mandelic and phenylglyoxylic acid urinary concentration)	COMET (alkaline)	67	↑	[53]
Boron (blood and urine)	COMET and TUNEL	103	=	[55]
Phthalate esters	Sperm nuclear chromatin decondensation test	53	↑	[65]
Phthalate and phthalate metabolites	COMET (neutral)	168	↑	[112]
Phthalate and phthalate metabolites	COMET (neutral)	379	↑	[43]
Phthalate and phthalate metabolites	SCSA	234	=	[74]
Phthalate and phthalate metabolites	SCSA	300	↑	[72]
Phthalate metabolites	SCSA	314	= DFI ↑ High DNA stainability	[75]
Phthalate metabolites (maternal sera—pregnancy)	SCSA	112	=	[76]
Acrylonitrile	COMET (alkaline)	60	↑	[113]
Lead	SCSA	503	= at blood Pb conc. <45 μg/dl	[57]
Lead	Nuclear chromatin decondensation (NCD) test	68	↑	[114]
Lead	SCSA	80	↑	[56]
Mercury	SCSA	195	= No synergism with PCB exposure	[115]

= No effect found

↑ Exposure-related increase in percentage of spermatozoa with DNA damage (Adapted from M Spanó, unpublished data)

Table 17.3 List of studies dealing with impact of pesticide exposure on sperm DNA integrity

Exposure	Assay used	No participants	Effect	Reference
p,p′-DDE	COMET (neutral)	212	=	[44]
p,p′-DDE	SCSA	176	=	[62]
p,p′-DDE	SCSA	707	=	[63]
p,p′-DDE	SCSA	680	↑ only in subjects with androgen receptor CAG repeat length of 21 or less	[95]
p,p′-DDE/DDT	SCSA	209	↑	[67]
p,p′-DDE	TUNEL	652	=	[64]
p,p′-DDE	Aniline blue	116	↑	[68]
Pesticides (occupation exposure)	SCSA	251	=	[77]
Pesticides (dietary intake)	SCSA	256	=	[78]
Pesticides	SCSA	256	=	[116]
Organophosphoric pesticides	SCSA	66	↑	[80]
Organophosphoric pesticides	ISNT	54	↑ paraoxonase: 192RR genotype more susceptible	[79]
Hexachlorobenzene	COMET (neutral)	212	=	[44]
Insecticides (fenvalerate)	COMET (alkaline) TUNEL	63	↑	[82]
Insecticides (chlorpyrifos, carbaryl)	COMET (neutral)	260	↑	[84]
Insecticides Pyrethroids	COMET (neutral)	207	↑	[83]
Insecticides (carbaryl)	TUNEL	46	↑	[81]
Insecticides (pyrethroids)	TUNEL	240	↑	[117]

= No effect found

↑ Exposure-related increase in percentage of spermatozoa with DNA damage (Adapted from M Spanó, unpublished data)

level of sperm anti-oxidative enzymes in smokers as compared to non-smokers, however, without any difference in the degree of sperm DNA damage between those two groups.

Two studies [47, 48] focused on effects of prenatal exposure to cigarette smoking, and although sons of mothers as well as fathers smoking during pregnancy presented with lower sperm counts, no difference in regard to sperm DNA integrity was seen.

Table 17.4 List of studies dealing with impact of PCB or bisphenol A exposure on sperm DNA integrity

Exposure	Assay used	No participants	Effect	Reference
PCB	NCD	53	↑	[65]
PCB	COMET (neutral)	212	=	[44]
PCB	SCSA	176	↑	[62]
PCB	SCSA	707	↑ In Caucasians but not in Inuits	[63]
PCB	TUNEL	652	↑ In Caucasians but not in Inuits	[64]
Bisphenol A	COMET (neutral)	190	↑	[85]
Bisphenol A	COMET (neutral)	132	↑	[86]

= No effect found

↑ Exposure-related increase in percentage of spermatozoa with DNA damage (Adapted from M Spanó, unpublished data)

Thus, although some studies might indicate a negative effect of cigarette smoking on sperm DNA integrity, the results are rather conflicting, the largest of them does not find a correlation between cigarette smoking and sperm DNA damage (Table 17.1).

Among other lifestyle-related factors, one study addressed the issue of coffee drinking in relation to the sperm DNA integrity. The authors reported that the major finding [49] was that using the COMET assay, men consuming more than three cups coffee per day have approximately 20% higher tail DNA—a measure of level of sperm DNA damage—under neutral but not alkaline conditions compared with men who consumed no caffeine ($P = 0.005$).

Although animal experiments have indicated that cocaine may induce increased apoptosis [50] as well as alteration of gene imprinting in germ cells [51], similar data in humans are lacking.

17.4.2 Occupational Exposure

Surprisingly few epidemiological studies have addressed the issue of occupational exposure in relation to sperm DNA integrity. Three studies dealing with impact of styrene exposure, two of them using COMET assay and one applying SCSA, found a statistically significant increase in the indices of impairment of DNA integrity in exposed workers as compared to unexposed subjects [52–54].

One study focused on occupational boron exposure and reported no significant correlations between blood and urine boron and adverse semen parameters including sperm DNA breaks and percentage of apoptotic cells [55].

Hsu et al. [56] reported on the effect of lead exposure on SCSA parameters in a group of battery factory workers in Taiwan and found a positive correlation between the blood levels of this metal and the percentage of sperm with DNA fragmentation.

An earlier study performed by Bonde et al. [57] only partly supported these results by reporting deterioration of sperm chromatin found in men with the highest concentrations of lead within spermatozoa.

17.4.3 Air Pollution

Animal studies have linked air pollution to the level of sperm DNA damage. Similar findings have also been done in Czech men, both in a cross-sectional [58] and a longitudinal [59] set-up. However, a study by Hansen et al. [60] based on a cohort of 228 fertile men could not find any association between the level of exposure to ozone and particulate matter (<2.5 μm in aerodynamic diameter) on sperm DNA indices as assessed by SCSA and by chromomycin A3 staining. On the other hand, Calogero et al. [61] reported a higher DFI in motorway tollgate workers as compared to controls.

17.4.4 Persistent Organohalogen Pollutants (POPs)

A number of studies have addressed the issue of the impact of exposure to POPs in relation to the sperm chromatin integrity. In a multicentre European Union-funded study (www.inuendo.dk), focus was given to association between serum levels of CB-153, a marker of exposure to polychlorinated biphenyls (PCBs), and concentrations of p,p′-DDE (dichlorodiphenyldichloroethylene), a metabolite of dichlorodiphenyltrichloroethane (DDT) and sperm parameters, including DNA integrity. Using both SCSA and TUNEL, high levels of PCB exposure were found to be associated with increased percentage of spermatozoa with DNA damage. However, interestingly these associations were found in Caucasian populations (Sweden, Ukraine, Poland) but not in Greenlandic Inuits, the latter—despite very high levels of CB-153—presenting with significantly lower DNA Fragmentation Index as compared to the European men [62–64]. This finding might indicate an interaction between POP exposure and genetic (see below) and/or other lifestyle or environmental factors in relation to the integrity of sperm DNA. The Inuendo findings seem to be in agreement with an earlier study by Rozati et al. [65] showing positive correlation between seminal PCB levels and percentage of spermatozoa with single-stranded DNA.

Study results on the impact of DDT exposure on sperm chromatin integrity are more diverging. No correlation between p,p′-DDE and TUNEL as well as SCSA parameters was found in the Inuendo study—if the impact of genetic polymorphisms was not taken into consideration (see below) [63]. However, it should be kept in mind that there was a high level of correlation between serum levels of CB-153 and the p,p′-DDE concentration, in an epidemiological set-up [66], making it impossible to detangle the biological effects of these two compounds. Thus, in a men living in areas with endemic malaria, where due to use of DDT the plasma levels of its metabolite can reach levels 1000-fold higher than in other populations, there was a positive correlation between SCSA DFI and the concentration of p,p′-DDE [67, 68].

Apart from the link between POPs and the extent of sperm DNA strand breaks, exposure to these compounds was also seen to be associated with sperm DNA hypomethylation, which may indicate epigenetic consequences of POP exposure leading to activation of genes which usually are silenced [69].

17.4.5 Phthalates

During the past few years, a lot of attention has been given to the potential endocrine disrupting effect of phthalates, chemicals believed to interfere with the Leydig cell function [70, 71] and thereby affect the levels of intra-testicular testosterone. A recent study has shown a positive correlation between the level of phthalate exposure and ROS production [72]. Therefore, these chemicals may exert a negative effect on sperm DNA integrity both by inducing high ROS levels and, through hormonal deregulation, by interfering with normal intra-testicular function of DNA repair enzymes.

Three studies on men attending infertility clinics found a positive association between at least some of the phthalate metabolites, and indices of sperm DNA damage, assessed by COMET [43, 73] or SCSA [72]. However, no such association was found in a younger group of Swedish military conscripts [74, 75]. In a recent study, no association between phthalate levels in maternal serum during early pregnancy and DFI of their sons was seen [76].

17.4.6 Insecticides and Pesticides Other Than DDT

Within this quite heterogeneous category of environmental toxicants, the studies have focused on either occupational exposure or consumption of food containing rests of such compounds.

Studies on effect of pesticides generated conflicting results. While no association between pesticide use and sperm DNA damage was demonstrated in the Danish agricultural workers, a positive correlation was observed in Mexico [77–80]. A number of reports related to exposure to insecticides have shown positive association between the levels of these chemicals and markers of sperm DNA damage. These findings have been rather consistent both in relation to occupational [81, 82] and environmental exposure [83, 84].

Also the exposure to organophosphoric pesticides (see Table 17.3) seems to have a negative impact on sperm DNA integrity [79, 80], whereas in two studies comparing organic and nonorganic farmers [77, 78], no such effect was found.

17.4.7 Other Exposures

There are a limited number of studies regarding the impact of exposure to bisphenol A—a high production volume chemical used in the manufacture of polycarbonate plastics, which can be used in baby and water bottles, and epoxy resins, used in food container linings and other applications. However, in two reports [85, 86], a positive association between the levels of this chemical and DFI was seen.

No indications for deleterious effects on sperm DNA integrity were reported in relation to exposure to perfluoroalkyl substances (PFAS) [87], polybrominated diphenyl esters [88], and hexachlorobenzene [89]. For PFAS, widely used in industrial processes and products, no consistent link with level of sperm DNA global methylation was seen. However, for some of the compounds belonging to the PFAS family, some statistically significant associations with DNA hypo- or hypermethylation were reported leaving the question of epigenetic alteration related to these compounds still unresolved [90]. Interestingly, when looking at subjects from geographical regions with differing profile of environmental load of chemical toxicants, significant discrepancies in the level of DNA global methylation were seen [91]. Furthermore, this parameter was not associated with any of the standard sperm indices indicated that normal semen quality is not a guarantee of sperm genome.

17.5 Gene-Environment Interaction and Sperm Chromatin

Impairment of sperm chromatin integrity due to lifestyle- or environment-related factors represents a unique form of "gene-environment interaction"—namely, environmental stress having a negative impact on the genome of the gamete and those changes being potentially transmittable to the following generation(s). The results of the study by Anway et al. [24], although focusing on epigenetic changes rather than direct DNA damage, illustrate that such scenario is not unlikely. However, in traditional terms, the term "gene-environment interaction" usually refers to interindividual variation in susceptibility to environmental/lifestyle factors based on genetic differences between the subjects. There are several indications of such mechanisms operating even in relation to impairment of sperm DNA integrity.

Thus, as already mentioned, in the Inuendo study, Inuits were found to have significantly lower DNA Fragmentation Index as compared to Caucasian men [63], the association between levels of PCB exposure being seen among the latter but not in the former ethnic group. Although nutritional or other environmental factors might be the cause of such difference, genetic diversity as a causative factor should not be overlooked.

Our research group has been focusing on polymorphisms in the androgen receptor gene (AR) as modifiers of the effect of endocrine disrupting chemicals, including POPs. One of the polymorphic regions in the AR is the glutamine encoding CAG repeats in the exon I of this gene [92]. It has been shown that the number of these repeats, which in a Caucasian normal population varies between 10 and 30 with a mean number of 22, has an impact on the receptor activity [92–94]. In the Inuendo study, we found that the association between p,p′-DDE, but not CB-153 levels, and the DFI depended on the CAG number [95]. For CAG lengths of 21 or less, those with high levels of the p,p′-DDE presented with 40% higher percentage of spermatozoa with impaired DNA integrity than those with low concentrations of this POP. Such association between exposure and sperm DNA damage was not seen for other CAG lengths. These findings might, at least partly, explain the robustness of Inuits to the deleterious effects of POP exposure. The mean CAG number is on average 1.5–2 higher in Inuits as compared to Caucasians, thus a lower proportion of men having the genotype encoding for higher level of susceptibility [96].

In same cohorts the association between POP exposure and sperm DNA integrity was also modified by genetic variations in gene encoding for the aryl hydrocarbon receptor (AHR) as well as in the AHR-repressor gene [97].

In the study of the impact of air pollution on sperm DNA integrity, this effect was shown to be modified by the polymorphisms in the glutathione-S-transferase M1 gene [98] as well as by variations in several DNA repair genes [99].

Therefore, it is to be expected that even for the other environmental and lifestyle factors shown to have an impact on sperm DNA integrity, the genetically determined susceptibility may vary between the individuals. Such gene-environment interaction might, at least partly, explain the mechanisms between the above-mentioned somewhat diverging results, when different population cohorts are investigated and/or several techniques for detection of sperm DNA damage are used.

17.6 Clinical Relevance

The issue of the possible effect of environment and lifestyle on sperm chromatin integrity is important from a clinical point of view. Infertility affects 15–20% of all couples and is a serious condition—both from a medical and also socio-economic point of view. In a large majority of cases, the causes are not or only poorly understood, and the treatment is purely symptomatic, based on assisted reproduction. It is now well established that at least certain types of sperm DNA damage may have a negative impact on the fertility of the subject in vivo and even in vitro.

Thus, we have reported that in subjects with normal standard sperm parameters, the odds ratio for spontaneous pregnancy significantly decreases when the DFI, as determined by the sperm chromatin structure assay (SCSA), exceeds the level of 20% [100]. However, this decrease in fertility in vivo is already seen at DFI above 10%, if one of standard sperm parameters is abnormal. Since many of the environmental toxicants may affect not only sperm DNA integrity but also concentration, motility, and/or morphology [101], a slight increase in percentage of sperms with abnormal DNA, combined with deterioration of some other semen characteristics, may lead to decrease in fertility.

The results of assisted reproduction seem to be dependent on the level of sperm DNA damage. For intrauterine insemination—similarly to what we see for spontaneous pregnancy—the chance of pregnancy starts to decline for DFI above 20% to approach the level of zero when DFI exceeds 30% [102].

Sperm DNA damage seems also to affect the results of in vitro fertilisation, although the impact is more pronounced in relation to standard in vitro fertilisation (IVF) than with respect to intracytoplasmic sperm injection (ICSI). For IVF the chance of live birth seems to decrease if the DFI is higher than 20% whereas such effects is not seen for ICSI. For both methods of fertilisation the risk of early miscarriage increases when DFI is above 40% [103].

As a consequence of these observations, a question arises: to which degree these DNA defects, which seem not to exclude child birth when ICSI is applied, are becoming repaired following the process of fertilisation. Unrepaired damaged sperm DNA introduced into the embryo might, in theory, impair foetal growth and induce congenital malformations and/or diseases arising during different phases of the postnatal life. These problems might not only occur in the offspring of the man exposed to such factors but might become manifest in the subsequent generation(s) [104].

The complexity of the question, the rather recent access to techniques for evaluation of sperm DNA integrity, and the relatively short follow-up of IVF and ICSI children do not allow a definite answer to be drawn at the moment. However, this issue should have a high priority on the future agenda of evaluating the potential risks of assisted reproduction.

Identification of environment- and lifestyle-related factors deleterious to sperm DNA does have implications in relation to the possibility of prevention and treatment of male-related infertility problems. Thus, once the implications of environment and lifestyle on sperm DNA integrity are understood, preventive measures can be taken. Furthermore, studying the mechanisms of environment-/lifestyle-related changes in the genome of the male gamete will also increase our level of understanding of the mechanisms involved in the impairment of testicular function. Such knowledge is crucial, not only for preservation of infertility but also for the development of specific drugs for treatment of fertility problems.

Therefore, studying and understanding the phenomenon involved in the effects of environmental and lifestyle factors on sperm DNA may be an important step in preventing and treating of infertility problems as well as other important diseases, not only in relation to the generation actually being exposed but also in their offspring and, possibly, even in the subsequent generations.

17.7 Conclusions

Available experimental and human data show that a number of lifestyle- and environment-related exposures may have negative effects on sperm DNA integrity. The extent of the sperm DNA damage seems to differ between different studies.

Such discrepancy may partly be due to use of several methods for assessment of sperm DNA integrity, these techniques not measuring exactly same characteristics of sperm DNA. Another contributing factor may be genetically determined variation in the individual susceptibility.

Sperm DNA damage due to environmental and lifestyle factors may have a negative impact on fertility, and there is a potential risk of transmission to the offspring. Therefore, it is of importance to focus on the association between environment and sperm DNA integrity in order to prevent male subfertility and to avoid potentially serious health effects in the next generation(s).

References

1. Giwercman A, Skakkebaek NE. The human testis—an organ at risk? Int J Androl. 1992;15(5):373–5.
2. Carlsen E, Giwercman A, Keiding N, Skakkeb'k NE. Evidence for decreasing quality of semen during past 50 years. Br Med J. 1992;305:609–13.
3. Carlsen E, Giwercman A, Skakkebk NE, Keiding N. Decreasing quality of semen (letter). Br Med J. 1993;306:461.
4. Toppari J, Larsen JC, Christiansen P, Giwercman A, Grandjean P, Guillette LJ Jr, et al. Male reproductive health and environmental xenoestrogens. Environ Health Perspect. 1996;104:741–803.
5. Richiardi L, Bellocco R, Adami HO, Torrang A, Barlow L, Hakulinen T, et al. Testicular cancer incidence in eight northern European countries: secular and recent trends. Cancer Epidemiol Biomark Prev. 2004;13(12):2157–66.
6. Aitken RJ, Krausz C. Oxidative stress, DNA damage and the Y chromosome. Reproduction. 2001;122(4):497–506.
7. Bannister LA, Schimenti JC. Homologous recombinational repair proteins in mouse meiosis. Cytogenet Genome Res. 2004;107(3–4):191–200.
8. Bench G, Corzett MH, De Yebra L, Oliva R, Balhorn R. Protein and DNA contents in sperm from an infertile human male possessing protamine defects that vary over time. Mol Reprod Dev. 1998;50(3):345–53.
9. de Yebra L, Ballesca JL, Vanrell JA, Bassas L, Oliva R. Complete selective absence of protamine P2 in humans. J Biol Chem. 1993;268(14):10553–7.
10. de Yebra L, Ballesca JL, Vanrell JA, Corzett M, Balhorn R, Oliva R. Detection of P2 precursors in the sperm cells of infertile patients who have reduced protamine P2 levels. Fertil Steril. 1998;69(4):755–9.
11. Carrell DT, Liu L. Altered protamine 2 expression is uncommon in donors of known fertility, but common among men with poor fertilizing capacity, and may reflect other abnormalities of spermiogenesis. J Androl. 2001;22(4):604–10.
12. Mengual L, Ballesca JL, Ascaso C, Oliva R. Marked differences in protamine content and P1/P2 ratios in sperm cells from percoll fractions between patients and controls. J Androl. 2003;24(3):438–47.
13. Nasr-Esfahani MH, Salehi M, Razavi S, Mardani M, Bahramian H, Steger K, et al. Effect of protamine-2 deficiency on ICSI outcome. Reprod BioMed Online. 2004;9(6):652–8.
14. Kierszenbaum AL. Transition nuclear proteins during spermiogenesis: unrepaired DNA breaks not allowed. Mol Reprod Dev. 2001;58(4):357–8.
15. Bakshi RP, Galande S, Bali P, Dighe R, Muniyappa K. Developmental and hormonal regulation of type II DNA topoisomerase in rat testis. J Mol Endocrinol. 2001;26(3):193–206.
16. Aitken RJ, De Iuliis GN. On the possible origins of DNA damage in human spermatozoa. Mol Hum Reprod. 2010;16(1):3–13.

17. O'Flaherty C. Iatrogenic genetic damage of spermatozoa. Adv Exp Med Biol. 2014;791:117–35.
18. Koppers AJ, De Iuliis GN, Finnie JM, McLaughlin EA, Aitken RJ. Significance of mitochondrial reactive oxygen species in the generation of oxidative stress in spermatozoa. J Clin Endocrinol Metab. 2008;93(8):3199–207.
19. Gavriliouk D, Aitken RJ. Damage to sperm DNA mediated by reactive oxygen species: its impact on human reproduction and the health trajectory of offspring. Adv Exp Med Biol. 2015;868:23–47.
20. Fraga CG, Motchnik PA, Wyrobek AJ, Rempel DM, Ames BN. Smoking and low antioxidant levels increase oxidative damage to sperm DNA. Mutat Res. 1996;351(2):199–203.
21. Aitken RJ, De Iuliis GN, McLachlan RI. Biological and clinical significance of DNA damage in the male germ line. Int J Androl. 2009;32(1):46–56.
22. Easley CA, Bradner JM, Moser A, Rickman CA, McEachin ZT, Merritt MM, et al. Assessing reproductive toxicity of two environmental toxicants with a novel in vitro human spermatogenic model. Stem Cell Res. 2015;14(3):347–55.
23. Trasler JM. Epigenetics in spermatogenesis. Mol Cell Endocrinol. 2009;306(1–2):33–6.
24. Anway MD, Cupp AS, Uzumcu M, Skinner MK. Epigenetic transgenerational actions of endocrine disruptors and male fertility. Science. 2005;308(5727):1466–9.
25. Cheng RY, Hockman T, Crawford E, Anderson LM, Shiao YH. Epigenetic and gene expression changes related to transgenerational carcinogenesis. Mol Carcinog. 2004;40(1):1–11.
26. Elshal MF, El-Sayed IH, Elsaied MA, El-Masry SA, Kumosani TA. Sperm head defects and disturbances in spermatozoal chromatin and DNA integrities in idiopathic infertile subjects: association with cigarette smoking. Clin Biochem. 2009;42(7–8):589–94.
27. Sorahan T, Lancashire RJ, Hulten MA, Peck I, Stewart AM. Childhood cancer and parental use of tobacco: deaths from 1953 to 1955. Br J Cancer. 1997;75(1):134–8.
28. Sorahan T, McKinney PA, Mann JR, Lancashire RJ, Stiller CA, Birch JM, et al. Childhood cancer and parental use of tobacco: findings from the inter-regional epidemiological study of childhood cancer (IRESCC). Br J Cancer. 2001;84(1):141–6.
29. Ji BT, Shu XO, Linet MS, Zheng W, Wacholder S, Gao YT, et al. Paternal cigarette smoking and the risk of childhood cancer among offspring of nonsmoking mothers. J Natl Cancer Inst. 1997;89(3):238–44.
30. Schuz J, Kaatsch P, Kaletsch U, Meinert R, Michaelis J. Association of childhood cancer with factors related to pregnancy and birth. Int J Epidemiol. 1999;28(4):631–9.
31. Aitken RJ. The Amoroso lecture. The human spermatozoon—a cell in crisis? J Reprod Fertil. 1999;115(1):1–7.
32. Sartorius GA, Nieschlag E. Paternal age and reproduction. Hum Reprod Update. 2010;16(1):65–79.
33. Whalley LJ, Thomas BM, McGonigal G, McQuade CA, Swingler R, Black R. Epidemiology of presenile Alzheimer's disease in Scotland (1974–88) I. Non-random geographical variation. Br J Psychiatry. 1995;167(6):728–31.
34. Marques CJ, Carvalho F, Sousa M, Barros A. Genomic imprinting in disruptive spermatogenesis. Lancet. 2004;363(9422):1700–2.
35. Marchetti F, Wyrobek AJ. Mechanisms and consequences of paternally-transmitted chromosomal abnormalities. Birth Defects Res C Embryo Today. 2005;75(2):112–29.
36. Shen HM, Chia SE, Ni ZY, New AL, Lee BL, Ong CN. Detection of oxidative DNA damage in human sperm and the association with cigarette smoking. Reprod Toxicol. 1997;11(5):675–80.
37. Shen H, Ong C. Detection of oxidative DNA damage in human sperm and its association with sperm function and male infertility. Free Radic Biol Med. 2000;28(4):529–36.
38. Sun JG, et al. Detection of deoxyribonucleic acid fragmentation in human sperm: correlation with fertilization in vitro. Biol Reprod. 1997;56:602–7.
39. Potts RJ, Newbury CJ, Smith G, Notarianni LJ, Jefferies TM. Sperm chromatin damage associated with male smoking. Mutat Res. 1999;423(1–2):103–11.

40. Sepaniak S, Forges T, Gerard H, Foliguet B, Bene MC, Monnier-Barbarino P. The influence of cigarette smoking on human sperm quality and DNA fragmentation. Toxicology. 2006;223(1–2):54–60.
41. Trisini AT, Singh NP, Duty SM, Hauser R. Relationship between human semen parameters and deoxyribonucleic acid damage assessed by the neutral comet assay. Fertil Steril. 2004;82(6):1623–32.
42. Viloria T, Meseguer M, Martinez-Conejero JA, O'Connor JE, Remohi J, Pellicer A, et al. Cigarette smoking affects specific sperm oxidative defense but does not cause oxidative DNA damage in infertile men. Fertil Steril. 2009;94:631.
43. Hauser R, Meeker JD, Singh NP, Silva MJ, Ryan L, Duty S, et al. DNA damage in human sperm is related to urinary levels of phthalate monoester and oxidative metabolites. Hum Reprod. 2007;22(3):688–95.
44. Hauser R, Singh NP, Chen Z, Pothier L, Altshul L. Lack of an association between environmental exposure to polychlorinated biphenyls and p,p′-DDE and DNA damage in human sperm measured using the neutral comet assay. Hum Reprod. 2003;18(12):2525–33.
45. Loft S, Kold-Jensen T, Hjollund NH, Giwercman A, Gyllemborg J, Ernst E, et al. Oxidative DNA damage in human sperm influences time to pregnancy. Hum Reprod. 2003;18(6):1265–72.
46. Saleh RA, Agarwal A, Sharma RK, Nelson DR, Thomas AJ Jr. Effect of cigarette smoking on levels of seminal oxidative stress in infertile men: a prospective study. Fertil Steril. 2002;78(3):491–9.
47. Storgaard L, Bonde JP, Ernst E, Spano M, Andersen CY, Frydenberg M, et al. Does smoking during pregnancy affect sons' sperm counts? Epidemiology. 2003;14(3):278–86.
48. Axelsson J, Rylander L, Rignell-Hydbom A, Silfver KA, Stenqvist A, Giwercman A. The impact of paternal and maternal smoking on semen quality of adolescent men. PLoS One. 2013;8(6):e66766.
49. Schmid TE, Eskenazi B, Baumgartner A, Marchetti F, Young S, Weldon R, et al. The effects of male age on sperm DNA damage in healthy non-smokers. Hum Reprod. 2007;22(1):180–7.
50. Yang GS, Wang W, Wang YM, Chen ZD, Wang S, Fang JJ. Effect of cocaine on germ cell apoptosis in rats at different ages. Asian J Androl. 2006;8(5):569–75.
51. He F, Lidow IA, Lidow MS. Consequences of paternal cocaine exposure in mice. Neurotoxicol Teratol. 2006;28(2):198–209.
52. Kolstad HA, Bonde JP, Spano M, Giwercman A, Zshiesche W, Kaae D, et al. Sperm chromatin structure and semen quality following occupational styrene exposure. Scand J Work Environ Health. 1999;25:70–3.
53. Migliore L, Colognato R, Naccarati A, Bergamaschi E. Relationship between genotoxicity biomarkers in somatic and germ cells: findings from a biomonitoring study. Mutagenesis. 2006;21(2):149–52.
54. Migliore L, Naccarati A, Zanello A, Scarpato R, Bramanti L, Mariani M. Assessment of sperm DNA integrity in workers exposed to styrene. Hum Reprod. 2002;17(11):2912–8.
55. Robbins WA, Xun L, Jia J, Kennedy N, Elashoff DA, Ping L. Chronic boron exposure and human semen parameters. Reprod Toxicol. 2010;29(2):184–90.
56. Hsu PC, Chang HY, Guo YL, Liu YC, Shih TS. Effect of smoking on blood lead levels in workers and role of reactive oxygen species in lead-induced sperm chromatin DNA damage. Fertil Steril. 2009;91(4):1096–103.
57. Bonde JP, Joffe M, Apostoli P, Dale A, Kiss P, Spano M, et al. Sperm count and chromatin structure in men exposed to inorganic lead: lowest adverse effect levels. Occup Environ Med. 2002;59(4):234–42.
58. Selevan SG, Borkovec L, Slott VL, Zudova Z, Rubes J, Evenson DP, et al. Semen quality and reproductive health of young Czech men exposed to seasonal air pollution. Environ Health Perspect. 2000;108(9):887–94.
59. Rubes J, Selevan SG, Evenson DP, Zudova D, Vozdova M, Zudova Z, et al. Episodic air pollution is associated with increased DNA fragmentation in human sperm without other changes in semen quality. Hum Reprod. 2005;20(10):2776–83.

60. Hansen C, Luben TJ, Sacks JD, Olshan A, Jeffay S, Strader L, et al. The effect of ambient air pollution on sperm quality. Environ Health Perspect. 2010;118(2):203–9.
61. Calogero AE, La Vignera S, Condorelli RA, Perdichizzi A, Valenti D, Asero P, et al. Environmental car exhaust pollution damages human sperm chromatin and DNA. J Endocrinol Investig. 2011;34(6):e139–43.
62. Rignell-Hydbom A, Rylander L, Giwercman A, Jonsson BA, Lindh C, Eleuteri P, et al. Exposure to PCBs and p,p′-DDE and human sperm chromatin integrity. Environ Health Perspect. 2005;113(2):175–9.
63. Spano M, Toft G, Hagmar L, Eleuteri P, Rescia M, Rignell-Hydbom A, et al. Exposure to PCB and p,p′-DDE in European and Inuit populations: impact on human sperm chromatin integrity. Hum Reprod. 2005;20(12):3488–99.
64. Stronati A, Manicardi GC, Cecati M, Bordicchia M, Ferrante L, Spano M, et al. Relationships between sperm DNA fragmentation, sperm apoptotic markers and serum levels of CB-153 and p,p′-DDE in European and Inuit populations. Reproduction. 2006;132(6):949–58.
65. Rozati R, Reddy PP, Reddanna P, Mujtaba R. Role of environmental estrogens in the deterioration of male factor fertility. Fertil Steril. 2002;78(6):1187–94.
66. Jonsson BA, Rylander L, Lindh C, Rignell-Hydbom A, Giwercman A, Toft G, et al. Inter-population variations in concentrations, determinants of and correlations between 2,2,′4,4,′5,5′-hexachlorobiphenyl (CB-153) and 1,1-dichloro-2,2-bis (p-chlorophenyl)-ethylene (p,p′-DDE): a cross-sectional study of 3161 men and women from Inuit and European populations. Environ Health. 2005;4:27.
67. de Jager C, Aneck-Hahn NH, Bornman MS, Farias P, Leter G, Eleuteri P, et al. Sperm chromatin integrity in DDT-exposed young men living in a malaria area in the Limpopo Province, South Africa. Hum Reprod. 2009;24(10):2429–38.
68. De Jager C, Farias P, Barraza-Villarreal A, Avila MH, Ayotte P, Dewailly E, et al. Reduced seminal parameters associated with environmental DDT exposure and p,p′-DDE concentrations in men in Chiapas, Mexico: a cross-sectional study. J Androl. 2006;27(1):16–27.
69. Consales C, Toft G, Leter G, Bonde JP, Uccelli R, Pacchierotti F, et al. Exposure to persistent organic pollutants and sperm DNA methylation changes in Arctic and European populations. Environ Mol Mutagen. 2016;57(3):200–9.
70. Scott HM, Mason JI, Sharpe RM. Steroidogenesis in the fetal testis and its susceptibility to disruption by exogenous compounds. Endocr Rev. 2009;30(7):883–925.
71. Svechnikov K, Svechnikova I, Soder O. Inhibitory effects of mono-ethylhexyl phthalate on steroidogenesis in immature and adult rat Leydig cells in vitro. Reprod Toxicol. 2008;25(4):485–90.
72. Pant N, Shukla M, Kumar Patel D, Shukla Y, Mathur N, Kumar Gupta Y, et al. Correlation of phthalate exposures with semen quality. Toxicol Appl Pharmacol. 2008;231(1):112–6.
73. Duty SM, Singh NP, Silva MJ, Barr DB, Brock JW, Ryan L, et al. The relationship between environmental exposures to phthalates and DNA damage in human sperm using the neutral comet assay. Environ Health Perspect. 2003;111(9):1164–9.
74. Jonsson BA, Richthoff J, Rylander L, Giwercman A, Hagmar L. Urinary phthalate metabolites and biomarkers of reproductive function in young men. Epidemiology. 2005;16(4):487–93.
75. Axelsson J, Rylander L, Rignell-Hydbom A, Jonsson BA, Lindh CH, Giwercman A. Phthalate exposure and reproductive parameters in young men from the general Swedish population. Environ Int. 2015;85:54–60.
76. Axelsson J, Rylander L, Rignell-Hydbom A, Lindh CH, Jonsson BA, Giwercman A. Prenatal phthalate exposure and reproductive function in young men. Environ Res. 2015;138:264–70.
77. Larsen SB, Giwercman A, Spano M, Bonde JP. A longitudinal study of semen quality in pesticide spraying Danish farmers. ASCLEPIOS Study Group. Reprod Toxicol. 1998;12(6):581–9.
78. Juhler RK, Larsen SB, Meyer O, Jensen ND, Spano M, Giwercman A, et al. Human semen quality in relation to dietary pesticide exposure and organic food. Arch Environ Contam Toxicol. 1999;37:415–23.
79. Perez-Herrera N, Polanco-Minaya H, Salazar-Arredondo E, Solis-Heredia MJ, Hernandez-Ochoa I, Rojas-Garcia E, et al. PON1Q192R genetic polymorphism modifies organophos-

phorus pesticide effects on semen quality and DNA integrity in agricultural workers from southern Mexico. Toxicol Appl Pharmacol. 2008;230(2):261–8.
80. Sanchez-Pena LC, Reyes BE, Lopez-Carrillo L, Recio R, Moran-Martinez J, Cebrian ME, et al. Organophosphorus pesticide exposure alters sperm chromatin structure in Mexican agricultural workers. Toxicol Appl Pharmacol. 2004;196(1):108–13.
81. Xia Y, Cheng S, Bian Q, Xu L, Collins MD, Chang HC, et al. Genotoxic effects on spermatozoa of carbaryl-exposed workers. Toxicol Sci. 2005;85(1):615–23.
82. Bian Q, Xu LC, Wang SL, Xia YK, Tan LF, Chen JF, et al. Study on the relation between occupational fenvalerate exposure and spermatozoa DNA damage of pesticide factory workers. Occup Environ Med. 2004;61(12):999–1005.
83. Meeker JD, Barr DB, Hauser R. Human semen quality and sperm DNA damage in relation to urinary metabolites of pyrethroid insecticides. Hum Reprod. 2008;23(8):1932–40.
84. Meeker JD, Singh NP, Ryan L, Duty SM, Barr DB, Herrick RF, et al. Urinary levels of insecticide metabolites and DNA damage in human sperm. Hum Reprod. 2004;19(11):2573–80.
85. Meeker JD, Ehrlich S, Toth TL, Wright DL, Calafat AM, Trisini AT, et al. Semen quality and sperm DNA damage in relation to urinary bisphenol A among men from an infertility clinic. Reprod Toxicol. 2010;30(4):532–9.
86. Meeker JD, Yang T, Ye X, Calafat AM, Hauser R. Urinary concentrations of parabens and serum hormone levels, semen quality parameters, and sperm DNA damage. Environ Health Perspect. 2011;119(2):252–7.
87. Specht IO, Hougaard KS, Spano M, Bizzaro D, Manicardi GC, Lindh CH, et al. Sperm DNA integrity in relation to exposure to environmental perfluoroalkyl substances—a study of spouses of pregnant women in three geographical regions. Reprod Toxicol. 2012;33(4):577–83.
88. Toft G, Lenters V, Vermeulen R, Heederik D, Thomsen C, Becher G, et al. Exposure to polybrominated diphenyl ethers and male reproductive function in Greenland, Poland and Ukraine. Reprod Toxicol. 2014;43:1–7.
89. Specht IO, Bonde JP, Toft G, Giwercman A, Spano M, Bizzaro D, et al. Environmental hexachlorobenzene exposure and human male reproductive function. Reprod Toxicol. 2015;58:8–14.
90. Leter G, Consales C, Eleuteri P, Uccelli R, Specht IO, Toft G, et al. Exposure to perfluoroalkyl substances and sperm DNA global methylation in Arctic and European populations. Environ Mol Mutagen. 2014;55(7):591–600.
91. Consales C, Leter G, Bonde JP, Toft G, Eleuteri P, Moccia T, et al. Indices of methylation in sperm DNA from fertile men differ between distinct geographical regions. Hum Reprod. 2014;29(9):2065–72.
92. Tut TG, Ghadessy FJ, Trifiro MA, Pinsky L, Young EL. Long polyglutamine tracts in the androgen receptor are associated with reduced trans-activation, impaired sperm production, and male infertility. JCEM. 1997;82:3777–82.
93. Eckardstein SV, Schmidt A, Kamischke A, Simoni M, Gromoll J, Nieschlag E. CAG repeat length in the androgen receptor gene and gonadotrophin suppression influence the effectiveness of hormonal male contraception. Clin Endocrinol. 2002;57(5):647–55.
94. Nenonen H, Bjork C, Skjaerpe PA, Giwercman A, Rylander L, Svartberg J, et al. CAG repeat number is not inversely associated with androgen receptor activity in vitro. Mol Hum Reprod. 2010;16(3):153–7.
95. Giwercman A, Rylander L, Rignell-Hydbom A, J"nsson BAG, Pedersen HS, Ludwicki JK, et al. Androgen receptor gene CAG repeat length as modifier of the association between persistent organohalogen pollutant exposure markers and semen characteristics. Pharmacogenet Genomics. 2007;17:391.
96. Giwercman C, Giwercman A, Pedersen HS, Toft G, Lundin K, Bonde JP, et al. Polymorphisms in genes regulating androgen activity among prostate cancer low-risk Inuit men and high-risk Scandinavians. Int J Androl. 2008;31(1):25–30.
97. Brokken LJ, Giwercman YL. Gene-environment interactions in male reproductive health: special reference to the aryl hydrocarbon receptor signaling pathway. Asian J Androl. 2014;16(1):89–96.

98. Rubes J, Selevan SG, Sram RJ, Evenson DP, Perreault SD. GSTM1 genotype influences the susceptibility of men to sperm DNA damage associated with exposure to air pollution. Mutat Res. 2007;625(1–2):20–8.
99. Rubes J, Rybar R, Prinosilova P, Veznik Z, Chvatalova I, Solansky I, et al. Genetic polymorphisms influence the susceptibility of men to sperm DNA damage associated with exposure to air pollution. Mutat Res. 2010;683(1–2):9–15.
100. Giwercman A, Lindstedt L, Larsson M, Bungum M, Spano M, Levine RJ, et al. Sperm chromatin structure assay as an independent predictor of fertility in vivo: a case-control study. Int J Androl. 2009;33:e221.
101. Toft G, Rignell-Hydbom A, Tyrkiel E, Shvets M, Giwercman A, Lindh CH, et al. Semen quality and exposure to persistent organochlorine pollutants. Epidemiology. 2006;17(4):450–8.
102. Bungum M, Humaidan P, Axmon A, Spano M, Bungum L, Erenpreiss J, et al. Sperm DNA integrity assessment in prediction of assisted reproduction technology outcome. Hum Reprod. 2007;22(1):174–9.
103. Oleszczuk K, Giwercman A, Bungum M. Sperm chromatin structure assay in prediction of in vitro fertilization outcome. Andrology. 2016;4(2):290–6.
104. Agarwal A, Said TM. Role of sperm chromatin abnormalities and DNA damage in male infertility. Hum Reprod Update. 2003;9(4):331–45.
105. Rubes J, Lowe X, Moore D 2nd, Perreault S, Slott V, Evenson D, et al. Smoking cigarettes is associated with increased sperm disomy in teenage men. Fertil Steril. 1998;70(4):715–23.
106. Spano M, Kolstad AH, Larsen SB, Cordelli E, Leter G, Giwercman A, et al. The applicability of the flow cytometric sperm chromatin structure assay as diagnostic and prognostic tool in then human fertility clinic. Hum Reprod. 1998;13:2495–505.
107. Sergerie M, Ouhilal S, Bissonnette F, Brodeur J, Bleau G. Lack of association between smoking and DNA fragmentation in the spermatozoa of normal men. Hum Reprod. 2000;15(6):1314–21.
108. Belcheva A, Ivanova-Kicheva M, Tzvetkova P, Marinov M. Effects of cigarette smoking on sperm plasma membrane integrity and DNA fragmentation. Int J Androl. 2004;27(5):296–300.
109. Smit M, Romijn JC, Wildhagen MF, Weber RF, Dohle GR. Sperm chromatin structure is associated with the quality of spermatogenesis in infertile patients. Fertil Steril. 2009;94:1748.
110. Hammiche F, Laven JS, Boxmeer JC, Dohle GR, Steegers EA, Steegers-Theunissen RP. Sperm quality decline among men below 60 years of age undergoing IVF or ICSI treatment. J Androl. 2011;32(1):70–6.
111. Hammadeh ME, Hamad MF, Montenarh M, Fischer-Hammadeh C. Protamine contents and P1/P2 ratio in human spermatozoa from smokers and non-smokers. Hum Reprod. 2010;25(11):2708–20.
112. Duty SM, Calafat AM, Silva MJ, Ryan L, Hauser R. Phthalate exposure and reproductive hormones in adult men. Hum Reprod. 2004;20:604.
113. Xu DX, Zhu QX, Zheng LK, Wang QN, Shen HM, Deng LX, et al. Exposure to acrylonitrile induced DNA strand breakage and sex chromosome aneuploidy in human spermatozoa. Mutat Res. 2003;537(1):93–100.
114. Hernandez-Ochoa I, Garcia-Vargas G, Lopez-Carrillo L, Rubio-Andrade M, Moran-Martinez J, Cebrian ME, et al. Low lead environmental exposure alters semen quality and sperm chromatin condensation in northern Mexico. Reprod Toxicol. 2005;20(2):221–8.
115. Rignell-Hydbom A, Axmon A, Lundh T, Jonsson BA, Tiido T, Spano M. Dietary exposure to methyl mercury and PCB and the associations with semen parameters among Swedish fishermen. Environ Health. 2007;6:14.
116. Larsen SB, Spano M, Giwercman A, Bonde JP. Semen quality and sex hormones among organic and traditional Danish farmers. ASCLEPIOS Study Group. Occup Environ Med. 1999;56(2):139–44.
117. Ji G, Xia Y, Gu A, Shi X, Long Y, Song L, et al. Effects of non-occupational environmental exposure to pyrethroids on semen quality and sperm DNA integrity in Chinese men. Reprod Toxicol. 2011;31(2):171–6.

Chapter 18
Sperm DNA Damage and Oocyte Repair Capability

Sezgin Gunes and Semra Sertyel

18.1 Introduction

Approximately one in every six couples suffers from infertility (17%), and male factor contributes to 40–50% of these cases [1, 2]. The causes of almost half of these male factor-associated infertilities are unexplained/idiopathic, and within this group, 5–10% men had high amount of sperm DNA fragmentation despite having normal semen parameters. In fact, DNA fragmentation is observed in 5–10% of infertile normozoospermic men [3–5]. Today, *routine* semen analysis is the "gold standard" test used in the evaluation of male infertility; however, it is unable to identify the causes of some of the cases [6]. Therefore, in order to distinguish infertile men from the fertile population and to predict the success of in vitro fertilization (IVF) cycle outcomes, a new diagnostic test is required. The use of DNA fragmentation tests as a part of the routine analysis in fertility investigation remains controversial [7–9], despite the fact that many research groups are greatly in favour of these test [10–13].

Some studies have shown that sperm DNA fragmentation is correlated with poor reproductive outcomes including miscarriages, chromosomal aberrations, congenital malformations, genetic disorders, neurological defects and cancer in offspring [14, 15]. Understanding the mechanisms after fertilization in the zygote is therefore important.

This chapter reviews closely the process of DNA damage in spermatozoa, origin of DNA damage, the effect of sperm DNA damage on reproductive outcomes and the selection methods for spermatozoa as well as the DNA repair mechanisms in the oocyte.

S. Gunes (✉)
Ondokuz Mayis University, Samsun, Turkey
e-mail: sgunes@omu.edu.tr

S. Sertyel
Embryology Laboratory, Centrum IVF Clinic, Ankara, Turkey
e-mail: semrasertyel@gmail.com

A. Zini, A. Agarwal (eds.), *A Clinician's Guide to Sperm DNA and Chromatin Damage*, https://doi.org/10.1007/978-3-319-71815-6_18

18.2 Sperm DNA Damage

Sperm DNA damage results from any modifications of the molecular structure of DNA, including a chemically changed base such as 8-OHdG, a base missing from the backbone of DNA or single-stranded DNA breaks (SSBs) and/or double-stranded DNA breaks (DSBs). DNA fragmentation of sperm has been assessed in epididymal, testicular and ejaculated sperm [16]. In male germ cells, DNA repair is highly effective during mitosis and meiosis until the last 3 weeks of spermatogenesis. Therefore, spermatozoa are very susceptible to DNA damage towards the end of spermatogenesis in the haploid and compacted nucleus of spermatid due to insufficient DNA repair system, and these lesions would be transmitted unrepaired into the egg [16, 17]. Errors in maternal repair of sperm DNA damage may, thus, lead to chromosomal abnormalities in zygotes [18].

In general, there are two pathways in which sperm DNA fragmentation is originated: intrinsic and extrinsic factors.

18.3 Origin of DNA Fragmentation in Sperm Nucleus

18.3.1 Intrinsic Factors

18.3.1.1 Aberrations in Recombination During Spermatogenesis

DSBs are formed by specific nucleases during meiotic crossing-over process. These breaks should be ligated prior to meiosis II. Generally, before the DNA is fully fixed, the recombination checkpoint of the prophase does not permit the cells to proceed to meiosis I [19]. However, the defects that occur or persist at the checkpoint may result in permanent DNA fragmentation in ejaculated spermatozoa [20].

18.3.1.2 Abnormal Spermatid Maturation (or Abnormal Protamination Defects) During Spermatogenesis

Both SSBs and DSBs occur during the maturation process of spermatozoa into spermatids. These breaks are necessary for the packaging of sperm DNA with protamines [21] and are usually repaired and restored prior to the epididymal transit [20].

18.3.1.3 Apoptosis During Spermatogenesis

Male germ cells are regulated by Sertoli cells; nearly half of them undergo apoptosis at meiosis I during spermatogenesis. These selected cells are labelled with the Fas-type apoptotic markers and should be phagocytosed and removed by the Sertoli cell [22].

18.3.1.4 Oxidative Stress

Reactive oxygen species (ROS) are extremely unstable particles that comprises of oxygen metabolites [23]. Sources of ROS can be exogenous or endogenous. Exogenous sources of ROS originate from outside of the cells/environment, including radiation (x-rays, UV light), cigarette smoking, herbicides, alcohol abuse, chronic stress, drugs (acetaminophen) and air pollution. On the other hand, the endogenous sources are those arise from within the cell, including mitochondrial respiration and enzymatic systems such as xanthine oxidase and NADPH oxidase [18].

18.3.2 Extrinsic Factors

18.3.2.1 Age

Some studies have indicated that men with advanced age have an elevated sperm DNA fragmentation, while DNA fragmentation is considerably lower in younger men (<35 years) [24, 25]. mtDNA is more vulnerable to ROS (generated by electron transport chain) than nuclear DNA. Mutations accumulate in mtDNA and result in mitochondrial dysfunction, which in turn causes an increase in ROS production and oxidative damage and decrease in ATP/ADP ratio. Elevated ROS production, decreased ATP production and apoptosis are three features of dysfunctional mitochondria disrupted by ageing. Some studies have indicated higher DNA fragmentation index (DFI) in older men. Furthermore, high oxidative stress leads to increased apoptosis and spermatozoal DNA damage. Although apoptosis is essential for spermatogenesis under normal conditions, the balance between proliferation of spermatogonia and apoptosis of different germ cell types appears to be disturbed with ageing. This is supported by recent histological and ultrastructural study showing increased apoptosis along with a reduced proliferation in germ cells of the ageing testes. Although the significant decrease in the number of germ cells was found at the late spermatid level, primary spermatocytes did show a numerical decrease in the elderly men compared with the young controls. As the effect of age on sperm DNA single- and double-strand breaks is well documented, the presence of DNA damage repair-associated proteins such as poly (ADP-ribose) polymerase 1 (PARP-1) was also investigated in testicular tissue samples from older men. Statistically significant differences in the expression of DNA repair proteins as well as apoptosis markers, such as active caspase-3 and cleaved PARP-1, were found most markedly in ageing spermatocytes [24].

18.3.2.2 Abstinence Time

Recent studies have claimed that short abstinence period between ejaculations may lead to lower levels of sperm DNA fragmentation (24 h and 3 h) [26]. Sperm DNA fragmentation appears to become considerably elevated during the transit in the seminiferous tubules towards the epididymis, possibly associated with oxidative stress, and as a result, DNA fragmentation levels rise within the sperm population because of the non-functional DNA repair pathways [27].

18.3.2.3 Scrotal Temperature

The scrotal temperature is 2–8 °C lower compared to the rest of the body, and this is essential for proper spermatogenesis in mammals. In a mouse model study, a high level of DNA fragmentation was observed in spermatocytes retrieved from testes exposed to 40–42 °C [28].

18.3.2.4 Response to Clinical Process, Medications, Environmental Pollutants and Smoking

Some environmental factors including radiation, smoking and alcohol consumption contribute to male infertility [29–31]. Untreated cancer patients [32] as well as those who have been exposed to chemotherapy and radiotherapy [33], environmental pollutants [34, 35] and certain cytotoxic medications [36] may be prone to sperm DNA fragmentation.

Tobacco smoke has known to have mutagenic effects and has been associated with a decrease in semen quality, fertilizing capacity and elevation in the quantity of abnormal cells [29, 37]. Smoking generates reactive intermediates, including reactive nitrogen species (RNS) and reactive oxygen species (ROS), which can induce various genetic and epigenetic alterations. Through the interaction of these intermediates, exposure to tobacco smoke can directly or indirectly cause the formation of DNA and protein adducts, mutations, promoter methylation, sister chromatid exchange (SCE), chromosomal abnormalities and micronucleus formation [29]. Additionally, several studies indicate that the sperm DNA fragmentation index is significantly elevated in fertile smokers [37, 38].

Various studies have demonstrated that alcohol consumption may change both spermatogenesis and the secretion of testosterone. Alcohol consumption produces notable morphological changes in spermatozoa including breakage of the sperm head, distention of the midsection and curled tails. Overall these effects may be based on alterations of the endocrine system controlling the hypothalamic–pituitary–testicular (HPT) axis function and/or testis and/or male accessory glands [30].

Ionizing radiation produces DNA lesions leading to DNA damage, and mutations result in genomic instability that is very harmful for fertility and/or the offspring in adult spermatogenic cells. Although the unique organization of spermatogenic cells within seminiferous tubules makes them less radiosensitive compared to somatic cells, DNA repair rate and frequency of unrepaired lesions are slower in spermatogenic cells compared to somatic cells. Therefore, the use of haploid cells with genomic instability in assisted reproduction could increase the hereditary risk [31, 39].

18.3.2.5 Varicocele

Varicocele affects approximately 15–20% of males and is one of the commonest causes of poor sperm quality (sperm concentration and motility). Significantly higher DNA fragmentation has been observed in patients with varicocele [40, 41] although the underlying mechanism still remains unclear.

18.3.2.6 Microbial Infections and Leucocytospermia

Elevated sperm DNA fragmentation has been found in some patients with genitourinary tract infection such as *Mycoplasma* and *Chlamydia trachomatis* in comparison to fertile controls [42, 43]. The presence of such genital tract infection is associated with a higher concentration of leucocytes and immature germ cell in semen [44] which could lead to the generation of ROS, leading to higher DNA damage. In addition, a higher level of DNA damaged cells were reported [45] in semen samples of leucocytospermic patients.

18.3.2.7 Sperm Preparation Techniques and Cryopreservation

Semen collection techniques and sperm preparation methods affect sperm DNA quality [46, 47]. To preserve spermatozoa with higher motility rates and lower sperm DNA fragmentation, density gradient and swim-up techniques have been suggested to be used for in vitro fertilization (IVF) [48, 49]. *Cryopreservation* of sperm is a useable method to preserve male fertility for utilization in artificial reproduction techniques (ART) in the future prior to chemotherapy, radio therapy, surgical treatments or vasectomy. However, some studies have demonstrated that this method might have a negative effect on sperm DNA stability [48, 50].

18.4 The Role of Sperm DNA Integrity on Reproductive Success

Model organism reports demonstrated the significance of sperm DNA integrity during prenatal development and implantation [51]. Following studies correlated the level of DNA damage and fertility indexes of the offspring including fertilization success, rate and quality of embryo cleavage, implantation, pregnancy, and live birth rates (Table 18.1).

Table 18.1 The association amongst sperm DNA damage, pregnancy and abortion rate

		High DNA damage			Low DNA damage			
Assay	Cut-off (%)	Pregnancy (%)	Abortion (%)	Total	Pregnancy (%)	Abortion (%)	Total	Reference
SCSA	27	50	0	10	29	0	24	[52]
Comet assay	NI	29	83	30	27	0	22	[53]
SCSA	30	28	NI	57	47	NI	107	[54]
TUNEL	15	32	36	44	36	8	258	[55]
TUNEL	30	27	26	201	30	23	797	[56]
SCSA	30	28	63	29	34	42	77	[57]
TUNEL	15	6	100	18	44	0	18	[58]
TUNEL	10	12	60	43	28	8	89	[59]
TUNEL	10	13	100	18	29	30	34	[60]
SCSA	27	28	NI	25	29	NI	61	[61]
Acridine orange	30	55	33	11	51	12	49	[62]
TUNEL	35	39	35	52	62	10	65	[63]
SCSA	27	51	27	43	52	10	180	[64]
TUNEL	36	42	46	26	56	11	135	[65]
Comet assay	50	19	14	192	33	17	147	[25]
Acridine orange	50	49	37	39	47	25	114	[66]

NI not indicated

18.4.1 Association Between DNA Damage and Basic Semen Criterion

Although a few reports have indicated a slight or non-significant association between semen parameters (sperm count, motility, progression and morphology) and sperm DNA damage, many studies show that sperm from men with abnormal sperm parameters have a higher percentage of DNA damage [52, 67–71] .

There are different causes of DNA damage during spermatogenesis. If sperm DNA damage arises from the failure of DNA break repair (DBR), it would also be correlated with other indications of spermatogenic failure including teratozoospermia and oligozoospermia.

Similarly, if the damage of sperm DNA is primarily a consequence of the negative effects of ROS, sperm motility will also be affected as ROS can induce lipid peroxidation in sperm membrane which contains high amount of unsaturated fatty acids [52, 67–71]. Unrepaired DSB can cause mutations as a result of fixed DNA fragmentation [72].

18.4.2 Natural Fertility

Recent studies have indicated an important relationship between IVF and the integrity of sperm DNA. A few reports have demonstrated significant variation in the degree of sperm DNA damage between infertile and fertile males by using different techniques [52, 71, 73–75]. If the level of spermatozoa with DNA fragmentation is higher than 30% detected by SCSA, the probability of natural conception is almost zero [3, 73]. Couples in whom the man has an elevated level of sperm DNA damage have low natural conception potential, with a long time to pregnancy. The sperm DNA integrity tests may be used to predict pregnancy outcomes of couples who do not know their fertility potential [71, 73].

18.4.3 Intrauterine Insemination

The fertilization potential by intrauterine insemination (IUI) is reportedly low if sperm DNA fragmentation is higher than 30% as detected by SCSA [56, 70]. In addition, sperm samples with sperm DNA fragmentation (SDF) index higher than 12% detected by TUNEL method have demonstrated that no pregnancies were achieved in insemination [76]. Sperm DNA stability and the level of fragmentation effected by insufficient maturation, oxidative damage, apoptosis and other causes may be a marker of poor IUI outcome. Thus, sperm DNA damage has a negative correlation with fertilization, and the evaluation of sperm DNA integrity can be used as a prognostic tool in predicting the outcomes of both natural conception and IUI [56].

18.4.4 In Vitro Fertilization

The correlation between high levels of sperm DNA damage and IVF and intracytoplasmic sperm injection (ICSI) outcomes remains questionable. A negative association between embryo development in IVF cycles and sperm DNA damage has been reported [77]. In addition, several reports have also shown an important relationship between sperm DNA integrity and fertilization success in IVF [15] and ICSI [78, 79]. It has been demonstrated that for a success in pregnancy both by ICSI and IVF, the predictive DFI cut-off value detected by SCSA was 27% [75]. On the other hand, an association between IVF rates and the low level of sperm DNA damage has been shown in several studies. Their results demonstrated that sperm DNA damage has a better prognostic value in IVF compared with ICSI [15, 75, 80]. A few studies reported that a successful pregnancy could still be achieved with severe poor sperm parameters and low sperm chromatin integrity by ICSI using testicular spermatozoa [81–84].

18.4.5 Embryo Growing Quality and Blastulation Rate

Results of several clinical reports have proposed an association between sperm DNA damage/poor sperm quality and embryo development/maturation [62, 72, 85]. The impact of DNA damage on the embryo seems to be related to the development of embryo more than the embryo quality [86]. Virro and colleagues have suggested that fertilization rate was not statistically distinctive between the patients groups with low and high DNA fragmentation level. However, high DNA fragmentation (> or =30% DFI) caused a lower blastocyst and pregnancy rates [54]. The blastocyst development is controlled by maternal genes during the first few steps of development, while paternal gene expression starts at four- to eight-cell stage (approximately 48–56 h after fertilization process) [85]. Thus, during this stage, fragmented DNA inherited by father may affect negatively on the embryo development and/or blastocyst formation. Interestingly, a study has demonstrated that the adverse paternal effect on development of embryo may occur at a later stage even if there are no morphological anomalies at the zygote stage [17]. Repeated failures of assisted reproduction without any evident defective zygote formation and cleavage of embryo are frequently correlated with high sperm DNA fragmentation levels.

18.4.6 The Role of DNA Damage on Embryo Progress After IVF

Blastocyst development is negatively affected by the degree of sperm DNA fragmentation in prepared ejaculated spermatozoa used in IVF. An important inverse relationship has been reported between the apoptotic activity of sperm specimens and blastocyst progress after either ICSI or IVF [77]. Second- and third-day embryo scoring was unaffected because the paternal genome is activated after the four-cell stage, until which point embryo development is mainly controlled by maternally inherited mRNA [17, 87].

The early paternal effects were not related with sperm DNA fragmentation; however, the late paternal effects were correlated with sperm DNA integrity; therefore, analysis of sperm DNA integrity may be helpful to predict late paternal effect. The early paternal effect has been suggested to be mediated by deficiency of oocyte-activating factors or centrosome dysfunction and commence at the four-cell stage [17]. It is well documented that the incidence of pronuclear stage defect is higher in couples with female factor infertility [88]. The late paternal effect may comprise sperm DNA damage, sperm aneuploidy or abnormal chromatin packaging of paternal genome, which can affect the proper activation of paternal gene expression [17]. The role of sperm DNA integrity on the embryo quality is reportedly less important during conventional IVF process compared to ICSI [86]. Sperm DNA repair in the oocyte and the natural selection that occurs during IVF may result in lack of influence of sperm DNA damage on IVF embryo quality. In fact, the sperm DNA integrity is associated with sperm membrane and motility; therefore, the chance of fertilization with DNA-fragmented sperm at conventional IVF is low compared to ICSI [89].

18.4.7 The Role of DNA Damage on Embryo Quality After ICSI

Highly fragmented sperm DNA can escape from the natural selection and fertilize the oocyte. Despite a range of DNA damage are repairable by the oocyte after fertilization, excessive damage may possibly cause poor embryo development. A study has shown that high levels of DNA damage were present in semen samples with teratozoospermia and also those with normal morphology [72, 90, 91]. The distinction between the IVF and ICSI studies has shown that the impact of sperm DNA fragmentation on embryo quality/growing rate is more remarkable with ICSI compared to conventional IVF [86].

18.4.8 The Impact of DNA Damage on Pregnancy and Pregnancy Loss

An inverse relationship has been reported between elevated sperm DNA fragmentation and pregnancy rate using SCSA [3, 75], TUNEL [3, 58, 59] and Comet assay [92], although a few reports have shown no relation between pregnancy and sperm DNA damage [74, 86]. Two systemic reviews have also shown an important correlation between high DNA damage and decreased pregnancy rate [93, 94]. The reported relationship between sperm DNA damage and pregnancy loss may be caused by abnormal embryo development as a result of abnormal paternal genome [59]. In fact, the oocyte can easily repair SSBs; however, the repair capability of high levels of DSBs is limited; therefore, these DSBs may lead to chromosomal rearrangements and mutations that may subsequently block or modify embryo development leading to pregnancy loss [87].

18.5 Management of Infertile Patients with Elevated Sperm DNA Fragmentation

The relationship between sperm DNA integrity and fertility potential is a growing interest amongst researchers [3]. As mentioned before, there are significant differences in the sperm DNA fragmentation levels between infertile and fertile men [71]. Both in vivo and in vitro, fertility capacity has been found to be lower in men with elevated level of DNA fragmentation [73, 95]. DNA fragmentation also has an impact on sperm parameters [96], embryonic development [17], chromosomal aneuploidy [97], implantation [11, 76, 98–100] and recurrent miscarriages [94, 101–103].

18.5.1 Antioxidant Treatment

The presence of high polyunsaturated fatty acids (PUFA) in the sperm membrane makes them highly susceptible to oxidative stress. Previous reports, using indirect assays, have demonstrated that oral antioxidant treatment could reduce the elevated levels of sperm DNA fragmentation in ejaculated spermatozoa [104, 105].

Harmful outcomes of ROS on sperm DNA have been reported in different studies [58, 106–109]. ROS generation can be controlled in some degree by the seminal plasma antioxidants. The favourable impact of antioxidants including reduction of DNA fragmentation level in ejaculated spermatozoa can be detected following 2 months of oral antioxidant therapy [109]. Additionally, dietary antioxidants are an appropriate therapeutic option to alleviate sperm DNA damage for infertile men [108].

18.6 The Use of Different Sperm Sources

18.6.1 The Use of Testicular Sperm

Two recent reports have indicated the lack of pregnancy and birth when the sperm subpopulation manifesting DNA fragmentation is higher than 20% and 15%, respectively, using TUNEL [55, 110]. When comparing testicular sperm samples to the ejaculate samples, a significantly decreased level of sperm DNA fragmentation was demonstrated in patients with fragmented sperm DNA (≥15%) during the treatment with ICSI. Additionally, high implantation, pregnancy and birth rates are reported in ICSI by using testicular spermatozoa [55, 110]. It has been shown that retrieved testicular spermatozoa have a reduced level of DNA damage than ejaculated sperm in men with continuously high DFI after previously ineffective oral antioxidant treatment [107]. Recently, we reported that ICSI using testicular spermatozoa retrieved by TESA appears to be an effective option for patients with elevated DNA fragmentation (>30%) and repeated pregnancy lost [111]. The reproductive outcomes of testicular and ejaculated spermatozoa were analysed using ICSI. The pregnancy rate using testicular and ejaculated spermatozoa was

44% and 6%, respectively. Implantation percentage was found as 22% and 2% using testicular spermatozoa and ejaculated spermatozoa, respectively [110, 112].

18.6.2 Utilization of the Second Ejaculation

An ongoing pregnancy rate of higher than 30% can be achieved by taking a second consecutive sperm ejaculate on the day of oocyte pick-up to increase the total motile sperm number for IVF treatment. Invasive sperm processing techniques and unnecessary micromanipulation can be avoided by this method [113].

Some studies have suggested that spermatozoa are significantly exposed to ROS and reactive nitrogen species (RNS) during epididymal transfer and storage; therefore, low intracellular ROS values may be an indication of efficient epididymal function and the short duration in the epididymis [114]. The reduction of intracellular ROS has been seen in samples received after only 1 day of abstinence; this can be explained by the fact that these spermatozoa spent a shorter period of time in the epididymis and that their intracellular antioxidants have not been fully consumed. Hence, recurrent ejaculations can potentially be an approach to reduce sperm DNA damage and improves IVF treatment success rate [26, 115]. Nevertheless, frequent daily ejaculation of 2 weeks has no major adverse effects on both conventional and functional sperm parameters. Therefore, frequent daily ejaculations can be utilized as an alternative treatment option in male infertility cases with high oxidative stress.

18.7 Sperm Preparation Techniques

18.7.1 Conventional Sperm Preparation Techniques

Different sperm centrifugation and sedimentation techniques are routinely used in the semen sample preparation for the ART for separating sperm from seminal plasma. Density gradient centrifugation and swim-up techniques have been used for separation of fragmented sperm DNA. Swim-up is a better sperm preparation method to eliminate fragmented sperm DNA. The fragmentation level reduced from 12% to 5.5% after swim-up [14, 77, 116]. Sperm DNA quality in neat sperm or prepared samples is important in the success of ARTs. The sperm obtained by density gradient separation provide spermatozoa with higher progressive motility, viability and lower fragmented DNA as compared to those which are prepared by the other conventional sperm separation techniques [117]. Consequently, a combination of swim-up and density gradient separation methods has been suggested to reduce sperm with damaged DNA during sperm preparation in IVF treatment [118].

18.7.2 Alternative Sperm Preparation Techniques Before ICSI

Magnetic-activated cell sorting (MACS) is a technique used in separation of apoptotic sperm [119] and reduction of sperm with fragmented DNA [120]. This method is based upon the property of spermatozoa in expressing the apoptotic signal phosphatidylserine that attached to annexin-V-combined micro-beads. Spermatozoa with apoptotic signal and fragmented DNA could be distinguished by a magnetic field to annexin-V-positive and annexin-V-negative fractions. This technique is recommended to use in IVF laboratories for sperm preparation [119]. The utilization of hyaluronic acid is another way of selection. The method is based on binding of spermatozoa with DNA fragmentation to hyaluronic acid [121]. Electrophoretic separation of spermatozoa for sperm selection is another advanced technique, which is based upon detection of mature spermatozoa because of the negatively charged glycocalyx rich in sialic acid remnants [122].

18.8 Advanced Sperm Selection for ICSI

18.8.1 Morphological Selection

Motile and morphologically normal sperm are selected for ICSI process; however, these sperms may have an elevated level of DNA fragmentation. Therefore, analysis of DNA fragmentation is suggested for motile and morphologically normal spermatozoa before ICSI procedure [67].

18.8.2 Sperm Selection Under High Magnification

Recently, to increase the reproductive outcomes of ICSI, non-invasive methods have been requested for patients with poor sperm quality [119, 122, 123], especially, selection of morphologically best sperm for injection based upon motility and morphology of organelles analysed at over 6000 magnification [124] to improve pregnancy and abortion rates. Intracytoplasmic morphologically selected sperm injection (IMSI) is a sperm selection method based on selection of motile spermatozoa without head vacuoles simultaneously under high magnification (>6000×). The presence of vacuoles in the nuclear region of the sperm head is one of the most prognostic indicators of poor sperm quality. These vacuoles seem to be related with fragmentation and/or denaturation of sperm DNA and lead to poor embryo development [125, 126].

18.8.3 Human Motile Sperm Head Birefringence

Sperm head birefringence (SHBF) is used as a criterion for the selection of best sperm to use in ICSI. A few studies reported a significant higher DNA fragmentation in spermatozoa with sperm head birefringence total (SHBF-T) than in those with sperm head birefringence partial (SHBF-P) [127].

18.9 DNA Repair Mechanisms

DNA damage/lesions arise as a result of spontaneous errors during DNA replication and spontaneous cellular metabolism. Approximately 105 DNA lesions are generated in a cell each day [128]. A number of mechanisms in our body are able to recognize and repair these DNA lesions. The DNA repair rate of these lesions is based on the cell types, the age of the cell and the extracellular environment of the cell. Following the DNA damage, the cell can enter one of three states, namely, (i) apoptosis, (ii) mutations or (iii) rearrangement and DNA repair (Fig. 18.1).

DNA repair mechanisms have evolved to compensate the DNA damage to maintain genomic integrity and stability. These mechanisms are base nucleotide excision repair (NER), excision repair (BER), mismatch repair (MMR), DSB repair (DSR) and post-replication repair. These mechanisms detect and correct the DNA lesions regardless of the cause (Fig. 18.2).

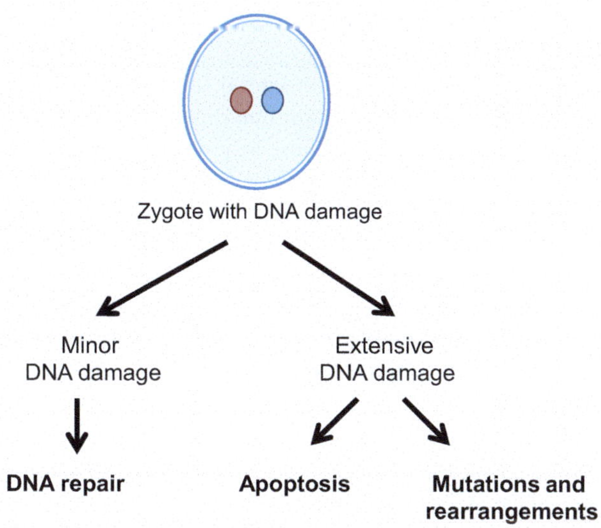

Fig. 18.1 Fate of DNA damage after zygote formation

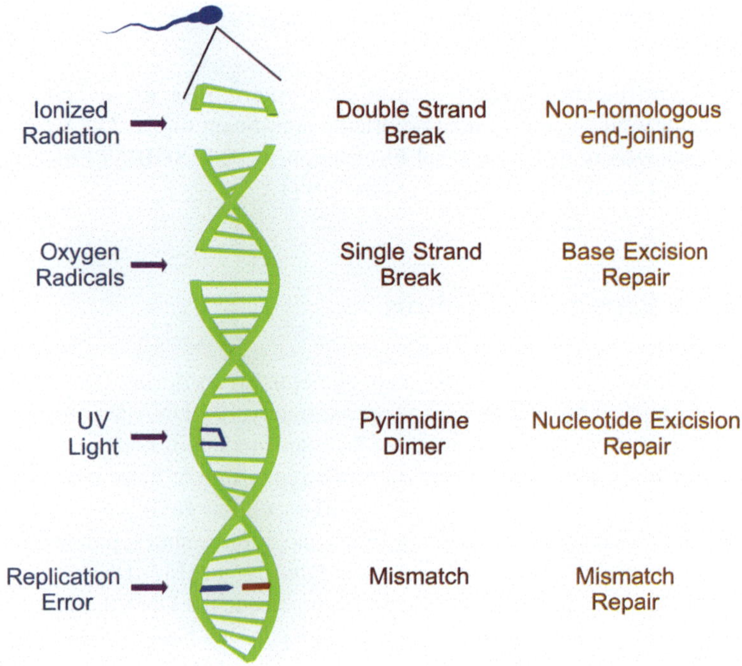

Fig. 18.2 DNA damage and DNA repair mechanisms

18.9.1 Nucleotide Excision Repair

NER mechanism repairs substantial lesions including oxidative damage and DNA intrastrand cross-links, pyrimidine dimers caused by the UV mismatched bases or bulky adducts [129, 130]. These lesions cause distortion of helical structure of DNA [131]. The DNA damage is scanned and detected by roughly 30 different proteins in the NER mechanism. Global genome NER (GG-NER) and transcription-coupled NER (TC-NER) are the two pathways of NER. Each pathway is liable for recognition of different types of damage [18]. GG-NER pathway repairs DNA damage throughout the whole genome [132], while TC-NER pathway is responsible for repairing lesions on the transcribed strand of DNA [130]. DNA damage is scanned and detected by XPC/RAD23B proteins in GG-NER pathway [130, 132–134]. XPC and RAD23B proteins are expressed highly in oocyte [18]. TC-NER activated by DNA distortions block the elongating RNA polymerase II complex [134, 135]. Following damage recognition, both of the pathways utilize the same repair machinery. Firstly, DNA helix unwinds to permit xeroderma pigmentosum (XP) complementation group A (XPA) binding by replication protein A (RPA) to DNA strand for secondary DNA damaged recognition. Subsequently, endonucleases XPG and XPF/

ERCC1 cleave the DNA, leading to removal of lesions [129]. Lastly, DNA polymerase fills the remaining gap and the remaining nick is sealed by DNA ligase. The expression of both XPA and RPA proteins is found at high levels in oocyte [18]. Defects in the NER mechanism may result in autosomal recessive diseases such as Cockayne syndrome (CS), xeroderma pigmentosum and trichothiodystrophy (TTD) [136, 137].

18.9.2 Base Excision Repair

BER is a highly coordinated mechanism in charge of the removal of non-helix-distorting base damages caused by different reactions/mechanisms such as oxidation or adduction [18, 138]. DNA glycosylases recognize specific base substitution in DNA helix and catalyse hydrolytic elimination of altered base [130]. *Uracil* DNA glycosylase (UNG) expression was reported to be high in the oocyte in germinal vesicle (GV) stage [139]. 8-Oxoguanine (80HdG) glycosylase 1 (OGG1) [140, 141] cuts the 80HdG residue and generates abasic sites. AP endonuclease 1 (APE1) incises phosphate backbone of DNA to insert unmodified nucleotide [141, 142]. The expression of OGG1 was found to be moderate; however, etheno-adenosine, 3-methyl adenine and N-methylpurine-DNA glycosylase (MPG) that distinguishes hypoxanthine are highly expressed in oocyte [139]. A recent study has demonstrated that post-translational modification to BER enzymes is initiated by conception such as OGG1 and X-ray repair cross-complementing protein 1 (XRCC1), causing nuclear localization and accelerated excision of 80HdG. The expression level of OGG1 in the oocyte is low compared to the male germ line where it is the only constituent of the BER pathway. Therefore, male germ line cooperates with female germ line to repair oxidative DNA damage, and oocytes are defenceless to high 80HdG levels being transmitted into the zygote by the fertilizing spermatozoon [143].

18.9.3 Mismatch Repair Mechanism

During DNA replication, mismatches occur as a consequence of tautomerization of the DNA strand bases due to inefficient proofreading by DNA polymerase [144]. Mismatches are base–base mismatches, for instance, G/T or A/C, and insertion–deletion loops [145]. MMR enhances fidelity of DNA replication about 100 times and suppresses the genomic instability of a cell. The mechanism is highly conserved evolutionarily to prevent genomic instability [142] in all living organisms. In order to repair the mismatch, MMR proteins first identify the mispaired nucleotides. The differentiation of parental and newly synthesized strands is performed through methylation, where the parental strand is methylated and the newly synthesized strand remains unmethylated in prokaryotes. However, in eukaryotes, MMR is associated with DNA replication machinery that facilitates discrimination via binding of *proliferating cell nuclear antigen* (PCNA) in the leading strand and free 5′ ends of Okazaki fragments at the lagging strand [130, 144]. MutS protein is responsible for the recognition and binding to mismatched base of the newly synthesized DNA strand. MutL is a latent clamp-structured molecule that binds at unmethylated sites along the newly synthesized strand to induce exonuclease activity of MutH in prokaryotes [146].

There are several homologs of the proteins MutS and MutL in eukaryotes. MutS homologs such as MSH1–MSH6 and MutL include MLH1–MLH3, PMS1 and PMS2 which form heterodimers [146, 147]. Maduro and colleagues showed genomic instability and defects of MLH1 or MSH2 in nonobstructive azoospermia [148]. In meiotic recombination process, MSH4 and MSH5 proteins are essential. There are two types of MutS homolog heterodimers. The first type is MutSa (MSH2/MSH6) which plays a role in DNA base–base mispairs. The second is MutSb (MSH2/MSH3) which is involved in insertion–deletion loop mispair repair [147]. The connection of MutL with MutS–DNA complex activates the MutH, which nicks the daughter strand and recruits DNA helicase II to disconnect the DNA double strands [149]. Germ line mutations of these proteins are related to hereditary nonpolyposis colorectal cancer (HNPC). Mutations or aberrant methylation of these genes is also related with sporadic cases [150, 151]. Exonucleases are recruited to digest the SSD tail followed by the formation of a gap. The gap is filled by DNA polymerase and sealed by an unidentified DNA ligase. MLH1 and MLH3 are essential to facilitate recombination and chiasmata separation during pachytene and diplotene.

18.9.4 DNA Double-Strand Repair

DSBs are caused by several factors including failed DNA replication through replication across a nick and DNA repair, ROS, recombination, meiosis, inadvertent action by nuclear enzymes on DNA including type II topoisomerases, chemotherapeutic agents and ionizing radiation [152]. Unrepaired DSBs can cause chromosomal instability through DNA fusions and chromosomal rearrangements, as well as cell death. Homologous recombination (HR) and non-homologous end-joining (NHEJ) repair are the two major pathways to repair DSBs [130].

18.9.4.1 Homologous Recombination

HR repair mechanism is an error-free repair mechanism that functions primarily during S and G2 phases of cell cycle [18, 130]. In this process, DSBs are protected from exonuclease activity, by the binding of RAD51 to the strands. Ataxia–telangiectasia mutated (ATM) and MRE11–RAD50–NBS1 (MRN) complex are the initiators of DSBs [129, 153], and 3′-ssDNA is generated by resecting the broken DNA ends through interactions with carboxy-terminal-binding protein (CtIP) [154]. The tail of the ssDNA is coated by replication protein A (RPA) to remove secondary disruptive structures; RPA are replaced with RAD51 homologous sequence on the sister chromatid [155]. RAD51C interacts with BRCA2 to form complexes for homologous pairing [156]. Few studies have suggested a relation between alterations of HR mechanism and infertility. A study conducted by Xu and Baltimore (1996) indicted that men with ataxia–telangiectasia (AT) have azoospermia and gonadal atrophy, due to the failure of primary spermatocytes at the leptotene–zygotene transition [157].

18.9.4.2 Non-homologous End-Joining

The Ku70/Ku80 heterodimers recognize and bind to DSBs in DNA and then recruit dependent protein kinase (DNA–PKcs) [129, 158]. The recruitment of DNA–PKcs induces the removal of non-ligatable termini by an inward translocation followed by replication of DNA polymerases and ligation to create compatible ends. Defects in this repair system, whether in non-homologous end-joining or homologous recombination, predispose a person to cancer and immunodeficiency syndromes [130, 159]. DNA repair proteins associated with germ cells are summarized in Table 18.2.

18.10 Conclusion

Sperm DNA damage has been shown to adversely associate with reduced male reproductive potential including natural fertilization, intrauterine insemination outcomes, IVF pregnancy rates, development of embryo and health of the offspring. However, the ASRM Practice Committee does not recommend routine use of sperm DNA tests [9]. In mice, sperm DNA damage has been found to be associated with chromosomal abnormalities, developmental loss, reduced longevity and birth defects [91]. Identification of a new tool that could help in predicting male fertilizing potential is one of the main areas of male infertility research nowadays. Several assessment techniques have been developed for evaluating sperm DNA damage and integrity [13, 112, 119]. Further studies are required to understand the molecular basis of sperm DNA damage repair and could provide better and tailor-made therapeutic options for couples.

It is well known that ART, especially ICSI, bypasses the natural selection mechanisms and leads to fertilization with spermatozoa with DNA damage, which is not compatible with fertilization under natural circumstances. However, in vivo improvement of spermatozoa before application of assisted reproductive techniques remains of ultimate importance. The repairing capacity of the human oocyte may be insufficient to overcome paternally transmitted damage. Deficiencies in DNA repair mechanisms in oocytes likely contribute to miscarriages, chromosomal aberrations, congenital malformations, genetic disorders, neurological defects and the

Table 18.2 DNA repair proteins associated with germ cells

Gene	Expression level	Phenotype	Reference
MLH1	Medium	Microsatellite instability Failure of crossing over and premature desynapsis of homologous chromosomes Male infertility	[147]
MSH2	High	Loss of germ cells MMR deficiency in somatic cells	[160]
MSH3	High	MMR deficiency in somatic cells Fertile	[161]
MSH4	Not expressed	Failure of spermatogonial maturation beyond zygonema Infertility	[39]
MSH5	Medium	Incomplete and non-homologous chromosomal pairing Infertility	[162]
MSH6	High	MMR deficiency in somatic cells Fertile	[39]
MLH3	Not expressed	Infertile	[161, 163]
PMS2	Medium	Genomic instability Disruption of normal chromosomal synapsis Infertility	[161]
UNG	High (in oocyte)	Removal of adducts	[18]
OGG1	Moderate (in oocyte)	Decrease the level of 80HdG	[143]

development cancer in offspring. However, further research is required to elucidate the precise underlying pathophysiologic mechanisms and thus in the development of potential treatments for DNA repair. The true clinical value of sperm DNA fragmentation and its impact on embryo quality and embryo development are critical areas that need further research.

References

1. Chung CC, Fleming R, Jamieson ME, Yates RW, Coutts JR. Randomized comparison of ovulation induction with and without intrauterine insemination in the treatment of unexplained infertility. Hum Reprod. 1995;10(12):3139–41.
2. Hamada A, Esteves SC, Nizza M, Agarwal A. Unexplained male infertility: diagnosis and management. Int Braz J Urol: Off J Braz Soc Urol. 2012;38(5):576–94.
3. Evenson DP, Jost LK, Marshall D, Zinaman MJ, Clegg E, Purvis K, et al. Utility of the sperm chromatin structure assay as a diagnostic and prognostic tool in the human fertility clinic. Hum Reprod. 1999;14(4):1039–49.
4. Venkatesh S, Shamsi MB, Deka D, Saxena V, Kumar R, Dada R. Clinical implications of oxidative stress & sperm DNA damage in normozoospermic infertile men. Indian J Med Res. 2011;134:396–8.
5. Shefi S, Turek PJ. Definition and current evaluation of subfertile men. Int Braz J Urol: Off J Braz Soc Urol. 2006;32(4):385–97.

6. Agarwal A, Allamaneni SS. Sperm DNA damage assessment: a test whose time has come. Fertil Steril. 2005;84(4):850–3.
7. Practice Committee of American Society for Reproductive M. The clinical utility of sperm DNA integrity testing. Fertil Steril. 2008;90(5 Suppl):S178–80.
8. Practice Committee of the American Society for Reproductive M. Effectiveness and treatment for unexplained infertility. Fertil Steril. 2006;86(5 Suppl 1):S111–4.
9. Practice Committee of the American Society for Reproductive M. The clinical utility of sperm DNA integrity testing: a guideline. Fertil Steril. 2013;99(3):673–7.
10. Abu DA, Franken DR, Hoffman B, Henkel R. Sequential analysis of sperm functional aspects involved in fertilisation: a pilot study. Andrologia. 2012;44(Suppl 1):175–81.
11. Bungum M. Sperm DNA integrity assessment: a new tool in diagnosis and treatment of fertility. Obstet Gynecol Int. 2012;2012:531042.
12. Giwercman A, Lindstedt L, Larsson M, Bungum M, Spano M, Levine RJ, et al. Sperm chromatin structure assay as an independent predictor of fertility in vivo: a case-control study. Int J Androl. 2010;33(1):e221–7.
13. Omran HM, Bakhiet M, Dashti MG. DNA integrity is a critical molecular indicator for the assessment of male infertility. Mol Med Rep. 2013;7(5):1631–5.
14. Gandini L, Lombardo F, Paoli D, Caruso F, Eleuteri P, Leter G, et al. Full-term pregnancies achieved with ICSI despite high levels of sperm chromatin damage. Hum Reprod. 2004;19(6):1409–17.
15. Hammadeh ME, Stieber M, Haidl G, Schmidt W. Association between sperm cell chromatin condensation, morphology based on strict criteria, and fertilization, cleavage and pregnancy rates in an IVF program. Andrologia. 1998;30(1):29–35.
16. Gonzalez-Marin C, Gosalvez J, Roy R. Types, causes, detection and repair of DNA fragmentation in animal and human sperm cells. Int J Mol Sci. 2012;13(11):14026–52.
17. Tesarik J, Greco E, Mendoza C. Late, but not early, paternal effect on human embryo development is related to sperm DNA fragmentation. Hum Reprod. 2004;19(3):611–5.
18. Menezo Y, Dale B, Cohen M. DNA damage and repair in human oocytes and embryos: a review. Zygote. 2010;18(4):357–65.
19. Bannister LA, Schimenti JC. Homologous recombinational repair proteins in mouse meiosis. Cytogenet Genome Res. 2004;107(3–4):191–200.
20. Erenpreiss J, Spano M, Erenpreisa J, Bungum M, Giwercman A. Sperm chromatin structure and male fertility: biological and clinical aspects. Asian J Androl. 2006;8(1):11–29.
21. Gunes S, Kulac T. The role of epigenetics in spermatogenesis. Turk J Urol. 2013;39(3):181–7.
22. Sakkas D, Mariethoz E, Manicardi G, Bizzaro D, Bianchi PG, Bianchi U. Origin of DNA damage in ejaculated human spermatozoa. Rev Reprod. 1999;4(1):31–7.
23. Aitken RJ, Gordon E, Harkiss D, Twigg JP, Milne P, Jennings Z, et al. Relative impact of oxidative stress on the functional competence and genomic integrity of human spermatozoa. Biol Reprod. 1998;59(5):1037–46.
24. Gunes S, Hekim GN, Arslan MA, Asci R. Effects of aging on the male reproductive system. J Assist Reprod Genet. 2016;33(4):441–54.
25. Simon L, Castillo J, Oliva R, Lewis SE. Relationships between human sperm protamines, DNA damage and assisted reproduction outcomes. Reprod BioMed Online. 2011;23(6):724–34.
26. Gosalvez J, Gonzalez-Martinez M, Lopez-Fernandez C, Fernandez JL, Sanchez-Martin P. Shorter abstinence decreases sperm deoxyribonucleic acid fragmentation in ejaculate. Fertil Steril. 2011;96(5):1083–6.
27. Gil-Guzman E, Ollero M, Lopez MC, Sharma RK, Alvarez JG, Thomas AJ Jr, et al. Differential production of reactive oxygen species by subsets of human spermatozoa at different stages of maturation. Hum Reprod. 2001;16(9):1922–30.
28. Paul C, Murray AA, Spears N, Saunders PT. A single, mild, transient scrotal heat stress causes DNA damage, subfertility and impairs formation of blastocysts in mice. Reproduction. 2008;136(1):73–84.

29. Harlev A, Agarwal A, Gunes SO, Shetty A, du Plessis SS. Smoking and male infertility: an evidence-based review. World J Men's Health. 2015;33(3):143–60.
30. La Vignera S, Condorelli RA, Balercia G, Vicari E, Calogero AE. Does alcohol have any effect on male reproductive function? A review of literature. Asian J Androl. 2013;15(2):221–5.
31. Marjault HB, Allemand I. Consequences of irradiation on adult spermatogenesis: between infertility and hereditary risk. Mutat Res. 2016;770(Pt B):340–8.
32. Kobayashi H, Larson K, Sharma RK, Nelson DR, Evenson DP, Toma H, et al. DNA damage in patients with untreated cancer as measured by the sperm chromatin structure assay. Fertil Steril. 2001;75(3):469–75.
33. Morris ID. Sperm DNA damage and cancer treatment. Int J Androl. 2002;25(5):255–61.
34. Specht IO, Hougaard KS, Spano M, Bizzaro D, Manicardi GC, Lindh CH, et al. Sperm DNA integrity in relation to exposure to environmental perfluoroalkyl substances – a study of spouses of pregnant women in three geographical regions. Reprod Toxicol. 2012;33(4):577–83.
35. Evenson DP, Wixon R. Environmental toxicants cause sperm DNA fragmentation as detected by the Sperm Chromatin Structure Assay (SCSA). Toxicol Appl Pharmacol. 2005;207(2 Suppl):532–7.
36. Tanrikut C, Feldman AS, Altemus M, Paduch DA, Schlegel PN. Adverse effect of paroxetine on sperm. Fertil Steril. 2010;94(3):1021–6.
37. Kunzle R, Mueller MD, Hanggi W, Birkhauser MH, Drescher H, Bersinger NA. Semen quality of male smokers and nonsmokers in infertile couples. Fertil Steril. 2003;79(2):287–91.
38. Sofikitis N, Miyagawa I, Dimitriadis D, Zavos P, Sikka S, Hellstrom W. Effects of smoking on testicular function, semen quality and sperm fertilizing capacity. J Urol. 1995;154(3):1030–4.
39. Gunes S, Al-Sadaan M, Agarwal A. Spermatogenesis, DNA damage and DNA repair mechanisms in male infertility. Reprod BioMed Online. 2015;31(3):309–19.
40. Talebi AR, Moein MR, Tabibnejad N, Ghasemzadeh J. Effect of varicocele on chromatin condensation and DNA integrity of ejaculated spermatozoa using cytochemical tests. Andrologia. 2008;40(4):245–51.
41. Zini A, Dohle G. Are varicoceles associated with increased deoxyribonucleic acid fragmentation? Fertil Steril. 2011;96(6):1283–7.
42. Gonzalez-Marin C, Roy R, Lopez-Fernandez C, Diez B, Carabano MJ, Fernandez JL, et al. Bacteria in bovine semen can increase sperm DNA fragmentation rates: a kinetic experimental approach. Anim Reprod Sci. 2011;123(3–4):139–48.
43. Gallegos G, Ramos B, Santiso R, Goyanes V, Gosalvez J, Fernandez JL. Sperm DNA fragmentation in infertile men with genitourinary infection by Chlamydia trachomatis and Mycoplasma. Fertil Steril. 2008;90(2):328–34.
44. Alvarez JG, Sharma RK, Ollero M, Saleh RA, Lopez MC, Thomas AJ Jr, et al. Increased DNA damage in sperm from leukocytospermic semen samples as determined by the sperm chromatin structure assay. Fertil Steril. 2002;78(2):319–29.
45. Sigman M, Lopes L. The correlation between round cells and white blood cells in the semen. J Urol. 1993;149(5 Pt 2):1338–40.
46. Rougier N, Uriondo H, Papier S, Checa MA, Sueldo C, Alvarez SC. Changes in DNA fragmentation during sperm preparation for intracytoplasmic sperm injection over time. Fertil Steril. 2013;100(1):69–74.
47. Mengual L, Ballesca JL, Ascaso C, Oliva R. Marked differences in protamine content and P1/P2 ratios in sperm cells from percoll fractions between patients and controls. J Androl. 2003;24(3):438–47.
48. Jackson RE, Bormann CL, Hassun PA, Rocha AM, Motta EL, Serafini PC, et al. Effects of semen storage and separation techniques on sperm DNA fragmentation. Fertil Steril. 2010;94(7):2626–30.
49. Jayaraman V, Upadhya D, Narayan PK, Adiga SK. Sperm processing by swim-up and density gradient is effective in elimination of sperm with DNA damage. J Assist Reprod Genet. 2012;29(6):557–63.

50. Gosalvez J, de la Torre J, Lopez-Fernandez C, Perez-Gutierrez L, Ortega L, Caballero P, et al. DNA fragmentation dynamics in fresh versus frozen thawed plus gradient-isolated human spermatozoa. Syst Biol Reprod Med. 2010;56(1):27–36.
51. Ahmadi A, Ng SC. Fertilizing ability of DNA-damaged spermatozoa. J Exp Zool. 1999;284(6):696–704.
52. Gandini L, Lombardo F, Paoli D, Caponecchia L, Familiari G, Verlengia C, et al. Study of apoptotic DNA fragmentation in human spermatozoa. Hum Reprod. 2000;15(4):830–9.
53. Morris ID, Ilott S, Dixon L, Brison DR. The spectrum of DNA damage in human sperm assessed by single cell gel electrophoresis (Comet assay) and its relationship to fertilization and embryo development. Hum Reprod. 2002;17(4):990–8.
54. Virro MR, Larson-Cook KL, Evenson DP. Sperm chromatin structure assay (SCSA) parameters are related to fertilization, blastocyst development, and ongoing pregnancy in in vitro fertilization and intracytoplasmic sperm injection cycles. Fertil Steril. 2004;81(5):1289–95.
55. Benchaib M, Braun V, Lornage J, Hadj S, Salle B, Lejeune H, et al. Sperm DNA fragmentation decreases the pregnancy rate in an assisted reproductive technique. Hum Reprod. 2003;18(5):1023–8.
56. Bungum M, Humaidan P, Spano M, Jepson K, Bungum L, Giwercman A. The predictive value of sperm chromatin structure assay (SCSA) parameters for the outcome of intrauterine insemination, IVF and ICSI. Hum Reprod. 2004;19(6):1401–8.
57. Check JH, Graziano V, Cohen R, Krotec J, Check ML. Effect of an abnormal sperm chromatin structural assay (SCSA) on pregnancy outcome following (IVF) with ICSI in previous IVF failures. Arch Androl. 2005;51(2):121–4.
58. Greco E, Romano S, Iacobelli M, Ferrero S, Baroni E, Minasi MG, et al. ICSI in cases of sperm DNA damage: beneficial effect of oral antioxidant treatment. Hum Reprod. 2005;20(9):2590–4.
59. Borini A, Tarozzi N, Bizzaro D, Bonu MA, Fava L, Flamigni C, et al. Sperm DNA fragmentation: paternal effect on early post-implantation embryo development in ART. Hum Reprod. 2006;21(11):2876–81.
60. Ozmen B, Caglar GS, Koster F, Schopper B, Diedrich K, Al-Hasani S. Relationship between sperm DNA damage, induced acrosome reaction and viability in ICSI patients. Reprod BioMed Online. 2007;15(2):208–14.
61. Boe-Hansen GB, Fedder J, Ersboll AK, Christensen P. The sperm chromatin structure assay as a diagnostic tool in the human fertility clinic. Hum Reprod. 2006;21(6):1576–82.
62. Zini A, Meriano J, Kader K, Jarvi K, Laskin CA, Cadesky K. Potential adverse effect of sperm DNA damage on embryo quality after ICSI. Hum Reprod. 2005;20(12):3476–80.
63. Frydman N, Prisant N, Hesters L, Frydman R, Tachdjian G, Cohen-Bacrie P, et al. Adequate ovarian follicular status does not prevent the decrease in pregnancy rates associated with high sperm DNA fragmentation. Fertil Steril. 2008;89(1):92–7.
64. Lin MH, Kuo-Kuang Lee R, Li SH, Lu CH, Sun FJ, Hwu YM. Sperm chromatin structure assay parameters are not related to fertilization rates, embryo quality, and pregnancy rates in in vitro fertilization and intracytoplasmic sperm injection, but might be related to spontaneous abortion rates. Fertil Steril. 2008;90(2):352–9.
65. Esbert M, Pacheco A, Vidal F, Florensa M, Riqueros M, Ballesteros A, et al. Impact of sperm DNA fragmentation on the outcome of IVF with own or donated oocytes. Reprod BioMed Online. 2011;23(6):704–10.
66. Dar S, Grover SA, Moskovtsev SI, Swanson S, Baratz A, Librach CL. In vitro fertilization-intracytoplasmic sperm injection outcome in patients with a markedly high DNA fragmentation index (>50%). Fertil Steril. 2013;100(1):75–80.
67. Avendano C, Oehninger S. DNA fragmentation in morphologically normal spermatozoa: how much should we be concerned in the ICSI era? J Androl. 2011;32(4):356–63.
68. Giwercman A, Richthoff J, Hjollund H, Bonde JP, Jepson K, Frohm B, et al. Correlation between sperm motility and sperm chromatin structure assay parameters. Fertil Steril. 2003;80(6):1404–12.

69. Oosterhuis GJ, Mulder AB, Kalsbeek-Batenburg E, Lambalk CB, Schoemaker J, Vermes I. Measuring apoptosis in human spermatozoa: a biological assay for semen quality? Fertil Steril. 2000;74(2):245–50.
70. Saleh RA, Agarwal A, Nada EA, El-Tonsy MH, Sharma RK, Meyer A, et al. Negative effects of increased sperm DNA damage in relation to seminal oxidative stress in men with idiopathic and male factor infertility. Fertil Steril. 2003;79(Suppl 3):1597–605.
71. Zini A, Bielecki R, Phang D, Zenzes MT. Correlations between two markers of sperm DNA integrity, DNA denaturation and DNA fragmentation, in fertile and infertile men. Fertil Steril. 2001;75(4):674–7.
72. Avendano C, Franchi A, Taylor S, Morshedi M, Bocca S, Oehninger S. Fragmentation of DNA in morphologically normal human spermatozoa. Fertil Steril. 2009;91(4):1077–84.
73. Spano M, Bonde JP, Hjollund HI, Kolstad HA, Cordelli E, Leter G. Sperm chromatin damage impairs human fertility. The Danish First Pregnancy Planner Study Team. Fertil Steril. 2000;73(1):43–50.
74. Host E, Lindenberg S, Kahn JA, Christensen F. DNA strand breaks in human sperm cells: a comparison between men with normal and oligozoospermic sperm samples. Acta Obstet Gynecol Scand. 1999;78(4):336–9.
75. Larson-Cook KL, Brannian JD, Hansen KA, Kasperson KM, Aamold ET, Evenson DP. Relationship between the outcomes of assisted reproductive techniques and sperm DNA fragmentation as measured by the sperm chromatin structure assay. Fertil Steril. 2003;80(4):895–902.
76. Duran EH, Morshedi M, Taylor S, Oehninger S. Sperm DNA quality predicts intrauterine insemination outcome: a prospective cohort study. Hum Reprod. 2002;17(12):3122–8.
77. Tomlinson MJ, Moffatt O, Manicardi GC, Bizzaro D, Afnan M, Sakkas D. Interrelationships between seminal parameters and sperm nuclear DNA damage before and after density gradient centrifugation: implications for assisted conception. Hum Reprod. 2001;16(10):2160–5.
78. Lopes S, Sun JG, Jurisicova A, Meriano J, Casper RF. Sperm deoxyribonucleic acid fragmentation is increased in poor-quality semen samples and correlates with failed fertilization in intracytoplasmic sperm injection. Fertil Steril. 1998;69(3):528–32.
79. Twigg JP, Irvine DS, Aitken RJ. Oxidative damage to DNA in human spermatozoa does not preclude pronucleus formation at intracytoplasmic sperm injection. Hum Reprod. 1998;13(7):1864–71.
80. Host E, Lindenberg S, Smidt-Jensen S. The role of DNA strand breaks in human spermatozoa used for IVF and ICSI. Acta Obstet Gynecol Scand. 2000;79(7):559–63.
81. Urman B, Alatas C, Aksoy S, Mercan R, Nuhoglu A, Mumcu A, et al. Transfer at the blastocyst stage of embryos derived from testicular round spermatid injection. Hum Reprod. 2002;17(3):741–3.
82. Vicdan K, Isik AZ, Delilbasi L. Development of blastocyst-stage embryos after round spermatid injection in patients with complete spermiogenesis failure. J Assist Reprod Genet. 2001;18(2):78–86.
83. Marh J, Tres LL, Yamazaki Y, Yanagimachi R, Kierszenbaum AL. Mouse round spermatids developed in vitro from preexisting spermatocytes can produce normal offspring by nuclear injection into in vivo-developed mature oocytes. Biol Reprod. 2003;69(1):169–76.
84. Khalili MA, Aflatoonian A, Zavos PM. Intracytoplasmic injection using spermatids and subsequent pregnancies: round versus elongated spermatids. J Assist Reprod Genet. 2002;19(2):84–6.
85. Seli E, Gardner DK, Schoolcraft WB, Moffatt O, Sakkas D. Extent of nuclear DNA damage in ejaculated spermatozoa impacts on blastocyst development after in vitro fertilization. Fertil Steril. 2004;82(2):378–83.
86. Zini A, Jamal W, Cowan L, Al-Hathal N. Is sperm DNA damage associated with IVF embryo quality? A systematic review. J Assist Reprod Genet. 2011;28(5):391–7.
87. Braude P, Bolton V, Moore S. Human gene expression first occurs between the four- and eight-cell stages of preimplantation development. Nature. 1988;332(6163):459–61.

88. Navot D, Bergh PA, Williams MA, Garrisi GJ, Guzman I, Sandler B, et al. Poor oocyte quality rather than implantation failure as a cause of age-related decline in female fertility. Lancet. 1991;337(8754):1375–7.
89. Huszar G, Jakab A, Sakkas D, Ozenci CC, Cayli S, Delpiano E, et al. Fertility testing and ICSI sperm selection by hyaluronic acid binding: clinical and genetic aspects. Reprod BioMed Online. 2007;14(5):650–63.
90. Cho C, Jung-Ha H, Willis WD, Goulding EH, Stein P, Xu Z, et al. Protamine 2 deficiency leads to sperm DNA damage and embryo death in mice. Biol Reprod. 2003;69(1):211–7.
91. Fernandez-Gonzalez R, Moreira PN, Perez-Crespo M, Sanchez-Martin M, Ramirez MA, Pericuesta E, et al. Long-term effects of mouse intracytoplasmic sperm injection with DNA-fragmented sperm on health and behavior of adult offspring. Biol Reprod. 2008;78(4):761–72.
92. Lewis SE, John Aitken R, Conner SJ, Iuliis GD, Evenson DP, Henkel R, et al. The impact of sperm DNA damage in assisted conception and beyond: recent advances in diagnosis and treatment. Reprod BioMed Online. 2013;27(4):325–37.
93. Robinson L, Gallos ID, Conner SJ, Rajkhowa M, Miller D, Lewis S, et al. The effect of sperm DNA fragmentation on miscarriage rates: a systematic review and meta-analysis. Hum Reprod. 2012;27(10):2908–17.
94. Zini A, Boman JM, Belzile E, Ciampi A. Sperm DNA damage is associated with an increased risk of pregnancy loss after IVF and ICSI: systematic review and meta-analysis. Hum Reprod. 2008;23(12):2663–8.
95. Benchaib M, Lornage J, Mazoyer C, Lejeune H, Salle B, Francois GJ. Sperm deoxyribonucleic acid fragmentation as a prognostic indicator of assisted reproductive technology outcome. Fertil Steril. 2007;87(1):93–100.
96. Cohen-Bacrie P, Belloc S, Menezo YJ, Clement P, Hamidi J, Benkhalifa M. Correlation between DNA damage and sperm parameters: a prospective study of 1,633 patients. Fertil Steril. 2009;91(5):1801–5.
97. Tang SS, Gao H, Zhao Y, Ma S. Aneuploidy and DNA fragmentation in morphologically abnormal sperm. Int J Androl. 2010;33(1):e163–79.
98. Speyer BE, Pizzey AR, Ranieri M, Joshi R, Delhanty JD, Serhal P. Fall in implantation rates following ICSI with sperm with high DNA fragmentation. Hum Reprod. 2010;25(7):1609–18.
99. Meseguer M, Santiso R, Garrido N, Garcia-Herrero S, Remohi J, Fernandez JL. Effect of sperm DNA fragmentation on pregnancy outcome depends on oocyte quality. Fertil Steril. 2011;95(1):124–8.
100. Henkel R, Hajimohammad M, Stalf T, Hoogendijk C, Mehnert C, Menkveld R, et al. Influence of deoxyribonucleic acid damage on fertilization and pregnancy. Fertil Steril. 2004;81(4):965–72.
101. Carrell DT, Liu L, Peterson CM, Jones KP, Hatasaka HH, Erickson L, et al. Sperm DNA fragmentation is increased in couples with unexplained recurrent pregnancy loss. Arch Androl. 2003;49(1):49–55.
102. Zhao J, Zhang Q, Wang Y, Li Y. Whether sperm deoxyribonucleic acid fragmentation has an effect on pregnancy and miscarriage after in vitro fertilization/intracytoplasmic sperm injection: a systematic review and meta-analysis. Fertil Steril. 2014;102(4):998–1005. e8
103. Osman A, Alsomait H, Seshadri S, El-Toukhy T, Khalaf Y. The effect of sperm DNA fragmentation on live birth rate after IVF or ICSI: a systematic review and meta-analysis. Reprod BioMed Online. 2015;30(2):120–7.
104. Comhaire FH, Christophe AB, Zalata AA, Dhooge WS, Mahmoud AM, Depuydt CE. The effects of combined conventional treatment, oral antioxidants and essential fatty acids on sperm biology in subfertile men. Prostaglandins Leukot Essent Fatty Acids. 2000;63(3):159–65.
105. Keskes-Ammar L, Feki-Chakroun N, Rebai T, Sahnoun Z, Ghozzi H, Hammami S, et al. Sperm oxidative stress and the effect of an oral vitamin E and selenium supplement on semen quality in infertile men. Arch Androl. 2003;49(2):83–94.
106. Aitken RJ, Clarkson JS, Fishel S. Generation of reactive oxygen species, lipid peroxidation, and human sperm function. Biol Reprod. 1989;41(1):183–97.

107. Moskovtsev SI, Jarvi K, Mullen JB, Cadesky KI, Hannam T, Lo KC. Testicular spermatozoa have statistically significantly lower DNA damage compared with ejaculated spermatozoa in patients with unsuccessful oral antioxidant treatment. Fertil Steril. 2010;93(4):1142–6.
108. Zini A, San Gabriel M, Baazeem A. Antioxidants and sperm DNA damage: a clinical perspective. J Assist Reprod Genet. 2009;26(8):427–32.
109. Greco E, Iacobelli M, Rienzi L, Ubaldi F, Ferrero S, Tesarik J. Reduction of the incidence of sperm DNA fragmentation by oral antioxidant treatment. J Androl. 2005;26(3):349–53.
110. Greco E, Scarselli F, Iacobelli M, Rienzi L, Ubaldi F, Ferrero S, et al. Efficient treatment of infertility due to sperm DNA damage by ICSI with testicular spermatozoa. Hum Reprod. 2005;20(1):226–30.
111. Pabuccu EG, Caglar GS, Tangal S, Haliloglu AH, Pabuccu R. Testicular versus ejaculated spermatozoa in ICSI cycles of normozoospermic men with high sperm DNA fragmentation and previous ART failures. Andrologia. 2016;49(2):609–614.
112. Nicopoullos JD, Gilling-Smith C, Almeida PA, Homa S, Norman-Taylor JQ, Ramsay JW. Sperm DNA fragmentation in subfertile men: the effect on the outcome of intracytoplasmic sperm injection and correlation with sperm variables. BJU Int. 2008;101(12):1553–60.
113. Zhai DM, Li MJ, Jiang L, Qin AP, Li LM, Hang F. Results of requesting a second consecutive sperm ejaculate on the day of oocyte pick-up in assisted reproductive technology. Zhonghua Nan Ke Xue = Natl J Androl. 2011;17(5):418–21.
114. Sharma RK, Agarwal A. Role of reactive oxygen species in male infertility. Urology. 1996;48(6):835–50.
115. Sanchez-Martin P, Sanchez-Martin F, Gonzalez-Martinez M, Gosalvez J. Increased pregnancy after reduced male abstinence. Syst Biol Reprod Med. 2013;59(5):256–60.
116. Younglai EV, Holt D, Brown P, Jurisicova A, Casper RF. Sperm swim-up techniques and DNA fragmentation. Hum Reprod. 2001;16(9):1950–3.
117. Amiri I, Ghorbani M, Heshmati S. Comparison of the DNA fragmentation and the sperm parameters after processing by the density gradient and the swim up methods. J Clin Diagn Res: JCDR. 2012;6(9):1451–3.
118. Ghumman S, Adiga SK, Upadhya D, Kalthur G, Jayaraman V, Rao SB, et al. Combination of swim-up and density gradient separation methods effectively eliminate DNA damaged sperm. J Turk Ger Gynecol Assoc. 2011;12(3):148–52.
119. Said TM, Agarwal A, Zborowski M, Grunewald S, Glander HJ, Paasch U. Utility of magnetic cell separation as a molecular sperm preparation technique. J Androl. 2008;29(2):134–42.
120. Rawe VY, Boudri HU, Alvarez Sedo C, Carro M, Papier S, Nodar F. Healthy baby born after reduction of sperm DNA fragmentation using cell sorting before ICSI. Reprod BioMed Online. 2010;20(3):320–3.
121. Parmegiani L, Cognigni GE, Bernardi S, Troilo E, Ciampaglia W, Filicori M. "Physiologic ICSI": hyaluronic acid (HA) favors selection of spermatozoa without DNA fragmentation and with normal nucleus, resulting in improvement of embryo quality. Fertil Steril. 2010;93(2):598–604.
122. Ainsworth C, Nixon B, Jansen RP, Aitken RJ. First recorded pregnancy and normal birth after ICSI using electrophoretically isolated spermatozoa. Hum Reprod. 2007;22(1):197–200.
123. Huszar G, Ozkavukcu S, Jakab A, Celik-Ozenci C, Sati GL, Cayli S. Hyaluronic acid binding ability of human sperm reflects cellular maturity and fertilizing potential: selection of sperm for intracytoplasmic sperm injection. Curr Opin Obstet Gynecol. 2006;18(3):260–7.
124. Bartoov B, Berkovitz A, Eltes F, Kogosowski A, Menezo Y, Barak Y. Real-time fine morphology of motile human sperm cells is associated with IVF-ICSI outcome. J Androl. 2002;23(1):1–8.
125. Garolla A, Fortini D, Menegazzo M, De Toni L, Nicoletti V, Moretti A, et al. High-power microscopy for selecting spermatozoa for ICSI by physiological status. Reprod BioMed Online. 2008;17(5):610–6.
126. Franco JG Jr, Baruffi RL, Mauri AL, Petersen CG, Oliveira JB, Vagnini L. Significance of large nuclear vacuoles in human spermatozoa: implications for ICSI. Reprod BioMed Online. 2008;17(1):42–5.

127. Petersen CG, Vagnini LD, Mauri AL, Massaro FC, Cavagna M, Baruffi RL, et al. Relationship between DNA damage and sperm head birefringence. Reprod BioMed Online. 2011;22(6):583–9.
128. Hoeijmakers JH. DNA damage, aging, and cancer. N Engl J Med. 2009;361(15):1475–85.
129. Mathews LA, Cabarcas SM. DNA repair pathways and mechanisms. DNA repair of cancer stem cells. Dordrecht: Springer.
130. Iyama T, Wilson DM 3rd. DNA repair mechanisms in dividing and non-dividing cells. DNA Repair. 2013;12(8):620–36.
131. Gillet LC, Scharer OD. Molecular mechanisms of mammalian global genome nucleotide excision repair. Chem Rev. 2006;106(2):253–76.
132. Fagbemi AF, Orelli B, Scharer OD. Regulation of endonuclease activity in human nucleotide excision repair. DNA Repair. 2011;10(7):722–9.
133. Sugasawa K, Ng JM, Masutani C, Iwai S, van der Spek PJ, Eker AP, et al. Xeroderma pigmentosum group C protein complex is the initiator of global genome nucleotide excision repair. Mol Cell. 1998;2(2):223–32.
134. Fousteri M, Mullenders LH. Transcription-coupled nucleotide excision repair in mammalian cells: molecular mechanisms and biological effects. Cell Res. 2008;18(1):73–84.
135. de Laat WL, Jaspers NG, Hoeijmakers JH. Molecular mechanism of nucleotide excision repair. Genes Dev. 1999;13(7):768–85.
136. Hanawalt PC, Spivak G. Transcription-coupled DNA repair: two decades of progress and surprises. Nat Rev Mol Cell Biol. 2008;9(12):958–70.
137. Vermeulen W, de Boer J, Citterio E, van Gool AJ, van der Horst GT, Jaspers NG, et al. Mammalian nucleotide excision repair and syndromes. Biochem Soc Trans. 1997;25(1):309–15.
138. Boiteux S, Radicella JP. Base excision repair of 8-hydroxyguanine protects DNA from endogenous oxidative stress. Biochimie. 1999;81(1–2):59–67.
139. Menezo Y Jr, Russo G, Tosti E, El Mouatassim S, Benkhalifa M. Expression profile of genes coding for DNA repair in human oocytes using pangenomic microarrays, with a special focus on ROS linked decays. J Assist Reprod Genet. 2007;24(11):513–20.
140. Maki H, Sekiguchi M. MutT protein specifically hydrolyses a potent mutagenic substrate for DNA synthesis. Nature. 1992;355(6357):273–5.
141. Aitken RJ, Smith TB, Jobling MS, Baker MA, De Iuliis GN. Oxidative stress and male reproductive health. Asian J Androl. 2014;16(1):31–8.
142. Shimura T, Inoue M, Taga M, Shiraishi K, Uematsu N, Takei N, et al. p53-dependent S-phase damage checkpoint and pronuclear cross talk in mouse zygotes with X-irradiated sperm. Mol Cell Biol. 2002;22(7):2220–8.
143. Lord T, Aitken RJ. Fertilization stimulates 8-hydroxy-2′-deoxyguanosine repair and antioxidant activity to prevent mutagenesis in the embryo. Dev Biol. 2015;406(1):1–13.
144. Champe PC, Harvey RA, Ferrier DR. DNA structure and replication. In: Harvey RA, Champe PC, editors. Biochemistry Lippincott's illustrated reviews. Philadelphia: Lippincott Williams & Wilkins; 2005.
145. Jiricny J. The multifaceted mismatch-repair system. Nat Rev Mol Cell Biol. 2006;7(5):335–46.
146. Gordon FKEA, Lamb DJ. DNA repair genes and genomic instability in severe male factor infertility. In: Carrell DT, editor. The genetics of male infertility. Totowa, New Jersey: Humana Press; 2006. p. 337.
147. Jun SH, Kim TG, Ban C. DNA mismatch repair system. Classical and fresh roles. FEBS J. 2006;273(8):1609–19.
148. Maduro MR, Lo KC, Chuang WW, Lamb DJ. Genes and male infertility: what can go wrong? J Androl. 2003;24(4):485–93.
149. Brierley DJ, Martin SA. Oxidative stress and the DNA mismatch repair pathway. Antioxid Redox Signal. 2013;18(18):2420–8.
150. Barnetson RA, Tenesa A, Farrington SM, Nicholl ID, Cetnarskyj R, Porteous ME, et al. Identification and survival of carriers of mutations in DNA mismatch-repair genes in colon cancer. N Engl J Med. 2006;354(26):2751–63.

151. Peltomaki P, Vasen H. Mutations associated with HNPCC predisposition – update of ICG-HNPCC/INSiGHT mutation database. Dis Markers. 2004;20(4–5):269–76.
152. Lieber MR. The mechanism of double-strand DNA break repair by the nonhomologous DNA end-joining pathway. Annu Rev Biochem. 2010;79:181–211.
153. Stracker TH, Petrini JH. The MRE11 complex: starting from the ends. Nat Rev Mol Cell Biol. 2011;12(2):90–103.
154. You Z, Bailis JM. DNA damage and decisions: CtIP coordinates DNA repair and cell cycle checkpoints. Trends Cell Biol. 2010;20(7):402–9.
155. Forget AL, Kowalczykowski SC. Single-molecule imaging brings Rad51 nucleoprotein filaments into focus. Trends Cell Biol. 2010;20(5):269–76.
156. Yoshida K, Miki Y. Role of BRCA1 and BRCA2 as regulators of DNA repair, transcription, and cell cycle in response to DNA damage. Cancer Sci. 2004;95(11):866–71.
157. Xu Y, Baltimore D. Dual roles of ATM in the cellular response to radiation and in cell growth control. Genes Dev. 1996;10(19):2401–10.
158. Getts RC, Stamato TD. Absence of a Ku-like DNA end binding activity in the xrs double-strand DNA repair-deficient mutant. J Biol Chem. 1994;269(23):15981–4.
159. Kohl KP, Sekelsky J. Meiotic and mitotic recombination in meiosis. Genetics. 2013;194(2):327–34.
160. Mukherjee S, Ridgeway AD, Lamb DJ. DNA mismatch repair and infertility. Curr Opin Urol. 2010;20(6):525–32.
161. Lipkin SM, Moens PB, Wang V, Lenzi M, Shanmugarajah D, Gilgeous A, et al. Meiotic arrest and aneuploidy in MLH3-deficient mice. Nat Genet. 2002;31(4):385–90.
162. de Vries SS, Baart EB, Dekker M, Siezen A, de Rooij DG, de Boer P, et al. Mouse MutS-like protein Msh5 is required for proper chromosome synapsis in male and female meiosis. Genes Dev. 1999;13(5):523–31.
163. Lipkin SM, Wang V, Jacoby R, Banerjee-Basu S, Baxevanis AD, Lynch HT, et al. MLH3: a DNA mismatch repair gene associated with mammalian microsatellite instability. Nat Genet. 2000;24(1):27–35.

Part IV
Clinical Studies on Utility of Sperm DNA Damage Tests

Chapter 19
Experimental Studies on Sperm DNA Fragmentation and Reproductive Outcomes

Serafín Perez-Cerezales, Priscila Ramos-Ibeas, Eva Pericuesta Camacho, Raul Fernández-González, Angela Patricia López-Cardona, Ricardo Laguna-Barraza, Noelia Fonseca Balvís, Alejandro Chacón de Castro, Benjamin Planells, and Alfonso Gutiérrez-Adan

19.1 Sperm Selection in the Female Genital Tract and DNA Fragmentation

Mammalian spermatozoa must overcome a number of obstacles along the female genital tract before reaching the fertilization site at the ampulla. The vaginal pH, the resistance by cervical mucus to sperm migration, the narrowness of the uterotubal junction, the tortuosity of the oviductal lumen, the response of the immune system, etc. are physio-anatomical conditions of the female genital tract that configure a stringent selection mechanism for those spermatozoa with certain features [1, 2]. In all mammalian species studied to date, among many millions of spermatozoa ejaculated only tens to hundreds reach the ampulla [3–6], where the fertilization occurs. Presumably, this is a select group of spermatozoa with higher fertilization capability and better characteristics for supporting embryo development. However, little is known about this sperm subpopulation and its relative effectiveness as well as about which are the characteristics that are selected in vivo (for a review see Sakkas et al.

S. Perez-Cerezales • P. Ramos-Ibeas • E.P. Camacho • R. Fernández-González
A.P. López-Cardona • B. Planells • A. Gutiérrez-Adan (✉)
Department of Animal Reproduction, Instituto Nacional de Investigación y Tecnología Agraria y Alimentaria (INIA), Madrid, Spain
e-mail: raulfg@inia.es

R. Laguna-Barraza
Veterinarian Science, Department of Animal Reproduction, Instituto Nacional de Investigación y Tecnología Agraria y Alimentaria (INIA), Madrid, Spain

N.F. Balvís
Veterinarian Science, Department of Animal Reproduction, Spanish National Institute for Agricultural and Food Research and Technology (INIA), Madrid, Spain

A.C. de Castro
Reproduction Department, Instituto Nacional de Investigación y Tecnología Agraria y Alimentaria (INIA), Madrid, Spain

A. Zini, A. Agarwal (eds.), *A Clinician's Guide to Sperm DNA and Chromatin Damage*, https://doi.org/10.1007/978-3-319-71815-6_19

[2]). In fact, if there is a mechanism for sperm selection that has evolved in mammalians through Darwinian forces, the genetic material ported in this sperm subpopulation should be of high integrity for ensuring a successful embryo development and a correct transmission of the genetic information. Unfortunately, only few studies have addressed directly or indirectly this hypothesis.

In the vagina, the first selective barrier encountered by spermatozoa is the viscosity of the cervical mucus. This secretion has been pointed to positively select motile spermatozoa exhibiting specific kinetics and normal motility to pass across the cervix to the uterus. Whereas the selective function of the cervical mucus has never been satisfactorily proven in vivo, the ability of spermatozoa to migrate within it has been correlated to sperm quality and selection [7], especially regarding sperm kinetics [8]. In a study conducted in mouse, Hourcade et al. [9] illustrated that the spermatozoa in the uterus show a higher level of fragmented DNA compared to spermatozoa retrieved from the epididymis, going against the selective function of the cervical mucus. It has been suggested that the fragmentation of the DNA might be provoked by the immune responses occurring in the cervix and uterus in response to the sperm migration [10] or because of the presence of nucleases in the seminal fluid affecting the spermatozoa in the uterus [11, 12]. Hourcade et al. [9] also demonstrated that there is a strong positive selection in the uterotubal junction for spermatozoa carrying low fragmented DNA. Thus, from all the highly DNA-damaged spermatozoa found in the uterus, this selective checkpoint allows only the sperm subpopulation containing DNA of high integrity to enter the oviduct. The selective function of the uterotubal junction in mouse has been also pointed by Nakanishi et al. [13], showing that from chimeric mice porting a sperm subpopulation lacking functional testis-specific putative chaperone, only the spermatozoa with the wild-type phenotype entered the oviduct. Furthermore, it has been postulated that the involvement of the sperm reservoir, present at this location, is important in aiding in the selection of spermatozoa able to interact with the epithelium [14].

Once in the oviduct, it is currently accepted that the spermatozoa must be actively guided in order to reach the fertilization site. To date, two sperm tropism mechanisms (sperm thermotaxis and rheotaxis), operating both as long-range guidance mechanisms within the oviduct, and a third one (chemotaxis) for guiding the spermatozoa in the proximity of the oocyte at the fertilization site have been proposed [15]. Thermotaxis has been described for human, mouse [16], and rabbit spermatozoa [17], whereas rheotaxis has been found in human and mouse spermatozoa [18] and chemotaxis in a large variety of species mammals [19]. The tropism shown as a response of the spermatozoa to the stimuli in vitro together with the existence of well-defined molecular mechanisms in the spermatozoa for each of them [16, 18, 20] points to their functioning in vivo. This hypothesis is reinforced by the use of mouse strains to which the receptors for thermotaxis was knocked out affecting the sperm migration in a temperature gradient. In addition the stimuli for each of the tropism (temperature gradient, oviductal fluid flow, and chemoattractants) have been found to exist in the oviduct [15]. Thus, the ability of the spermatozoa to direct their swimming direction in response to these guidance stimuli could provide a sort of selective mechanisms that could be also linked to the genomic integrity of the spermatozoa. This is a very interesting hypothesis that however no one has ever approached.

When spermatozoa encounter the oocyte, they have to penetrate the zona pellucida (ZP). Thus, the ZP could function as a last selective barrier. Accordingly, two investigations on in vitro fertilization (IVF) have reported that mouse and human spermatozoa attached to the ZP exhibit lower level of DNA fragmentation compared to the nonattached spermatozoa [9, 21]. Furthermore, when the ZP-attached spermatozoa were used for ICSI, they failed to generate viable blastocysts [9]. Together these results indicate a fine-tuned selection process occurring during ZP penetration of spermatozoa able to support embryo development. This ZP-mediated selection seems to be linked to the source and type of sperm damage because experiments performed by Hourcade et al. [9] in mouse show that when the sperm DNA fragmentation was generated by ɣ[gamma]-radiation during spermatogenesis, there were a decrease in the production of blastocysts by IVF and a reduction in the percentage of implantations in vivo. Conversely, following the same experiment but generating the DNA fragmentation by heat shock, the blastocyst production by IVF and the percentage of implantation in vivo were similar to the control using undamaged spermatozoa [9]. This discrimination of the sperm damage is possibly related to the effect of the heat shock on different structures of the spermatozoa that then are negatively selected by the female genital tract. On the other hand, the ɣ[gamma]-radiation affects mainly the DNA leaving the rest of the sperm structures undamaged.

Since the female reproductive tract cannot get direct access to the sperm nucleus for assessing directly the DNA quality of the spermatozoa, the selection has to be based in other sperm features linked to the integrity of the genetic material. Consistently, also Hourcade et al. [9] showed that the subpopulation of mouse spermatozoa with the highest velocities separated in vitro contained lower level of fragmented DNA than the whole sperm population. Other studies have shown a negative correlation between various sperm quality parameters and DNA fragmentation levels in humans [22, 23] and in other animals such as turkey [24] and ram [25]. Kasimanickam et al. [26], employing heterospermic doses of bulls for the insemination of receptive cows, showed that the female genital tract selected the spermatozoa from those bulls reporting lower DNA fragmentation and higher plasma membrane integrity. As suggested by Holt and Fazeli [27], these results point to a connection between the status of the DNA integrity and externally exposed characteristics of the spermatozoa, for example, some plasma membrane components that could be "read" at the surface of the spermatozoa as a "passport" by the female genital tract. These authors gone even further in their hypothesis of the "cryptic female choice" suggesting a connection between the spermatozoa features and the genotype contained in its nucleus over which the female genital tract could select the spermatozoa containing specific sets of genes.

Sperm selection is a challenging field of research that still needs to address basic questions for a deeper understanding of the fundamental mechanism involved in the selection of the spermatozoa within the female genital tract. Animal experiments will certainly contribute to the discovery of the sperm characteristics that are selected, their linkage to the DNA integrity and to the reproductive outcome. This basic knowledge would be of great interest for designing procedures for the in vitro selection of spermatozoa that eventually could improve the outcomes of the currently poorly efficient assisted reproductive technologies (ARTs).

19.2 Long-Term Effects of Mouse Intracytoplasmic Sperm Injection with DNA-Fragmented Sperm on Health and Behavior of Adult Offspring

Nowadays 1% of babies born in the first world are conceived using assisted reproductive techniques (ART). Except for artificial insemination, ARTs bypass the sperm selection occurring within the female genital tract. This is especially relevant in case of the intracytoplasmic sperm injection (ICSI) and could explain the low efficiency of ART in general [28]. Nearly half of the male patients diagnosed as infertile show high levels of sperm DNA damage [29], and most patients subjected to fertility treatments show alterations in the sperm chromatin [30–33]. Moreover, low sperm counts have been related to higher presence of chromosomal aberrations in the spermatozoa. Azoospermic males show a higher frequency of numerical sex chromosome alterations such as XXY or XYY [34] and oligozoospermic have a higher frequency of translocations at autosomal chromosomes [35]. It has also been reported that mutations causing infertility could be transmitted to the male descendants, such as Y-chromosome deletions [36, 37]. Therefore, when applying ICSI, the probability of choosing a sperm with damaged chromatin, fragmented DNA, or any kind of genetic alteration should not be neglected. This is especially important considering that using ICSI, the DNA-fragmented spermatozoa (DFS) are able to fertilize oocyte resulting in pronucleus formation, chromatin decondensation, and embryos developing to blastocyst stage as was shown in mouse [38]. But human oocyte can partially repair low DNA fragmentation levels before cleavage leading to a viable embryo to blastocyst, the fertilization with spermatozoa containing highly fragmented DNA reduces pregnancy rates [39]. Furthermore, abnormal fetal karyotypes have been found in the offspring of spermatozoa containing aberrant DNA and processed by ICSI, resulting from numerical or structural sex chromosomal anomalies and autosomal anomalies both inherited and de novo [40]. It is known that all these aberrations in the DNA produce alterations on fertility and failures, affecting pregnancy rates and the health of the adult descendants. Since the first humans born from ICSI procedures are nearly 25 years old, the long-term effects in adulthood remain unknown. That is why it is important to study the possible consequences on the health of ICSI offspring with DNA-fragmented sperm through animal models.

Using epididymal mouse spermatozoa, Yamauchi et al. [41] demonstrated that sperm DNA damage induced by various treatments persists after ICSI without changes. Epididymal mouse spermatozoa were either frozen without cryoprotectant or treated with Triton X-100 together with dithiothreitol to induce DNA damage. Both treatment groups showed increased sperm DNA fragmentation when compared to untreated group used as control. After ICSI, chromosome analysis demonstrated paternal DNA damage in those oocytes injected with both sperm-treated groups, frozen-thawed, or Triton X-100 but not with fresh sperm. However, there were no differences in the incidence of abnormal paternal karyoplates prior and after DNA synthesis in all the examined groups. Fernández-Gonzalez et al. [38]

analyzed the short- and long-term effects of ICSI using DFS in a mouse model. In their work, DNA fragmentation was produced by freezing and thawing epididymal spermatozoa retrieved from B6D2F1 males. In addition to the DNA damage, telomere loss was also observed. Oocytes were then injected with fresh- or frozen-thawed spermatozoa, and the resultant two-cell embryos were transferred to pseudopregnant CD1 females. The first notorious effect noticed was a delay of 2 h on the active demethylation of male pronucleus in those embryos produced by ICSI with DFS. Furthermore, when ICSI-DFS was performed, both the rate of preimplantation embryo development and litter size were reduced, and the transcription and methylation of epigenetically regulated genes were altered. In addition, adult animals produced by ICSI showed behavioral alterations as well as abnormal weight gain and anatomopathological alterations including solid tumors in the lungs and dermis and premature aging symptoms. Moreover, surviving rates of mice generated with ICSI-DFS were reduced dramatically compared with in vivo controls. This work concluded that depending on the level of DFS, oocytes may either repair fragmented DNA, producing blastocysts able to implant and produce live offspring, or partially repair DNA damage leading to short- and long-term alterations or completely fail on repairing DNA aberrations producing the death of the embryo.

19.3 Effects of Intracytoplasmic Sperm Injection Using DNA-Fragmented Spermatozoa on Embryo-Derived Embryonic Stem Cells and on Transgenerational Heritability of Epiallele in Mice

Embryonic stem cells (ESCs) are commonly used as a valuable model to analyze embryonic development. Thus, Moreira et al. [42] reported that mouse embryos produced by DFS-ICSI show a reduced efficiency for ESC derivation that was suggested to be related to the low quality of the DFI-ICSI-derived embryos. Consistently, these embryos show low implantation and development rates. In another study, Yamagata et al. [43] reported that 40% of DFI-ICSI-generated mouse embryos show abnormal chromosome segregation and chromosome fragmentation. Although these embryos developed to normal-looking blastocysts, almost all of them were lost shortly after implantation, and embryos with abnormal karyotype are less capable of generating ESC lines. Furthermore, alterations of the gene expression in the ESCs lines generated with DFS-ICSI embryos were found at early passages: abnormalities at the cellular level were associated with embryo performance and offspring health. The genetic alterations described in the ESC lines include alterations in DNA methylation and histone acetylation, on pluripotency, on epigenetic gene silencing, as well as on DNA damage and genes related to its reparation. However, these alterations were not maintained in the long-term culture [44]. Interestingly, males of the offspring produced by DFS-ICSI showed alterations in the testes, including low weight, reduced spermatogenesis, morphological abnormalities in the seminiferous tubules, and an increased number of apoptotic cells [44]. Sperm quantity, vaginal plug detection, and pregnancy rates after mating were also significantly lower in these animals, while the number of females showing resorptions was higher. Moreover, a significant decrease in pregnancy rates and an increase in the resorptions rate related to the age were reported. These results suggest a deleterious effect of the DNA damage when DFS-ICSI is used in the resultant embryos that affects the male germ line and could transmit genetic alterations toward following generations. Consistently, it has been reported that DFS-ICSI induces epigenetic modifications that are transmitted to the progeny. Axin1Fu allele is a locus very sensitive to epigenetic alterations which regulates embryonic axis formation in vertebrates. In mice the Axin1Fu phenotype consists of kinks in the tail, which are determined by the DNA methylation pattern. Modifications in this allele may persist across several generations because its methylation state in mature spermatozoa is identical to somatic cells, indicating that it is not epigenetically reprogrammed during gametogenesis [45]. Using spermatozoa retrieved from Axin1Fu/+ mice in ICSI revealed a higher proportion of pups in the second generation expressing the active kinky-tail epiallele, indicating that this procedure affected the postnatal expression of Axin1Fu and that this modification was inherited across generations [44].

The experiments in animal models conducted to date reveal that the analyses of sperm DNA damage are critical when ARTs are applied. This is especially relevant for ICSI because all the barriers of sperm selection operating along the female genital tract are being bypassed. In an era in which advanced forms of ART are frequently used in clinical treatments of fertility, it is essential to apply protocols and methodologies for preselecting the sperm samples or for the separation of spermatozoa carrying the genetic material integral in order to avoid deleterious effects in the offspring.

19.4 Cryopreservation and Damage of the Sperm DNA

Cryopreservation of gametes has been widely used over the last century in human assisted reproduction, animal breeding, and conservation programs for endangered species. Although several protocols have been developed for both male and female gametes, sperm cryopreservation is the most extensively used technique. The limited volume of spermatozoa cytoplasm, together with their small size, makes sperm particularly suitable for cryopreservation. Moreover, some protocols, coupled to recently developed ARTs, permit long-term storage of freeze-dried sperm, even at room temperature, capable of producing live offspring [46]. However, cryopreservation is not completely effective in stopping sperm degradation because its quality declines with storage time [47]. The effects of DNA fragmentation after sperm cryopreservation are also a controversial issue as it adversely affects early embryonic development and results in reduced implantation rates and pregnancy outcomes [48]. Fluctuation of media pH [49], osmotic stress [50, 51] or the cryoprotectant used [52, 53] may increase the amount of reactive oxygen species (ROS) inside the cell or activate endonucleases that ultimately lead to breaks in the sperm DNA. Interestingly, cryopreservation seems to cause more DNA fragmentation to subfertile or infertile males [54], so perhaps inherent defects in the spermatozoa could enhance cryodamage. This also points to the need for evaluating the DNA integrity of the cryopreserved spermatozoa of this type of patients when subjected to fertility treatments involving ARTs and for the improvement of the sperm cryopreservation procedures.

Conventional cryopreservation (also known as slow-freezing) results in slowly lowering cell temperature until enzymatic reactions cannot take place within the cytoplasm. As intracellular milieu is an aqueous environment, ice crystals are formed inside the cells during freezing process, and this causes deleterious effects on sperm, like membrane damage, leading to decreased motility and viability. To avoid ice crystal formation, cryoprotectants are added to sperm prior to freezing in order to diminish water content of the cells. Cryoprotectants are usually small molecules with a high solubility in water at low temperatures. The presence of these small molecules in the freezing solution generates an osmotic pressure that forces intracellular water to leave the cell and, as a consequence, solutes concentrate in the cytoplasm. At the same time, cryoprotectants slowly diffuse through the plasma membrane and substitute intracellular water, impeding ice crystal formation diminishing osmotic shock after thawing due to high salt concentration in the cytoplasm. However, slow-freezing physically damages sperm to some extent in a variety of ways: decreased motility, alterations of the plasma membrane and mitochondrial activity, or degradation of acrosomes [55].

Besides the physical damages that ice crystals can cause on membranes, cryopreservation can also compromise sperm DNA integrity. Spermatozoa are highly specialized haploid cells in which DNA is tightly packaged in order to reduce cell size and to protect DNA from fragmentation. In many species, most of the nuclear histones are exchanged for protamines during spermiogenesis [56]. DNA forms loops that attach to the membrane and progressively compact around protamines forming toroids (donut-loop model, reviewed in Ward and Ward [57]). Although disulfide bridges between protamines reinforce the stability of the DNA [58], it can be attacked by endonucleases at toroid linker regions [59]. One interesting finding is that some endonucleases are actually packaged inside sperm heads [60]. After cryopreservation, these enzymes can be released from damaged spermatozoa and activated by cations present in the media [61]. Using mouse spermatozoa, Szczygiel and Ward [62] demonstrated that adding chelating factors to the media improves chromosome stability after freezing-thawing processes, even when sperm is intentionally damaged with detergents and DTT. However, some fragmentation persists, suggesting that other mechanisms also cause sperm DNA degradation. For example, an investigation performed with koala spermatozoa demonstrated that extreme osmotic changes during cryopreservation can also disturb the tertiary structure of the DNA so the chromatin relaxes and becomes more prone to DNA degradation [63].

Oxidative stress has also been shown to produce DNA fragmentation during cryopreservation. It is caused by an imbalance between the production of ROS and the ability of the sample to detoxify or to repair the damages in DNA [64]. ROS are very reactive free radicals and oxidizing subproducts of metabolism capable of reacting with the DNA and producing breaks in the double chain. Damaged spermatozoa produce a greater amount of ROS compared to normal ones [65], but both sperm and seminal plasma contain antioxidant systems that prevent genetic and cellular damage [66]. Unfortunately, cryopreservation can lead to an imbalance in the ratio between ROS and antioxidants promoting DNA fragmentation [67] and ejaculated sperm lack DNA repair mechanisms, so they are highly vulnerable to oxidative stress. Studies conducted in bulls and stallions have shown that ROS production increases immediately after thawing slow-frozen sperm samples [55, 68] inducing DNA fragmentation [69]. Oxidative stress also triggers apoptosis of damaged spermatozoa (reviewed in Said et al. [70]). Therefore, identification of apoptotic markers in individual spermatozoa could be used to determine the overall quality of sperm or even to preselect only spermatozoa suitable for ARTs.

In the last decades, some new cryopreservation techniques, like vitrification or freeze-drying (FD), have been developed in order to overcome the potential deleterious effects of cryopreservation. Vitrification consists of ultra-quick freezing using liquid nitrogen resuspended in an aqueous solution with high concentrations of cryoprotectants [71]. Cooling is so quick that cryoprotectants effectively prevent ice crystal nucleation, and the solution becomes viscous and solidifies into a glassy state without forming ice. Despite this apparent advantage, vitrification seems to damage human sperm as much as the conventional slow-freezing protocol [72, 73]. In mouflon spermatozoa, for example, vitrification has been reported to generate damage at a greater extent than freezing-thawing [74]. As an alternative to cryoprotectants, it has been suggested that some components present in the seminal fluid could exert cryoprotective characteristics in boar [75], bull [76], and dog [77] and act like an important factor for pregnancy success (reviewed in Schjenken and Robertson [78]). Actually, artificial solutions have been developed based on seminal fluid composition, and they are already achieving good results in terms of sperm motility in human [79]. On the other hand, FD or lyophilization is a method in which frozen material is dried by sublimation of ice [46]. Due to lack of water molecules, enzymatic reactions cannot take place even though sperm is stored at 4° or transported at room temperature. This feature makes FD really attractive for long-term storage of sperm, as liquid nitrogen is not needed. Freeze-dried sperm can then be rehydrated by adding pure water to the original volume of the sample, and then it can be diluted with a suitable physiological saline buffer. The main drawback of FD is that membranes are destroyed during the process, so sperm is dead after rehydration. However, sperm heads retain their fertilizing capacity if they are used for ICSI procedure, and sperm DNA integrity seem to be less compromised compared to conventional freezing as was demonstrated in mouse [46] and later in humans [80].

Cryopreservative techniques have improved greatly in the last decades in terms of designing procedures that are easy to perform and increasing the time that the samples can be stored. However, DNA fragmentation caused by cryopreservation and inherent to the quality of the sperm sample can result in poor-quality spermatozoa and ultimately in a low pregnancy success. Animal experimentation can contribute to the basic knowledge about the cryobiology of spermatozoa and help improve this important methodology for reproductive medicine.

19.5 Sperm DNA Damage and Repair in Fish: A Useful Model

From the shape of the cell to the highly compacted status of its chromatin, the architecture of the sperm cell has been designed through natural selection for an effective transportation and protection of the paternal genetic information. However, once delivered spermatozoa encounter a hostile environment through which they migrate. Thus, spermatozoa are exposed to different agents that could provoke damage to their DNA with effects the reproductive outcomes. As mentioned earlier, it has been demonstrated in mouse that despite the strong sperm selection occurring within the female genital tract, spermatozoa porting damaged DNA are able to fertilize, potentially affecting the embryo production [9]. In addition, the use of artificial reproductive techniques overcomes this selective process suggesting that the study of the paternal contribution to the embryo development deserves more attention.

Studying the paternal effects on mammalian embryo development in detail has the significant restriction of an internal location of the embryo, rendering difficult the monitoring of in vivo development. Thus, for the following reasons, external fertilizers are excellent models for studying embryo development. First, the external location of the embryo allows real-time monitoring of the development. Second, embryos are more resistant to manipulation facilitating the in vivo study of developmental processes. Third, a high number of embryos can be obtained from each mating minimizing the variability related to the individual. Fourth, for studying the paternal effect on embryo development, the weaker sperm selection in contrast to mammals allows for easy fertilization with damaged or altered spermatozoa [81, 82].

Pérez-Cerezales et al. [82] were the first to show unequivocally the ability of trout spermatozoa porting damaged DNA to fertilize the egg. In this work, the authors reported a direct relationship between the level of fragmented DNA and the percentage of abortions during development. Furthermore, they demonstrated for first time in a fish specie the ability of the egg to repair the sperm DNA by the base scission repair (BER) pathway. Due to the limited capacity of the spermatozoa to repair DNA [83, 84], the repairmen of the paternal DNA relies on the oocyte after fertilization occurring in the zygote and in the first developmental stages [85]. Consequently, like in mammals, the fish oocyte contains the elements of the BER pathway for repairing simple-strand breaks of the DNA [86] as well as the homologous end-joining (HR) and nonhomologous end-joining (NHEJ) pathways for repairing double-stand breaks [85, 87]. However, these systems are limited in that they can only repair a certain level of damaged DNA. In trout, the zygote can repair around 10% of the damaged DNA by the BER [82], a similar percentage to that reported in mice by Ahmadi and Ng [88]. In addition, these repair systems can introduce errors in the DNA sequence and provoke mutations with consequences of different magnitude potentially affecting offspring performance [38].

In an earlier work, Pérez-Cerezales et al. [89] similarly demonstrated in trout that fertilization with damaged DNA spermatozoa provokes genetic alterations in offspring survival after hatching. These authors found overexpression of genes related to growth and development in the larvae obtained using spermatozoa with cryodamaged DNA. Moreover, whereas cryodamage provoked a reduction in the telomere length of the spermatozoa, the resultant embryos showed higher telomere length. To explain these surprising findings, the authors also found an overexpression of the telomerase reverse transcriptase (TERT), a subunit of the telomerase which function is to increase the telomere length in the larvae [90]. In accordance with these results, Fernández-Díez et al. [91], using microarrays from BER repaired trout embryos, reported that 810 genes were differentially expressed after hatching. Their results point to long-term effects of fertilizing with DNA-damaged spermatozoa due to an impaired DNA damage signalization and repair in the oocyte possibly introducing punctual mutations. These results are in agreement with the ones reported by Fernández-González et al. [38], showing the negative effects of DNA-fragmented spermatozoa used for ICSI in the pre-implantational development, implantation rates and embryo development to term as well as provoking abnormal behavior, diverse anatomopathologies, and higher incidence of cancer in the adulthood in a mouse model.

19.6 Conclusions

Altogether, studies in fish, mouse, and other animals have demonstrated the importance and implications of sperm DNA damage in reproductive outcomes and offspring performance. Understanding the origin of the sperm DNA damage, the mechanisms and dynamics for its reparation, the effects on embryo development, as well as the long-term effects on the offspring are questions that are being explored and need to get more attention by the scientific community, especially in the context of ARTs in the clinical treatment of human fertility.

References

1. Suarez SS, Pacey AA. Sperm transport in the female reproductive tract. Hum Reprod Update. 2006;12:23–37.
2. Sakkas D, Ramalingam M, Garrido N, Barratt CL. Sperm selection in natural conception: what can we learn from mother nature to improve assisted reproduction outcomes? Hum Reprod Update. 2015;21:711–26.
3. Timothy T, Koyanagi F, Yanagimachi R. Distribution and number of spermatozoa in the oviduct of the golden after natural mating and artificial insemination & hamster. Biol Reprod. 1987;37:225–34.
4. Williams M, Hill CJ, Scudamore I, Dunphy B, Cooke ID, Barratt CL. Sperm numbers and distribution within the human fallopian tube around ovulation. Hum Reprod. 1993;8:2019–26.
5. Hino T, Muro Y, Tamura-Nakano M, Okabe M, Tateno H, Yanagimachi R. The behavior and acrosomal status of mouse spermatozoa in vitro, and within the oviduct during fertilization after natural mating. Biol Reprod. 2016;95:50.

6. Muro Y, Hasuwa H, Isotani A, Miyata H, Yamagata K, Ikawa M, Yanagimachi R, Okabe M. Behavior of mouse spermatozoa in the female reproductive tract from soon after mating to the beginning of fertilization. Biol Reprod. 2016;94:80.
7. Ola B, Afnan M, Papaioannou S, Sharif K, Björndahl L, Coomarasamy A. Accuracy of sperm–cervical mucus penetration tests in evaluating sperm motility in semen: a systematic quantitative review. Hum Reprod. 2003;18:1037–46.
8. Aitken RJ, Bowie H, Buckingham D, Harkiss D, Richardson DW, West KM. Sperm penetration into a hyaluronic acid polymer as a means of monitoring functional competence. J Androl. 1992;13:44–54.
9. Hourcade JD, Pérez-Crespo M, Fernández-González R, Pintado B, Gutiérrez-Adán A. Selection against spermatozoa with fragmented DNA after postovulatory mating depends on the type of damage. Reprod Biol Endocrinol. 2010;8:9.
10. Schuberth HJ, Taylor U, Zerbe H, Waberski D, Hunter R, Rath D. Immunological responses to semen in the female genital tract. Theriogenology. 2008;70:1174–81.
11. Sakkas D, Moffatt O, Manicardi GC, Mariethoz E, Tarozzi N, Bizzaro D. Nature of DNA damage in ejaculated human spermatozoa and the possible involvement of apoptosis. Biol Reprod. 2002;66:1061–7.
12. Sullivan R, Saez F. Epididymosomes, prostasomes, and liposomes: their roles in mammalian male reproductive physiology. Reproduction. 2013;146:R21.
13. Nakanishi T, Isotani A, Yamaguchi R, Ikawa M, Baba T, Suarez SS, Okabe M. Selective passage through the uterotubal junction of sperm from a mixed population produced by chimeras of calmegin-knockout and wild-type male mice. Biol Reprod. 2004;71:959–65.
14. Talevi R, Gualtieri R. Molecules involved in sperm-oviduct adhesion and release. Theriogenology. 2010;73:796–801.
15. Perez-Cerezales S, Boryshpolets S, Eisenbach M. Behavioral mechanisms of mammalian sperm guidance. Asian J Androl. 2015;17:628–32.
16. Pérez-Cerezales S, Boryshpolets S, Afanzar O, Brandis A, Nevo R, Kiss V, Eisenbach M. Involvement of opsins in mammalian sperm thermotaxis. Sci Rep. 2015;5:16146.
17. Bahat A, Tur-Kaspa I, Gakamsky A, Giojalas LC, Breitbart H, Eisenbach M. Thermotaxis of mammalian sperm cells: a potential navigation mechanism in the female genital tract. Nat Med. 2003;9:149–50.
18. Miki K, Clapham DE. Rheotaxis guides mammalian sperm. Curr Biol. 2013;23:443–52.
19. Sugiyama H, Chandler DE. Sperm guidance to the egg finds calcium at the helm. Protoplasma. 2014;251:461–75.
20. Alvarez L, Friedrich BM, Gompper G, Kaupp UB. The computational sperm cell. Trends Cell Biol. 2014;24:198–207.
21. Liu DY, Baker HWG. Human sperm bound to the zona pellucida have normal nuclear chromatin as assessed by acridine orange fluorescence. Hum Reprod. 2007;22:1597–602.
22. Ramos L, Wetzels AM. Low rates of DNA fragmentation in selected motile human spermatozoa assessed by the TUNEL assay. Hum Reprod. 2001;16:1703–7.
23. Huang CC, Lin DP, Tsao HM, Cheng T-C, Liu CH, Lee MS. Sperm DNA fragmentation negatively correlates with velocity and fertilization rates but might not affect pregnancy rates. Fertil Steril. 2005;84:130–40.
24. Kotłowska M, Dietrich G, Wojtczak M, Karol H, Ciereszko A. Effects of liquid storage on amidase activity, DNA fragmentation and motility of turkey spermatozoa. Theriogenology. 2000;67:276–86.
25. Kasimanickam R, Pelzer KD, Kasimanickam V, Swecker WS, Thatcher CD. Association of classical semen parameters, sperm DNA fragmentation index, lipid peroxidation and antioxidant enzymatic activity of semen in ram-lambs. Theriogenology. 1980;65:1407–21.
26. Kasimanickam R, Nebel RL, Peeler ID, Silvia WL, Wolf KT, McAllister AJ, Cassell BG. Breed differences in competitive indices of Holstein and Jersey bulls and their association with sperm DNA fragmentation index and plasma membrane integrity. Theriogenology. 1997;66:1307–15.
27. Holt WV, Fazeli A. Do sperm possess a molecular passport? Mechanistic insights into sperm selection in the female reproductive tract. Mol Hum Reprod. 2015;21:491–501.

28. Yanagimachi R. Intracytoplasmic injection of spermatozoa and spermatogenic cells: its biology and applications in humans and animals. Reprod Biomed Online. 2005;10:247–88.
29. Lopes S, Sun JG, Jurisicova A, Meriano J, Casper RF. Sperm deoxyribonucleic acid fragmentation is increased in poor-quality semen samples and correlates with failed fertilization in intracytoplasmic sperm injection. Fertil Steril. 1998;69:528–32.
30. Saleh RA, Agarwal A, Sharma RK, Said TM, Sikka SC, Thomas AJ. Evaluation of nuclear DNA damage in spermatozoa from infertile men with varicocele. Fertil Steril. 2003;80:1431–6.
31. Enciso M, Muriel L, Fernández JL, Goyanes V, Segrelles E, Marcos M, Montejo JM, Ardoy M, Pacheco A, Gosálvez J. Infertile men with varicocele show a high relative proportion of sperm cells with intense nuclear damage level, evidenced by the sperm chromatin dispersion test. J Androl. 2006;27:106–11.
32. Zini A, Libman J. Sperm DNA damage: importance in the era of assisted reproduction. Curr Opin Urol. 2006;16:428–34.
33. Ozmen B, Caglar GS, Koster F, Schopper B, Diedrich K, Al-Hasani S. Relationship between sperm DNA damage, induced acrosome reaction and viability in ICSI patients. Reprod Biomed Online. 2007;15:208–14.
34. Yoshida A, Nakahori Y, Kuroki Y, Miura K, Shirai M. An azoospermic male with an unbalanced autosomal-Y translocation. Jpn J Hum Genet. 1997;42:451–5.
35. Van Assche E, Bonduelle M, Tournaye H, Joris H, Verheyen G, Devroey P, Van Steirteghem A, Liebaers I. Cytogenetics of infertile men. Hum Reprod. 1996;11(Suppl 4):1–24. 6
36. Kent-First MG, Kol S, Muallem A, Blazer S, Itskovitz-Eldor J. Infertility in intracytoplasmic-sperm-injection-derived sons. Lancet. 1996;348:332.
37. Silber SJ, Repping S. Transmission of male infertility to future generations: lessons from the Y chromosome. Hum Reprod Update. 2002;8:217–29.
38. Fernández-Gonzalez R, Moreira PN, Pérez-Crespo M, Sánchez-Martín M, Ramirez MA, Pericuesta E, Bilbao A, Bermejo-Alvarez P, de Dios HJ, de Fonseca FR, Gutiérrez-Adán A. Long-term effects of mouse intracytoplasmic sperm injection with DNA-fragmented sperm on health and behavior of adult offspring. Biol Reprod. 2008;78:761–72.
39. Benchaib M, Braun V, Lornage J, Hadj S, Salle B, Lejeune H, Guérin JF. Sperm DNA fragmentation decreases the pregnancy rate in an assisted reproductive technique. Hum Reprod. 2003;18:1023–8.
40. Devroey P, Van Steirteghem A. A review of ten years experience of ICSI. Hum Reprod Update. 2004;10:19–28.
41. Yamauchi Y, Riel JM, Ward MA. Paternal DNA damage resulting from various sperm treatments persists after fertilization and is similar before and after DNA replication. J Androl. 2012;33:229–38.
42. Moreira PN, Pérez-Crespo M, Ramírez MA, Pozueta J, Montoliu L, Gutiérrez-Adán A. Effect of transgene concentration, flanking matrix attachment regions, and RecA-coating on the efficiency of mouse transgenesis mediated by intracytoplasmic sperm injection. Biol Reprod. 2007;76:336–43.
43. Yamagata K, Suetsugu R, Wakayama T. Assessment of chromosomal integrity using a novel live-cell imaging technique in mouse embryos produced by intracytoplasmic sperm injection. Hum Reprod. 2009;24:2490–9.
44. Ramos-Ibeas P, Calle A, Fernández-González R, Laguna-Barraza R, Pericuesta E, Calero A, Ramírez MA, Gutiérrez-Adán A. Intracytoplasmic sperm injection using DNA Fragmented sperm in mice negatively affects embryo-derived embryonic stem cells, reduces the fertility of male offspring and induces heritable changes in epialleles. PLoS One. 2014;9:e95625.
45. Rakyan VK, Chong S, Champ ME, Cuthbert PC, Morgan HD, Luu KV, Whitelaw E. Transgenerational inheritance of epigenetic states at the murine Axin(Fu) allele occurs after maternal and paternal transmission. Proc Natl Acad Sci U S A. 2003;100:2538–43.
46. Wakayama T, Yanagimachi R. Development of normal mice from oocytes injected with freeze-dried spermatozoa. Nat Biotechnol. 1998;16:639–41.
47. Fraser L, Strzeżek J, Kordan W. Post-thaw sperm characteristics following long-term storage of boar semen in liquid nitrogen. Anim Reprod Sci. 2014;147:119–27.

48. Simon L, Murphy K, Shamsi MB, Liu L, Emery B, Aston KI, Hotaling J, Carrel DT. Paternal influence of sperm DNA integrity on early embryonic development. Hum Reprod. 2014;29:2402–12.
49. Kaneko T, Whittingham DG, Overstreet JW, Yanagimachi R. Tolerance of the mouse sperm nuclei to freeze-drying depends on their disulfide status. Biol Reprod. 2003;69:1859–62.
50. Yildiz C, Law N, Ottaviani P, Jarvi K, McKerlie C. Comparison of sperm quality and DNA integrity in mouse sperm exposed to various cooling velocities and osmotic stress. Theriogenology. 2010;74:1420–30.
51. McCarthy MJ, Baumber J, Kass PH, Meyers SA. Osmotic stress induces oxidative cell damage to rhesus macaque spermatozoa. Biol Reprod. 2010;82:644–51.
52. Yildiz C, Ottaviani P, Law N, Ayearst R, Liu L, McKerlie C. Effects of cryopreservation on sperm quality, nuclear DNA integrity, in vitro fertilization, and in vitro embryo development in the mouse. Reproduction. 2007;133:585–95.
53. Taşdemir U, Büyükleblebici S, Tuncer PB, Coşkun E, Ozgürtaş T, Aydın FN, Büyükleblebici O, Gürcan IS. Effects of various cryoprotectants on bull sperm quality, DNA integrity and oxidative stress parameters. Cryobiology. 2013;66:38–42.
54. Donnelly ET, Steele EK, McClure N, Lewis SE. Assessment of DNA integrity and morphology of ejaculated spermatozoa from fertile and infertile men before and after cryopreservation. Hum Reprod. 2001;16:1191–9.
55. Gürler H, Malama E, Heppelmann M, Calisici O, Leiding C, Kastelic JP, Bollwein H. Effects of cryopreservation on sperm viability, synthesis of reactive oxygen species, and DNA damage of bovine sperm. Theriogenology. 2016;86:562–71.
56. Balhorn R. A model for the structure of chromatin in mammalian sperm. J Cell Biol. 1982;93:298–305.
57. Ward MA, Ward WS. A model for the function of sperm DNA degradation. Reprod Fertil Dev. 2004;16:547–54.
58. Evenson DP, Jost LK, Varner DD. Relationship between sperm nuclear protamine free -SH status and susceptibility to DNA denaturation. J Reprod Fertil Suppl. 2000:14(3):199–204.
59. Sotolongo B, Lino E, Ward WS. Ability of hamster spermatozoa to digest their own DNA. Biol Reprod. 2003;69:2029–35.
60. Maione B, Pittoggi C, Achene L, Lorenzini R, Spadafora C. Activation of endogenous nucleases in mature sperm cells upon interaction with exogenous DNA. DNA Cell Biol. 1997;16:1087–97.
61. Kusakabe H, Szczygiel MA, Whittingham DG, Yanagimachi R. Maintenance of genetic integrity in frozen and freeze-dried mouse spermatozoa. Proc Natl Acad Sci U S A. 2001;98:13501–6.
62. Szczygiel MA, Ward WS. Combination of dithiothreitol and detergent treatment of spermatozoa causes paternal chromosomal damage. Biol Reprod. 2002;67:1532–7.
63. Johnston SD, Satake N, Zee Y, López-Fernández C, Holt WV, Gosálvez J. Osmotic stress and cryoinjury of koala sperm: an integrative study of the plasma membrane, chromatin stability and mitochondrial function. Reproduction. 2012;143:787–97.
64. Amidi F, Pazhohan A, Shabani Nashtaei M, Khodarahmian M, Nekoonam S. The role of antioxidants in sperm freezing: a review. Cell Tissue Bank. 2016;17:745–56.
65. Sikka SC. Oxidative stress and role of antioxidants in normal and abnormal sperm function. Front Biosci. 1996;1:e78–86.
66. Peeker R, Abramsson L, Marklund SL. Superoxide dismutase isoenzymes in human seminal plasma and spermatozoa. Mol Hum Reprod. 1997;3:1061–6.
67. Bansal AK, Bilaspuri GS. Impacts of oxidative stress and antioxidants on semen functions. Vet Med Int. 2010;2010:686137.
68. Ortega Ferrusola C, González Fernández L, Macías García B, Salazar-Sandoval C, Morillo Rodríguez A, Rodríguez Martinez H, Tapia JA, Peña FJ. Effect of cryopreservation on nitric oxide production by stallion spermatozoa. Biol Reprod. 2009;81:1106–11.
69. Baumber J, Ball BA, Linfor JJ, Meyers SA. Reactive oxygen species and cryopreservation promote DNA fragmentation in equine spermatozoa. J Androl. 2003;24:621–8.

70. Said TM, Gaglani A, Agarwal A. Implication of apoptosis in sperm cryoinjury. Reprod Biomed Online. 2010;21:456–62.
71. Rall WF, Fahy GM. Ice-free cryopreservation of mouse embryos at −196 °C by vitrification. Nature. 1985;313:573–5.
72. Ali Mohamed MS. Slow cryopreservation is not superior to vitrification in human spermatozoa; an experimental controlled study. Iran J Reprod Med. 2015;13:633–44.
73. Valcarce DG, Cartón-García F, Riesco MF, Herráez MP, Robles V. Analysis of DNA damage after human sperm cryopreservation in genes crucial for fertilization and early embryo development. Andrology. 2013;1:723–30.
74. Pradiee J, Esteso MC, Castaño C, Toledano-Díaz A, Lopez-Sebastián A, Guerra R, Santiago-Moreno J. Conventional slow freezing cryopreserves mouflon spermatozoa better than vitrification. Andrologia. 2017;49(3):e12629.
75. Fernández-Gago R, Álvarez-Rodríguez M, Alonso ME, González JR, Alegre B, Domínguez JC, Martínez-Pastor F. Thawing boar semen in the presence of seminal plasma improves motility, modifies subpopulation patterns and reduces chromatin alterations. Reprod Fertil Dev. 2017;29(8):1576–1584.
76. Patel M, Gandotra VK, Cheema RS, Bansal AK, Kumar A. Seminal plasma heparin binding proteins improve semen quality by reducing oxidative stress during cryopreservation of cattle bull semen. Asian-Australasian J Anim Sci. 2016;29:1247–55.
77. Treulen F, Sánchez R, Risopatrón J. Effects of seminal fluid fractions on plasma and acrosome membrane integrity and mitochondrial membrane potential determined by flow cytometry in chilled canine spermatozoa. Reprod Domest Anim. 2012;47:1043–8.
78. Schjenken JE, Robertson SA. Seminal fluid signalling in the female reproductive tract: implications for reproductive success and offspring health. Adv Exp Med Biol. 2015;868:127–58.
79. Agha-Rahimi A, Khalili MA, Nottola SA, Miglietta S, Moradi A. Cryoprotectant-free vitrification of human spermatozoa in new artificial seminal fluid. Andrology. 2016;4(6):1037–1044.
80. Gianaroli L, Magli MC, Stanghellini I, Crippa A, Crivello AM, Pescatori ES, Ferraretti AP. DNA integrity is maintained after freeze-drying of human spermatozoa. Fertil Steril. 2012;97:1067–73. e1
81. Holt WV, Van Look KJ. Concepts in sperm heterogeneity, sperm selection and sperm competition as biological foundations for laboratory tests of semen quality. Reproduction. 2004;127:527–35.
82. Pérez-Cerezales S, Martínez-Páramo S, Beirão J, Herráez MP. Fertilization capacity with rainbow trout DNA-damaged sperm and embryo developmental success. Reproduction. 2010;139:989–97.
83. Reinardy HC, Syrett JR, Jeffree RA, Henry TB, Jha AN. Cobalt-induced genotoxicity in male zebrafish (Danio rerio), with implications for reproduction and expression of DNA repair genes. Aquat Toxicol. 2013;126:224–30.
84. Smith TB, Dun MD, Smith ND, Curry BJ, Connaughton HS, Aitken RJ. The presence of a truncated base excision repair pathway in human spermatozoa that is mediated by OGG1. J Cell Sci. 2013;126:1488–97.
85. Derijck A, van der Heijden G, Giele M, Philippens M, de Boer P. DNA double-strand break repair in parental chromatin of mouse zygotes, the first cell cycle as an origin of de novo mutation. Hum Mol Genet. 2008;17:1922–37.
86. Mitra S, Boldogh I, Izumi T, Hazra TK. Complexities of the DNA base excision repair pathway for repair of oxidative DNA damage. Environ Mol Mutagen. 2001;38:180–90.
87. Bladen CL, Lam WK, Dynan WS, Kozlowski DJ. DNA damage response and Ku80 function in the vertebrate embryo. Nucleic Acids Res. 2005;33:3002–10.
88. Ahmadi A, Ng SC. Fertilizing ability of DNA-damaged spermatozoa. J Exp Zool. 1999;284:696–704.
89. Pérez-Cerezales S, Gutiérrez-Adán A, Martínez-Páramo S, Beirão J, Herráez MP. Altered gene transcription and telomere length in trout embryo and larvae obtained with DNA cryodamaged sperm. Theriogenology. 2011;76:1234–45.

90. Ocalewicz K, Babiak I, Dobosz S, Nowaczyk J, Goryczko K. The stability of telomereless chromosome fragments in adult androgenetic rainbow trout. J Exp Biol. 2004;207:2229–36.
91. Fernández-Díez C, González-Rojo S, Montfort J, Le Cam A, Bobe J, Robles V, Pérez-Cerezales S, Herráez MP. Inhibition of zygotic DNA repair: transcriptome analysis of the offspring in trout (Oncorhynchus mykiss). Reproduction. 2015;149:101–11.

Chapter 20
Sperm DNA and Natural Pregnancy

Marcello Spanò and Aleksander Giwercman

20.1 Introduction

Infertility is defined as a reproductive disease in which a couple desiring a child is unable to conceive after 12 consecutive months of regular, unprotected sexual intercourse. Estimates on the responsibilities of the partners are almost equally distributed: 35–40% of infertility cases are due to a solely female factor, pure male factor accounts for 20–25% of the problem, and the remaining 30–40% is due to a combination of both male and female factors, and unexplained couple infertility is confined to some 10% [1]. Thus, a male factor is implicated in almost 50% of the cases, either solely or in combination with female factors. Male (and couple) infertility must be considered as a multifactorial disease generally resulting from the entanglement of a variety of genetic, epigenetic, environmental, and lifestyle factors. The start-up of the male infertility diagnosis is the semen quality analysis performed according to the procedures outlined in the latest WHO guidelines [2, 3] which can detect radical forms of sperm dysfunction (e.g. azoospermia or globozoospermia) and, more commonly, can provide useful information regarding the male fertility potential and causes of its impairment. Nevertheless, the presence of values below the WHO thresholds per se might not preclude the possibility of starting an in vivo pregnancy, or, contrastingly, a "normal" spermiogram does not necessarily guarantee a satisfactory fertilizing potential. Actually, it is estimated that roughly 15% of men with normal basic semen analysis profiles have nonetheless been associated

M. Spanò (Deceased)
Laboratory of Biosafety and Risk Assessment, Division of Technologies and Methodologies for Health Protection, ENEA (Italian National Agency for New Technologies, Energy and Sustainable Economic Development), Rome, Italy
e-mail: marcello.spano@enea.it

A. Giwercman (✉)
Lund University, Malmö, Sweden
e-mail: Aleksander.Giwercman@med.lu.se

A. Zini, A. Agarwal (eds.), *A Clinician's Guide to Sperm DNA and Chromatin Damage*, https://doi.org/10.1007/978-3-319-71815-6_20

with infertility [4]. Thus, even though WHO conventional semen analysis is a cornerstone examination, limitation exists in the diagnostic potential of the traditional spermiogram, and there is a substantial overlap in semen parameters among men who did achieve a pregnancy or not [5, 6]. Furthermore, its predictive power in the context of medically assisted reproductive technologies (ARTs) is even more limited. WHO parameters do not provide information about one of the most important players of the reproductive outcome, i.e. paternal DNA. In the last decades, a variety of potential semen biomarkers to be used diagnostically or prognostically have been studied and proposed. We will concentrate here on biomarkers based on sperm DNA/chromatin, which have demonstrated their clinical utility and have gained scientific popularity and acceptance.

Our view that sperm cell is a mere vehicle for commuting the male genomic material to the oocyte, embedded into an inert, highly condensed chromatin, is rapidly fading. On the other hand, the integrity of the sperm cell, of its genome, and of its epigenome represents essential requirements for a successful fertilization and embryo development [7–10]. DNA defects that can be found in the sperm and that the father can pass to the zygote include microscopy visible karyotype changes, DNA sequence, and chemical modifications. These defects can arise spontaneously during chromatin remodelling or can be induced by the action of reactive oxygen species (ROS) or by compounds capable to modify nucleotides and DNA-associated proteins [11, 12]. DNA damage is quite a common feature in human sperm, and each man has his own fraction of DNA-defective sperm. This personal burden can increase with ageing, because of some pathological condition and some medical treatment, due to a variety of exogenous toxic compounds present in the environment we live in often exacerbated by individual negative lifestyles, or due to dangerous occupational exposures [13–15]. DNA damage may decrease the fertility potential or, most worryingly, may increase the sperm mutational load. Normally, DNA brought into the zygote is effectively repaired by the oocyte. But when the egg's repair capacity is occasionally defective or overwhelmed by a high level of damage, paternal DNA may either remain unrepaired or be aberrantly repaired creating mutations, which can have a significant impact on the viability of the embryo and on the health of the progeny. Thus, sperm DNA damage can have different and multifactorial origins, but the underlying processes are probably not necessarily mutually exclusive and somehow entangled. Unified theories integrating into a coherent framework reactive oxygen species (ROS), oxidative stress, apoptosis, chromatin compaction, oxidative DNA damage, and DNA fragmentation have been put forward [11, 12, 16, 17].

Whatever the origin, DNA damage in spermatozoa seems linked to impaired embryonic development, pregnancy loss, and birth defects. Therefore, sperm DNA damage assessment can provide information on both spermatogenesis quality and about the risk that defective genetic material will be transmitted to the progeny. Even though the clinical significance of sperm DNA damage has been and continues to be a highly debated topic [18–21], a bulk of data has accumulated demonstrating an association between genetic damage and subfertility or progeny outcome [reviewed in 16, 20, 22, 23, 24, 25, 26, 27, 28, 29, 30, 31, 32, 33]. Being that sperm DNA integrity is an essential prerequisite for successful embryo development, it has been proposed as a supplement to the traditional sperm parameters used to assess semen quality. This chapter will deal mainly with the effects of unspecific and non-positional DNA breaks and the objects detected by a variety of sperm DNA damage techniques described in detail in other chapters in this book and in other reviews [16, 20, 22, 24, 27, 29, 33]. The most common assays are the SCSA (sperm chromatin structure assay) [34, 35], the Comet (single-cell gel electrophoresis) assay [36, 37], the TUNEL (terminal deoxynucleotidyl transferase-mediated dUTP nick end labelling) assay [38, 39], and the SCD (sperm chromatin dispersion) assay [40, 41]. All these tests are able to detect the fraction of DNA/chromatin-defective sperm within a given ejaculate, often expressed in terms of DNA fragmentation index (DFI). To a certain extent, these tests may complement each other as, working according to different strategies of damage detection, they may have different accessibility to DNA-damaged sites and/or may preferentially recognize some kind of DNA lesions. Furthermore, we can reasonably assume that the DNA damage itself can be heterogeneous in nature (single-stranded/double-stranded DNA breaks, damage to nucleotides, damage to introns, exons, or regulatory regions) and such heterogeneity can impact on the clinical relevance and predictive power of the assay. By and large, these assays have shown a moderate level of correlation with each other, according to the results provided by several studies on fertile and subfertile men where at least two different approaches could be compared [42–47]. Interestingly, these tests have also shown a good correlation with the level of 8-hydroxy-2′-deoxyguanosine (8-OHdG) evaluated by HPLC (high-performance liquid chromatography) considered a reliable biomarker of oxidative damage [46, 48–51]. One thing not to be overlooked is the lower variability (and higher intra-sample, inter-sample, inter-laboratory repeatability) of sperm DNA damage tests as compared with other semen quality variables [52–58].

20.2 Factors Potentially Impacting Sperm DNA Integrity

Semen quality in adult men can be affected by a variety of lifestyle, environmental, and occupational factors [reviewed in 13, 14, 59, 60, 61, 62, 63, 64, 65]. The personal burden of sperm DNA fragmentation can increase under the influence of some of these external stressors as exposures can directly target DNA or can indirectly impact DNA integrity by the induction of oxidative stress. Reproductive epidemiological studies where sperm DNA/chromatin integrity has been associated to exposures to physical agents and chemicals including therapeutic drugs, pesticides, metals, air pollutants, and recreational drugs will be reported in other chapters of this book. As well, other important pathological conditions, like cancer and varicocele, which have been considered for their impact on the fraction of DNA-defective sperm in the ejaculate will be discussed in other sections of this book. Here we briefly review the scientific evidence about the impact of a few important determinants of the chance of natural pregnancy related with lifestyle and habits, pathological conditions, and ageing, as the impairment of sperm DNA integrity might be a part of the pathogenetic mechanism.

20.2.1 Prenatal Determinants

For some reproductive problems manifest during adult life, such as male infertility and testicular cancer, it has been speculated that they might have a foetal origin [66, 67]. However, the literature on whether prenatal exposures could impact sperm DNA integrity in the adult is quite scanty. In a population-based cohort study of 337 young men in Denmark, the potential association between several prenatal and preconceptional exposures (maternal smoking during pregnancy, maternal alcohol intake during pregnancy, parental overweight, maternal coffee intake during pregnancy, parental waiting time to pregnancy, parental treatment for infertility) and sperm DNA integrity has been investigated [68]. The results indicated that SCSA-derived DFI can be affected by prenatal exposures, such as parental obesity, and is also associated with a prolonged time to pregnancy (TTP), but confidence limits were wide and results statistically insignificant.

20.2.2 Smoking

Tobacco smoking is one of the greatest risk factors of more than 60% of non-communicable diseases, among them decreased male (and female) fertility [69, 70]. Even if the relationship between smoking habits and sperm DNA damage remains to be clarified, it has been reported that tobacco smoke can increase the level of sperm oxidative stress, the level of DNA oxidative lesions, and DNA damage [64, 71, 72]. Inefficient or aberrant repair of such premutational sperm DNA lesions by the oocyte could account for genomic instability [73] and increased cancer risk in the children of smoking fathers.

20.2.3 Obesity

In addition to tobacco smoking, another worldwide epidemic is obesity, also known to be associated with the induction of systemic oxidative stress [64]. Recent studies have indicated an association between obesity, generally evaluated from the individual body mass index (BMI), and reduced semen quality [74–77]. More conflicting results about the impact of obesity on sperm DNA fragmentation have been reported. With some notable exception [78–82], the majority of studies do not indicate that overweight and obesity per se have a negative impact on sperm DNA integrity [68, 76, 83–89]. A synopsis of studies (with cohorts of at least 100 men) in which BMI has been associated with DNA fragmentation is shown in Table 20.1. Even if the issue of obesity and sperm DNA integrity remains open, a program of body weight loss among the

Table 20.1 Association between BMI and sperm DNA integrity (only studies with >100 men)

Cohort	Assay	Country	Reference
Positive studies			
520 healthy patients undergoing semen analysis	SCSA	USA	[78]
483 male partners in subfertile couples	Comet (neutral)	USA	[79]
305 male patients presenting for clinical evaluation	Comet (alkaline)	Brazil	[80]
150 healthy non-smoking men from general population	FCM TUNEL	Italy	[81]
330 male partners in subfertile couples	Fl M TUNEL	France	[82]
Negative studies			
279 men from infertile couples	SCSA	The Netherlands	[83]
227 men from infertile couples undergoing ART	SCSA	The Netherlands	[84]
153 men from infertile couples	SCSA	Czech Republic	[85]
337 men from general population	SCSA	Denmark	[68]
612 men from infertile couples undergoing ART	SCSA	Denmark	[88]
468 men from infertile couples	SCSA	USA	[76]
1503 men from general population	SCSA	Sweden, Greenland, Poland, Ukraine, Norway	[89]

ART assisted reproductive technology, *BMI* body mass index, *FCM TUNEL* flow cytometry TUNEL assay, *Fl M TUNEL* fluorescence microscopy TUNEL assay, *SCSA* sperm chromatin structure assay

therapeutic repertoire for male (and couple) infertility is suggested, and pilot studies showed that weight reduction programs could be of benefit for semen quality recovery [85].

20.2.4 Abstinence

Several studies have reported that the higher the abstinence period, the higher the fraction of DNA-defective sperm. It seems likely that this correlation stems from a longer exposure of sperm to ROS attacks. By and large, with a few exceptions [52, 90, 91], weak positive correlations have been found, using a variety of techniques, both in the general population and in infertile patients [54, 68, 92–102]. The results of studies where potential associations between abstinence time and sperm DNA integrity have been considered are reported in Table 20.2. Interestingly, reduced male abstinence periods are associated with a reduced fraction of DNA-defective sperm and a significant increase in pregnancy rate when using ICSI (IntraCytoplasmic Sperm Injection) [102].

Table 20.2 Association between abstinence time and sperm DNA integrity

Cohort	Assay	Country	Reference
Positive studies			
277 men from general population	SCSA	Denmark	[92]
215 young men first-pregnancy planners	SCSA	Denmark	[93]
503 men from general population	SCSA	Italy, UK, Belgium	[95]
278 young men from general population	SCSA	Sweden	[96]
449 young men from general population	SCSA	Denmark, Sweden	[54]
707 fertile men from general population	SCSA	Sweden, Greenland, Poland, Ukraine	[94]
282 men from infertile couples undergoing ART	SCSA	Sweden	[97]
88 non-smoking men from general population	SCSA	USA	[98]
337 men from general population	SCSA	Denmark	[68]
113 men from infertile couples undergoing ART	Fl M TUNEL	Australia	[99]
1633 men undergoing infertility investigation	FCM TUNEL	France	[100]
33 normozoospermic men	SCD	Spain	[101]
190 men from infertile couples undergoing ART	SCD	Spain	[102]
Negative studies			
45 men from general population	SCSA	USA	[52]
11 men from infertile couples	SCSA	USA	[91]
148 men from infertile couples undergoing ART	FCM TUNEL	Canada	[90]

ART assisted reproductive technology, *FCM TUNEL* flow cytometry TUNEL assay, *Fl M TUNEL* fluorescence microscopy TUNEL assay, *SCD* sperm chromatin dispersion assay, *SCSA* sperm chromatin structure assay

20.2.5 Ageing

In contrast to women, there is no abrupt loss of fertility as men age, and reproductive capability can be retained till old age. However, the quality of male gametes deteriorates with time, starting at around the age of 35 [103]. An age-associated decline in androgen levels, semen volume, percentage motility, progressive motility, and normal morphology and an increase in the fraction of sperm with damaged DNA have been reported [104, 105]. The older the father, the higher the risk of miscarriage, and, if the pregnancies carry to term, the higher are the chances of disease in the offspring [64]. The mechanisms that are behind this paternal age-dependent rise in mutational load carried by children are complex and likely involve an array of factors (replication error, accumulation of mutations, de novo mutation, coupled with aberrant repair of sperm DNA damage in the oocyte immediately after fertilization). Increased life expectancy, advanced age of marriage, and various socio-economic factors have led couples to start their family at a later age delaying reproduction. It is well documented that there is a continuing rise in the age of fathers in most regions of the world [106]. The increased accessibility to ART has increased the chance of older parents with poor pregnancy outcomes to conceive children, hence, increasing the average paternal age at first childbirth. The age-related increase of damage in male germ cells raises substantial health concerns regarding the possible long-term consequences of increasing paternal ages on the viability and genetic health of the offspring [107]. The issue of deterioration of sperm DNA integrity with ageing is discussed in detail in another part of this book. By and large, with few exceptions [108], in accordance with the age-dependent decline in standard semen parameters, several studies, carried out all over the world with different sperm DNA integrity tests, have demonstrated that sperm DNA damage is associated with advanced paternal age either in men from general population [92, 94, 98, 109–113] or in male partners of infertile couples [57, 83, 84, 86, 100, 114–124]. The potential clinical importance of these results is obvious and strongly suggests that DNA fragmentation should at least be routinely screened for men of advanced age and counselling should be offered about the potential risks.

20.2.6 Other Pathological Conditions

Some specific clinical conditions have been associated with a higher prevalence of elevated sperm DNA fragmentation. Usually, a higher percentage of defective sperm is found in varicocele patients, probably attributable to oxidative stress [119, 125–131]. In many cases, sperm chromatin quality was improved after surgery [132–134] or by antioxidant therapy [135, 136]. As far as microorganism-associated pathologies are concerned, patients with infectious diseases like genitourinary infection by *Chlamydia trachomatis* or *Mycoplasma* showed an increased fraction of DNA-damaged sperm in comparison with fertile controls, and antibiotic therapy was shown to ameliorate infection-induced high DNA fragmentation levels [137]. This is consistent with the results from another study where patients with bacteriospermia had improvement in DFI after antibiotic treatment [135]. On the other hand, the concomitant occurrence of viruses (i.e. herpes, papilloma) in the ejaculate seemed not affecting the fraction of DNA-defective sperm [138]. A higher fraction of DNA-defective sperm has repeatedly observed in men with spinal cord injury [139–141]. In a case-control study among infertile patients, diabetes mellitus was found to be associated with a higher DNA-defective sperm fraction [142]. Finally, it has been occasionally observed that high fever can impact markedly on both the conventional semen parameters and sperm DNA integrity with a recovery to normal values in the next spermatogenic cycles [143, 144].

20.3 Male Infertility and Sperm Chromatin Damage

20.3.1 Association with the Traditional WHO Sperm Parameters and Sexual Hormones

Several studies have demonstrated a weak-to-moderate inverse correlation, if any, between sperm DNA fragmentations measured by the various sperm integrity assays and the traditional semen parameters. As shown in Table 20.3, the correlation levels among different studies can vary even for the same sperm DNA/chromatin integrity assay when looking at population groups representative of the general population or of infertile patient cohorts [45, 47, 54, 83, 90, 92–94, 96, 100, 116, 118, 119, 124, 145–150]. The variable degree of association probably reflects the different methods used for DNA integrity testing, the variability in the conventional semen quality analyses, and the lack of uniformity of the population groups involved [4]. Motility has generally been the parameter with the highest degree of association to sperm DNA defects, probably because both sperm chromatin compaction and acquisition of motility are parallel differentiation processes culminating during the passage of the maturing male gamete in the epididymal tract [54, 57, 151, 152]. Swim-up prepared motile sperm cells are characterized by a lower fraction of DNA-defective sperm as compared to that initially present in the neat semen [153, 154], whereas morphologically normal human sperm can carry fragmented DNA [155]. Few studies have tried to assess the relation between the fractions of DNA-defective sperm and blood concentration of sexual hormones and other biomarkers of the sexual accessory glands. In a study involving 278 young men with no knowledge of their fertility status [96], the SCSA DFI was weakly inversely correlated with oestradiol and free testosterone and positively correlated with the seminal concentration of zinc and fructose. In another study of 279 men from infertile couples, the SCSA DFI was positively associated with the level of FSH, but not with the levels of inhibin B and LH [83]. Finally, in a study involving 362 male partners of infertile couples [156], the fraction of sperm with high DNA damage, evaluated by the neutral Comet assay, resulted positively associated with free thyroxine and total triiodothyronine.

20.3.2 Prevalence of Sperm DNA Fragmentation in Fertile and Infertile Men

Sperm cells with DNA breaks are always present in the ejaculate although the levels will vary from one man to another. There is an extensive literature where the average frequency of DNA-defective sperm has been measured and compared between infertile patients and a control population represented by healthy, normozoospermic men [55, 157–159], proven fertile men [41, 42, 44, 57, 83, 160–182], or unselected men from general population [9, 48, 183]. In almost all studies, carried out in

Table 20.3 Correlation between sperm DNA integrity and WHO parameters (only from studies with >200 men)

Technique	*N* and country		WHO parameter Concentration	Morphology	Motility	Reference
	General population	Infertile patients				
SCSA	277 (Denmark)		−0.31	−0.38	–	[92]
SCSA	215 (Denmark)		−0.23	−0.25	–	[93]
SCSA	278 (Sweden)		−0.12	–	–	[96]
SCSA	449 (Denmark, Sweden)		−0.12/−0.26	–	−0.25/−0.43	[54]
SCSA		201 (UK)	−0.22	−0.46	−0.56	[145]
SCSA		249 (USA)	−0.12	−0.13	−0.17	[146]
SCSA	707 (Greenland, Sweden, Ukraine, Poland)		N.S.	−0.17	−0.23	[94]
SCSA		234 (Denmark)		N.S.		[147]
SCSA	209 (South Africa)		N.S.	−0.22	−0.19	[148]
SCSA		2586 (Canada)	−0.219	−0.39	−0.61	[118]
SCSA		279 (Netherlands)	−0.41	−0.35	−0.50	[83]
SCSA		288 (Canada)	N.S.	−0.38	−0.50	[119]
SCSA		277 (Canada)	N.S.	N.S.	−0.16	[124]
SCSA		212 (USA)	−0.34	N.S.	−0.45	[47]
M TUNEL		332 (France)		−0.2	−0.2	[149]
Fl M TUNEL		262 (Germany)	N.S.	−0.44	−0.60	[150]
Fl M TUNEL		235 (USA)	−0.13	−0.21	−0.16	[45]
Fl M TUNEL		212 (USA)	N.S.	N.S.	N.S.	[47]
FCM TUNEL		298 (Canada)	−0.18	−0.34	−0.12	[90]
FCM TUNEL		1633 (France)	N.S.	Inverse	Inverse	[100]
FCM TUNEL		1974 (France)	N.S.	N.S.	−0.26	[57]
COMET (alkaline)		238 (USA)	N.S.	N.S.	N.S.	[45]
COMET (neutral)		257 (USA)	−1.42	−0.05	−0.43	[116]

FCM TUNEL flow cytometry TUNEL assay, *Fl M TUNEL* flucrescence microscopy TUNEL assay, *M TUNEL* bright-field microscopy TUNEL assay, *N.S.* statistically not significant, *SCSA* sperm chromatin structure assay several parts of the world with a variety of assays, the infertile population was characterized by significantly higher mean values of the DNA-defective sperm fraction and by a higher incidence of men with high DFI. Even the Practice Committee of the American Society for Reproductive Medicine [19], which does not endorse sperm DNA integrity testing in the clinical setting to predict pregnancy rates in ART, states that "sperm DNA damage is more common in infertile men and may contribute to poor reproductive performance". There is an overwhelming evidence showing that even within the group of men with subfertility problem, the DFI is significantly lower among those with normal standard semen parameters as compared to those having one or more abnormal WHO sperm parameters [41, 57, 118, 147, 165, 167, 184–189]. As shown in Table 20.4, in studies where subfertile patients have been discriminated between normozoospermic (idiopathic male infertility) and dyspermic men, the relative incidence of men characterized by a high DFI fraction is generally lower in men having WHO parameters in the normal range [55, 57, 100, 118, 165, 189–191]. A notable concern is that a large fraction of infertile patients possess high levels of sperm DNA damage. A lower rate of men with high level of DNA fragmentation emerged also from studies where cohorts of fertile men with normal semen parameters were compared with men from unexplained infertility couples [176, 191]. It is important to stress that, for almost all these studies, the values of normality for standard semen quality parameters have been considered the ones proposed by the WHO manual, 1999 edition [192]. As the latest WHO manual has revised some reference values as compared to the previous editions, for example, setting the lower limit for sperm concentration at 15 million/mL, the risk of

Table 20.4 Incidence of patients characterized by a high level of sperm DNA fragmentation (DFI ≥30%) in cohorts of male partners of infertility couples discriminated as normozoospermic or dyspermic (non-azoospermic) men

Assay	Country	Normozoospermic men		Dyspermic men		Reference
		N	% of men with DFI ≥30%	*N*	% of men with DFI ≥30%	
SCSA	Canada	13	8%	75	17%	[165]
SCSA	USA	25	12%	50	52%	[190]
SCSA	Sweden	126	5%	224	16%	[189]
SCSA	Canada	408	0.5%	1652	29%	[118]
SCSA	Netherlands	20	10%			[83]
SCSA	Sweden	119	8.4%			[191]
FCM TUNEL	France			1633	30.7%	[100]
FCM TUNEL	USA			194	44.8%	[55]
FCM TUNEL	France	1974	11%	2371	20%[a]	[57]

DFI DNA fragmentation index, *FCM TUNEL* flow cytometry TUNEL assay, *SCSA* sperm chromatin structure assay
[a]Value referred to the entire cohort of 4345 infertile men

including more subfertile men as normal controls in epidemiological studies and the risk that a large number of couples previously diagnosed with male factor infertility will now be classified as having unexplained infertility (with normozoospermia) have been put forward [57, 193–196]. As such, a critical reexamination of the association between the results of sperm DNA integrity tests and the new evidence-based WHO reference values will be necessary.

20.3.3 Intra-individual Variation of Sperm Chromatin Parameters

It is known that traditional semen parameters, even if assessed under highly standardized conditions, usually exhibit a high intra-individual variability [197–199] and coefficients of variation (CV) as high as 54% have been reported [200]. On the other hand, sperm DNA integrity parameters seem characterized by a higher level of repeatability. Time-related intra-individual changes of sperm DNA/chromatin parameters have specifically been addressed by different groups, with consistent results. In a study of 45 men who delivered eight monthly semen samples, the average within-donor CV of DFI as measured by SCSA was around 23% [52]. These results were confirmed by other SCSA studies. Zini et al. [53] measured the DFI in 21 men who provided two semen samples, 2–6 weeks apart, and observed a within-subject CV of 21%. In another study, involving 277 men, semen was measured twice during 6 months, and a within-subject CV of 23% for DFI was obtained [92]. In another study on 282 patients undergoing ARTs (assisted reproductive technologies) with repeated (between two and five) SCSA measurements, CV of DFI resulted about 29% [97]. Similar mean DFI CV values of 30% were recently obtained after repeated SCSA analyses on 616 samples from men from infertile couples between 18 and 66 years of age [56]. Altogether, these data from quite large studies point to a lower level of intra-individual variation for SCSA measurements as compared to the standard sperm parameters. Notably, SCSA DFI was not significantly affected during a 2-week period of daily ejaculations [201].

Time stability of sperm DNA integrity was assessed both by the SCSA and the TUNEL assays in a healthy non-smoking fertile volunteer, characterized by a low DFI, over a 10-year period. Compared with TUNEL data, SCSA measurements showed less variation over the data collection period with a DFI within-subject CV of 47.4% and 22.3%, respectively. DFI remained normal, and no trend was observed over the period of observation [202]. The stability over time of the flow cytometry TUNEL assay, during a 6-month period, was tested in a longitudinal study using 15 donors who provided monthly semen samples. A good reproducibility of the assay was obtained: individual CVs for sperm DFI ranged from 12.9% to 43.9%, whereas parallel measurements on cell counts showed within-donor CVs ranging from 16.7% up to 63.2% [203]. The results of a recent study involving up to 70 men with the flow cytometry TUNEL assay corroborated the previous findings as repeated measurements at 100 days, 1 and 2 years apart, gave mean CVs ranging from 9.2% to 14% [58].

Stability along time of sperm DNA integrity tests has obvious clinical implications for those tests that have a threshold for the choice of ART treatment. A recent study involving 616 men from infertile couples evaluated whether SCSA test results could switch from being above to below a defined sperm DFI threshold of 30% (or vice versa) over a 30-month period. The results were quite reassuring as, compared with the first measurement, 85% of the men remained on the same side of the DFI cutoff point of 30% [56]. Thus, a single SCSA measure remains a reliable (reproducible) marker of male fertility potential in vivo.

20.3.4 Impact of Sperm DNA Damage on Fecundity in General Population

Almost all we know about the predictive power of sperm DNA damage on fecundity in general population comes from a few studies, carried out with the same SCSA approach, which produced remarkably homogeneous and consistent results. In this context, fecundity, which is the demographic term corresponding to the term fertility in reproductive medicine, refers to the ability to conceive and have children, given unprotected intercourse. Whether sperm chromatin integrity parameters, independently from the WHO parameters, could predict the chances of spontaneous pregnancy was a question addressed at the turn of the century by two almost concomitant studies, one carried out in the USA (the Georgetown study, 165 couples) and the other carried out in Europe (the Danish first-pregnancy planners study, 215 couples). Both studies demonstrated that in couples from the general population, the chance of spontaneous pregnancy, measured by the TTP, decreases when DFI increases, and this happens independently of sperm concentration (as defined by the WHO 1999 edition). In the Georgetown study [183], SCSA DFI values from the male partners of couples not achieving pregnancy were higher than values in men of couples achieving pregnancy in months 4–12 and even much higher with respect to couples achieving pregnancy after 1–3 months; no couples achieving fast pregnancy had a DFI ≥30%. In the Danish study [93], fecundability progressively decreased as a function of the percentage of DNA-defective sperm, starting at DFI >20%, and, for DFI ≥30%, the chances of spontaneous pregnancies were quite negligible with TTP tending to become infinite. These two studies showed that the pregnancy rates after normal intercourse are significantly higher (6.5 times) for the group with DFI below the threshold of 30% [204]. Thus, from these studies, the fraction of sperm with defective DNA seems the best predictor for a couple's probability to achieve pregnancy, and a threshold value of 30% coherently emerges as the DFI value above which the man's fertility potential markedly deteriorates. Interestingly, in the same population of Danish first-pregnancy planners [93], the likelihood of pregnancy during the six-menstrual cycle follow-up was inversely associated with the level of 8OHdG [205]. This observation corroborated the result of the previous SCSA analysis and reinforced the notion that oxidative DNA damage can play a major role in the genesis of DNA breaks [11]. The risk for infertility has also been calculated in a Swedish cohort of 264 men (of which 127 from infertile couples with no known female factor) in relation to SCSA-determined DFI fraction [176]. As compared with men with a DFI <10%, men with a DFI between 10% and 20% had a 2.5-fold increased risk for infertility. The risk rose to 8.4 for men with a DFI >20%. In men with normal standard sperm parameters, the odd ratios (OR) for infertility were 5.1 higher for DFI >20%, whereas if at least one of the WHO semen parameters was abnormal, the OR for infertility was 16 already at DFI >10%. These results reinforce previous observation on infertile patients where it was noted that men with low sperm motility and abnormal morphology had significantly higher OR for having a DFI >20% (4.0 for motility and 1.9 for morphology) and DFI >30% (6.2 for motility and 2.8 for morphology) compared with men with normal sperm motility and morphology [189]. Further, a significant proportion of men (almost 30%) diagnosed as having unexplained infertility according to traditional diagnostic methods can have SCSA-determined DFI above 20% indicating reduced chances of fathering a child naturally [191]. Thus, SCSA DFI seems to add to the value of semen analysis in predicting the chance of natural conception, and a high fraction of sperm with abnormal DNA/chromatin makes individuals at higher risk of not fathering a child. The obvious clinical implication is that couples with a high sperm DFI should avoid prolonged attempts to achieve pregnancy by normal intercourse and take into consideration other strategies to have children.

20.3.5 Clinically Operative Threshold Values

Any sperm DNA damage test to be useful diagnostically or prognostically must have cutoff levels that can provide adequate discriminatory power in the clinical situation [20]. All sperm DNA integrity tests can define thresholds that mirror, in a probabilistic perspective, the fertility potential of an individual, especially when integrated with the result of WHO assessment. We have already seen that the various sperm DNA integrity tests may complement each other as they may have different accessibility to DNA damage and may preferentially recognize different kinds of DNA lesions. Thus, we can choose among a variety of assays, often proposing some variations of the published protocol, but, so far, we cannot comfortably decide which is the most robust and why. Often the choice is dictated more by logistic problems (accessibility to sophisticated laboratory equipment, self-confidence with a technology) than driven by scientific reasons. Cost is another variable, but it can change, at least for patients, in different countries according to the specific health system. Statistically validated threshold values could be of help in the future clinical applications of sperm DNA integrity tests. So far, SCSA has been the only method providing thresholds of clinical relevance for in vivo and in vitro conception based on repeated large-scale studies performed in different centres.

Operative, clinical SCSA threshold values able to reasonably predict whether a man has chances to father a child naturally are well documented. The chance of pregnancy in vivo decreases when the DFI exceeds the level of 20%, the probability of spontaneous pregnancy being close to zero for DFI >30% [93, 183]. Similar figures emerged with IUI (intrauterine insemination) [206] and for the risk of miscarriages [183]. Men seeking treatment for infertility may have normal standard sperm characteristics but a DFI >20%, indicating that the impairment of sperm DNA integrity is an independent predictor of male fertility status [206]. Proposed TUNEL assay thresholds for very low chance of natural pregnancy are more variable. In a Canadian study involving 47 proven fertile men and 66 infertile patients, the calculated threshold value for TUNEL assay to distinguish between fertile and infertile men was 20% [170]. A very similar value was obtained in an American study involving 25 healthy male volunteers (controls) and 194 infertile men (with male factor infertility), where a TUNEL assay cutoff of 19.3% with observed 100% specificity could differentiate infertile men with DNA damage from healthy men [55]. In an Australian study involving a cohort of 50 random patients undergoing ART treatments and a cohort of 36 unselected healthy donors of unknown fertility status [49], values of 40% for neat samples and of 25% following Percoll centrifugation were established using a modified flow cytometry TUNEL assay [207]. Finally, in a recent Italian study, another modified version of the TUNEL assay was adopted able to distinguish specific subfractions of DNA-damaged cells and improve the predictive value of the analysis. This method was applied to a cohort of 348 unselected patients and 86 proven fertile men; a threshold value of 36% emerged when referred to the whole population of DNA-damaged sperm, and a value of 22.4% was found when a particular subpopulation of brighter cells was considered [58]. In a Northern Irish study on 75 male partners of couples undergoing IVF (in vitro fertilization) and 28 fertile donors and employing the alkaline Comet assay, it was observed that a fraction of defective sperm ≥25% was able to discriminate between patients and donors and that men with semen samples above this threshold had a ninefold higher risk of infertility; the risk of failure to achieve a pregnancy (in IVF) increased when sperm DNA fragmentation exceeded a prognostic threshold value of 52% evaluated on the neat semen (and 42% if assessed on sperm separated after discontinuous gradient centrifugation) [181].

Therefore, by and large, when a fraction of DNA aberrant sperm around 30% is detected, whatever the technique of damage assessment, human fertility seems at stake. On the other hand, it should be kept in mind that whereas high DFI is a good predictor of severe subfertility, the normal value of this parameter does not guarantee normal male fertility. It looks like that all these tests can detect only a subgroup of the possible alterations of the DNA molecule and, likely, only a "tip of the iceberg" of the overall DNA damage is measured [34]. Unravelling unknown factors such as the extent of DNA damage per sperm, the type and location of DNA damage, and if it is clinically important or irrelevant, the association of DNA breaks to other types of DNA lesions, and how much and what kind of sperm DNA damage an oocyte can cope with, will require a much deeper investigation, and further fundamental research is mandatory to solve these key questions.

20.3.6 *Strategies Aimed at Reducing Sperm DNA Damage*

Cause-related therapy is almost non-existing in male subfertility. As oxidative damage is considered one of the main, if not the most important, factors underlying the induction of sperm DNA damage, potential benefits of an antioxidant therapy for sperm DNA quality have been exploited to treat subfertile patients. However, the few studies so far have been small and conflicting, and there are no convincing data that these treatments improve pregnancy rates by an amelioration of the level of DNA fragmentation. Further trials are needed to investigate whether such therapy and other types of causal treatment are effective. Standardized, well-designed clinical trials should be undertaken to address the effectiveness of antioxidant therapies [17].

20.3.7 *Clinical Application of Sperm DNA Integrity Testing in Relation to Natural Pregnancy*

Having in mind that the assessment of sperm DFI is a powerful tool in the prediction of in vivo subfertility, in our opinion this analysis has an important role in managing clinical issues related to fertility. The figures below refer to SCSA analysis, but the threshold values can be adjusted to other measurement techniques.

20.3.7.1 In Managing Infertility Patients

Explaining the cause of infertility is an important part of the management of this serious clinical problem. DFI above 20% indicates reduced male fertility, even though the standard WHO parameters may be within normal range. If the DFI is higher than 30%, the chance of obtaining pregnancy, by intercourse or IUI, is close to zero. Further management is dependent on the female age and fertility status:

- If the female partner is above 35 years and/or has an untreatable cause of infertility, a DFI above 20% should lead to immediate referral for in vitro infertility treatment, preferably ICSI [33].
- In case the partner is 35 or younger and has no known cause of subfertility, for those men having DFI >20%, changes in lifestyle and/or treatment with antioxidants can be considered. If no effect on DFI is seen following 3–6 months of intervention, the same recommendations as those mentioned above should be applied.

20.3.7.2 In Fertility Counselling

Since more and more couples postpone the childbearing, there is a growing demand of “fertility counselling” identifying couples for which relatively high age at the time of attempting to become pregnant may be associated with high risk of infertility [208]. Even in this scenario, DFI assessment plays an important role due to the association between sperm DNA integrity and lifestyle factors, intake of pharmaceuticals drugs, as well as age. Finding of DFI >20% should be followed by repeated testing and counselling regarding possible lifestyle changes and the consequences that the delayed attempt of parenthood may have for the chance of achieving natural pregnancy.

20.4 Conclusions

The fraction of sperm with damaged DNA is generally higher in infertile men and is predictive of chances of natural conception. Although an indiscriminate application of sperm nuclear integrity testing in the infertility work-up has been argued, there are specific conditions where men would certainly benefit from this analysis. DNA fragmentation assays measure strand breaks as an end point. While it provides data on the level of breakage, it provides little-to-no insights into the origin of the damage. Biochemical characterization of the DNA adducts present in human spermatozoa could provide additional clues to the DNA damage aetiology supplementing the data generated by DNA fragmentation assays.

So far, matters of particular urgency to be addressed are the delay in standardization of some of the techniques and the definitions of clinical thresholds for the various assays. These shortcomings have certainly hampered the adoption of the sperm DNA damage assessment as a routine test in the couple infertility work-up [209]. From a clinical long-term perspective, we cannot overlook the message from extensive animal experiments providing unequivocal links between DNA damage in spermatozoa and defects in embryonic development or in the health of the offspring. The results of an impressive amount of data from animal experiments demonstrate that DNA-damaged sperm have the ability to fertilize the oocyte but that embryonic development can be derailed depending on the gravity and degree of DNA damage [210, 211]. Deleterious effects on reproduction can be dramatic, including increase in embryo lethality, heritable translocations, malformations, and cancer in the offspring. This can happen either after normal mating [212–214] or after ICSI with DNA-defective sperm [215, 216]. Therefore, a sort of a "precautionary principle" should be adopted deploying all possible strategies aiming at reducing the involvement of defective sperm in the fertilization process.

Finally, the future of a holistic, system biology-based approach for diagnosis of male infertility will ultimately rely on the efficient combination of information derived from the conventional semen parameters, from the sperm genomic integrity assessment, and from the results of other -omics approaches [9, 217, 218]. Large-scale targeted studies are necessary to standardize the variables determining the specific traits and reference values that will aid the optimized diagnosis, treatment, and prevention of specific aspects of male factor infertility. A more precise diagnosis would enable clinicians to better counsel the infertile couple and may also result in improvement and further development of cause-related therapy.

References

1. Thonneau P, Marchand S, Tallec A, Ferial ML, Ducot B, Lansac J, et al. Incidence and main causes of infertility in a resident population (1,850,000) of three French regions (1988–1989). Hum Reprod. 1991;6:811–6.
2. Cooper TG, Noonan E, von Eckardstein S, Auger J, Baker HW, Behre HM, et al. World Health Organization reference values for human semen characteristics. Hum Reprod Update. 2010;16:231–45.
3. World Health Organization. WHO laboratory manual for the examination and processing of human semen. 5th ed. Geneva: World Health Organization; 2010.
4. Evgeni E, Charalabopoulos K, Asimakopoulos B. Human sperm DNA fragmentation and its correlation with conventional semen parameters. J Reprod Infertil. 2014;15:2–14.
5. Bonde JPE, Ernst E, Jensen TK, Hjollund NHI, Kolstad H, Henriksen TB, et al. Relation between semen quality and fertility: a population-based study of 430 first-pregnancy planners. Lancet. 1998;352:1172–7.
6. Guzick DS, Overstreet JW, Factor-Litvak P, Brazil CK, Nakajima ST, Coutifaris C, et al. Sperm morphology, motility, and concentration in fertile and infertile men. N Engl J Med. 2001;345:1388–93.
7. Miller D, Brinkworth M, Iles D. Paternal DNA packaging in spermatozoa: more than the sum of its parts? DNA, histones, protamines and epigenetics. Reproduction. 2010;139:287–301.
8. Ward WS. Function of sperm chromatin structural elements in fertilization and development. Mol Hum Reprod. 2010;16:30–6.
9. Castillo J, Estanyol JM, Ballescá JL, Oliva R. Human sperm chromatin epigenetic potential: genomics, proteomics, and male infertility. Asian J Androl. 2015;17:601–9.
10. Carrell DT. Epigenetics of the male gamete. Fertil Steril. 2012;97:267–74.
11. Aitken RJ, De Iuliis GN. On the possible origins of DNA damage in human spermatozoa. Mol Hum Reprod. 2010;16:3–13.
12. Aitken RJ, Bronson R, Smith TB, De Iuliis GN. The source and significance of DNA damage in human spermatozoa; a commentary on diagnostic strategies and straw man fallacies. Mol Hum Reprod. 2013;19:475–85.
13. Sharpe RM. Environmental/lifestyle effects on spermatogenesis. Philos Trans R Soc Lond Ser B Biol Sci. 2010;365:1697–712.
14. Giwercman A, Giwercman YL. Environmental factors and testicular function. Best Pract Res Clin Endocrinol Metab. 2011;25:391–402.
15. Sharma R, Biedenharn KR, Fedor JM, Agarwal A. Lifestyle factors and reproductive health: taking control of your fertility. Reprod Biol Endocrinol. 2013;11:66.
16. Sakkas D, Alvarez JG. Sperm DNA fragmentation: mechanisms of origin, impact on reproductive outcome, and analysis. Fertil Steril. 2010;93:1027–36.
17. Gharagozloo P, Aitken RJ. The role of sperm oxidative stress in male infertility and the significance of oral antioxidant therapy. Hum Reprod. 2011;26:1628–40.
18. Zini A, Sigman M. Are tests of sperm DNA damage clinically useful? Pros Cons J Androl. 2009;30:219–29.
19. Practice Committee of the American Society for Reproductive Medicine. The clinical utility of sperm DNA integrity testing: a guideline. Fertil Steril. 2013;99:673–7.
20. Lewis SE, Aitken JR, Conner SJ, Iuliis GD, Evenson DP, Henkel R, et al. The impact of sperm DNA damage in assisted conception and beyond: recent advances in diagnosis and treatment. Reprod Biomed Online. 2013;27:325–37.
21. Palermo GD, Neri QV, Cozzubbo T, Rosenwaks Z. Perspectives on the assessment of human sperm chromatin integrity. Fertil Steril. 2014;102:1508–17.
22. Erenpreiss J, Spano M, Erenpreisa J, Bungum M, Giwercman A. Sperm chromatin structure and male fertility: biological and clinical aspects. Asian J Androl. 2006;8:11–29.
23. Zini A, Boman JM, Belzile E, Ciampi A. Sperm DNA damage is associated with an increased risk of pregnancy loss after IVF and ICSI: systematic review and meta-analysis. Hum Reprod. 2008;23:2663–8.

24. Barratt CL, Aitken RJ, Björndahl L, Carrell DT, de Boer P, Kvist U, et al. Sperm DNA: organization, protection and vulnerability: from basic science to clinical applications—a position report. Hum Reprod. 2010;25:824–38.
25. Lewis SE, Simon L. Clinical implications of sperm DNA damage. Hum Fertil (Camb). 2010;13:201–7.
26. Bungum M, Bungum L, Giwercman A. Sperm chromatin structure assay (SCSA): a tool in diagnosis and treatment of infertility. Asian J Androl. 2011;13:69–75.
27. Shamsi MB, Imam SN, Dada R. Sperm DNA integrity assays: diagnostic and prognostic challenges and implications in management of infertility. J Assist Reprod Genet. 2011;28:1073–85.
28. Zini A. Are sperm chromatin and DNA defects relevant in the clinic? Syst Biol Reprod Med. 2011;57:78–85.
29. Bungum M. Sperm DNA integrity assessment: a new tool in diagnosis and treatment of fertility. Obstet Gynecol Int. 2012;2012:531042.
30. Robinson L, Gallos ID, Conner SJ, Rajkhowa M, Miller D, Lewis S, et al. The effect of sperm DNA fragmentation on miscarriage rates: a systematic review and meta-analysis. Hum Reprod. 2012;27:2908–17.
31. Simon L, Proutski I, Stevenson M, Jennings D, McManus J, Lutton D, et al. Sperm DNA damage has a negative association with live-birth rates after IVF. Reprod Biomed Online. 2013;26:68–78.
32. Ioannou D, Miller D, Griffin DK, Tempest HG. Impact of sperm DNA chromatin in the clinic. J Assist Reprod Genet. 2016;33:157–66.
33. Oleszczuk K, Giwercman A, Bungum M. Sperm chromatin structure assay in prediction of in vitro fertilization outcome. Andrology. 2016;4:290–6.
34. Evenson DP, Larson KL, Jost LK. Sperm chromatin structure assay: its clinical use for detecting sperm DNA fragmentation in male infertility and comparisons with other techniques. J Androl. 2002;23:25–43.
35. Evenson DP, Darzynkiewicz Z, Melamed MR. Relationship of mammalian sperm chromatin heterogeneity to fertility. Science. 1980;240:1131–3.
36. Singh NR, Danner DB, Tice RR, McCoy MT, Collins GD, Schneider EL. Abundant alkali labile sites in DNA of human and mouse sperm. Exp Cell Res. 1989;184:461–70.
37. Singh NP, Stephens RE. X-ray induced DNA double-strand breaks in human sperm. Mutagenesis. 1998;13:75–9.
38. Gorczyca W, Traganos F, Jesionowska H, Darzynkiewicz Z. Presence of DNA strand breaks and increased sensitivity of DNA in situ to denaturation in abnormal human sperm cells: analogy to apoptosis of somatic cells. Exp Cell Res. 1993;207:202–5.
39. Sharma R, Masaki J, Agarwal A. Sperm DNA fragmentation analysis using the TUNEL assay. Methods Mol Biol. 2013;927:121–36.
40. Fernández JL, Muriel L, Rivero MT, Goyanes V, Vazquez R, Alvarez JG. The sperm chromatin dispersion test: a simple method for the determination of sperm DNA fragmentation. J Androl. 2003;24:59–66.
41. Fernández JL, Muriel L, Goyanes V, Segrelles E, Gosálvez J, Enciso M, et al. Simple determination of human sperm DNA fragmentation with an improved sperm chromatin dispersion test. Fertil Steril. 2005;84:833–42.
42. Chohan KR, Griffin JT, Lafromboise M, De Jonge CJ, Carrell DT. Comparison of chromatin assays for DNA fragmentation evaluation in human sperm. J Androl. 2006;27:53–9.
43. Ståhl O, Eberhard J, Jepson K, Spanò M, Cwikiel M, Cavallin-Ståhl E, et al. Sperm DNA integrity in testicular cancer patients. Hum Reprod. 2006;21:3199–205.
44. Ribas-Maynou J, García-Peiró A, Fernández-Encinas A, Abad C, Amengual MJ, Prada E, et al. Comprehensive analysis of sperm DNA fragmentation by five different assays: TUNEL assay, SCSA, SCD test and alkaline and neutral Comet assay. Andrology. 2013;1:715–22.
45. Simon L, Liu L, Murphy K, Ge S, Hotaling J, Aston KI, et al. Comparative analysis of three sperm DNA damage assays and sperm nuclear protein content in couples undergoing assisted reproduction treatment. Hum Reprod. 2014;29:904–17.

46. Jeng HA, Pan CH, Chao MR, Lin WY. Sperm DNA oxidative damage and DNA adducts. Mutat Res Genet Toxicol Environ Mutagen. 2015;794:75–82.
47. Stahl PJ, Cogan C, Mehta A, Bolyakov A, Paduch DA, Goldstein M. Concordance among sperm deoxyribonucleic acid integrity assays and semen parameters. Fertil Steril. 2015;104:56–61.e1.
48. De Iuliis GN, Thomson LK, Mitchell LA, Finnie JM, Koppers AJ, Hedges A, et al. DNA damage in human spermatozoa is highly correlated with the efficiency of chromatin remodeling and the formation of 8-hydroxy-2′-deoxyguanosine, a marker of oxidative stress. Biol Reprod. 2009;81:517–24.
49. Aitken RJ, De Iuliis GN, Finnie JM, Hedges A, McLachlan RI. Analysis of the relationships between oxidative stress, DNA damage and sperm vitality in a patient population: development of diagnostic criteria. Hum Reprod. 2010;25:2415–26.
50. Thomson LK, Fleming SD, Aitken RJ, De Iuliis GN, Zieschang JA, Clark AM. Cryopreservation-induced human sperm DNA damage is predominantly mediated by oxidative stress rather than apoptosis. Hum Reprod. 2009;24:2061–70.
51. Thomson LK, Zieschang JA, Clark AM. Oxidative deoxyribonucleic acid damage in sperm has a negative impact on clinical pregnancy rate in intrauterine insemination but not intracytoplasmic sperm injection cycles. Fertil Steril. 2011;96:843–7.
52. Evenson DP, Jost LK, Baer RK, Turner TW, Schrader SM. Individuality of DNA denaturation patterns in human sperm as measured by the sperm chromatin structure assay. Reprod Toxicol. 1991;5:115–25.
53. Zini A, Kamal K, Phang D, Willis J, Jarvi K. Biologic variability of sperm DNA denaturation in infertile men. Urology. 2001;58:258–61.
54. Giwercman A, Richthoff J, Hjøllund H, Bonde JP, Jepson K, Frohm B, et al. Correlation between sperm motility and sperm chromatin structure assay parameters. Fertil Steril. 2003;80:1404–12.
55. Sharma RK, Sabanegh E, Mahfouz R, Gupta S, Thiyagarajan A, Agarwal A. TUNEL as a test for sperm DNA damage in the evaluation of male infertility. Urology. 2010;76:1380–6.
56. Oleszczuk K, Giwercman A, Bungum M. Intra-individual variation of the sperm chromatin structure assay DNA fragmentation index in men from infertile couples. Hum Reprod. 2011;26:3244–8.
57. Belloc S, Benkhalifa M, Cohen-Bacrie M, Dalleac A, Amar E, Zini A. Sperm deoxyribonucleic acid damage in normozoospermic men is related to age and sperm progressive motility. Fertil Steril. 2014;101:1588–93.
58. Muratori M, Marchiani S, Tamburrino L, Cambi M, Lotti F, Natali I, et al. DNA fragmentation in brighter sperm predicts male fertility independently from age and semen parameters. Fertil Steril. 2015;104:582–90.e4.
59. Jurewicz J, Hanke W, Radwan M, Bonde JP. Environmental factors and semen quality. Int J Occup Med Environ Health. 2009;22:305–29.
60. Bonde JP. Male reproductive organs are at risk from environmental hazards. Asian J Androl. 2010b;12:152–6.
61. Delbès G, Hales BF, Robaire B. Toxicants and human sperm chromatin integrity. Mol Hum Reprod. 2010;16:14–22.
62. Meeker JD. Exposure to environmental endocrine disrupting compounds and men's health. Maturitas. 2010;66:236–41.
63. Pacey AA. Environmental and lifestyle factors associated with sperm DNA damage. Hum Fertil (Camb). 2010;13:189–93.
64. Aitken RJ. Age, the environment and our reproductive future: bonking baby boomers and the future of sex. Reproduction. 2014;147:S1–S11.
65. Vested A, Giwercman A, Bonde JP, Toft G. Persistent organic pollutants and male reproductive health. Asian J Androl. 2014;16:71–80.
66. Juul A, Almstrup K, Andersson AM, Jensen TK, Jørgensen N, Main KM, et al. Possible fetal determinants of male infertility. Nat Rev Endocrinol. 2014;10:553–62.

67. Skakkebaek NE, Rajpert-De Meyts E, Buck Louis GM, Toppari J, Andersson AM, Eisenberg ML, et al. Male reproductive disorders and fertility trends: influences of environment and genetic susceptibility. Physiol Rev. 2016;96:55–97.
68. Håkonsen LB, Spanò M, Bonde JP, Olsen J, Thulstrup AM, Ernst E, et al. Exposures that may affect sperm DNA integrity: two decades of follow-up in a pregnancy cohort. Reprod Toxicol. 2012;33:316–21.
69. Dai JB, Wang ZX, Qiao ZD. The hazardous effects of tobacco smoking on male fertility. Asian J Androl. 2015;17:954–60.
70. Harlev A, Agarwal A, Gunes SO, Shetty A, du Plessis SS. Smoking and male infertility: an evidence-based review. World J Mens Health. 2015;33:143–60.
71. Fraga CG, Motchnik PA, Wyrobek AJ, Rempel DM, Ames BN. Smoking and low antioxidant levels increase oxidative damage to sperm DNA. Mutat Res. 1996;351:199–203.
72. Zenzes MT. Smoking and reproduction: gene damage to human gametes and embryos. Hum Reprod Update. 2000;6:122–31.
73. Laubenthal J, Zlobinskaya O, Poterlowicz K, Baumgartner A, Gdula MR, Fthenou E, et al. Cigarette smoke-induced transgenerational alterations in genome stability in cord blood of human F1 offspring. FASEB J. 2012;26:3946–56.
74. Macdonald AA, Stewart AW, Farquhar CM. Body mass index in relation to semen quality and reproductive hormones in New Zealand men: a cross-sectional study in fertility clinics. Hum Reprod. 2013;28:3178–87.
75. Sermondade N, Faure C, Fezeu L, Shayeb AG, Bonde JP, Jensen TK, et al. BMI in relation to sperm count: an updated systematic review and collaborative meta-analysis. Hum Reprod Update. 2013;19:221–31.
76. Eisenberg ML, Kim S, Chen Z, Sundaram R, Schisterman EF, Buck Louis GM. The relationship between male BMI and waist circumference on semen quality: data from the LIFE study. Hum Reprod. 2014;29:193–200.
77. Andersen JM, Herning H, Aschim EL, Hjelmesæth J, Mala T, Hanevik HI, et al. Body Mass Index is associated with impaired semen characteristics and reduced levels of anti-Müllerian hormone across a wide weight range. PLoS One. 2015;10:e0130210.
78. Kort HI, Massey JB, Elsner CW, Mitchell-Leef D, Shapiro DB, Witt MA, et al. Impact of body mass index values on sperm quantity and quality. J Androl. 2006;27:450–2.
79. Chavarro JE, Toth TL, Wright DL, Meeker JD, Hauser R. Body mass index in relation to semen quality, sperm DNA integrity, and serum reproductive hormone levels among men attending an infertility clinic. Fertil Steril. 2010;93:2222–31.
80. Fariello RM, Pariz JR, Spaine DM, Cedenho AP, Bertolla RP, Fraietta R. Association between obesity and alteration of sperm DNA integrity and mitochondrial activity. BJU Int. 2012;110:863–7.
81. La Vignera S, Condorelli RA, Vicari E, Calogero AE. Negative effect of increased body weight on sperm conventional and nonconventional flow cytometric sperm parameters. J Androl. 2012;33:53–8.
82. Dupont C, Faure C, Sermondade N, Boubaya M, Eustache F, Clément P, et al. Obesity leads to higher risk of sperm DNA damage in infertile patients. Asian J Androl. 2013;15:622–5.
83. Smit M, Romijn JC, Wildhagen MF, Weber RF, Dohle GR. Sperm chromatin structure is associated with the quality of spermatogenesis in infertile patients. Fertil Steril. 2010;94:1748–52.
84. Hammiche F, Laven JS, Boxmeer JC, Dohle GR, Steegers EA, Steegers-Theunissen RP. Sperm quality decline among men below 60 years of age undergoing IVF or ICSI treatment. J Androl. 2011;32:70–6.
85. Håkonsen LB, Thulstrup AM, Aggerholm AS, Olsen J, Bonde JP, Andersen CY, et al. Does weight loss improve semen quality and reproductive hormones? Results from a cohort of severely obese men. Reprod Health. 2011;8:24.
86. Rybar R, Kopecka V, Prinosilova P, Markova P, Rubes J. Male obesity and age in relationship to semen parameters and sperm chromatin integrity. Andrologia. 2011;43:286–91.
87. Tunc O, Bakos HW, Tremellen K. Impact of body mass index on seminal oxidative stress. Andrologia. 2011;43:121–8.

88. Thomsen L, Humaidan P, Bungum L, Bungum M. The impact of male overweight on semen quality and outcome of assisted reproduction. Asian J Androl. 2014;16:749–54.
89. Bandel I, Bungum M, Richtoff J, Malm J, Axelsson J, Pedersen HS, et al. No association between body mass index and sperm DNA integrity. Hum Reprod. 2015;30:1704–13.
90. Sun JG, Jurisicova A, Casper RF. Detection of deoxyribonucleic acid fragmentation in human sperm: correlation with fertilization in vitro. Biol Reprod. 1997;56:602–7.
91. De Jonge C, LaFromboise M, Bosmans E, Ombelet W, Cox A, Nijs M. Influence of the abstinence period on human sperm quality. Fertil Steril. 2004;82:57–65.
92. Spanò M, Kolstad AH, Larsen SB, Cordelli E, Leter G, Giwercman A, et al. The applicability of the flow cytometric sperm chromatin structure assay in epidemiological studies. Asclepios Hum Reprod. 1998;13:2495–505.
93. Spanò M, Bonde JP, Hjøllund HI, Kolstad HA, Cordelli E, Leter G. Sperm chromatin damage impairs human fertility. The Danish First Pregnancy Planner Study Team. Fertil Steril. 2000;73:43–50.
94. Spanò M, Toft G, Hagmar L, Eleuteri P, Rescia M, Rignell-Hydbom A, et al. Exposure to PCB and p, p′-DDE in European and Inuit populations: impact on human sperm chromatin integrity. Hum Reprod. 2005;20:3488–99.
95. Bonde JP, Joffe M, Apostoli P, Dale A, Kiss P, Spanò M, et al. Sperm count and chromatin structure in men exposed to inorganic lead: lowest adverse effect levels. Occup Environ Med. 2002;59:234–42.
96. Richthoff J, Spanò M, Giwercman YL, Frohm B, Jepson K, Malm J, et al. The impact of testicular and accessory sex gland function on sperm chromatin integrity as assessed by the sperm chromatin structure assay (SCSA). Hum Reprod. 2002;17:3162–9.
97. Erenpreiss J, Bungum M, Spanò M, Elzanaty S, Orbidans J, Giwercman A. Intra-individual variation in sperm chromatin structure assay parameters in men from infertile couples: clinical implications. Hum Reprod. 2006;21:2061–4.
98. Wyrobek AJ, Eskenazi B, Young S, Arnheim N, Tiemann-Boege I, Jabs EW, et al. Advancing age has differential effects on DNA damage, chromatin integrity, gene mutations, and aneuploidies in sperm. Proc Natl Acad Sci U S A. 2006;103:9601–6.
99. Bakos HW, Thompson JG, Feil D, Lane M. Sperm DNA damage is associated with assisted reproductive technology pregnancy. Int J Androl. 2008;31:518–26.
100. Cohen-Bacrie P, Belloc S, Ménézo YJ, Clement P, Hamidi J, Benkhalifa M. Correlation between DNA damage and sperm parameters: a prospective study of 1,633 patients. Fertil Steril. 2009;91:1801–5.
101. Gosálvez J, González-Martínez M, López-Fernández C, Fernández JL, Sánchez-Martín P. Shorter abstinence decreases sperm deoxyribonucleic acid fragmentation in ejaculate. Fertil Steril. 2011;96:1083–6.
102. Sánchez-Martín P, Sánchez-Martín F, González-Martínez M, Gosálvez J. Increased pregnancy after reduced male abstinence. Syst Biol Reprod Med. 2013;59:256–60.
103. Stone BA, Alex A, Werlin LB, Marrs RP. Age thresholds for changes in semen parameters in men. Fertil Steril. 2013;100:952–8.
104. Johnson SL, Dunleavy J, Gemmell NJ, Nakagawa S. Consistent age-dependent declines in human semen quality: a systematic review and meta-analysis. Ageing Res Rev. 2015;19:22–33.
105. Sharma R, Agarwal A, Rohra VK, Assidi M, Abu-Elmagd M, Turki RF. Effects of increased paternal age on sperm quality, reproductive outcome and associated epigenetic risks to offspring. Reprod Biol Endocrinol. 2015;13:35.
106. Sartorius GA, Nieschlag E. Paternal age and reproduction. Hum Reprod Update. 2010;16:65–79.
107. Kong A, Frigge ML, Masson G, Besenbacher S, Sulem P, Magnusson G, et al. Rate of de novo mutations and the importance of father's age to disease risk. Nature. 2012;488:471–5.
108. Nijs M, De Jonge C, Cox A, Janssen M, Bosmans E, Ombelet W. Correlation between male age, WHO sperm parameters, DNA fragmentation, chromatin packaging and outcome in assisted reproduction technology. Andrologia. 2011;43:174–9.

109. Migliore L, Naccarati A, Zanello A, Scarpato R, Bramanti L, Mariani M. Assessment of sperm DNA integrity in workers exposed to styrene. Hum Reprod. 2002;17:2912–8.
110. Singh NP, Muller CH, Berger RE. Effects of age on DNA double-strand breaks and apoptosis in human sperm. Fertil Steril. 2003;80:1420–30.
111. Rignell-Hydbom A, Rylander L, Giwercman A, Jönsson BA, Lindh C, Eleuteri P, et al. Exposure to PCBs and p,p′-DDE and human sperm chromatin integrity. Environ Health Perspect. 2005;113:175–9.
112. Schmid TE, Eskenazi B, Baumgartner A, Marchetti F, Young S, Weldon R, et al. The effects of male age on sperm DNA damage in healthy non-smokers. Hum Reprod. 2007;22:180–7.
113. Horta F, Madariaga M, García A, Hartel S, Smith R. Association of age with sperm DNA fragmentation. Rev Med Chil. 2011;139:306–12.
114. Morris ID, Ilott S, Dixon L, Brison DR. The spectrum of DNA damage in human sperm assessed by single cell gel electrophoresis (Comet assay) and its relationship to fertilization and embryo development. Hum Reprod. 2002;17:990–8.
115. Hauser R, Singh NP, Chen Z, Pothier L, Altshul L. Lack of an association between environmental exposure to polychlorinated biphenyls and p,p′-DDE and DNA damage in human sperm measured using the neutral comet assay. Hum Reprod. 2003;18:2525–33.
116. Trisini AT, Singh NP, Duty SM, Hauser R. Relationship between human semen parameters and deoxyribonucleic acid damage assessed by the neutral comet assay. Fertil Steril. 2004;82:1623–32.
117. Moskovtsev SI, Willis J, Mullen JB. Age-related decline in sperm deoxyribonucleic acid integrity in patients evaluated for male infertility. Fertil Steril. 2006;85:496–9.
118. Moskovtsev SI, Willis J, White J, Mullen JB. Sperm DNA damage: correlation to severity of semen abnormalities. Urology. 2009;74:789–93.
119. Moskovtsev SI, Mullen JB, Lecker I, Jarvi K, White J, Roberts M, et al. Frequency and severity of sperm DNA damage in patients with confirmed cases of male infertility of different aetiologies. Reprod Biomed Online. 2010;20:759–63.
120. Plastira K, Msaouel P, Angelopoulou R, Zanioti K, Plastiras A, Pothos A, et al. The effects of age on DNA fragmentation, chromatin packaging and conventional semen parameters in spermatozoa of oligoasthenoteratozoospermic patients. J Assist Reprod Genet. 2007;24:437–43.
121. Vagnini L, Baruffi RL, Mauri AL, Petersen CG, Massaro FC, Pontes A, et al. The effects of male age on sperm DNA damage in an infertile population. Reprod Biomed Online. 2007;15:514–9.
122. Belloc S, Benkhalifa M, Junca AM, Dumont M, Bacrie PC, Ménézo Y. Paternal age and sperm DNA decay: discrepancy between chromomycin and aniline blue staining. Reprod Biomed Online. 2009;19:264–9.
123. Silva LF, Oliveira JB, Petersen CG, Mauri AL, Massaro FC, Cavagna M, et al. The effects of male age on sperm analysis by motile sperm organelle morphology examination (MSOME). Reprod Biol Endocrinol. 2012;10:19.
124. Das M, Al-Hathal N, San-Gabriel M, Phillips S, Kadoch IJ, Bissonnette F, et al. High prevalence of isolated sperm DNA damage in infertile men with advanced paternal age. J Assist Reprod Genet. 2013;30:843–8.
125. Saleh RA, Agarwal A, Sharma RK, Said TM, Sikka SC, Thomas AJ Jr. Evaluation of nuclear DNA damage in spermatozoa from infertile men with varicocele. Fertil Steril. 2003;80:1431–6.
126. Enciso M, Muriel L, Fernández JL, Goyanes V, Segrelles E, Marcos M, et al. Infertile men with varicocele show a high relative proportion of sperm cells with intense nuclear damage level, evidenced by the sperm chromatin dispersion test. J Androl. 2006;27:106–11.
127. Smith R, Kaune H, Parodi D, Madariaga M, Rios R, Morales I, et al. Increased sperm DNA damage in patients with varicocele: relationship with seminal oxidative stress. Hum Reprod. 2006;21:986–93.
128. Bertolla RP, Cedenho AP, Hassun Filho PA, Lima SB, Ortiz V, Srougi M. Sperm nuclear DNA fragmentation in adolescents with varicocele. Fertil Steril. 2006;85:625–8.

129. Blumer CG, Fariello RM, Restelli AE, Spaine DM, Bertolla RP, Cedenho AP. Sperm nuclear DNA fragmentation and mitochondrial activity in men with varicocele. Fertil Steril. 2008;90:1716–22.
130. Blumer CG, Restelli AE, Giudice PT, Soler TB, Fraietta R, Nichi M, et al. Effect of varicocele on sperm function and semen oxidative stress. BJU Int. 2012;109:259–65.
131. Cho CL, Esteves SC, Agarwal A. Novel insights into the pathophysiology of varicocele and its association with reactive oxygen species and sperm DNA fragmentation. Asian J Androl. 2016;18:186–93.
132. Zini A, Blumenfeld A, Libman J, Willis J. Beneficial effect of microsurgical varicocelectomy on human sperm DNA integrity. Hum Reprod. 2005;20:1018–21.
133. Werthman P, Wixon R, Kasperson K, Evenson DP. Significant decrease in sperm deoxyribonucleic acid fragmentation after varicocelectomy. Fertil Steril. 2008;90:1800–4.
134. Nasr-Esfahani MH, Abasi H, Razavi S, Ashrafi S, Tavalaee M. Varicocelectomy: semen parameters and protamine deficiency. Int J Androl. 2009;32:115–22.
135. Moskovtsev SI, Lecker I, Mullen JB, Jarvi K, Willis J, White J, et al. Cause-specific treatment in patients with high sperm DNA damage resulted in significant DNA improvement. Syst Biol Reprod Med. 2009b;55:109–15.
136. Barekat F, Tavalaee M, Deemeh MR, Bahreinian M, Azadi L, Abbasi H, et al. A preliminary study: N-acetyl-L-cysteine improves semen quality following varicocelectomy. Int J Fertil Steril. 2016;10:120–6.
137. Gallegos G, Ramos B, Santiso R, Goyanes V, Gosálvez J, Fernández JL. Sperm DNA fragmentation in infertile men with genitourinary infection by Chlamydia trachomatis and Mycoplasma. Fertil Steril. 2008;90:328–34.
138. Kaspersen MD, Bungum M, Fedder J, Bonde J, Larsen PB, Ingerslev JH, et al. No increased sperm DNA fragmentation index in semen containing human papillomavirus or herpesvirus. Andrology. 2013;1:361–4.
139. Brackett NL, Ibrahim E, Grotas JA, Aballa TC, Lynne CM. Higher sperm DNA damage in semen from men with spinal cord injuries compared with controls. J Androl. 2008;29:93–9.
140. Restelli AE, Bertolla RP, Spaine DM, Miotto A Jr, Borrelli M Jr, Cedenho AP. Quality and functional aspects of sperm retrieved through assisted ejaculation in men with spinal cord injury. Fertil Steril. 2009;91:819–25.
141. Qiu Y, Wang LG, Zhang LH, Zhang AD, Wang ZY. Quality of sperm obtained by penile vibratory stimulation and percutaneous vasal sperm aspiration in men with spinal cord injury. J Androl. 2012;33:1036–46.
142. Agbaje IM, Rogers DA, McVicar CM, McClure N, Atkinson AB, Mallidis C, et al. Insulin dependant diabetes mellitus: implications for male reproductive function. Hum Reprod. 2007;22:1871–7.
143. Evenson DP, Jost LK, Corzett M, Balhorn R. Characteristics of human sperm chromatin structure following an episode of influenza and high fever: a case study. J Androl. 2000;21:739–46.
144. Sergerie M, Mieusset R, Croute F, Daudin M, Bujan L. High risk of temporary alteration of semen parameters after recent acute febrile illness. Fertil Steril. 2007;88:970.e1–7.
145. Apedaile AE, Garrett C, Liu DY, Clarke GN, Johnston SA, Baker HW. Flow cytometry and microscopic acridine orange test: relationship with standard semen analysis. Reprod Biomed Online. 2004;8:398–407.
146. Virro MR, Larson-Cook KL, Evenson DP. Sperm chromatin structure assay (SCSA) parameters are related to fertilization, blastocyst development, and ongoing pregnancy in in vitro fertilization and intracytoplasmic sperm injection cycles. Fertil Steril. 2004;81:1289–95.
147. Boe-Hansen GB, Fedder J, Ersbøll AK, Christensen P. The sperm chromatin structure assay as a diagnostic tool in the human fertility clinic. Hum Reprod. 2006;21:1576–82.
148. de Jager C, Aneck-Hahn NH, Bornman MS, Farias P, Leter G, Eleuteri P, et al. Sperm chromatin integrity in DDT-exposed young men living in a malaria area in the Limpopo Province. S Afr Hum Reprod. 2009;24:2429–38.
149. Benchaib M, Lornage J, Mazoyer C, Lejeune H, Salle B, François GJ. Sperm deoxyribonucleic acid fragmentation as a prognostic indicator of assisted reproductive technology outcome. Fertil Steril. 2007;87:93–100.

150. Henkel R, Kierspel E, Hajimohammad M, Stalf T, Hoogendijk C, Mehnert C, et al. DNA fragmentation of spermatozoa and assisted reproduction technology. Reprod Biomed Online. 2003;7:477–84.
151. Bungum M, Spano M, Humaidan P, Eleuteri P, Rescia M, Giwercman A. Sperm chromatin structure assay parameters measured after density gradient centrifugation are not predictive for the outcome of ART. Hum Reprod. 2008;23:4–10.
152. Simon L, Lewis SEM. Sperm DNA damage or progressive motility: which one is the better predictor of fertilization in vitro? Syst Biol Reprod Med. 2011;57:133–8.
153. Spanò M, Cordelli E, Leter G, Lombardo F, Lenzi A, Gandini L. Nuclear chromatin variations in human spermatozoa undergoing swimming up and cryoconservation evaluated by the flow cytometric sperm chromatin structure assay. Mol Hum Reprod. 1999;5:29–37.
154. Jackson RE, Bormann CL, Hassun PA, Rocha AM, Motta EL, Serafini PC, et al. Effects of semen storage and separation techniques on sperm DNA fragmentation. Fertil Steril. 2010;94:2626–30.
155. Avendaño C, Oehninger S. DNA fragmentation in morphologically normal spermatozoa: how much should we be concerned in the ICSI era? J Androl. 2011;32:356–63.
156. Meeker JD, Singh NP, Hauser R. Serum concentrations of estradiol and free T4 are inversely correlated with sperm DNA damage in men from an infertility clinic. J Androl. 2008;29:379–88.
157. Irvine DS, Twigg JP, Gordon EL, Fulton N, Milne PA, Aitken RJ. DNA integrity in human spermatozoa: relationships with semen quality. J Androl. 2000;21:33–44.
158. de Paula TS, Bertolla RP, Spaine DM, Cunha MA, Schor N, Cedenho AP. Effect of cryopreservation on sperm apoptotic deoxyribonucleic acid fragmentation in patients with oligozoospermia. Fertil Steril. 2006;86:597–600.
159. Mehdi M, Khantouche L, Ajina M, Saad A. Detection of DNA fragmentation in human spermatozoa: correlation with semen parameters. Andrologia. 2009;41:383–6.
160. Høst E, Lindenberg S, Smidt-Jensen S. The role of DNA strand breaks in human spermatozoa used for IVF and ICSI. Acta Obstet Gynecol Scand. 2000;79:559–63.
161. Hammadeh ME, Zeginiadov T, Rosenbaum P, Georg T, Schmidt W, Strehler E. Predictive value of sperm chromatin condensation (aniline blue staining) in the assessment of male fertility. Arch Androl. 2001;46:99–104.
162. Zini A, Nam RK, Mak V, Phang D, Jarvi K. Influence of initial semen quality on the integrity of human sperm DNA following semen processing. Fertil Steril. 2000;74:824–7.
163. Zini A, Bielecki R, Phang D, Zenzes MT. Correlations between two markers of sperm DNA integrity, DNA denaturation and DNA fragmentation, in fertile and infertile men. Fertil Steril. 2001;75:674–7.
164. Zini A, Kamal KM, Phang D. Free thiols in human spermatozoa: correlation with sperm DNA integrity. Urology. 2001;58:80–4.
165. Zini A, Fischer MA, Sharir S, Shayegan B, Phang D, Jarvi K. Prevalence of abnormal sperm DNA denaturation in fertile and infertile men. Urology. 2002;60:1069–72.
166. Fischer MA, Willis J, Zini A. Human sperm DNA integrity: correlation with sperm cytoplasmic droplets. Urology. 2003;61:207–11.
167. Saleh RA, Agarwal A, Nada EA, El-Tonsy MH, Sharma RK, Meyer A, Nelson DR, Thomas AJ. Negative effects of increased sperm DNA damage in relation to seminal oxidative stress in men with idiopathic and male factor infertility. Fertil Steril. 2003;79(Suppl 3):1597–605.
168. Schmid TE, Kamischke A, Bollwein H, Nieschlag E, Brinkworth MH. Genetic damage in oligozoospermic patients detected by fluorescence in-situ hybridization, inverse restriction site mutation assay, sperm chromatin structure assay and the Comet assay. Hum Reprod. 2003;18:1474–80.
169. McVicar CM, McClure N, Williamson K, Dalzell LH, Lewis SE. Incidence of Fas positivity and deoxyribonucleic acid double-stranded breaks in human ejaculated sperm. Fertil Steril. 2004;81(Suppl 1):767–74.
170. Sergerie M, Laforest G, Bujan L, Bissonnette F, Bleau G. Sperm DNA fragmentation: threshold value in male fertility. Hum Reprod. 2005a;20:3446–51.

171. Aoki VW, Emery BR, Liu L, Carrell DT. Protamine levels vary between individual sperm cells of infertile human males and correlate with viability and DNA integrity. J Androl. 2006;27:890–8.
172. Nicopoullos JD, Gilling-Smith C, Almeida PA, Homa S, Norman-Taylor JQ, Ramsay JW. Sperm DNA fragmentation in subfertile men: the effect on the outcome of intracytoplasmic sperm injection and correlation with sperm variables. BJU Int. 2008;101:1553–60.
173. Shamsi MB, Venkatesh S, Tanwar M, Talwar P, Sharma RK, Dhawan A, et al. DNA integrity and semen quality in men with low seminal antioxidant levels. Mutat Res. 2009;665:29–36.
174. Tsarev I, Bungum M, Giwercman A, Erenpreisa J, Ebessen T, Ernst E, et al. Evaluation of male fertility potential by Toluidine Blue test for sperm chromatin structure assessment. Hum Reprod. 2009;24:1569–74.
175. Bellver J, Meseguer M, Muriel L, García-Herrero S, Barreto MA, Garda AL, et al. Y chromosome microdeletions, sperm DNA fragmentation and sperm oxidative stress as causes of recurrent spontaneous abortion of unknown etiology. Hum Reprod. 2010;25:1713–21.
176. Giwercman A, Lindstedt L, Larsson M, Bungum M, Spano M, Levine RJ, et al. Sperm chromatin structure assay as an independent predictor of fertility in vivo: a case-control study. Int J Androl. 2010;33:e221–7.
177. Tang SS, Gao H, Zhao Y, Ma S. Aneuploidy and DNA fragmentation in morphologically abnormal sperm. Int J Androl. 2010;33:e163–79.
178. Zhang LH, Qiu Y, Wang KH, Wang Q, Tao G, Wang LG. Measurement of sperm DNA fragmentation using bright-field microscopy: comparison between sperm chromatin dispersion test and terminal uridine nick-end labeling assay. Fertil Steril. 2010;94:1027–32.
179. Brahem S, Mehdi M, Elghezal H, Saad A. Detection of DNA fragmentation and meiotic segregation in human with isolated teratozoospermia. J Assist Reprod Genet. 2011;28:41–8.
180. García-Peiró A, Oliver-Bonet M, Navarro J, Abad C, Guitart M, Amengual MJ, et al. Dynamics of sperm DNA fragmentation in patients carrying structurally rearranged chromosomes. Int J Androl. 2011;34:e546–53.
181. Simon L, Lutton D, McManus J, Lewis SE. Sperm DNA damage measured by the alkaline Comet assay as an independent predictor of male infertility and in vitro fertilization success. Fertil Steril. 2011;95:652–7.
182. Faduola P, Kolade CO. Sperm chromatin structure assay results in Nigerian men with unexplained infertility. Clin Exp Reprod Med. 2015;42:101–5.
183. Evenson DP, Jost LK, Marshall D, Zinaman MJ, Clegg E, Purvis K, et al. Utility of the sperm chromatin structure assay as a diagnostic and prognostic tool in the human fertility clinic. Hum Reprod. 1999;14:1039–49.
184. Filatov MV, Semenova EV, Vorob'eva OA, Leont'eva OA, Drobchenko EA. Relationship between abnormal sperm chromatin packing and IVF results. Mol Hum Reprod. 1999;5:825–30.
185. Tomlinson MJ, Moffatt O, Manicardi GC, Bizzaro D, Afnan M, Sakkas D. Interrelationships between seminal parameters and sperm nuclear DNA damage before and after density gradient centrifugation: implications for assisted conception. Hum Reprod. 2001;16:2160–5.
186. Erenpreisa J, Erenpreiss J, Freivalds T, Slaidina M, Krampe R, Butikova J, et al. Toluidine blue test for sperm DNA integrity and elaboration of image cytometry algorithm. Cytometry A. 2003;52:19–27.
187. Liu CH, Tsao HM, Cheng TC, Wu HM, Huang CC, Chen CI, et al. DNA fragmentation, mitochondrial dysfunction and chromosomal aneuploidy in the spermatozoa of oligoasthenoteratozoospermic males. J Assist Reprod Genet. 2004;21:119–26.
188. Huang CC, Lin DP, Tsao HM, Cheng TC, Liu CH, Lee MS. Sperm DNA fragmentation negatively correlates with velocity and fertilization rates but might not affect pregnancy rates. Fertil Steril. 2005;84:130–40.
189. Erenpreiss J, Elzanaty S, Giwercman A. Sperm DNA damage in men from infertile couples. Asian J Androl. 2008;10:786–90.
190. Song GJ, Norkus EP, Lewis V. Relationship between seminal ascorbic acid and sperm DNA integrity in infertile men. Int J Androl. 2006;29:569–75.

191. Oleszczuk K, Augustinsson L, Bayat N, Giwercman A, Bungum M. Prevalence of high DNA fragmentation index in male partners of unexplained infertile couples. Andrology. 2013;1:357–60.
192. World Health Organization. WHO laboratory manual for the examination of human semen and sperm–cervical mucus interaction. 5th ed. Cambridge: Cambridge University Press; 1999.
193. Bonde JPE. Semen analysis from an epidemiologic perspective. Asian J Androl. 2010;12:91–4.
194. Skakkebaek NE. Normal reference ranges for semen quality and their relations to fecundity. Asian J Androl. 2010;12:95–8.
195. Esteves SC, Zini A, Aziz N, Alvarez JG, Sabanegh ES, Agarwal A. Critical appraisal of World Health Organization's new reference values for human semen characteristics and effect on diagnosis and treatment of subfertile men. Urology. 2012;79:16–22.
196. Murray KS, James A, McGeady JB, Reed ML, Kuang WW, Nangia AK. The effect of the new 2010 World Health Organization criteria for semen analyses on male infertility. Fertil Steril. 2012;98:1428–31.
197. Auger J, Eustache F, Ducot B, Blandin T, Daudin M, Diaz I, et al. Intra- and inter-individual variability in human sperm concentration, motility and vitality assessment during a workshop involving ten laboratories. Hum Reprod. 2000;15:2360–8.
198. Francavilla F, Barbonetti A, Necozione S, Santucci R, Cordeschi G, Macerola B, et al. Within-subject variation of seminal parameters in men with infertile marriages. Int J Androl. 2007;30:174–81.
199. Leushuis E, van der Steeg JW, Steures P, Repping S, Bossuyt PM, Blankenstein MA, et al. Reproducibility and reliability of repeated semen analyses in male partners of subfertile couples. Fertil Steril. 2010;94:2631–5.
200. Keel BA. Within- and between-subject variation in semen parameters in infertile men and normal semen donors. Fertil Steril. 2006;85:128–34.
201. Mayorga-Torres BJ, Camargo M, Agarwal A, du Plessis SS, Cadavid ÁP, Cardona Maya WD. Influence of ejaculation frequency on seminal parameters. Reprod Biol Endocrinol. 2015;13:47.
202. Sergerie M, Mieusset R, Daudin M, Thonneau P, Bujan L. Ten-year variation in semen parameters and sperm deoxyribonucleic acid integrity in a healthy fertile man. Fertil Steril. 2006;86:1513.e11–8.
203. Sergerie M, Laforest G, Boulanger K, Bissonnette F, Bleau G. Longitudinal study of sperm DNA fragmentation as measured by terminal uridine nick end-labelling assay. Hum Reprod. 2005;20:1921–7.
204. Evenson DP, Wixon R. Data analysis of two in vivo fertility studies using Sperm Chromatin Structure Assay-derived DNA fragmentation index vs. pregnancy outcome. Fertil Steril. 2008;90:1229–31.
205. Loft S, Kold-Jensen T, Hjollund NH, Giwercman A, Gyllemborg J, Ernst E, Olsen J, Scheike T, Poulsen HE, Bonde JP. Oxidative DNA damage in human sperm influences time to pregnancy. Hum Reprod. 2003;18:1265–72.
206. Bungum M, Humaidan P, Axmon A, Spano M, Bungum L, Erenpreiss J, et al. Sperm DNA integrity assessment in prediction of assisted reproduction technology outcome. Hum Reprod. 2007;22:174–9.
207. Mitchell LA, De Iuliis GN, Aitken RJ. The TUNEL assay consistently underestimates DNA damage in human spermatozoa and is influenced by DNA compaction and cell vitality: development of an improved methodology. Int J Androl. 2011;34:2–13.
208. Birch Petersen K, Hvidman HW, Forman JL, Pinborg A, Larsen EC, Macklon KT, et al. Ovarian reserve assessment in users of oral contraception seeking fertility advice on their reproductive lifespan. Hum Reprod. 2015;30:2364–75.
209. Zini A, Albert O, Robaire B. Assessing sperm chromatin and DNA damage: clinical importance and development of standards. Andrology. 2014;2:322–5.
210. González-Marín C, Gosálvez J, Roy R. Types, causes, detection and repair of DNA fragmentation in animal and human sperm cells. Int J Mol Sci. 2012;13:14026–52.

211. Anderson D, Schmid TE, Baumgartner A. Male-mediated developmental toxicity. Asian J Androl. 2014;16:81–8.
212. Marchetti F, Wyrobek AJ. Mechanisms and consequences of paternally-transmitted chromosomal abnormalities. Birth Defects Res C Embryo Today. 2005;75:112–29.
213. Marchetti F, Essers J, Kanaar R, Wyrobek AJ. Disruption of maternal DNA repair increases sperm-derived chromosomal aberrations. Proc Natl Acad Sci U S A. 2007;104:17725–9.
214. Marchetti F, Bishop J, Gingerich J, Wyrobek AJ. Meiotic interstrand DNA damage escapes paternal repair and causes chromosomal aberrations in the zygote by maternal misrepair. Sci Rep. 2015;5:768.
215. Fernández-Gonzalez R, Moreira PN, Pérez-Crespo M, Sánchez-Martín M, Ramirez MA, Pericuesta E, et al. Long-term effects of mouse intracytoplasmic sperm injection with DNA-fragmented sperm on health and behavior of adult offspring. Biol Reprod. 2008;78:761–72.
216. Pérez-Crespo M, Moreira P, Pintado B, Gutiérrez-Adán A. Factors from damaged sperm affect its DNA integrity and its ability to promote embryo implantation in mice. J Androl. 2008;29:47–54.
217. Sakkas D, Ramalingam M, Garrido N, Barratt CL. Sperm selection in natural conception: what can we learn from Mother Nature to improve assisted reproduction outcomes? Hum Reprod Update. 2015;21:711–26.
218. Carrell DT, Aston KI, Oliva R, Emery BR, De Jonge CJ. The "omics" of human male infertility: integrating big data in a systems biology approach. Cell Tissue Res. 2016;363:295–312.

Chapter 21
Sperm DNA and ART (IUI, IVF, ICSI) Pregnancy

Mona Bungum and Krzysztof Oleszczuk

21.1 Introduction

Up to one fourth of all couples in reproductive age are seeking medical help for involuntary childlessness. However, by the use of assisted reproductive techniques (ART), intrauterine insemination (IUI), in vitro fertilization (IVF) or intracytoplasmic sperm injection (ICSI) now, almost every involuntarily childless couple has a realistic hope of parenting. In 1992, the introduction of ICSI represented a breakthrough in the treatment of infertility [1, 2]. The indication of ICSI has been expanding from treatment for severe male factor infertility to, nowadays, couples without a significant male factor. However, despite all the advancement, ART results have been relatively stable rate during the last decades. One reason for this can be a lack of methods to identify the most effective type of ART treatment in a given couple.

Traditionally, diagnosis of male infertility is based on the conventional sperm parameters including concentration, motility and morphology. The criteria for normality, set by the WHO [3], are however claimed to be poorly standardized, subjective and not good predictors of fertility. A search for better predictors of male fertility has led to a growing focus on the genomic integrity of sperm. Several methods to assess sperm DNA damage have been developed. Although many questions remain unanswered, it is now well documented that sperm DNA integrity is a good marker of male fertility, alone or in combination with the traditional semen parameters, in natural conception as well as in ART. During the present chapter, the role of sperm chromatin integrity in ART will be reviewed.

M. Bungum (✉)
Reproductive Medicine Centre, Malmö University Hospital, Malmö, Sweden
e-mail: mona.bungum@med.lu.se

K. Oleszczuk
Reproductive Medicine Centre, Skåne University Hospital, Malmö, Sweden

A. Zini, A. Agarwal (eds.), *A Clinician's Guide to Sperm DNA and Chromatin Damage*, https://doi.org/10.1007/978-3-319-71815-6_21

21.2 Assisted Reproductive Techniques (ART)

The term ART covers medical treatments where gametes are handled outside the body, either sperm alone as in IUI or oocytes, spermatozoa and embryos as in IVF and ICSI [4]. The simplest and often first choice of ART treatment used in unexplained infertility, ovulatory dysfunction and milder forms of male subfertility is IUI. Following hormone stimulation of the female partner, prepared spermatozoa is inseminated into the women's uterus. IVF or ICSI is used in other indications [5]. Oocytes are fertilized by sperm in vitro, either by co-incubating around 25,000–150,000 sperm together with the oocytes as in IVF or by injecting one single spermatozoon directly into the cytoplasm of the oocyte as in ICSI. Two to 5 days later, the pre-embryo(s) is transferred to the woman's uterus. Around 25–30% of the couples per cycle will succeed having a child.

21.3 Traditional Predictors of ART Outcome

The best predictor of ART outcome is female age [6, 7]. There has been a continuous search for other parameters able to assess fertility capacity; however, none have been shown to be powerful. For instance, a panel of other sperm function tests have been suggested, such as antisperm antibody test, vitality staining, hypoosmotic swelling test, biochemical analysis, sperm penetration assay, hemizona assay, reactive oxygen species (ROS) tests and computer-assisted sperm analysis (CASA). However, the clinical value of all these tests has been questioned [5].

In ART, semen samples are normally prepared by a swim-up or density gradient centrifugation to sort out populations of spermatozoa with the highest fertilization potential. Unfortunately, none of these procedures is sufficient for the prediction of male fertility capacity [8]. The parameters are found to be subjective, poorly standardized [9] and not powerful predictors of fertility [10, 11]. However, traditionally, concentration and motility after sperm preparation have been used by clinicians in deciding the choice of ART method for a given couple. However, in many cases this is not sufficient for assessing the fertilizing capacity and the quality of a sperm, and, as a consequence, the criteria for IVF and ICSI as well as the ratio between the two methods vary tremendously between countries as well as between clinics.

21.4 Sperm DNA Integrity Testing

During the last decades, a growing focus on sperm chromatin integrity testing in prediction of fertility is seen. It is well documented that infertile men have more sperm DNA damage than fertile men and that in order to predict fertility capacity, sperm DNA integrity testing can be used in addition to the traditional sperm parameters [12].

A number of techniques to assess sperm DNA integrity are available [13]. Principles, procedures and more specific aspects of the different tests are described in detail in other chapters of this book. Briefly, four DNA damage tests are used, namely, the Comet assay (single cell gel electrophoresis) [14], the TUNEL (terminal deoxynucleotidyl transferase-mediated dUTP nick end labelling) assay [15], the Sperm Chromatin Structure assay (SCSA) [16] and the sperm chromatin dispersion test (SCD) [17, 18].

In the Comet assay, spermatozoa are mixed with melted agarose and then placed on a glass slide. Thereafter, the spermatozoa are lysed and DNA visualized with the help of a DNA-specific fluorescent dye. By electrophoresis technique, potential DNA damage is quantified by measuring the displacement of the fragmented DNA (tail) away from the intact DNA at the comet head.

The TUNEL assay can be run both by use of bright-field/fluorescence microscopy and by flow cytometry. In the TUNEL assay, terminal deoxynucleotidyl transferase (TdT) incorporates labelled nucleotides to 3′-OH at single- and double-strand DNA breaks to create a signal, which increases with the number of DNA breaks. On a glass slide, sperm are scored and classified positive or negative depending whether they are labelled or not. In flow cytometry, the fraction of positive sperm is represented by the cells above a threshold channel value on a relative fluorescence intensity scale.

SCSA is a flow cytometric test that measures the susceptibility of sperm DNA to acid-induced DNA denaturation in situ, followed by staining with acridine orange. The level of DNA denaturation is determined by measuring the shift from green fluorescence (double-stranded, native DNA) to red fluorescence (single-stranded, denatured DNA) in a flow cytometer, followed by further analysis by a specific SCSA-software. The extent of DNA denaturation is expressed as DNA fragmentation index (DFI) [19]. The fraction of high DNA stainable (HDS) cells, thought to represent immature spermatozoa, is also recorded [20]. However, HDS has not been shown to be of clinical value.

Infertile men have significantly more sperm DNA damage compared to fertile men, and sperm DNA fragmentation was found to be an independent predictor of time to pregnancy in spontaneous pregnancy as well as an independent predictor of success in couples undergoing intrauterine insemination (IUI) [21].

In parallel to the SCSA test, the fluorescence/light microscopic SCD test determines the susceptibility of sperm DNA to acid denaturation. Spermatozoa are first mixed with agarose, then placed on a slide, treated with a low pH solution to denature fragmented or broken DNA and finally treated with lysis buffer to remove membranes and proteins. Removal of nuclear proteins results in nucleoids with a central core and a peripheral halo of dispersed DNA loops. Sperm nuclei with elevated DNA fragmentation produce very small or no halos of DNA dispersion, whereas those sperm with low levels of DNA fragmentation release their DNA loops forming large halos. The sperm nucleoids may be visualized using fluorescence microscopy, after staining with a DNA-specific fluorochrome or by bright-field microscopy.

Moderate-to-high correlations between the different tests have been reported, indicating that, very likely, they are addressing different aspects of DNA damage [22]. The tests that have been most extensively tested clinically and found to have the most stable clinical threshold values are the SCSA and the Comet assays.

21.5 Sperm DNA Integrity Testing in ART

21.5.1 Intrauterine Insemination (IUI)

Duran and co-workers published the first study indicating an association between sperm DNA damage and reduced pregnancy chances after IUI [23]. In a retrospective study of 154 IUI cycles, they assessed sperm DNA damage by the TUNEL assay and reported no pregnancies when DFI was above the level of 12%. Thereafter, Saleh et al. performed a small study where 12 of 19 couples had a DFI value as measured by SCSA above the level of 28%. None of these couples achieved a pregnancy [24]. A Danish study including 48 IUI couples reported no pregnancies for those with a high DFI above 30%. In another larger Danish study of 387 IUI cycles, where SCSA was used to assess DNA damage, it was shown that DFI can be used as an independent predictor of fertility. Whilst the baby take-home rate was 19.0% when the DFI value was below 30%, it was only 1.5% for those with a DFI above 30% [25]. In a recent meta-analysis, Castilla and colleagues found that the clinical value of sperm DNA damage detected with SCSA was more than three times higher than that of sperm morphology [26]. In another meta-analysis, Evenson and Wixon found that patients with a DFI below 30% (assessed by SCSA) were 7.3 times more likely to achieve a pregnancy than patients with a DFI >30% ($n = 518$, $P = 0.0001$) [27].

These IUI results are in good accordance with those results reported from natural conception. Both Evenson and Spano demonstrated that time to pregnancy increased when the proportion of sperm with abnormal chromatin measured by the SCSA was high [25, 28]. In contrast, one single study of 100 Spanish IUI patients has reported no correlation found between SCD results and pregnancy outcome [29].

For an overview of IUI papers, see Table 21.1.

21.5.2 In Vitro Fertilization (IVF) and Intracytoplasmic Sperm Injection (ICSI)

A number of retrospective studies as well as meta-analyses have examined the role of sperm chromatin damage in IVF and ICSI.

In Table 21.2 an overview of IVF and ICSI studies using SCSA, TUNEL, Comet or SCD assays is presented.

In Table 21.3 an overview of relevant published meta-analyses of IVF and ICSI is presented.

Table 21.1 Impact of sperm DNA damage on pregnancy rates in IUI treatment

First author year of publication	Patients (*n*)	Pregnancy rates affected	Test applied	DFI threshold suggested (%)
Duran et al. (2002) [23]	154	Yes	TUNEL	12
Saleh et al. (2003) [30]	19	Yes	SCSA	30
Bungum et al. (2004) [31]	131	Yes	SCSA	27
Muriel et al. (2006) [29]	100	No	SCD	–
Bungum et al. (2007) [32]	387	Yes	SCSA	30

IUI intrauterine insemination, *SCSA* sperm chromatin structure assay, *TUNEL* terminal deoxynucleotidyl transferase dUTP nick end labelling, *SCD* sperm chromatin dispersion test

21.5.3 Pregnancy Outcome

Larson and Evenson suggested early that a DFI above 27% as measured by SCSA could be used as a cutoff value for infertility [39]. They reported that in couples with a DFI above 27%, no pregnancy could be obtained, regardless of the type of ART used. However, in 2004 three other individual groups demonstrated that a DFI level above 27% (by SCSA) was indeed compatible with pregnancy and delivery after IVF as well as after ICSI demonstrating that ART can compensate for poor sperm chromatin quality [31–41].

In a study of 34 IVF and ICSI couples, Gandini found no difference in DNA damage level between patients obtaining pregnancies or not and found normal pregnancies with levels of DFI up to 66.3%. In a study by Bungum and co-workers including 109 IVF and 66 ICSI patients, no statistically significant difference in the pregnancy outcome was seen when dividing patients according to the previously suggested DFI level of 27%. However, in the group with a high DFI (above 27%), the pregnancy and delivery outcome of ICSI were significantly better than those of IVF, clinical pregnancy (CP) (52.9 vs. 22.2%), implantation (37.5 vs. 19.4%) and delivery (D) (47.1 vs. 22.2%). Virro also studied 249 couples undergoing IVF/ICSI and found that those with DFI below 33% had significantly better chances to give rise to a pregnancy, lower risk of miscarriages and an increased probability of ongoing pregnancy at 12 weeks (47 versus 28%) compared to men with a DFI above 33%.

These data were in agreement with reports using TUNEL or Comet assays [34, 71], reporting that sperm DNA damage is more predictive in IVF treatment than in ICSI. Two other very large datasets confirmed these findings [72, 73]. In a study including close to 1000 men in IUI, IVF or ICSI treatment using DFI 30% as threshold level, no statistically significant difference between the outcomes of ICSI versus IVF in the group with DFI ≤30% was seen. However, in the DFI >30% group, the results of ICSI were significantly better than those of IVF with odds ratios (ORs) for biochemical pregnancy (BP), CP and D of 3.0 (95% CI: 1.4–6.2), 2.3 (5% CI: 1.1–4.6) and 2.2 (95% CI: 1.0–4.5), respectively. In the ICSI group, also a tendency towards higher rates of BP, CP and D and implantation with a DFI >30% versus a

Table 21.2 Impact of sperm DNA damage on fertilization, embryo development and pregnancy rates in IVF and ICSI

First author year of publication	IVF (*n*)	ICSI (*n*)	Fertilization rates impaired	Embryo development impaired	Pregnancy rates impaired	Test applied
Tomsu et al. (2002) [33]	40	0	No	Yes	Yes	Comet
Morris et al. (2002) [34]	20	40	No	Yes	NA	Comet
Caglar et al. (2007) [35]	0	56	No	No	No	Comet
Lewis et al. (2004) [36]	0	77	No	NA	Yes	Comet
Nasr-Esfahani (2005) [37]	0	28	No	No	NA	Comet
Larson-Cook et al. (2003) [38]	55	34	No	No	Yes	SCSA
Larson et al. (2000) [39]	24 IVF/ ICSI	NA	No	No	Yes	SCSA
Saleh et al. (2003) [30]	10	4	Yes	Yes	Yes	SCSA
Bungum et al. (2004) [31]	109	66	No	No	Yes	SCSA
Gandini et al. (2004) [40]	12	24	No	Yes (blastocysts)	Yes	SCSA
Virro et al. (2004) [41]	249 IVF/ ICSI	NA	No	No	Yes	SCSA
Check et al. (2005) [42]	0	106	No	No	Yes	SCSA
Payne et al. (2005) [43]	46	54	No	No	No	SCSA
Boe-Hansen et al. (2006) [44]	139	47	No	No	Yes	SCSA
Bungum et al. (2007) [32]	388	223	No	No	Yes	SCSA
Oleszczuk et al. (2016) [45]	516	1117	Yes	Yes	Yes	SCSA
Sun et al. (1997) [46]	143	0	Yes	Yes	NA	TUNEL
Lopes et al. (1998) [47]	0	150	Yes	No	NA	TUNEL
Høst et al. (2000) [48]	50	61	Yes	NA	NA	TUNEL
Tomlinson et al. (2001) [49]	140	0	No	No	Yes	TUNEL

(continued)

Table 21.2 (continued)

First author year of publication	IVF (*n*)	ICSI (*n*)	Fertilization rates impaired	Embryo development impaired	Pregnancy rates impaired	Test applied
Benchaib et al. (2003) [50]	50	54	Yes	No	Yes	TUNEL
Henkel et al. (2003) [51]	208	54	No	No	No	TUNEL
Huang et al. (2005) [52]	217	86	Yes	No	No	TUNEL
Seli et al. (2004) [53]	49	NA	NA	Yes	No	TUNEL
Henkel et al. (2004) [54]	208	54	No	No	No	TUNEL
Hammadeh et al. (2006) [55]	26	22	NA	NA	No	TUNEL
Borini et al. (2006) [56]	82	50	NA	NA	Only for ICSI	TUNEL
Benchaib et al. (2007) [57]	88	234	Only for ICSI	Only for ICSI	No	TUNEL
Bakos et al. (2008) [58]	45	68	Only for IVF	No	Only for ICSI	TUNEL
Frydman et al. (2008) [59]	117	0	NA	NA	Yes	TUNEL
Tarozzi et al. (2009) [60]	82	50	NA	NA	Only for ICSI	TUNEL
Muriel et al. (2006) [29]	85 IVF/ ICSI	NA	NA	NA	No	SCD
Velez de la Calle et al. (2008) [61]	622 IVF/ ICSI	NA	No	Yes	No	SCD
Tavalace et al. (2009) [62]	92 IVF/ ICSI	NA	Only for ICSI	NA	No	SCD

IVF in vitro fertilization, *ICSI* intracytoplasmic sperm injection, *SCSA* sperm chromatin structure assay, TUNEL terminal deoxynucleotidyl transferase dUTP nick end labelling, SCD sperm chromatin dispersion test, *NA* not applicable

DFI ≤30% were found. The most recent study by Oleszczuk and colleagues included 1633 IVF and ICSI cycles and categorized DFI values into four intervals: DFI ≤ 10% (reference group), 10% < DFI ≤ 20%, 20% < DFI ≤ 30% and DFI > 30%. OR for live birth calculated per oocyte retrieval was significantly lower in the standard IVF group if DFI > 20% (OR 0.61; 95% CI: 0.38–0.97; $p = 0.04$). No such associations were seen in the ICSI group. OR for live birth by ICSI compared to IVF was statistically significantly higher for DFI > 20% (OR 1.7; 95% CI: 1.0–2.9; $p = 0.05$). Also these results suggested that ICSI should be a preferred method of in vitro treatment in cases with high DFI [45].

Table 21.3 Impact of sperm DNA damage on pregnancy rates in IVF/ICSI (meta-analyses and systematic reviews)

Reference	Method	Result significant(s)/not significant (ns)	Technique
Evenson and Wixon et al. (2006) [63]	IUI/IVF/ICSI	s-IUI, IVF ns-ICSI	SCSA
Li et al. (2006) [64]	IVF/ICSI	s-TUNEL ns-SCSA	SCSA/TUNEL
Agarwal et al. (2007) [65]	Infertile men	s	SCSA/TUNEL/Comet/CMA3
Zini et al. (2008) [66]	Miscarriage after IVF/ICSI	s	SCSA/TUNEL
Castilla et al. (2010) [26]	IUI/spontaneous	s	SCSA/CSP
Zini et al. (2011) [67]	IVF/ICSI	ns	SCSA/TUNEL/Comet/CC
Osman et al. (2015) [68]	IVF/ICSI	s	SCSA/TUNEL/Comet
Zhang et al. (2015) [69]	IVF/ICSI	ns	SCSA/TUNEL/AOT
Simon et al. (2017) [70]	IVF/ICSI	s	SCSA/TUNEL/SCD/Comet

IUI intrauterine insemination, *SCSA* sperm chromatin structure assay, *TUNEL* terminal deoxynucleotidyl transferase dUTP nick end labelling, *SCD* sperm chromatin dispersion test

In contrast, one single study reported that the poorer the integrity of sperm nuclear DNA, the better the pregnancy outcome. However, with only 100 IVF/ICSI treatments, the power of the study was weak [43].

Chohan did not observe any significant relationship between sperm chromatin damage and fertilization rate, embryo quality and pregnancy rate after IVF/ICSI [74]. Regarding embryo quality, a TUNEL-based study by Benchaib and colleagues did not show any association [50]. The same was shown by Henkel in relation to fertilization rate [51]. However, both studies reported a negative impact of sperm DNA damage on the chance of pregnancy.

Despite convincing data from several authors, some reports have challenged the predictive value of sperm DNA integrity testing. The studies differ, however, in study design, are mixing ART procedures and are using various techniques for sperm DNA integrity assessment. One example is the position paper from the Practice Committee of the American Society for Reproductive Medicine [75] recognized that fragmented sperm DNA is more frequent in infertile than in fertile men and may contribute to poor reproductive performance; they concluded that, so far, there was no proven role for routine DNA integrity testing in the evaluation of infertility. The ASRM followed up their report with similar conclusions in 2008 and 2014 [76, 77].

Another two meta-analyses including studies using either TUNEL or SCSA assays also questioned the predictive value of DNA integrity test in IVF/ICSI outcomes. Both Collins and co-workers, who considered 13 IVF/ICSI studies (9 carried by SCSA and 4 by the TUNEL assay, in total 2162 cycles) [78], and Zini and co-workers [66], who included 9 IVF (6 carried out by TUNEL assay and 3 by SCSA) and 11 ICSI studies (6 SCSA and 5 TUNEL assay), found only small associations between sperm DNA integrity test results and pregnancy in IVF and ICSI.

Two other meta-analyses including only SCSA studies have been performed. Based on 14 papers, Evenson and Wixon [63] reported that in IVF and ICSI, CP was closely related to DFI. In contrast, based on three papers, Li and colleagues found that DFI had no effect on the chance of CP after IVF or ICSI [64]. Overall, a significant increase was observed in life birth rate (LBR) in couples with low compared with those with high sperm DNA fragmentation (RR 1.17, 95% CI 1.07–1.28; $P = 0.0005$). In IVF treatments the LBR results of the four studies were pooled, and the three assays combined together ($n = 553$). Significantly higher LBR was seen after IVF in men with low compared with those with high sperm DNA fragmentation (RR 1.27, 95% CI 1.05–1.52; $P = 0.01$). When the LBR results of the five ICSI studies were pooled ($n = 445$), a marginally significant difference was seen in LBR in men with low compared to those with high sperm DNA fragmentation (RR 1.11, 95% CI 1.00–1.23, $P = 0.04$). Similar conclusions were found in a recent meta-analysis [68]. The detrimental effect of high DNA damage on LBR was seen in the IVF group but not when ICSI was used.

In a more recent meta-analysis of mixed DNA fragmentation methods, the 15 included studies were divided into 3 groups according to the DFI cutoff value (>27%, 15–27%, ≤15%). Within each group, subgroup analysis was performed by the type of fertilization (IVF or ICSI) and sperm DNA integrity method. When the studies with a DFI cutoff value >27% were pooled, the OR demonstrated that the couples were more likely to achieve CP if the DFI was <27% (OR (95%CI) = 1.437 (1.186–1.742), $p = 0.000$). For the IVF group, the pooled OR indicated a similar result (OR (95%CI) = 1.742 (1.382–2.195), $p = 0.000$). However, in the ICSI group, the result was not statistically significant (OR (95%CI) = 0.895 (0.629–1.273), $p = 0.537$). Separate analysis by detection method (SCSA and TUNEL) revealed a higher chance to obtain CP if DFI <27% in the TUNEL group (OR (95% CI) = 1.87 (1.36–2.58), $p = 0.000$), whilst DFI was not associated with clinical pregnancy in SCSA subgroup (OR (95% CI) = 1.24 (0.98–1.58), $p = 0.076$) [69].

The largest and most recent meta-analysis published so far by Simon and colleagues included 56 studies with a total of 8068 ART cycles including 16 IVF studies, 24 ICSI studies and 16 mixed (IVF + ICSI) studies [70]. These studies measured DNA damage by 1 of 4 assays: 23 SCSA, 18 TUNEL, 8 SCD and 7 Comet assay. The combined OR of 1.68 (95% CI: 1.49–1.89; $P < 0.0001$) indicated that sperm DNA damage may influence CP following IVF and/or ICSI treatment. In addition, the combined OR estimates of IVF (OR = 1.65; 95% CI: 1.34–2.04; $P < 0.0001$), ICSI (OR = 1.31; 95% CI: 1.08–1.59; $P = 0.0068$) and mixed IVF + ICSI studies (OR = 2.37; 95% CI: 1.89–2.97; $P < 0.0001$) were also statistically significant. Thus, the authors observed a strong negative association between sperm DNA damage and clinical pregnancy after ART and also separately for IVF and/or ICSI. Here the TUNEL, Comet and SCD assays were applied. They concluded that there is sufficient evidence in the existing literature to suggest that sperm DNA damage has a negative effect on clinical pregnancy following IVF and/or ICSI treatment.

21.5.4 Sperm DNA Damage in Relation to Fertilization

Whether there is a relationship between sperm DNA damage and fertilization rates after ART is also debatable. Using a mouse model, Ahmadi and Ng demonstrated that spermatozoa with DNA damage were able to fertilize. Also, several human studies have shown that men with high number of sperm with damaged DNA have the same ability to fertilize in vitro as men with a low number of sperm with DNA damage. However, there are contrasting findings even in ICSI [79].

HDS (an SCSA parameter thought to represent immature spermatozoa with incomplete protamination) was found to be related to IVF but not ICSI fertilization rates. Consequently, the authors suggested that men with HDS >15% should be treated with ICSI. However, this finding has not been confirmed by others, and HDS does not appear to have importance in clinical practice [32].

In a cross-sectional study where Comet assay was used to assess DNA damage, the low DNA damage group had a higher percentage of good-quality embryos ($P < 0.05$) and lower percentage of poor-quality embryos ($P < 0.05$) compared with the high DNA damage group. Implantation was lower in the high DNA damage (33.33%) compared with intermediate (55.26%; $P < 0.001$) and low DNA damage groups (65.00%; $P < 0.001$) [80].

The most recent and largest study so far by Oleszczuk and colleagues included 1633 IVF and ICSI cycles [45]. In this study, DFI values as assessed by SCSA were categorized into four intervals: DFI ≤ 10% (reference group), 10% < DFI ≤ 20%, 20% < DFI ≤ 30% and DFI > 30%. In the standard IVF group, a significant negative association between DFI and fertilization rate was found. This was not the case for ICSI patients.

21.5.5 Sperm DNA Damage in Relation to Pre-embryo Development

Several investigators have explored the potential impact of sperm DNA damage on human embryo development and offspring health. Based on data from mice, Ahmadi and Ng first reported that sperm DNA damage is related to poor embryo development. Corresponding studies in human are somewhat conflicting. Whilst some authors have reported similar cleavage stage embryo developmental rates between high and low DFI groups, others have shown that sperm DNA damage is negatively correlated with embryo quality after IVF and ICSI. Two studies have also reported that men with high levels of DNA fragmentation are at increased risk of low blastocyst formation compared to men with a low DFI.

In the recent published paper by Oleszczuk et al., DFI values were categorized into four intervals: DFI ≤10% (reference group), 10% < DFI ≤ 20%, 20% < DFI ≤ 30% and DFI > 30% [45]. When calculated per ovum pick-up (OPU), ORs for at least one good-quality embryo (GQE) were significantly lower in the standard IVF group if DFI was >20%. OR for live birth calculated per OPU was significantly lower in the standard IVF group if DFI was above 20% (OR 0.61; 95% CI: 0.38–0.97; $p = 0.04$). No such associations were seen in the ICSI group. The authors suggested that ICSI might be a preferred method of in vitro treatment in cases with high DFI.

Embryo development is a highly dynamic process, and with the use of traditional embryo scoring, it is impossible to precisely time the different developmental stages. However, the new time-lapse technology represents a new tool in IVF by providing digital images of embryos at continuous time intervals as well as providing a more stable, undisturbed environment for the embryos [81]. Thus far, only one published work on the association between morphokinetic parameters and sperm DNA damage exists [82]. Analysing only transferred embryos from 165 couples undergoing ICSI, the investigators found that a low DFI implied that embryos reached the blastocyst stage at a faster rate as compared to cases with a high DFI. Another retrospective study based on 6117 oocytes from 639 ART treatments (256 IVF and 383 ICSI) (Oleszczuk et al., submitted) found that in the ICSI group, the mean time of appearance of pronuclei was significantly lower for 10%<DFI ≤20% and DFI >20, as compared to the DFI ≤10% as the reference group. The effect of reduced mean time in ICSI relative to IVF was observed for pronuclei fading and early cleavage. However, the significance was achieved only for DFI >20. Also, the mean time for starting blastulation was significantly longer in the ICSI group for DFI ≤20 as compared to IVF, but no such association was observed within the IVF/ICSI group.

In a recent meta-analysis, Zini and co-workers included 28 studies (8 IVF, 12 ICSI and 8 mixed IVF-ICSI studies), in total 3226 treatment cycles [67]. Sperm DNA integrity was assessed with SCSA, TUNEL, Comet, chromatin compaction test, aniline blue test, SCD and DNA oxidation test. Of the 28 studies, 16 reported on embryo quality, 11 reported on embryo development and 1 reported on both embryo quality and embryo development. Eleven of the 28 studies reported a significant inverse relationship between sperm DNA damage and embryo quality and/or embryo development. Of the 17 studies that evaluated embryo quality, 5 reported a significant association between sperm DNA damage and embryo quality.

To conclude, sperm DNA integrity seems to have an impact on embryo quality and development; however, more research is needed.

21.6 Neat Versus Prepared Semen

In order to separate the most normal, motile spermatozoa from lymphocytes, epithelial cells, abnormal or immature sperm, cell debris, bacteria and seminal fluid, sperm samples used for ART are normally prepared by density gradient centrifugation or swim-up. When comparing neat semen samples and samples prepared for ART, several authors have reported an improvement in DFI after preparation [83]. However, others show unchanged or worse results [84].

When analysing semen samples before and after density gradient centrifugation in 510 consecutive ART cycles, no predictive value of DFI assessed by SCSA could be seen. This finding is in contrast to what has been reported for raw semen in relation to ART pregnancy outcome. These data supported the two first SCSA–ART studies where the SCSA parameters were analysed also on prepared semen in 24 and 34 patients, respectively. Borini and colleagues found a DFI >10% in density gradient centrifuged semen as measured by the TUNEL assay to be discriminative for ICSI pregnancy [56]. Duran's group tested washed semen samples and found no IUI pregnancy if DFI (by TUNEL assay) exceeded the level of 12%. Duran et al. suggested that a high DFI in neat semen may reflect chromatin or other abnormalities within the entire sperm population interfering with the ability of the sperm to fertilize, but that is not completely eliminated by the sperm preparation procedure [23].

21.7 Intra-individual Variation of DFI in Relation to ART

One of the obstacles of the traditional WHO sperm parameters is the huge intra-individual variation reported. In contrast, a lower intra-individual variation for DFI measures is seen for SCSA. Erenpreiss et al. reported a day-to-day variation of DFI with a mean coefficient of variation (CV) of 29% [85], and in the study by Oleszczuk et al., it was shown that among 616 men who had their semen analysed by SCSA both in infertility workup and in the actual ART cycle, 85% of the men remained in the same DFI category, <30% or >30% from measurement 1 to 2. Clinically, it means that only 15% will have a clinically relevant change if a repeat SCSA measurement is obtained [86].

21.8 Conclusions

Sperm DNA integrity assessment and conventional semen analysis can be, to a certain degree, complementary to each other. The combination of these two methods can be helpful both during the diagnostic process and therapeutic procedure. It can differentiate more effectively men with reduced fertilizing ability and put the right diagnosis of "male factor" to the couples classified before as "unexplained infertile". It's apparently profitable to the patients. Infertile couples can get more proper information about their status and can react more accurately – either continue with the most correct treatment method or contrary, depending on other biological, economic or social reason, continue attempts to conceive spontaneously. Also on the later stage of the process, when in vitro procedure is already begun, the better assessment of sperm fertilizing potential help to reduce the dilemma which fertilization method should be adopted. This enables to use preferable standard IVF as wide as possible and, in the same way, minimalizes risk of decreased fertilization rate and complete fertilization failure, in extreme cases.

Men with high numbers of DNA-fragmented sperm have similar chances of obtaining pregnancy by IVF and ICSI as men with low sperm DNA fragmentation. However, the group of men who will benefit from sperm DNA integrity assessment is those diagnosed with unexplained infertility. Roughly, one out of four, with normal WHO sperm parameters, will have a SCSA–DFI above 20–30%, which is the DFI level where the chance of giving rise to a spontaneous or IUI-induced pregnancy reduces significantly. In order to find these men with sperm DNA damage as hidden causes to their childlessness, those where the traditional semen analysis shows one or no abnormality should be offered sperm DNA testing using a validated assay. In men where all standard parameters are normal, chances of in vivo pregnancy start reducing for DFI above 20%. In the presence of one abnormal semen quality parameter, the chance of spontaneous pregnancy is significantly reduced already at DFI above 10%. Thus, in such couples, DFI should be taken into consideration, and the couple should consider a more advanced ART such as IVF/ICSI.

In some studies, the SCSA and the Comet assays have provided the most stable clinical threshold values in relation to infertility. It is evident that the relevance of sperm DNA integrity testing concerns, first of all, in vivo fertilization. In addition to being a predictor of natural conception, DFI can be used as an independent predictor of success in couples undergoing IUI. However, the predictive value of sperm DNA damage in IVF and ICSI needs to be further investigated by prospective, randomized studies.

The correlation between sperm DNA damage and fertilization rates remains controversial. However, a large SCSA dataset recently showed that IVF but not ICSI fertilization rates are correlated with the level of sperm DNA fragmentation. The same study also demonstrated that the chance of having at least one GQE was significantly lower in the standard IVF group if DFI >20%. However, no such associations were seen in the ICSI group. Studies also suggest that high levels of DNA fragmentation are associated with low blastocyst formation.

More research is needed to improve our understanding of DNA damage in spermatozoa. A better standardization of the methods of DNA damage evaluation is necessary. Moreover, a better insight into the causes of sperm DNA damage should help us develop treatment strategies for men with sperm DNA damage and contribute to improved assisted reproduction outcome.

References

1. Palermo G, Joris H, Devroey P, Van Steirteghem AC. Pregnancies after intracytoplasmic injection of single spermatozoon into an oocyte. Lancet. 1992;340(8810):17–8.
2. de Kretser DM. Male infertility. Lancet. 1997;349(9054):787–90.
3. World Health Organization. WHO laboratory manual for the examination and processing of human semen. 5th ed. Geneva: WHO Press; 2010.
4. Andersen AN, Gianaroli L, Felberbaum R, de Mouzon J, Nygren KG, European IVF-monitoring programme (EIM), European Society of Human Reproduction and Embryology (ESHRE). Assisted reproductive technology in Europe, 2001. Results generated from European registers by ESHRE. Hum Reprod. 2005;20(5):1158–76.

5. Auger J, Eustache F, Ducot B, Blandin T, Daudin M, Diaz I, Matribi SE, Gony B, Keskes L, Kolbezen M, Lamarte A, Lornage J, Nomal N, Pitaval G, Simon O, Virant-Klun I, Spira A, Jouannet P. Intra- and inter-individual variability in human sperm concentration, motility and vitality assessment during a workshop involving ten laboratories. Hum Reprod. 2000;15(11):2360–8.
6. Dunson DB, Baird DD, Colombo B. Increased infertility with age in men and women. Obstet Gynecol. 2004;103(1):51–6.
7. Hull MG, Fleming CF, Hughes AO, McDermott A. The age-related decline in female fecundity: a quantitative controlled study of implanting capacity and survival of individual embryos after in vitro fertilization. Fertil Steril. 1996;65(4):783–90.
8. Edwards RG, Brody SA. Principles and practice of assisted human reproduction. Philadelphia: W.B Saunders Company; 1995.
9. Jørgensen N, Auger J, Giwercman A, Irvine DS, Jensen TK, Jouannet P, Keiding N, Le Bon C, MacDonald E, Pekuri AM, Scheike T, Simonsen M, Suominen J, Skakkeboek NE. Semen analysis performed by different laboratory teams: an intervariation study. Int J Androl. 1997;20(4):201–8.
10. Bonde JP, Ernst E, Jensen TK, Hjollund NH, Kolstad H, Henriksen TB, Scheike T, Giwercman A, Olsen J, Skakkebaek NE. Relation between semen quality and fertility: a population-based study of 430 first-pregnancy planners. Lancet. 1998;352(9135):1172–7.
11. DS G, Overstreet JW, Factor-Litvak P, Brazil CK, Nakajima ST, Coutifaris C, Carson SA, Cisneros P, Steinkampf MP, Hill JA, Xu D, Vogel DL, National Cooperative Reproductive Medicine Network. Sperm morphology, motility, and concentration in fertile and infertile men. N Engl J Med. 2001;345(19):1388–93.
12. Agarwal A, Said TM. Role of sperm chromatin abnormalities and DNA damage in male infertility. Hum Reprod Update. 2003;9(4):331–45.
13. Erenpreiss J, Spano M, Erenpreisa J, Bungum M, Giwercman A. Sperm chromatin structure and male fertility: biological and clinical aspects. Asian J Androl. 2006;8(1):11–29.
14. Ostling O, Johanson KJ. Microelectrophoretic study of radiation-induced DNA damages in individual mammalian cells. Biochem Biophys Res Commun. 1984;123(1):291–8.
15. Gorczyca W, Gong J, Darzynkiewicz Z. Detection of DNA strand breaks in individual apoptotic cells by the in situ terminal deoxynucleotidyl transferase and nick translation assays. Cancer Res. 1993;53(8):1945–51.
16. Evenson DP, Darzynkiewicz Z, Melamed MR. Relation of mammalian sperm chromatin heterogeneity to fertility. Science. 1980;210(4474):1131–3.
17. Fernández JL, Muriel L, Rivero MT, Goyanes V, Vazquez R, Alvarez JG. The sperm chromatin dispersion test: a simple method for the determination of sperm DNA fragmentation. J Androl. 2003;24(1):59–66.
18. Fernández JL, Muriel L, Goyanes V, Segrelles E, Gosálvez J, Enciso M, LaFromboise M, De Jonge C. Simple determination of human sperm DNA fragmentation with an improved sperm chromatin dispersion test. Fertil Steril. 2005;84(4):833–42.
19. Aitken RJ. Sperm function tests and fertility. Int J Androl. 2006;29(1):69–75. discussion 105–108
20. Muller CH. Rationale, interpretation, validation, and uses of sperm function tests. J Androl. 2000;21(1):10–30.
21. Giwercman A, Lindstedt L, Larsson M, Bungum M, Spano M, Levine RJ, Rylander L. Sperm chromatin structure assay as an independent predictor of fertility in vivo: a case-control study. Int J Androl. 2010;33(1):e221–7.
22. Boomsma CM, Heineman MJ, Cohlen BJ, Farquhar C. Semen preparation techniques for intrauterine insemination. Cochrane Database Syst Rev. 2007;4:CD004507.
23. Duran EH, Morshedi M, Taylor S, Oehninger S. Sperm DNA quality predicts intrauterine insemination outcome: a prospective cohort study. Hum Reprod. 2002;17(12):3122–8.
24. Saleh RA, Agarwal A, Nelson DR, Nada EA, El-Tonsy MH, Alvarez JG, Thomas AJ Jr, Sharma RK. Increased sperm nuclear DNA damage in normozoospermic infertile men: a prospective study. Fertil Steril. 2002;78(2):313–8.

25. Spanò M, Bonde JP, Hjøllund HI, Kolstad HA, Cordelli E, Leter G. Sperm chromatin damage impairs human fertility. The Danish First Pregnancy Planner Study Team. Fertil Steril. 2000;73(1):43–50.
26. Castilla JA, Zamora S, Gonzalvo MC, Luna Del Castillo JD, Roldan-Nofuentes JA, Clavero A, Björndahl L, Martínez L. Sperm chromatin structure assay and classical semen parameters: systematic review. Reprod Biomed Online. 2010;20(1):114–24.
27. Evenson D, Wixton R. Meta-analysis of sperm DNA fragmentation using the sperm chromatin structure assay. Reprod Biomed Online. 2006;12:466–72.
28. Evenson DP, Jost LK, Marshall D, Zinaman MJ, Clegg E, Purvis K, de Angelis P, Claussen OP. Utility of the sperm chromatin structure assay as a diagnostic and prognostic tool in the human fertility clinic. Hum Reprod. 1999;14(4):1039–49.
29. Muriel L, Meseguer M, Fernández JL, Alvarez J, Remohí J, Pellicer A, Garrido N. Value of the sperm chromatin dispersion test in predicting pregnancy outcome in intrauterine insemination: a blind prospective study. Hum Reprod. 2006;21(3):738–44.
30. Saleh RA, Agarwal A, Nada EA, El-Tonsy MH, Sharma RK, Meyer A, Nelson DR, Thomas AJ. Negative effects of increased sperm DNA damage in relation to seminal oxidative stress in men with idiopathic and male factor infertility. Fertil Steril. 2003;79(Suppl 3):1597–605.
31. Bungum M, Humaidan P, Spano M, Jepson K, Bungum L, Giwercman A. The predictive value of sperm chromatin structure assay (SCSA) parameters for the outcome of intrauterine insemination, IVF and ICSI. Hum Reprod. 2004;19(6):1401–8.
32. Bungum M, Humaidan P, Axmon A, Spano M, Bungum L, Erenpreiss J, Giwercman A. Sperm DNA integrity assessment in prediction of assisted reproduction technology outcome. Hum Reprod. 2007;22(1):174–9.
33. Tomsu M, Sharma V, Miller D. Embryo quality and IVF treatment outcomes may correlate with different sperm comet assay parameters. Hum Reprod. 2002;17(7):1856–62.
34. Morris ID, Ilott S, Dixon L, Brison DR. The spectrum of DNA damage in human sperm assessed by single cell gel electrophoresis (Comet assay) and its relationship to fertilization and embryo development. Hum Reprod. 2002;17(4):990–8.
35. Caglar GS, Köster F, Schöpper B, Asimakopoulos B, Nehls B, Nikolettos N, Diedrich K, Al-Hasani S. Semen DNA fragmentation index, evaluated with both TUNEL and Comet assay, and the ICSI outcome. In Vivo. 2007;21(6):1075–80.
36. Lewis SE, O'Connell M, Stevenson M, Thompson-Cree L, McClure N. An algorithm to predict pregnancy in assisted reproduction. Hum Reprod. 2004;19(6):1385–94.
37. Nasr-Esfahani MH, Salehi M, Razavi S, Anjomshoa M, Rozbahani S, Moulavi F, Mardani M. Effect of sperm DNA damage and sperm protamine deficiency on fertilization and embryo development post-ICSI. Reprod Biomed Online. 2005;11(2):198–205.
38. Larson-Cook KL, Brannian JD, Hansen KA, Kasperson KM, Aamold ET, Evenson DP. Relationship between the outcomes of assisted reproductive techniques and sperm DNA fragmentation as measured by the sperm chromatin structure assay. Fertil Steril. 2003;80(4):895–902.
39. Larson KL, DeJonge CJ, Barnes AM, Jost LK, Evenson DP. Sperm chromatin structure assay parameters as predictors of failed pregnancy following assisted reproductive techniques. Hum Reprod. 2000;15(8):1717–22.
40. Gandini L, Lombardo F, Paoli D, Caruso F, Eleuteri P, Leter G, Ciriminna R, Culasso F, Dondero F, Lenzi A, Spanò M. Full-term pregnancies achieved with ICSI despite high levels of sperm chromatin damage. Hum Reprod. 2004;19(6):1409–17.
41. Virro MR, Larson-Cook KL, Evenson DP. Sperm chromatin structure assay (SCSA) parameters are related to fertilization, blastocyst development, and ongoing pregnancy in in vitro fertilization and intracytoplasmic sperm injection cycles. Fertil Steril. 2004;81(5):1289–95.
42. Check JH, Graziano V, Cohen R, Krotec J, Check ML. Effect of an abnormal sperm chromatin structural assay (SCSA) on pregnancy outcome following (IVF) with ICSI in previous IVF failures. Arch Androl. 2005;51(2):121–4.
43. Payne JF, Raburn DJ, Couchman GM, Price TM, Jamison MG, Walmer DK. Redefining the relationship between sperm deoxyribonucleic acid fragmentation as measured by the sperm

chromatin structure assay and outcomes of assisted reproductive techniques. Fertil Steril. 2005;84(2):356–64.
44. Boe-Hansen GB, Fedder J, Ersbøll AK, Christensen P. The sperm chromatin structure assay as a diagnostic tool in the human fertility clinic. Hum Reprod. 2006;21(6):1576–82.
45. Oleszczuk K, Giwercman A, Bungum M. Sperm chromatin structure assay in prediction of in vitro fertilization outcome. Andrology. 2016;4(2):290–6.
46. Sun JG, Jurisicova A, Casper RF. Detection of deoxyribonucleic acid fragmentation in human sperm: correlation with fertilization in vitro. Biol Reprod. 1997;56(3):602–7.
47. Lopes S, Sun JG, Jurisicova A, Meriano J, Casper RF. Sperm deoxyribonucleic acid fragmentation is increased in poor-quality semen samples and correlates with failed fertilization in intracytoplasmic sperm injection. Fertil Steril. 1998;69(3):528–32.
48. Høst E, Lindenberg S, Smidt-Jensen S. The role of DNA strand breaks in human spermatozoa used for IVF and ICSI. Acta Obstet Gynecol Scand. 2000;79(7):559–63.
49. Tomlinson MJ, Moffatt O, Manicardi GC, Bizzaro D, Afnan M, Sakkas D. Interrelationships between seminal parameters and sperm nuclear DNA damage before and after density gradient centrifugation: implications for assisted conception. Hum Reprod. 2001;16(10):2160–5.
50. Benchaib M, Braun V, Lornage J, Hadj S, Salle B, Lejeune H, Guérin JF. Sperm DNA fragmentation decreases the pregnancy rate in an assisted reproductive technique. Hum Reprod. 2003;18(5):1023–8.
51. Henkel R, Kierspel E, Hajimohammad M, Stalf T, Hoogendijk C, Mehnert C, Menkveld R, Schill WB, Kruger TF. DNA fragmentation of spermatozoa and assisted reproduction technology. Reprod Biomed Online. 2003;7(4):477–84.
52. Huang CC, Lin DP, Tsao HM, Cheng TC, Liu CH, Lee MS. Sperm DNA fragmentation negatively correlates with velocity and fertilization rates but might not affect pregnancy rates. Fertil Steril. 2005;84(1):130–40.
53. Seli E, Gardner DK, Schoolcraft WB, Moffatt O, Sakkas D. Extent of nuclear DNA damage in ejaculated spermatozoa impacts on blastocyst development after in vitro fertilization. Fertil Steril. 2004;82(2):378–83.
54. Henkel R, Hajimohammad M, Stalf T, Hoogendijk C, Mehnert C, Menkveld R, Gips H, Schill WB, Kruger TF. Influence of deoxyribonucleic acid damage on fertilization and pregnancy. Fertil Steril. 2004;81(4):965–72.
55. Hammadeh ME, Radwan M, Al-Hasani S, Micu R, Rosenbaum P, Lorenz M, Schmidt W. Comparison of reactive oxygen species concentration in seminal plasma and semen parameters in partners of pregnant and non-pregnant patients after IVF/ICSI. Reprod Biomed Online. 2006;13(5):696–706.
56. Borini A, Tarozzi N, Bizzaro D, Bonu MA, Fava L, Flamigni C, Coticchio G. Sperm DNA fragmentation: paternal effect on early post-implantation embryo development in ART. Hum Reprod. 2006;21(11):2876–81.
57. Benchaib M, Lornage J, Mazoyer C, Lejeune H, Salle B, François GJ. Sperm deoxyribonucleic acid fragmentation as a prognostic indicator of assisted reproductive technology outcome. Fertil Steril. 2007;87(1):93–100.
58. Bakos HW, Thompson JG, Feil D, Lane M. Sperm DNA damage is associated with assisted reproductive technology pregnancy. Int J Androl. 2008;31(5):518–26.
59. Frydman N, Prisant N, Hesters L, Frydman R, Tachdjian G, Cohen-Bacrie P, Fanchin R. Adequate ovarian follicular status does not prevent the decrease in pregnancy rates associated with high sperm DNA fragmentation. Fertil Steril. 2008;89(1):92–7.
60. Tarozzi N, Nadalini M, Stronati A, Bizzaro D, Dal Prato L, Coticchio G, Borini A. Anomalies in sperm chromatin packaging: implications for assisted reproduction techniques. Reprod Biomed Online. 2009;18(4):486–95.
61. Velez de la Calle JF, Muller A, Walschaerts M, Clavere JL, Jimenez C, Wittemer C, Thonneau P. Sperm deoxyribonucleic acid fragmentation as assessed by the sperm chromatin dispersion test in assisted reproductive technology programs: results of a large prospective multicenter study. Fertil Steril. 2008;90(5):1792–9.

62. Tavalaee M, Razavi S, Nasr-Esfahani MH. Influence of sperm chromatin anomalies on assisted reproductive technology outcome. Fertil Steril. 2009;91(4):1119–26.
63. Evenson DP, Wixon R. Clinical aspects of sperm DNA fragmentation detection and male infertility. Theriogenology. 2006;65(5):979–91.
64. Li Z, Wang L, Cai J, Huang H. Correlation of sperm DNA damage with IVF and ICSI outcomes: a systematic review and meta-analysis. J Assist Reprod Genet. 2006;23(9–10):367–76.
65. Agarwal A, Deepinder F, Cocuzza M, Agarwal R, Short RA, Sabanegh E, Marmar JL. Efficacy of varicocelectomy in improving semen parameters: new meta-analytical approach. Urology. 2007;70(3):532–8.
66. Zini A, Boman JM, Belzile E, Ciampi A. Sperm DNA damage is associated with an increased risk of pregnancy loss after IVF and ICSI: systematic review and meta-analysis. Hum Reprod. 2008;23(12):2663–8.
67. Zini A, Jamal W, Cowan L, Al-Hathal N. Is sperm DNA damage associated with IVF embryo quality? A systematic review. J Assist Reprod Genet. 2011;28(5):391–7.
68. Osman A, Alsomait H, Seshadri S, El-Toukhy T, Khalaf Y. The effect of sperm DNA fragmentation on live birth rate after IVF or ICSI: a systematic review and meta-analysis. Reprod Biomed Online. 2015;30(2):120–7.
69. Zhang Z, Zhu L, Jiang H, Chen H, Chen Y, Dai Y. Sperm DNA fragmentation index and pregnancy outcome after IVF or ICSI: a meta-analysis. J Assist Reprod Genet. 2015;32(1):17–26.
70. Simon L, Zini A, Dyachenko A, Ciampi A, Carrell DT. A systematic review and meta-analysis to determine the effect of sperm DNA damage on in vitro fertilization and intracytoplasmic sperm injection outcome. Asian J Androl. 2017;19(1):80–90.
71. Sharma RK, Sabanegh E, Mahfouz R, Gupta S, Thiyagarajan A, Agarwal A. TUNEL as a test for sperm DNA damage in the evaluation of male infertility. Urology. 2010;76(6):1380–6.
72. Aravindan GR, Bjordahl J, Jost LK, Evenson DP. Susceptibility of human sperm to in situ DNA denaturation is strongly correlated with DNA strand breaks identified by single-cell electrophoresis. Exp Cell Res. 1997;236(1):231–7.
73. Erenpreiss J, Jepson K, Giwercman A, Tsarev I, Erenpreisa J, Spano M. Toluidine blue cytometry test for sperm DNA conformation: comparison with the flow cytometric sperm chromatin structure and TUNEL assays. Hum Reprod. 2004;19(10):2277–82.
74. Chohan KR, Griffin JT, Lafromboise M, De Jonge CJ, Carrell DT. Sperm DNA damage relationship with embryo quality and pregnancy outcome in IVF patients. Fertil Steril. 2004;82:S55–6.
75. Practice Committee of the American Society for Reproductive Medicine. The clinical utility of sperm DNA integrity testing. Fertil Steril. 2006;86(5 Suppl 1):35–7. Review
76. Practice Committee of the American Society for Reproductive Medicine. The clinical utility of sperm DNA integrity testing. Fertil Steril. 2008;90(5 Suppl):178–80. Review
77. Practice Committee of the American Society for Reproductive Medicine. The clinical utility of sperm DNA integrity testing : a guideline. Fertil Steril. 2013;99(3):673–7. https://doi.org/10.1016/j.fertnstert.2012.12.049. Epub 2013 Feb 1. Erratum in: Fertil Steril. 2014 Mar;101(3):884. Review
78. Collins JA, Barnhart KT, Schlegel PN. Do sperm DNA integrity tests predict pregnancy with in vitro fertilization? Fertil Steril. 2008;89(4):823–31.
79. Evenson DP, Larson KL, Jost LK. Sperm chromatin structure assay: its clinical use for detecting sperm DNA fragmentation in male infertility and comparisons with other techniques. J Androl. 2002;23(1):25–43.
80. Simon L, Murphy K, Shamsi MB, Liu L, Emery B, Aston KI, Hotaling J, Carrell DT. Paternal influence of sperm DNA integrity on early embryonic development. Hum Reprod. 2014;29(11):2402–12.
81. Kirkegaard K, Agerholm IE, Ingerslev HJ. Time-lapse monitoring as a tool for clinical embryo assessment. Hum Reprod. 2012;27(5):1277–85.
82. Wdowiak A, Bakalczuk S, Bakalczuk G. The effect of sperm DNA fragmentation on the dynamics of the embryonic development in intracytoplasmatic sperm injection. Reprod Biol. 2015;15(2):94–100.

83. Muratori M, Maggi M, Spinelli S, Filimberti E, Forti G, Baldi E. Spontaneous DNA fragmentation in swim-up selected human spermatozoa during long term incubation. J Androl. 2003;24(2):253–62.
84. Bungum M, Spanò M, Humaidan P, Eleuteri P, Rescia M, Giwercman A. Sperm chromatin structure assay parameters measured after density gradient centrifugation are not predictive for the outcome of ART. Hum Reprod. 2008;23(1):4–10.
85. Erenpreiss J, Bungum M, Spano M, Elzanaty S, Orbidans J, Giwercman A. Intra-individual variation in sperm chromatin structure assay parameters in men from infertile couples: clinical implications. Hum Reprod. 2006;21(8):2061–4.
86. Oleszczuk K, Giwercman A, Bungum M. Intra-individual variation of the sperm chromatin structure assay DNA fragmentation index in men from infertile couples. Hum Reprod. 2011;26(12):3244–8.

Chapter 22
Sperm DNA and Pregnancy Loss After IVF and ICSI

Nirlipta Swain, Gayatri Mohanty, and Luna Samanta

22.1 Introduction

The relative rate of success of reproduction in humans is extremely low with only 30% of all conceptions resulting in live birth [1]. Assisted reproductive technologies (ART) are the treatment of choice for many couples facing infertility issues, be it due to male or female factor or idiopathic [2, 3]. Every year there is an increase by 4% in the number of couples seeking ART for conception. ART involves procedures like fertility medication, artificial insemination, in vitro fertilization (IVF), micromanipulation of gametes, and surrogacy as well. It is well established that high-quality gametes are required to produce high-quality embryos and that both the sperm and oocyte genomes contribute to the embryonic genome [4]. In contrast to natural selection of the male gametes that occurs during transit in the female genital tracts, in the ART laboratory healthy spermatozoa are selected with routine separation techniques. Despite the advancement in ART during the last 30 years, the rate of pregnancy failures post ART being high (about 70%), thus warrants further improvements [5, 6].

ART bypass the natural selection barrier which would compromise the quality of the fittest sperm selected for fertilization. There is a chance that a normal-looking sperm with abnormal genomic material, which naturally may be incompetent for

N. Swain
School of Life Sciences, Redox Biology Laboratory, Department of Zoology, Ravenshaw University, Cuttack, India

G. Mohanty
Redox Biology Laboratory, Department of Zoology, Ravenshaw University, Cuttack 753003, India

L. Samanta (✉)
Redox Biology Laboratory, Department of Zoology, School of Life Sciences, Ravenshaw University, Cuttack, India
e-mail: lsamanta@ravenshawuniversity.ac.in

A. Zini, A. Agarwal (eds.), *A Clinician's Guide to Sperm DNA and Chromatin Damage*, https://doi.org/10.1007/978-3-319-71815-6_22

impregnation, may still be utilized for ART [7]. In such a scenario, concern over the use of the damaged DNA for artificial fertilization is growing. With the success rate of pregnancy using ART remains comparatively low and somewhat unpredictable, the identification of perfect sperm is an area of active research. Procedures for detection of suitable spermatozoa having strong prognostic power in predicting successful IVF and ICSI outcomes are mostly aimed at techniques for determination of sperm DNA quality. However, the true clinical significance of sperm DNA damage assays remains to be established since the available studies are few and heterogeneous.

Several studies have shown the role of paternal genomic alterations in predicting the success rates of ART [8, 9]. Not only fertilization rates and embryo quality but also subsequent 'embryo viability' and progression of pregnancy would be affected by the status of sperm DNA integrity [10]. When spermatozoa with extensive DNA damage are used, the embryo may fail to develop or implant in the uterus or it may be naturally aborted at a later stage [11]. It could be suggested that functional spermatozoon with intact DNA may have higher chances of successfully delivering a healthy progeny. In this chapter the primary focus is on the role of a fertilizing spermatozoon carrying DNA damage on pregnancy outcome. The ability of DNA tests assessing different aspects of DNA damage, in predicting IVF or ICSI outcome, is discussed with consistent proofs and meta-analysis studies. Moreover, the chapter gives an insight into the late paternal effect and repair capability of oocytes of damaged sperm DNA. In an era where ART are frequently used, study of the influence of sperm DNA damage on embryonic development holds a pivotal role for improvement of success rate.

22.2 DNA Damage and Sperm

DNA damage refers to alterations in the chemical structure of DNA, namely, DNA strand breaks, a base missing from the backbone of DNA (depurination or depyrimidination), and a chemically changed base such as 8-oxoguanine (8-oxoGua), 5-hydroxymethyluracil (5-hmUra), 6-methylguanine, and deaminated cytosine. Most of these changes are attributed to oxidative stress since despite extensive DNA repair oxidatively, damaged DNA are abundant in many human tissues, and these modified bases are potential mutagens [12]. Thus, it will not be out of context to mention that spermatozoa, devoid of substantial cytoplasm, lack effective antioxidants within the cell making them more prone to oxidative DNA damage. When the oxidative DNA damage occurs in the germ cells of the testis, it will result in the production of spermatozoa laden with damaged DNA and/or mutated DNA, and if inseminated with these spermatozoa, the ART outcome will be severely affected.

The aetiology of DNA damage is multifactorial (Fig. 22.1) and categorized as (i) primary (i.e. testicular) or secondary (i.e. environmental) [13]. Single and double DNA strand breaks resulting in abnormal sperm chromatin/DNA structure are thought to arise from four potential sources, namely, (i) strand breaks during

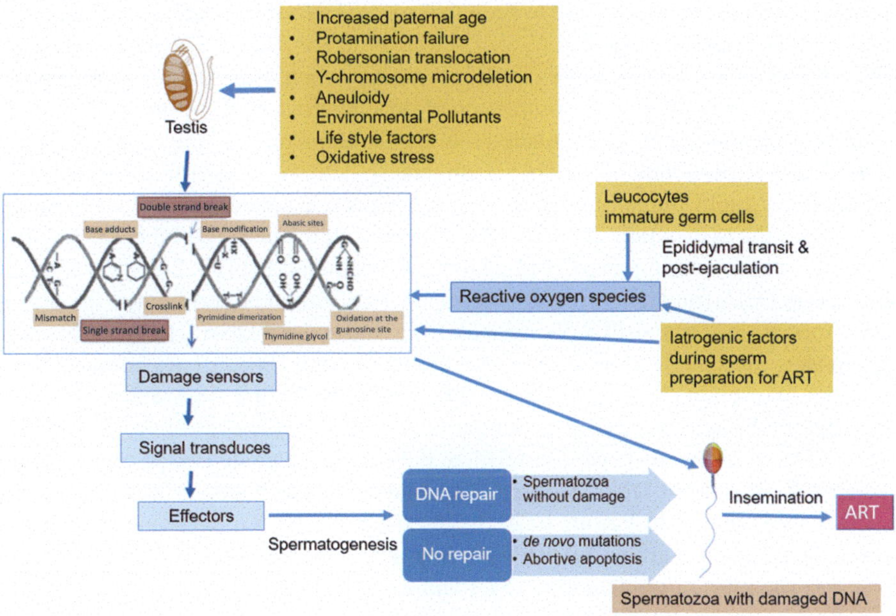

Fig. 22.1 Sources of DNA damage in spermatozoa used in assisted reproductive technologies

chromatin remodelling in the processes of spermiogenesis, (ii) abnormal spermatid maturation (disturbances in protamination), (iii) abortive apoptosis during spermatogenesis, and (iv) oxidative stress [14–16]. Moreover, the damage can be induced and aggravated by exogenous factors like environmental conditions, toxins, pathological diseases [17], and iatrogenic (e.g. ART preparation protocols) [9].

Damaged DNA has been observed in testicular, epididymal, and ejaculated human spermatozoa. Single-strand breaks are a direct result of oxidative damage on sperm DNA, while double-strand breaks may arise from exposure to 4-hydroxyl-2-nonenal, a major product of lipid peroxidation [18]. Two types of DNA adducts, namely, 8-hydroxy-2-deoxyguanosine and two ethenonucleosides (1, N6-ethenoadenosine and 1, N6-ethenoguanosine), are found in human spermatozoa, both of which have been considered key biomarkers of DNA damage caused by oxidative stress [19].

22.3 Effect of Sperm DNA Damage on Fertilization Rate and Embryogenesis

Depending on the level of DNA fragmentation, a sperm may lose its fertilizing ability and developmental potential. Analysis of 170 non-fertilized oocytes from couples attending an IVF programme showed that sperm with a high degree of defective chromatin packaging would lead to probable sperm DNA decondensation failure in oocytes [20]. Similarly, Sakkas et al. [21] have demonstrated that spermatozoon with a high level of abnormalities in the chromatin when used for ICSI apparently would impede the initiation or completion of decondensation, therefore leading to a failed fertilization. It can be postulated that DNA fragmentation, improper chromatin packaging (protamine deficiency), epigenetic defects, or sperm chromosomal aneuploidies might impair fertilization [22]. However, studies on animal models have shown the association of sperm DNA damage with abnormal embryo development and subsequent impaired implantation. Ahmadi and Ng [23, 24] showed that high sperm DNA fragmentation did not impair fertilization but prohibited the blastocyst formation. They artificially created different levels of DNA damage in sperm by exposing the sample to different doses (5, 10, 50, and 100 GY) of gamma radiation prior to insemination. Fertilization rates (FR) of 64.3, 59.9, 58.5, and 61.1% for the different dosages were seen as compared to 53.2% in the control group, implying that DNA-damaged sperm can fertilize the oocytes at a rate comparable to that of sperm having intact DNA. However, the blastocyst development was decreased from 49.8% in the control group to 20.3, 7.8, 3.4, and 2.3%. Of the transferred blastocysts in the control group, 69.8% were implanted and 33.9% developed into live foetuses. The rates of implantation (57.1 and 21.4%) and live foetuses (20 and 0%) were decreased significantly when spermatozoa were exposed to doses of 5 and 10 GY, respectively. Higher dosages of gamma radiation, resulting in severe DNA damage, reduced blastocyst formation to less than 5%. Furthermore, none of these could reach full term.

Recently, Wdowiak et al. [25] reported that higher sperm genomic damage can also slow down embryo morphokinetic parameters such as attaining the blastocyst stage much later, thus affecting ICSI outcome. Tesarik et al. [26] have reported that with pre-damaged paternal genome, high proportions of zygotes would be formed with abnormal pronuclear morphology. These zygotes would cleave slowly and show extensive fragmentation and blastomere irregularities resulting in arrested growth even before blastocyst formation. An early transcriptional activity of human male pronucleus is essential for early embryonic development. A weak transcriptional activity detected in defective male pronucleus would lead to retarded male pronuclear development in comparison to female pronucleus, thus impairing amphimixis. Furthermore, Speyer et al. [27] postulated that strand breaks in the sperm DNA may not affect early embryo growth but begin to have an effect at the stage of blastocyst development and then have a very marked effect on implantation of the embryo. A late paternal effect [11] has been mainly attributed to anomalies in the organization of the sperm chromatin (i.e. reduced chromatin condensation, chromosome anomalies, and increased DNA strand breaks or fragmentation). The embryonic genome is demonstrated to be activated on day 3 [28], and blastocyst shows the earliest expression of an 'errant paternal genome' [29]. A negative effect of high DNA fragmentation index (DFI) on the formation of blastocysts has been reported [30–32]. If critical genes are damaged when the paternal genome is activated at day 3 (four- to eight-cell stage), then sensitive developmental programme of embryo is badly affected [33]. Tesarik et al. [11] have demonstrated that a (late) adverse

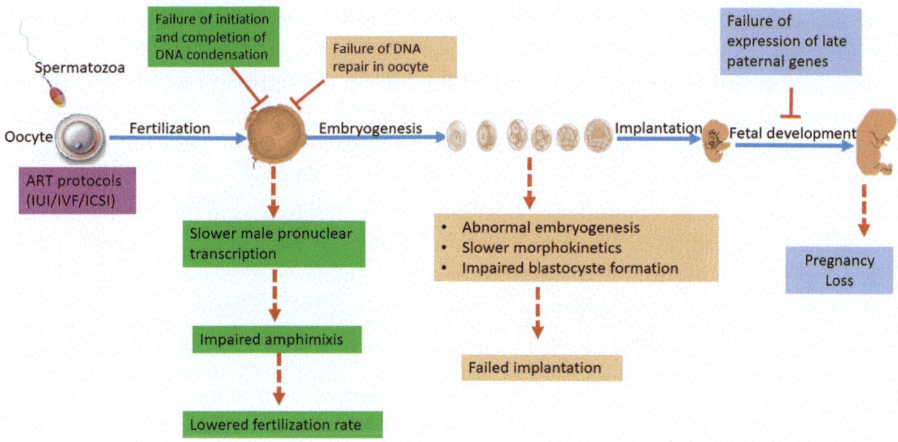

Fig. 22.2 Effect of sperm DNA damage and failure of its repair on different stages of development from fertilization to live birth. Blue solid arrows: normal development; red broken arrows: impaired development leading to pregnancy loss

paternal effect on embryo development can be existent even in the absence of any morphological abnormalities at the zygote stage. Thus, embryos with extensive paternal DNA damage may reach the blastocyst stage. Nevertheless, only those embryos without extensively compromised parental genetic material can progress to full term (Fig. 22.2).

22.4 Failure of DNA Damage Repair by Oocyte: A Confounding Factor

One of the limiting factors in analysing the adverse effect of sperm DNA fragmentation on pregnancy rates following ART is its dependency on both male factors (extent of DNA damage) and female factors (capacity to repair DNA) [34]. This might be the rationale underlying the disparity between the correlations of sperm DNA damage and fertility reported by different studies (Fig. 22.2). Experimental evidence in a number of in vivo and in vitro systems demonstrated the repair ability of vertebrate oocyte of both endogenous and exogenous DNA damage [19]. DNA repair can occur either during or post-fertilization in the oocyte and the developing zygote. Expression of genes and maternal mRNA in human oocytes and blastocysts involved in DNA repair have been detected suggesting the existence of potentially functional DNA repair systems [35, 36]. Ahmadi and Ng [23] suggested that the oocyte repair machinery may not be sufficient to repair DNA damage of sperm >8%. Studies have indicated that implantation of embryos with a normal karyotype may be impaired if there is the presence of unrepaired DNA damage above a critical threshold. Therefore, the varying quality of the oocyte would represent a major potential confounding variable when making fertility predictions based solely on sperm DNA damage. This favours the use of high-quality oocytes from proven donors as a useful strategy for controlling female factor contribution [37]. The quality and competence of the oocyte especially depends on female age, as the innate capacity to repair sperm DNA damage may be weaker in eggs from older women (>35 years) [38]. Moreover, when DNA damage is extensive, some lesions remain unrepaired or are mis-repaired, and the embryo may fail to develop or implant in the uterus or may be aborted naturally at a later stage (uncompensable damage) [19]. The factors affecting this inadequate repair are female age, ovarian environment, and level of fertility as evident from donated oocytes [34].Therefore, several studies have used young healthy egg donors to obtain embryos and to acknowledge the effect of sperm DNA damage on implantation and pregnancy rates which reduces the variability of associated oocyte quality [37, 39–41].

22.5 Iceberg Effect

The discrepancies between the studies to support the predictive value of sperm DNA damage in ART can also be explained by the 'iceberg effect' [9, 42]. The first level of iceberg corresponded to easily detectable sperm cells with high sperm DNA fragmentation (SDF), using current available technologies, while the second level includes the sperm with undetectable, cryptic SDF within the population with a high possibility that this cryptic population would contain sufficient DNA damage to have a detrimental effect on embryonic development, especially if the oocyte is not capable of DNA repair. The bottom layer of the 'iceberg' model represents the spermatozoa with minimal damage; however, current methodologies are difficult to isolate them from the rest. Gosalvez [37] proposed a strong correlation between spermatozoa found in the tip of the 'iceberg' and the proportion of spermatozoa in level 2 under the surface. For example, it is possible that a patient may have a high underlying undetectable population of sperm with a predisposition for DNA damage but has a low detectable level of DFI. On the other hand, a patient might have a low underlying subpopulation of sperm with a predisposition for DNA damage but may have a high detectable level of DFI. The situation may also exist where a similar detectable level of SDF is present in two individuals, but differences in the underlying undetectable population are present. Therefore, the variability in the amount, quality, and distribution of DNA damage among the different spermatozoa in the ejaculate explains the possibility of successful pregnancies despite a high DFI in sperm [43]. Besides DNA damage, protamination failure is another compounding factor leading to defective chromatin condensation affecting FR and embryo development. In spontaneous recurrent pregnancy loss, the number of spermatozoa having intermediate acidic aniline blue staining were significantly higher than their fertile counterparts [44], suggesting that spermatozoa with intermediate defect are equally responsible for successful pregnancy.

22.6 The ART Protocol and Sperm DNA Damage

The ART procedures involve extensive sperm handling and processing that increase the potential risk of damaging paternal DNA material (Table 22.1). These procedures utilize sperm sorting methods (swim-up and density-gradient centrifugation) to select viable sperm from the semen. These methods use multiple centrifugation steps, which have been shown to generate reactive oxygen species (ROS) affecting DNA integrity. Exposure to artificial media and light during ART protocols are also examples of non-natural environment that has no equivalent when fertilization is natural. As spermatozoa get exposed to conditions that are contrary to physiological state, it can be hypothesized that all these procedures could damage sperm DNA. However, studies have found that the percentage of spermatozoa with fragmented DNA and the degree of fragmentation within these cells in prepared spermatozoa are significantly less than in neat semen [45–48]. Sperm preparation can enrich the sperm population by eliminating defective sperm with nicked DNA and poorly condensed chromatin, which is likely to improve the chances of achieving a viable pregnancy [49–51]. Moreover Zini et al. [52] reported that in comparison to density-gradient centrifugation, spermatozoa recovered after swim-up possess higher DNA integrity. But Hammadeh et al. [53] observed that the fertilization, implantation, and pregnancy rates were similar in both semen preparation methods. Moreover, arguments were put forth to justify the effectiveness of DFI in neat semen as better predictors of pregnancy outcome post ART as compared to DFI in processed semen [54]. Tomlinson et al. [55] propose the ‘normalizing’ effect of density-gradient preparations as the reason for the little prognostic value of DFI in processed semen. Nevertheless, if the DFI is high in both neat and processed semen, both fertilization rate and embryo quality are adversely affected [48, 56]. It is presumed that advanced techniques (motile sperm organelle morphology examination: MSOME) [57], electrophoresis [58], microfluidics [59], zeta potential [60, 61], and birefringence [62]) that eliminate the centrifugation steps of conventional sperm preparation (Table 22.1) may improve the selection of sperm with higher DNA integrity, normal morphology, and motility resulting in improved ART outcomes (as reviewed by Rappa et al. [63]).

22.7 In Vitro Fertilization and Pregnancy Loss

Conventional IVF involves ovarian hyperstimulation to generate and collect multiple eggs, preparation and co-incubation of gametes, and fertilization, culture, and selection of resultant embryos before embryo transfer into a uterus. In congruence to natural conception, IVF allows naturally selected best sperm to compete and reach the oocyte in artificial media unlike ICSI [64]. Studies have reported a significant adverse effect of defective DNA structural integrity and breakage on different parameters of reproductive outcome post IVF (Table 22.2).

Table 22.1 Effect of sperm processing in ART on DNA integrity

Sperm processing technique	Outcome	Limitations	References
Conventional swim-up Direct swim-up/ density-gradient centrifugation	Mean numbers and percentage of structurally normal spermatozoa with less DNA damage can be selected by swim-up	Immature sperm with elliptical or roundish nuclei, distorted acrosomes, and uncondensed chromatin remain part of fertilizing pool	[50]
	Density-gradient-prepared spermatozoa have significantly less DNA damage than in neat semen ($P < 0.005$)	Generated ROS during processing may cause sperm DNA damage	[45, 46]
	Both PureSperm® and Percoll® density-gradient-prepared spermatozoa have less nicked DNA than swim-up preparation	–	[49]
Zeta potential	Larger percentages of mature sperm, intact DNA, strict normal morphology, hyperactivation, and progressive motility	Recovery rate only 8.8% Not suitable for oligozoospermic samples	[60, 61]
Magnetic-assisted cell sorting (MACS) system	Selects higher proportion of sperm with normal protamine content and lesser DNA fragmentation	–	[61]
Electrophoresis (microflow)	Less oxidative DNA damage due to decrease in exposure to ROS	–	[58]
Motile sperm organellar morphology examination (MSOME)	Sperm with more than 50% vacuolated nuclei are associated with DNA fragmentation	Incubation of sperm for longer time compromises quality	[57]
Microfluidics	In comparison to swim-up, a microfluidic device resulted in a significantly lower rate of DNA damage (16.4% swim-up vs. 8.4% MF)	–	[59]
Birefringence	Partial birefringence had a significant lower proportion of DNA fragmentation compared to total birefringence (7.3% vs. 19.5%)	–	[62]

Table 22.2 Effect of sperm DNA damage on IVF outcome

DFI assay undertaken	Study population	Sample size	Results after IVF	References
TUNEL	Canada	298	Fertilization failure	[65]
	France	111		[64]
	Italy	82		[71]
	Denmark	50		[56]
	Australia	45		[66]
Alkaline COMET	Ireland	73		[48]
SCD	China	136		[70]
	Slovenia(Europe)	113		[69]
AOT	China	302		[65]
	South Africa	76		[74]
CA3	South Africa	72		[20]
TUNEL	USA	49	Impaired blastocyst formation	[31]
SCSA	South Dakota	63		[30]
TUNEL	Germany	249	Lower pregnancy rates	[77]
COMET	Ireland	203		[79]
	England	40		[80]
SCD	Spain	152		[78]
	Croatia (Europe)	88		[64]
NT and CA3	England	140		[55]

22.7.1 Fertilization Rate

Studies have shown that high DFI may impair FR in IVF procedures, resulting in poor embryo quality (EQ) and higher pregnancy loss (PL). A negative correlation between the percentage of sperm with high DFI (TUNEL assay) and FR in couples undergoing IVF was reported [65–67]. It was proposed that FR was more likely to be adversely affected by high DNA damage in a sample with abnormal chromatin packaging [68, 69]. Studies have shown a negative correlation between FR and sperm chromatin defects (as detected by staining methods such as chromomycin A3 [70, 71] or ethidium bromide [72]). Moreover, underprotamination would also adversely affect the FR [73]. A higher level of intact DNA with an acridine orange test (AOT) score of >24% results in a better FR [74]. Similarly Liu et al. [75] reported that the percentage of sperm bound to zona pellucida had low amounts of DNA damage and good IVF rates.

22.7.2 *Pregnancy and Live-Birth Rates*

Several studies have shown that a compromised sperm DNA would reduce the chances of positive pregnancy outcome. The blastocyst formation rate is significantly lower in couples with severely impaired sperm DNA [76]. Cut-off scores as determined by different DFI analysis assays could be associated with higher probability of IVF failure. Cut-off DFI values as measured by microscopy-based TUNEL were reported to be 20% [31], FACS-based TUNEL to be 36.5% [77], SCSA to be 30% [30], and SCD to be 25.5% [78]. Similarly, couples with sperm DFI >50% (Comet assay) had 13% live-birth rate, while sperm DFI <25% had a live-birth rate of 33% [79]. Another study has shown that both Comet head DNA damage and tail damage can be used as good predictors of successful pregnancy or failure [80]. Recently Tandara et al. [64] argued the suitability of measuring the percentage of spermatozoa with undamaged DNA as better prognostic parameter of embryo quality and pregnancy achieved by conventional IVF rather than DFI. Samples with AOT score of ≥12% [77] and big halo % of >38% have lower blastocyst rates and pregnancy failure.

22.8 ICSI and Pregnancy Loss

In intra-cytoplasmic sperm injection (ICSI), a single sperm is selected and injected directly into oocyte. The results of a meta-analysis support the use of ICSI over IVF in men with high sperm DNA fragmentation [81]. The rationale advocated that ICSI involves selection of morphologically normal motile sperm which is believed to have lower DNA fragmentation. The stratified analysis by type of procedure (IVF vs. ICSI) revealed that sperm with high DNA damage have higher pregnancy rate in ICSI, while the rate of miscarriage is similar in both IVF and ICSI [38]. Table 22.3 summarizes the studies correlating sperm DNA integrity and ICSI outcome.

Table 22.3 Effect of sperm DNA damage on ICSI outcome at different stages

DFI assay	Study population	Sample size	Results after ICSI	References
TUNEL	Canada	150	Lowered fertilization rate	[82]
	France	54		[32]
SCD	Iran	92		[22]
AOT	Turkey	56		[83]
TUNEL	Italy	50	Lowered pregnancy rate	[84]
	Virginia	36		[33]
SCSA	Poland	60		[85]
AOT	Italy	50		[86]
FISH	Italy	48		[89]
	Spain	19		[87]
	Italy	18		[88]
	USA	9		[90]

22.8.1 *Pregnancy Rate*

Paternal genomic alterations may compromise not only fertilization and embryo quality [82, 83] but also 'embryo viability' and progression of pregnancy, resulting in spontaneous miscarriage. Avendano et al. [33] investigated the percentage of morphologically normal sperm with fragmented DNA and observed a negative association with mean embryo score. The study showed that when the percentage of normal sperm DNA fragmentation was ≤17.6%, the likelihood of pregnancy was 3.5 times higher. Another study reported a threshold TUNEL score of 20% as cut-off for miscarriage [84]. Similarly, a reduction in pregnancy rates was observed with samples having DFI of 23% as determined by SCSA [85]. Dar et al. [86] found a close relationship between DNA fragmentation and post-implantation development in ICSI by comparing the miscarriage rates between two groups with low DFI (<15%) and with high DFI (>50%). The study detected a trend toward a higher miscarriage rate in high DFI group.

Couples with a clinical background of recurrent miscarriages of unknown aetiology or implantation failure after ICSI were also characterized for abnormal sperm aneuploidy by FISH [87]. Higher rates of miscarriage were obtained in patients with abnormal sperm FISH results. Calogero et al. [88] reported that unselected patients undergoing ICSI had an elevated sperm aneuploidy rate related to subsequent pregnancy failure. Similarly, Burrello et al. [89] focussed on role of sperm aneuploidy on ICSI outcome in patients with male factor infertility. Taking a cut-off value of aneuploidy as >1.55%, lower pregnancy and implantation rates were observed. Targeting the recurrent miscarriages post ICSI in oligoasthenozoospermic sample, FISH, using directly labelled (fluorochrome-dUTP) satellite or contig DNA probes specific for chromosomes 4, 6, 7, 8, 9, 10, 11, 12, 13, 17, 18, 21, X, and Y, was performed on decondensed spermatozoa [90]. Significantly elevated frequencies of diploidy, autosomal disomy and nullisomy, sex chromosome aneuploidy, and total aneuploidy in these patients suggest increased risk of abortion.

22.9 Effect of DNA Damage on Outcome of IVF and ICSI: A Comparison

In patients with poor spermiogram, ICSI is the treatment of choice, as it is assumed that DFI has a minimal effect on ICSI outcome [91]. However, the chances of selecting a normal sperm with fragmented DNA for oocyte injection put every ICSI cycle at high risk. Thus it warrants finding a threshold value of DFI which determines the type of ART treatment to be chosen. Nonetheless, the heterogeneity of the threshold value set among the various studies is due to difference in methods used for sperm preparation and assessment of DNA damage.

Sergerie et al. [92] proposed a pathological DFI threshold of 20% (TUNEL) for fertility status in vivo; however, a threshold for IVF and ICSI failures is controversial.

Taking 15% as TUNEL threshold score, the risk of non-transfer due to blocked embryo development increased, more so for ICSI (18.2%) than that for IVF (4.2%) with an odds ratio of 5.05 [93]. Similarly, the miscarriage risk increased fourfold (37.5% for ICSI vs. 8.8% for IVF) with ≥15% DFI. The threshold DFI (SCSA) for better pregnancy rates is higher in case of IVF (≤ 30%), in comparison to ICSI (≤19%) [27]. Bungum et al. [94] found that in the patients with the SCSA score >30%, the pregnancy results of ICSI were significantly better than those of IVF. It is advocated that in vitro ART is able to bypass the impairment of sperm chromatin, in particular if ICSI is chosen as a fertilization method. So, when DFI exceeded a level of 30%, ICSI is a more efficient treatment option. However, another study reported a DFI value of 30% (AOT) as threshold for decreasing FR, cleavage, implantation, and pregnancy in ICSI cycles but not significantly in IVF cycles [95]. The biological rationale explained is that in IVF mostly sperm with higher DNA integrity are naturally selected for oocyte penetration and fertilization [96].

Irrespective of ART technique used, FR were affected when TUNEL score was >10% [97]. The effect on FR was more pronounced in IVF than ICSI. Similarly, above a threshold SCD score of 18%, EQ and FR can also be adversely affected [98]. Muriel et al. [10] proposed that higher DNA fragmentation determined by SCD would produce an increased proportion of zygotes showing asynchrony between the nucleolar precursor bodies of zygote pronuclei (73.8% vs. 28.8% $P < 0.001$). Moreover, slower embryo development and reduced implantation rate in IVF/ICSI were also associated with higher sperm DNA fragmentation. Similarly, no patients achieved clinical pregnancy after ART, if SCSA values exceeded 27% ($P < 0.01$) [99]. Henkel et al. [100] observed a significantly reduced pregnancy rate in both IVF and ICSI patients inseminated with TUNEL-positive spermatozoa. It could be inferred here that although patients may be able to conceive via ART, sperm DNA damage might be a limiting factor, and severe damage would lead to increase in abortion rates [101].

22.10 Inference Drawn from Meta-analysis Studies

Evenson et al. [9] carried out comparative meta-analyses taking 17 studies to compare the effect of sperm DNA damage on pregnancy outcome after IVF and ICSI. Using the Cochran–Mantel–Haenszel (CMH) statistic, the meta-analysis results found that patients using in vivo fertilization were 7.0 times (CI 3.17, 17.7) more likely to achieve a pregnancy/delivery if the DFI was <30% ($n = 362$, $P = 0.0001$). In comparison, infertile couples were approximately 2.0 times (CI 1.02, 2.84) more likely to become pregnant with IVF treatment if their DFI was <30% ($n = 381$, $P = 0.03$). For ICSI, the results indicated 1.6 times (CI 0.92, 2.94) higher possibility to achieve a pregnancy/delivery if the DFI was <30% ($n = 323$, $P = 0.06$). A MEDLINE and bibliographic search (from Jan 1978 to Apr 2006) resulted in selection of eight articles based on inclusion/exclusion criteria [102]. RevMan software was used, and the relative likelihood of DNA damage effect on

IVF/ICSI outcomes was expressed as a risk ratio (RR). About five studies which measured DFI by TUNEL assay revealed that there is 32% (CI 0.54–0.85, $P = 0.0006$) and 24% (CI 0.55–1.04, $P = 0.09$) reduction, respectively, in the odds of having pregnancy for IVF and ICSI patients ($n = 816$), with high degree of sperm DNA damage compared with those with low degree of sperm DNA damage. However, 3 studies that used the SCSA assay and took 299 subjects indicated there are no significant effects of sperm DNA damage on the clinical pregnancy rate after IVF (RR 0.58, 95% CI 0.25–1.31, $P = 0.19$) or ICSI (RR 1.18, 95% CI 0.81–1.74, $P = 0.38$). Thus, the above study favours TUNEL assay over SCSA as a better predictor of ART outcome.

Zini et al. [8] carried out meta-analysis looking at 11 studies that involve 1549 cycles of treatment (808 IVF and 741 ICSI) with 640 pregnancies (345 IVF and 295 ICSI) and 122 pregnancy losses. Six (6) studies measured DFI using SCSA and estimated OR of 1.77 for pregnancy loss (95% CI, 1.01–3.13; $P = 0.05$); five studies measured DFI by TUNEL and estimated OR of 7.04 (95% CI, 2.81–17.67; $P = 0.001$). The fixed effects model combined OR of 2.48 (95% CI 1.52–4.04, $P < 0.0001$) indicates that sperm DNA damage is predictive of pregnancy loss after IVF and ICSI. Similarly another systemic review and meta-analysis were carried out on 16 cohort studies (2969 couples), 14 of which were prospective [103]. Searches were conducted on MEDLINE, EMBASE, and the Cochrane Library from database inception to January 2012. Meta-analysis of relative risks of miscarriage was performed with a random effects model. A cumulative risk ratio of 2.16 (1.54–3.03; $P = 0.00001$) indicates a significant increase in miscarriage in patients with high DNA damage compared with those with low DNA damage. About six studies used TUNEL assay and had the strongest miscarriage association (RR = 3.94, 95% CI 2.45–6.32; $P < 0.00001$). While the summary RR estimate of studies using SCSA (six studies) was 3.94 (95% CI, 2.45–6.32; $P = 0.00001$), using the Comet assay (two studies) was 1.43 (95% CI, 0.4–5.14; $P = 0.58$), and using the AOT assay (one study) was 2.78 (95% CI, 0.59–13.11; $P = 0.20$). A subgroup analysis showed a strong association of the prepared semen with high DNA damage and miscarriage (RR = 3.47, 95% CI: 2.13 t–5.63; $P = 0.00001$) than the raw semen group (RR = 1.50, 95% CI: 1.11–2.01; $P = 0.007$).

An exhaustive electronic literature search from database inception to October 2013 included 16 cohort studies (3106 couples) and examined the influence of sperm DNA damage on pregnancy and miscarriage following IVF/ICSI [38]. A meta-analysis showed that high-level sperm DNA fragmentation is detrimental to IVF/ICSI outcome, with decreased pregnancy rate (OR = 0.81, 95% CI:0.70–0.95; $P = 0.008$) and increased miscarriage rate (OR = 2.28, 95%CI:1.55–3.35; $P < 0.0001$). The stratified analysis by type of procedure (IVF vs. ICSI) indicated that high sperm DNA damage was related to lower pregnancy rates in IVF with OR of 0.66 (95% CI: 0.48–0.90; $P = 0.008$) but not in ICSI cycles, whereas it was significantly associated with higher miscarriage rates in ICSI cycles (OR 2.68; 95% CI:1.40–5.14; $P = 0.003$). Furthermore, the study also observes significant OR when DFI was measured by TUNEL as compared to SCSA. Osman et al. [81] conducted a meta-analysis of six studies to evaluate the relationship between the extent of sperm DNA damage and live-birth rate (LBR) per couple. Overall, they found a significant increase in LBR (RR 1.17, 95% CI 1.07–1.28; $P = 0.0005$) in couples with low sperm DNA fragmentation compared to those with high sperm DNA fragmentation. After IVF and ICSI, men with low sperm DNA fragmentation had significantly higher LBR (RR 1.27, 95% CI 1.05–1.52; $P = 0.01$) and (RR 1.11, 95% CI 1.00–1.23, $P = 0.04$), respectively. A sensitivity analysis observed no statistically significant difference in LBR between low and high sperm DNA fragmentation when ICSI treatment was used (RR 1.08, 95% CI 0.39–2.96; $P = 0.88$). High sperm DNA fragmentation in couples undergoing ART is associated with lower LBR. The most recent and extensive meta-analytical report [104] identified 41 articles (with a total of 56 studies) including 16 IVF studies, 24 ICSI studies, and 16 mixed (IVF + ICSI) studies. These studies measured DNA damage (by one of four assays: 23 SCSA, 18 TUNEL, 8 SCD, and 7 Comet) and included a total of 8068 treatment cycles (3734 IVF, 2282 ICSI, and 2052 mixed IVF + ICSI). The combined OR of 1.68 (95% CI: 1.49–1.89; $P < 0.0001$) indicates that sperm DNA damage affects clinical pregnancy following IVF and/or ICSI treatment. In addition, the combined OR estimates of IVF (16 estimates, OR = 1.65; 95% CI: 1.34–2.04; $P < 0.0001$), ICSI (24 estimates, OR = 1.31; 95% CI: 1.08–1.59; $P = 0.0068$), and mixed IVF + ICSI studies (16 estimates, OR = 2.37; 95% CI: 1.89–2.97; $P < 0.0001$) were also statistically significant. Moreover, a strong negative association was observed between sperm DNA damage and clinical pregnancy (with a statistically significant combined OR estimate) utilizing assays that measure sperm DNA damage directly (TUNEL and Comet assays) than those measured indirectly (SCSA and SCD assay).

Contrary to the above studies, a systematic review and meta-analysis [105] evaluated 13 relevant studies with 18 estimates of the diagnostic test properties of sperm DNA integrity tests in 2162 cycles of treatment. The summary diagnostic OR was 1.44 (95% CI, 1.03, 2.03), but the likelihood ratios (LR) were not predictive of pregnancy outcome (LR+ = 1.23; 95% CI, 0.98, 1.54; LR− = 0.81; 95%CI, 0.67, 0.98). Thus, the above meta-analysis shows that neither SCSA, NT, nor TUNEL was predictive of IVF/ICSI outcome. Recently, Zhang et al. [106] included about 20 studies for a meta-analysis and proposed that infertile couples were more likely to get pregnant if DFI was less than threshold value (i.e. >27% and 15–27% group, combined overall OR (95% CI) = 1.437 (1.186–1.742), 1.639 (1.093–2.459) respectively). However, the predication value of DFI for IVF or ICSI outcome could not be confirmed.

22.11 Making the Right Choice

With a handful of DNA assessment assays with different levels of efficacy to identify sperm DNA damage, both the patient and physician can be frustrated. It is still noteworthy to mention that irrespective of the low predictive power of sperm DNA testing, clinicians counsel their patients depending upon the knowledge gained through several clinical trials. That is, for couples planning their first pregnancy, test of sperm DNA damage (especially SCSA) is a good predictor of negative pregnancy outcome. The level of DNA fragmentation would help them to know their potential for natural fertility and opt for ART if needed [7]. Moreover, if evaluated in men before ART, sperm DNA abnormalities would likely identify the cause of infertility in a large percentage of patients. DNA tests like SCSA would help the infertile couples to go for intrauterine insemination (IUI) as the first-line treatment for unexplained infertility [96]. However, if the male partner has high levels of sperm DNA damage, the couples should consider advanced forms of assisted reproduction (IVF or ICSI) to achieve a pregnancy. Moreover, couples facing recurrent miscarriages post ART should be advised to check their sperm DNA integrity. When high DFI is detected (>30%), ICSI using testicular spermatozoa was an effective option particularly for those with repeated ART failures in terms of clinical, ongoing pregnancies and miscarriages even though conventional sperm parameters are within normal range. Recently, Pabuccu et al. [107] took normozoospermic subjects with high sperm DFI facing previous ART failures. They studied the pregnancy rates of testicular aspirated sperm (TESA sample) vs. ejaculated spermatozoa (EJ) in those subjects. They found that clinical (41.9% versus 20%) and ongoing pregnancy rates (38.7% versus 15%) were significantly better and miscarriages were lower in TESA group when compared to EJ group. The authors recommended sperm DFI to be a part of male partner's evaluation following unsuccessful ART attempts.

22.12 Conclusion

Conventional semen parameters remain the epitome for assessment of the fertility potential in males opting for ART. However, their utility in predicting reproductive success is questionable. In contrast, sperm DNA damage has been associated with a significantly increased risk of pregnancy loss post IVF and ICSI, as evidenced from the documented literature. Ambiguity over the influence of female factors can be minimized by ovum donation. Despite our limited knowledge about the possible mechanisms involved in miscarriage caused by DNA damage, the contribution of the paternal genome in miscarriages cannot be underestimated. Studies have shown that when the paternal genes are 'switched on', the deleterious consequences of fragmented paternal DNA became evident pausing further embryonic development.

Moreover, the ability of the oocyte to repair DNA damage in the fertilizing spermatozoon is going to depend not only on the severity but also on the type of damage. In general, single-stranded DNA damage is easier to repair than double-stranded DNA damage [19]. The failure of meta-analysis interpretations to address the controversial association between DFI and ART outcome could be based on the rationale that mostly the assays for sperm DNA fragmentation were performed on raw semen samples. These samples would contain a high percentage of immotile, nonviable, or degenerated sperm with abnormal chromatin. On the contrary, the procedures followed for sperm preparation may not directly affect the integrity of the DNA but increase the susceptibility of the DNA to damage. The significant limitations (methodological and design weakness) of the sperm DNA studies warrant further research on the predictive value of sperm DNA fragmentation on pregnancy outcomes after ART.

References

1. Macklon NS, Geraedts JP, Fauser BC. Conception to ongoing pregnancy: the 'black box' of early pregnancy loss. Hum Reprod Update. 2002;8(4):333–43.
2. Swain N, et al. Proteomics and male infertility, in proteomics in human reproduction: biomarkers for millennials. Cham: Springer International Publishing; 2016. p. 21–43.
3. Swain N, Cirenza C, Samanta L. Role of proteomics in female infertility, in proteomics in human reproduction: biomarkers for millennials. Cham: Springer International Publishing; 2016. p. 45–63.
4. Marteil G, Richard-Parpaillon L, Kubiak JZ. Role of oocyte quality in meiotic maturation and embryonic development. Reprod Biol. 2009;9(3):203–24.
5. Coughlan C, et al. Sperm DNA fragmentation, recurrent implantation failure and recurrent miscarriage. Asian J Androl. 2015;17(4):681–5.
6. Bach PV, Schlegel PN. Sperm DNA damage and its role in IVF and ICSI. Basic Clin Androl. 2016;26:15.
7. Zini A, Libman J. Sperm DNA damage: clinical significance in the era of assisted reproduction. CMAJ. 2006;175(5):495–500.
8. Zini A, et al. Sperm DNA damage is associated with an increased risk of pregnancy loss after IVF and ICSI: systematic review and meta-analysis. Hum Reprod. 2008;23(12):2663–8.
9. Evenson D, Wixon R. Meta-analysis of sperm DNA fragmentation using the sperm chromatin structure assay. Reprod Biomed Online. 2006;12(4):466–72.
10. Muriel L, et al. Value of the sperm deoxyribonucleic acid fragmentation level, as measured by the sperm chromatin dispersion test, in the outcome of in vitro fertilization and intracytoplasmic sperm injection. Fertil Steril. 2006;85(2):371–83.
11. Tesarik J, Greco E, Mendoza C. Late, but not early, paternal effect on human embryo development is related to sperm DNA fragmentation. Hum Reprod. 2004;19(3):611–5.
12. De Bont R, van Larebeke N. Endogenous DNA damage in humans: a review of quantitative data. Mutagenesis. 2004;19(3):169–85.
13. Zini A, Sigman M. Are tests of sperm DNA damage clinically useful? Pros and cons. J Androl. 2009;30(3):219–29.
14. Irvine DS, et al. DNA integrity in human spermatozoa: relationships with semen quality. J Androl. 2000;21(1):33–44.
15. Sakkas D, Alvarez JG. Sperm DNA fragmentation: mechanisms of origin, impact on reproductive outcome, and analysis. Fertil Steril. 2010;93(4):1027–36.
16. Aitken RJ, De Iuliis GN. On the possible origins of DNA damage in human spermatozoa. Mol Hum Reprod. 2010;16(1):3–13.
17. Evenson D. Reply to: 'The predictive value of the sperm chromatin structure assay (SCSA)' – a response from the SCSA inventor. Hum Reprod. 2006;21(2):570–2.
18. Samanta L, Mohanty G, Agarwal A. Male factors in recurrent pregnancy loss, in recurrent pregnancy loss. New York: Springer; 2016. p. 109–29.
19. Gonzalez-Marin C, Gosalvez J, Roy R. Types, causes, detection and repair of DNA fragmentation in animal and human sperm cells. Int J Mol Sci. 2012;13(11):14026–52.
20. Esterhuizen AD, et al. Defective sperm decondensation: a cause for fertilization failure. Andrologia. 2002;34(1):1–7.
21. Sakkas D, et al. Sperm chromatin anomalies can influence decondensation after intracytoplasmic sperm injection. Hum Reprod. 1996;11(4):837–43.

22. Tavalaee M, Razavi S, Nasr-Esfahani MH. Influence of sperm chromatin anomalies on assisted reproductive technology outcome. Fertil Steril. 2009;91(4):1119–26.
23. Ahmadi A, Ng SC. Fertilizing ability of DNA-damaged spermatozoa. J Exp Zool. 1999;284(6):696–704.
24. Ahmadi A, Ng SC. Developmental capacity of damaged spermatozoa. Hum Reprod. 1999;14(9):2279–85.
25. Wdowiak A, Bakalczuk S, Bakalczuk G. The effect of sperm DNA fragmentation on the dynamics of the embryonic development in intracytoplasmatic sperm injection. Reprod Biol. 2015;15(2):94–100.
26. Tesarik J, Mendoza C, Greco E. Paternal effects acting during the first cell cycle of human preimplantation development after ICSI. Hum Reprod. 2002;17(1):184–9.
27. Speyer BE, et al. Fall in implantation rates following ICSI with sperm with high DNA fragmentation. Hum Reprod. 2010;25(7):1609–18.
28. Braude P, Bolton V, Moore S. Human gene expression first occurs between the four-and eight-cell stages of preimplantation development. Nature. 1988;332(6163):459–61.
29. Banerjee S, et al. Does blastocyst culture eliminate paternal chromosomal defects and select good embryos?: inheritance of an abnormal paternal genome following ICSI. Hum Reprod. 2000;15(12):2455–9.
30. Virro MR, Larson-Cook KL, Evenson DP. Sperm chromatin structure assay (SCSA) parameters are related to fertilization, blastocyst development, and ongoing pregnancy in in vitro fertilization and intracytoplasmic sperm injection cycles. Fertil Steril. 2004;81(5):1289–95.
31. Seli E, et al. Extent of nuclear DNA damage in ejaculated spermatozoa impacts on blastocyst development after in vitro fertilization. Fertil Steril. 2004;82(2):378–83.
32. Benchaib M, et al. Sperm DNA fragmentation decreases the pregnancy rate in an assisted reproductive technique. Hum Reprod. 2003;18(5):1023–8.
33. Avendano C, et al. DNA fragmentation of normal spermatozoa negatively impacts embryo quality and intracytoplasmic sperm injection outcome. Fertil Steril. 2010;94(2):549–57.
34. Marchetti F, et al. Disruption of maternal DNA repair increases sperm-derived chromosomal aberrations. Proc Natl Acad Sci U S A. 2007;104(45):17725–9.
35. Menezo Y Jr, et al. Expression profile of genes coding for DNA repair in human oocytes using pangenomic microarrays, with a special focus on ROS linked decays. J Assist Reprod Genet. 2007;24(11):513–20.
36. Jaroudi S, et al. Expression profiling of DNA repair genes in human oocytes and blastocysts using microarrays. Hum Reprod. 2009;24(10):2649–55.
37. Gosalvez J, et al. Can DNA fragmentation of neat or swim-up spermatozoa be used to predict pregnancy following ICSI of fertile oocyte donors? Asian J Androl. 2013;15(6):812–8.
38. Zhao J, et al. Whether sperm deoxyribonucleic acid fragmentation has an effect on pregnancy and miscarriage after in vitro fertilization/intracytoplasmic sperm injection: a systematic review and meta-analysis. Fertil Steril. 2014;102(4):998–1005. e8
39. Esbert M, et al. Impact of sperm DNA fragmentation on the outcome of IVF with own or donated oocytes. Reprod Biomed Online. 2011;23(6):704–10.
40. Meseguer M, et al. Effect of sperm DNA fragmentation on pregnancy outcome depends on oocyte quality. Fertil Steril. 2011;95(1):124–8.
41. Nunez-Calonge R, et al. An improved experimental model for understanding the impact of sperm DNA fragmentation on human pregnancy following ICSI. Reprod Sci. 2012;19(11):1163–8.
42. Alvarez JG. The predictive value of sperm chromatin structure assay. Hum Reprod. 2005;20(8):2365–7.
43. Payne JF, et al. Redefining the relationship between sperm deoxyribonucleic acid fragmentation as measured by the sperm chromatin structure assay and outcomes of assisted reproductive techniques. Fertil Steril. 2005;84(2):356–64.
44. Mohanty G, et al. Histone retention, protein carbonylation, and lipid peroxidation in spermatozoa: possible role in recurrent pregnancy loss. Syst Biol Reprod Med. 2016;62(3):201–12.

45. Donnelly ET, et al. Differences in nuclear DNA fragmentation and mitochondrial integrity of semen and prepared human spermatozoa. Hum Reprod. 2000;15(7):1552–61.
46. Morrell JM, et al. Reduced senescence and retained nuclear DNA integrity in human spermatozoa prepared by density gradient centrifugation. J Assist Reprod Genet. 2004;21(6):217–22.
47. Caglar GS, et al. Semen DNA fragmentation index, evaluated with both TUNEL and Comet assay, and the ICSI outcome. In Vivo. 2007;21(6):1075–80.
48. Simon L, et al. Sperm DNA damage measured by the alkaline Comet assay as an independent predictor of male infertility and in vitro fertilization success. Fertil Steril. 2011;95(2):652–7.
49. Sakkas D, et al. The use of two density gradient centrifugation techniques and the swim-up method to separate spermatozoa with chromatin and nuclear DNA anomalies. Hum Reprod. 2000;15(5):1112–6.
50. Piomboni P, et al. Ultrastructural and DNA fragmentation analyses in swim-up selected human sperm. Arch Androl. 2006;52(1):51–9.
51. Jayaraman V, et al. Sperm processing by swim-up and density gradient is effective in elimination of sperm with DNA damage. J Assist Reprod Genet. 2012;29(6):557–63.
52. Zini A, et al. Influence of semen processing technique on human sperm DNA integrity. Urology. 2000;56(6):1081–4.
53. Hammadeh ME, et al. Comparison of sperm preparation methods: effect on chromatin and morphology recovery rates and their consequences on the clinical outcome after in vitro fertilization embryo transfer. Int J Androl. 2001;24(6):360–8.
54. Bungum M, et al. Sperm chromatin structure assay parameters measured after density gradient centrifugation are not predictive for the outcome of ART. Hum Reprod. 2008;23(1):4–10.
55. Tomlinson MJ, et al. Interrelationships between seminal parameters and sperm nuclear DNA damage before and after density gradient centrifugation: implications for assisted conception. Hum Reprod. 2001;16(10):2160–5.
56. Host E, Lindenberg S, Smidt-Jensen S. The role of DNA strand breaks in human spermatozoa used for IVF and ICSI. Acta Obstet Gynecol Scand. 2000;79(7):559–63.
57. Oliveira JB, et al. Correlation between semen analysis by motile sperm organelle morphology examination and sperm DNA damage. Fertil Steril. 2010;94(5):1937–40.
58. Aitken RJ, Hanson AR, Kuczera L. Electrophoretic sperm isolation: optimization of electrophoresis conditions and impact on oxidative stress. Hum Reprod. 2011;26(8):1955–64.
59. Wang W, et al. Effects of a microfluidic sperm sorter on sperm routine parameters and DNA integrity. Zhonghua Nan Ke Xue. 2011;17(4):301–4.
60. Kheirollahi-Kouhestani M, et al. Selection of sperm based on combined density gradient and Zeta method may improve ICSI outcome. Hum Reprod. 2009;24(10):2409–16.
61. Zahedi A, et al. Zeta potential vs apoptotic marker: which is more suitable for ICSI sperm selection? J Assist Reprod Genet. 2013;30(9):1181–6.
62. Petersen CG, et al. Relationship between DNA damage and sperm head birefringence. Reprod Biomed Online. 2011;22(6):583–9.
63. Rappa KL, et al. Sperm processing for advanced reproductive technologies: where are we today? Biotechnol Adv. 2016;34(5):578–87.
64. Tandara M, et al. Sperm DNA integrity testing: big halo is a good predictor of embryo quality and pregnancy after conventional IVF. Andrology. 2014;2(5):678–86.
65. Sun JG, Jurisicova A, Casper RF. Detection of deoxyribonucleic acid fragmentation in human sperm: correlation with fertilization in vitro. Biol Reprod. 1997;56(3):602–7.
66. Bakos HW, et al. Sperm DNA damage is associated with assisted reproductive technology pregnancy. Int J Androl. 2008;31(5):518–26.
67. Marchetti C, et al. Study of mitochondrial membrane potential, reactive oxygen species, DNA fragmentation and cell viability by flow cytometry in human sperm. Hum Reprod. 2002;17(5):1257–65.
68. Zhang X, et al. Localization of single-stranded DNA in human sperm nuclei. Fertil Steril. 2007;88(5):1334–8.
69. Pregl Breznik B, Kovacic B, Vlaisavljevic V. Are sperm DNA fragmentation, hyperactivation, and hyaluronan-binding ability predictive for fertilization and embryo development in in vitro fertilization and intracytoplasmic sperm injection? Fertil Steril. 2013;99(5):1233–41.

70. Gu LJ, et al. Sperm chromatin anomalies have an adverse effect on the outcome of conventional in vitro fertilization: a study with strictly controlled external factors. Fertil Steril. 2009;92(4):1344–6.
71. Tarozzi N, et al. Anomalies in sperm chromatin packaging: implications for assisted reproduction techniques. Reprod Biomed Online. 2009;18(4):486–95.
72. Filatov MV, et al. Relationship between abnormal sperm chromatin packing and IVF results. Mol Hum Reprod. 1999;5(9):825–30.
73. Haidl G, Schill WB. Assessment of sperm chromatin condensation: an important test for prediction of IVF outcome. Arch Androl. 1994;32(3):263–6.
74. Claassens OE, et al. The Acridine Orange test: determining the relationship between sperm morphology and fertilization in vitro. Hum Reprod. 1992;7(2):242–7.
75. Liu DY, Baker HW. Sperm nuclear chromatin normality: relationship with sperm morphology, sperm-zona pellucida binding, and fertilization rates in vitro. Fertil Steril. 1992;58(6):1178–84.
76. Janny L, Menezo YJ. Evidence for a strong paternal effect on human preimplantation embryo development and blastocyst formation. Mol Reprod Dev. 1994;38(1):36–42.
77. Henkel R, et al. Influence of deoxyribonucleic acid damage on fertilization and pregnancy. Fertil Steril. 2004;81(4):965–72.
78. Lopez G, et al. Diagnostic value of sperm DNA fragmentation and sperm high-magnification for predicting outcome of assisted reproduction treatment. Asian J Androl. 2013;15(6):790–4.
79. Simon L, et al. Sperm DNA damage has a negative association with live-birth rates after IVF. Reprod Biomed Online. 2013;26(1):68–78.
80. Tomsu M, Sharma V, Miller D. Embryo quality and IVF treatment outcomes may correlate with different sperm comet assay parameters. Hum Reprod. 2002;17(7):1856–62.
81. Osman A, et al. The effect of sperm DNA fragmentation on live birth rate after IVF or ICSI: a systematic review and meta-analysis. Reprod Biomed Online. 2015;30(2):120–7.
82. Lopes S, et al. Sperm deoxyribonucleic acid fragmentation is increased in poor-quality semen samples and correlates with failed fertilization in intracytoplasmic sperm injection. Fertil Steril. 1998;69(3):528–32.
83. Cebesoy FB, Aydos K, Unlu C. Effect of sperm chromatin damage on fertilization ratio and embryo quality post-ICSI. Arch Androl. 2006;52(5):397–402.
84. Borini A, et al. Sperm DNA fragmentation: paternal effect on early post-implantation embryo development in ART. Hum Reprod. 2006;21(11):2876–81.
85. Micinski P, et al. The sperm chromatin structure assay (SCSA) as prognostic factor in IVF/ICSI program. Reprod Biol. 2009;9(1):65–70.
86. Dar S, et al. In vitro fertilization-intracytoplasmic sperm injection outcome in patients with a markedly high DNA fragmentation index (>50%). Fertil Steril. 2013;100(1):75–80.
87. Rubio C, et al. Incidence of sperm chromosomal abnormalities in a risk population: relationship with sperm quality and ICSI outcome. Hum Reprod. 2001;16(10):2084–92.
88. Calogero AE, et al. High sperm aneuploidy rate in unselected infertile patients and its relationship with intracytoplasmic sperm injection outcome. Hum Reprod. 2001;16(7):1433–9.
89. Burrello N, et al. Lower sperm aneuploidy frequency is associated with high pregnancy rates in ICSI programmes. Hum Reprod. 2003;18(7):1371–6.
90. Pang MG, et al. Detection of aneuploidy for chromosomes 4, 6, 7, 8, 9, 10, 11, 12, 13, 17, 18, 21, X and Y by fluorescence in-situ hybridization in spermatozoa from nine patients with oligoasthenoteratozoospermia undergoing intracytoplasmic sperm injection. Hum Reprod. 1999;14(5):1266–73.
91. Nicopoullos JD, et al. Sperm DNA fragmentation in subfertile men: the effect on the outcome of intracytoplasmic sperm injection and correlation with sperm variables. BJU Int. 2008;101(12):1553–60.
92. Sergerie M, et al. Sperm DNA fragmentation: threshold value in male fertility. Hum Reprod. 2005;20(12):3446–51.
93. Benchaib M, et al. Sperm deoxyribonucleic acid fragmentation as a prognostic indicator of assisted reproductive technology outcome. Fertil Steril. 2007;87(1):93–100.

94. Bungum M, et al. Sperm DNA integrity assessment in prediction of assisted reproduction technology outcome. Hum Reprod. 2007;22(1):174–9.
95. Jiang H, et al. The relationship of sperm DNA fragmentation index with the outcomes of in-vitro fertilisation-embryo transfer and intracytoplasmic sperm injection. J Obstet Gynaecol. 2011;31(7):636–9.
96. Bungum M, et al. The predictive value of sperm chromatin structure assay (SCSA) parameters for the outcome of intrauterine insemination IVF and ICSI. Hum Reprod. 2004;19(6):1401–8.
97. Huang CC, et al. Sperm DNA fragmentation negatively correlates with velocity and fertilization rates but might not affect pregnancy rates. Fertil Steril. 2005;84(1):130–40.
98. Velez de la Calle JF, et al. Sperm deoxyribonucleic acid fragmentation as assessed by the sperm chromatin dispersion test in assisted reproductive technology programs: results of a large prospective multicenter study. Fertil Steril. 2008;90(5):1792–9.
99. Larson-Cook KL, et al. Relationship between the outcomes of assisted reproductive techniques and sperm DNA fragmentation as measured by the sperm chromatin structure assay. Fertil Steril. 2003;80(4):895–902.
100. Henkel R, et al. DNA fragmentation of spermatozoa and assisted reproduction technology. Reprod Biomed Online. 2003;7(4):477–84.
101. Kennedy C, et al. Sperm chromatin structure correlates with spontaneous abortion and multiple pregnancy rates in assisted reproduction. Reprod Biomed Online. 2011;22(3):272–6.
102. Li Z, et al. Correlation of sperm DNA damage with IVF and ICSI outcomes: a systematic review and meta-analysis. J Assist Reprod Genet. 2006;23(9–10):367–76.
103. Robinson L, et al. The effect of sperm DNA fragmentation on miscarriage rates: a systematic review and meta-analysis. Hum Reprod. 2012;27(10):2908–17.
104. Simon L, et al. A systematic review and meta-analysis to determine the effect of sperm DNA damage on in vitro fertilization and intracytoplasmic sperm injection outcome. Asian J Androl. 2017;19(1):80–90.
105. Collins JA, Barnhart KT, Schlegel PN. Do sperm DNA integrity tests predict pregnancy with in vitro fertilization? Fertil Steril. 2008;89(4):823–31.
106. Zhang Z, et al. Sperm DNA fragmentation index and pregnancy outcome after IVF or ICSI: a meta-analysis. J Assist Reprod Genet. 2015;32(1):17–26.
107. Pabuccu EG, et al. Testicular versus ejaculated spermatozoa in ICSI cycles of normozoospermic men with high sperm DNA fragmentation and previous ART failures. Andrologia. 2017;49(2):e12609.

Chapter 23
Sperm DNA Tests Are Clinically Useful: Pro

Luke Simon, Douglas T. Carrell, and Armand Zini

23.1 Introduction

Sperm is a vehicle that aids the transport of the haploid paternal genome to the oocyte. The delivery of intact and complete genetic material to the oocyte is required for normal embryonic development [1]. To facilitate this process, the sperm nucleus is equipped with a unique design of nuclear architecture, where the nuclear proteins are replaced by smaller and positively charged protamines that allow the chromatin to form a compact structure [2]. During sperm nuclear structural reorganization, the sperm loses its cytoplasm, which provides the sperm its streamline nature and facilitates movement through the male and female reproductive tract. On the other hand, the lack of cytoplasm leaves the nucleus vulnerable and unprotected against the free radicals [3]. The seminal plasma not only acts as a medium for the sperm to swim in but also scavenges the free radicals to minimize the effect of oxidative stress-mediated DNA damage [4].

Despite such precaution, DNA fragmentation is common and is believed to be a property of all sperm. However, the level of DNA damage may vary from one sperm to another [5]. DNA damage occurring in sperm can be the result of

L. Simon
Department of Surgery (Urology), University of Utah, Salt Lake City, UT, USA

D.T. Carrell
Department of Surgery (Urology), Department of Human Genetics,
Department of Obstetrics and Gynecology, University of Utah School of Medicine,
Salt Lake City, UT, USA

A. Zini (✉)
Department of Surgery, Division of Urology, McGill University, Montreal, QC, Canada
e-mail: ziniarmand@yahoo.com

A. Zini, A. Agarwal (eds.), *A Clinician's Guide to Sperm DNA and Chromatin Damage*, https://doi.org/10.1007/978-3-319-71815-6_23

intrinsic factors where poor organization of sperm chromatin leaves the sperm vulnerable to oxidative stress-mediated DNA damage [1]. Studies have suggested that there may be a cascade of events that starts with seminal oxidative stress leading to DNA base modifications and DNA fragmentation resulting in apoptosis of sperm [6, 7]. Other factors such as medication, heat, radiation, etc. are some of the extrinsic factors also known to cause sperm DNA damage [8–11]. Either way, sperm lacks any DNA repair mechanism to fix the fragmented DNA, and therefore the damage occurring to sperm DNA is believed to be an irreversible process.

Most commonly studied damage to the sperm chromatin are the single- and double-strand breaks, commonly known as DNA fragmentation. A number of tests are now available to measure the level of sperm DNA fragmentation rates. Of these methods, the single-cell gel electrophoresis (commonly called as the comet assay) and the terminal deoxynucleotide transferase-mediated dUTP nick-end labeling (TUNEL) assays more directly measure the level of DNA fragmentation. Whereas, the sperm chromatin dispersion (SCD) assay (commonly called as the halo test) and sperm chromatin structure assay (SCSA) are known to indirectly measure the level of DNA fragmentation in sperm. Each of these tests measure different aspects of DNA fragmentation in sperm.

23.2 Effect of Sperm DNA Fragmentation on Clinical Outcomes: Literature Review

The comprehensive review of the published literature yielded 88 articles for systematic review, following exclusion of overlapping data, inappropriate sampling method, assays that are less commonly used (neutral comet assay, in situ nick translation assay and acridine orange slide-based staining method), and studies with insufficient data. The studies included for systematic review involved DNA fragmentation assays using TUNEL assay (34 studies), SCSA (31 studies), comet assay (12 studies), and SCD assay (11 studies). Based on the treatment types, these studies involve IUI (11 studies), IVF (28 studies), ICSI (33 studies), and IVF+ICSI mixed (17 studies). 42 studies were identified that compared fertile and infertile men using the abovementioned assays. Sixty-seven of the abovementioned studies provided sufficient data to construct two-by-two table to perform a meta-analysis, and the data of meta-analysis was recently published [12]. Among these studies, there were differences in definition of threshold values for DNA damage assays, study design, lack of control for female factors, small sample size, diverse patient group, insufficient statistical power, non-consecutive recruitment of patients, and variations in the protocols used to measure DNA fragmentation, and in some studies the selection of subjects were not clearly stated.

23.2.1 Is Sperm DNA Fragmentation Associated with Male Fertility?

A number of studies have compared DNA fragmentation between fertile and infertile men [13–21]. Overall, DNA fragmentation is more prevalent in the sperm of infertile men and may contribute to their declined fertility status. In addition, chromosomal abnormalities were shown to be increased in these patients [22, 23]. An increase in the level of DNA fragmentation in infertile men can be attributed to abnormal histone to protamine exchange [24], abnormal protamine content and ratio [25], and reduced antioxidant activity in the seminal plasma [26, 27]. A study examining the effect of DNA fragmentation on male fertility among first-pregnancy planners with no previous knowledge of their fertility capability suggested that fecundity declined with an increase in sperm DNA fragmentation, indicating the necessity of normal sperm chromatin for the expression of full male fertility potential [28]. Overall, the existing literature suggests a negative impact of sperm DNA fragmentation on male reproductive health.

23.2.2 Can Sperm DNA Fragmentation Predict Intrauterine Insemination (IUI) Success?

We identified ten studies that analyzed the association between sperm DNA fragmentation with IUI outcome. A total of 1673 IUI cycles were analyzed using SCSA (seven studies), TUNEL (two studies), and SCD (one study) assays. The results from five of the seven studies by SCSA [18, 29–32] and one study using the TUNEL assay [33] suggested a significant statistical difference in the level of sperm DNA fragmentation between the clinically pregnant and nonpregnant groups. Conclusive results were not reported in two studies using SCSA [34, 35], while no correlations were reported in two studies: using TUNEL assay [36] and using SCD assay [37].

Data was available to construct a two-by-two table from six of the seven studies performed using SCSA (except for Alkhayal et al. [35]—data not available). A meta-analysis was performed on five studies (Bungum et al. [29]—overlapping study was excluded) consisting of 1135 IUI cycles and with an overall pregnancy rate of 18.23%, resulted in an odds ratio of 5.61 (CI: 2.59–12.16; Z statistics: 4.37; $p < 0.0001$) and relative risk of 1.17 (CI: 1.12–1.22; $p < 0.0001$) indicating a strong association between sperm DNA fragmentation and IUI outcome (unpublished data). The positive and negative predictive values were 96.0% and 15.9%, respectively. This model provided a low sensitivity (16%) but high specificity (93%) values. In conclusion, this meta-analysis showed a slight but significant predictive ability of DNA fragmentation assay (SCSA) to predict IUI success, and this is in contrast to recommendations provided by the Practice Committee of the American Society for Reproductive Medicine [38], which included four of the ten studies presented above for their analysis.

23.2.3 *Is Sperm DNA Fragmentation Associated with Fertilization In Vitro?*

We identified 67 eligible articles that analyzed sperm DNA fragmentation with assisted reproductive treatment (ART) outcomes, of which 15 did not have data associating fertilization rate with sperm DNA fragmentation. The 52 eligible articles included 73 studies (25 IVF, 31 ICSI, and 17 mixed IVF+ICSI studies) and involved 8590 treatment cycles (2997 IVF, 2470 ICSI, and 3123 mixed IVF+ICSI cycles). Twenty-eight of the 73 studies (13 TUNEL, 5 SCSA, 6 SCD, and 4 comet) reported a significant inverse relationship between sperm DNA damage and fertilization rate, whereas the other 45 studies (16 TUNEL, 18 SCSA, 6 SCD, and 5 comet) showed no significant relationship between these parameters (Table 23.1).

Although we did not perform a formal meta-analysis, our systematic review of studies on sperm DNA fragmentation and fertilization rate after IVF and/or ICSI demonstrated that 38% (28/73) of the studies reported a significant inverse relationship between the two parameters. We found that a higher proportion of the IVF studies (60% or 16/25) reported a significant inverse relationship between sperm DNA fragmentation and fertilization rate than the ICSI (23% or 7/31) and mixed IVF+ICSI studies (35% or 6/17) (Table 23.1). A complete description of studies associating sperm DNA fragmentation with fertilization rate is presented in Table 23.2.

It is known that sperm progressive motility and sperm DNA fragmentation are the two most important sperm factors to affect IVF rate [39]. Indeed, there is an association between sperm DNA fragmentation and progressive motility [40–45], and this may explain the influence of these two parameters on IVF rates. A possible explanation for fertilization failure could be that sperm with abnormal chromatin may not properly decondense after penetrating the oocyte, and this can prevent development of the pronuclear stage [46–48]. The differential adverse effect of sperm DNA frag-

Table 23.1 Summary of studies associating sperm DNA fragmentation with fertilization rate

Fertilization rate	IVF Studies (*n*)	IVF Cycles (*n*)	ICSI Studies (*n*)	ICSI Cycles (*n*)	IVF+ICSI Studies (*n*)	IVF+ICSI Cycles (*n*)
Studies reporting no effect	10	1327	24	1831	11	1640
TUNEL	5	461	9	460	2	291
SCSA	5	866	8	805	5	811
SCD	0	0	3	323	3	478
Comet	0	0	4	243	1	60
Studies reporting adverse effect	15	1670	7	639	6	1483
TUNEL	7	810	5	543	1	238
SCSA	1	111	2	96	2	300
SCD	4	387	0	0	2	707
Comet	3	362	0	0	1	238

Table 23.2 Description of studies associating sperm DNA fragmentation with fertilization rate and embryo quality

Study	ART	DD test	(*n*)	Fertilization rate	Day of ET	EQ marker	DD vs. EQ	FF inclusion	FF controlled (Y/N)
Anifandis et al. (2015) [44]	IVF+ICSI	SCD	139	Non-significant	2 or 3	Grade	Significant	Unspecified	No
Avendano et al. (2010) [108]	ICSI	TUNEL	36	NA	3	Grade	Significant	Unspecified	No
Bakos et al. (2007) [118]	IVF	TUNEL	45	Significant	2 or 3	Grade	Non-significant	Unspecified	Yes
	IVF+ICSI	TUNEL	113	Non-significant	2 or 3	Grade	Non-significant	Unspecified	Yes
	ICSI	TUNEL	68	Non-significant	2 or 3	Grade	Non-significant	Unspecified	Yes
Benchaib et al. (2003) [52]	IVF	TUNEL	50	Significant	2, 3, and 5	Grade	Non-significant	Unspecified	No
	ICSI	TUNEL	54	Significant	2, 3, & 5	Grade	Non-significant	Unspecified	No
Benchaib et al. (2007) [41]	IVF	TUNEL	84	Non-significant	5	Development	Non-significant	Unspecified	Yes
	ICSI	TUNEL	218	Significant	5	Development	Significant	Unspecified	Yes
Boe-Hansen et al. (2006) [34]	IVF	SCSA	139	NA	NA		NA	Unspecified	No
	ICSI	SCSA	47	NA	NA		NA	Unspecified	No
Borini et al. (2006) [40]	IVF	TUNEL	82	Significant	2		NA	Unspecified	No
	ICSI	TUNEL	50	Non-significant	2		NA	Unspecified	No

(continued)

Table 23.2 (continued)

Study	ART	DD test	(*n*)	Fertilization rate	Day of ET	EQ marker	DD vs. EQ	FF inclusion	FF controlled (Y/N)
Breznik et al. (2013) [175][a]	IVF	SCD	133	Significant	NA	Development	Significant	Female age <37, normal female	Yes
	ICSI	SCD	133	Non-significant	NA	Development	Non-significant	Female age <37, normal female	Yes
Bungum et al. (2007) [30]	IVF	SCSA	388	Non-significant	2, 3, and 5	Grade	Non-significant	Female age <40, BMI <30, FSH <12	Yes
	ICSI	SCSA	223	Non-significant	2, 3, and 5	Grade	Non-significant	Female age <40, BMI <30, FSH <12	Yes
Caglar et al. (2007) [42]	ICSI	TUNEL	56	Non-significant	2	Grade	Non-significant	Unspecified	No
Check et al. (2005) [85]	ICSI	SCSA	106	NA	3	Grade	Significant	Unspecified	No
Dar et al. (2013) [164]	ICSI	SCSA	153	Non-significant	NA		NA	Unspecified	No
Daris et al. (2010) [176]	ICSI	TUNEL	20	Non-significant	NA		NA	Unspecified	No
Esbert et al. (2011) [90]	IVF+ICSI	TUNEL	178	Non-significant	3	Grade	Non-significant	Unspecified	No
Fang et al. (2011) [43]	IVF	SCSA	111	Significant	2 or 3	Grade	Non-significant	Unspecified	No
Frydman et al. (2008) [81]	IVF	TUNEL	117	Non-significant	NA	Grade	Non-significant	Female age <38, FSH <10	Yes
Gandini et al. (2004) [85]	IVF	SCSA	12	Non-significant	2		NA	Unspecified	No
	ICSI	SCSA	22	Non-significant	2	Grade	NA	Unspecified	Yes

Study	ART	DD test	(*n*)	Fertilization rate	Day of ET	EQ marker	DD vs. EQ	FF inclusion	FF controlled (Y/N)
Gosalvez et al. (2013) [177]	ICSI	SCD	81	NA	NA		NA	Unspecified	No
Gu et al. (2009) [106]	IVF	SCD	136	Significant	2 or 3		NA	Normal female or oviduct obstruction	Yes
Gu et al. (2011) [107]	IVF	SCD	67	Significant	3	Grade	Non-significant	Unspecified	No
Guerin et al. (2005) [178]	IVF+ICSI	SCSA	100	Non-significant	NA	Development	Non-significant	Unspecified	No
Hammadeh et al. (2006) [179]	IVF	TUNEL	26	Non-significant	NA		NA	Unspecified	No
	ICSI	TUNEL	22	Non-significant	NA		NA	Unspecified	No
Hammadeh et al. (2008) [128]	IVF	TUNEL	26	Non-significant	NA		NA	Unspecified	No
	ICSI	TUNEL	22	Non-significant	NA		NA	Unspecified	No
Henkel et al. (2003) [53]	IVF	TUNEL	208	Non-significant	NA	Fragmentation	Non-significant	Unspecified	No
	ICSI	TUNEL	54	Significant	NA	Fragmentation	Non-significant	Unspecified	No
Host et al. (2000) [125]	IVF	TUNEL	175	Significant	3	Grade	Significant	Unspecified	Yes
	ICSI	TUNEL	60	Non-significant	3	Grade	Non-significant	Unspecified	Yes

(continued)

Table 23.2 (continued)

Study	ART	DD test	(*n*)	Fertilization rate	Day of ET	EQ marker	DD vs. EQ	FF inclusion	FF controlled (Y/N)
Huang et al. (2005) [54]	IVF	TUNEL	204	Significant	3	Grade	Non-significant	Unspecified	No
	ICSI	TUNEL	86	Significant	3	Grade	Non-significant	Unspecified	No
Jiang et al. (2011) [127]	IVF	SCSA	137	Non-significant	2 or 3	Grade	Non-significant	Female age <37 years, BMI <25, FSH <10	Yes
	ICSI	SCSA	50	Non-significant	2 or 3	Grade	Non-significant	Female age <37 years, BMI <25, FSH <10	Yes
Kennedy et al. (2011) [180]	ICSI	SCSA	233	NA	NA		NA	Unspecified	Yes
Larson-Cook et al. (2003) [117]	IVF+ICSI	SCSA	82	Non-significant	3	Development	Non-significant	Unspecified	Yes
Lazaros et al. (2013) [181]	ICSI	SCSA	36	Significant	3	Fragmentation	Significant	Male factor only	Yes
Lewis et al. (2004) [182]	ICSI	Comet	77	Non-significant	2		NA	Unspecified	No
Lin et al. (2008) [55]	IVF	SCSA	137	Non-significant	3	Grade	Non-significant	Female age <40, FSH <15	Yes
	ICSI	SCSA	86	Non-significant	3	Grade	Non-significant	Female age <40, FSH <15	Yes
Lopes et al. (1998a) [47]	ICSI	TUNEL-M	131	Significant	NA	Development	Non-significant	Unspecified	No
Lopez et al. (2013) [151]	IVF+ICSI	SCD	152	NA	NA		NA	Female age <42 years, FSH <10	Yes
Marchetti et al. (2002) [183]	IVF	TUNEL	111	Significant	NA		NA	Unspecified	No

Study	ART	DD test	(*n*)	Fertilization rate	Day of ET	EQ marker	DD vs. EQ	FF inclusion	FF controlled (Y/N)
Meseguer et al. (2011) [82]	IVF+ICSI	SCD	210	NA	NA		NA	Unspecified	No
Micinski et al. (2009) [165]	ICSI	SCSA	60	Significant	2	Development	Non-significant	Female age <38	No
Morris et al. (2002) [65]	IVF+ICSI	Comet	60	Non-significant	2	Development	Significant	Female age <40	No
Muriel et al. (2006) [37]	IVF+ICSI	Halo	85	Significant	3 and 5	Development	Significant	Unspecified	No
Na and Li et al. (2011) [184]	IVF	SCD	51	Significant	3	Grade and development	Non-significant	Female age <35 years	Yes
Nasr-Esfahan et al. (2005) [185]	ICSI	Comet	28	Non-significant	2	Development	Significant	Unspecified	No
Ni et al. (2014) [105]	IVF	SCD	1380	NA	2 or 3	Development	Non-significant	Normal female	Yes
	ICSI	SCD	355	NA	2 or 3	Development	Non-significant	Normal female	Yes
Nicopoullos et al. (2008) [186]	ICSI	SCSA	56	Non-significant	2 or 3	Grade	NA	Unspecified	No
Nijs et al. (2009) [56]	IVF+ICSI	SCSA	205	Significant	3, 4 or 5	Grade	NA	Unspecified	No
Nijs et al. (2011) [187]	IVF+ICSI	SCSA	278	Non-significant	3, 4 or 5		NA	Female age ≤34, 35–39 or ≥40	Yes
Nunez-Calonge et al. (2012) [188]	ICSI	SCD	70	Non-significant	2 or 3	Grade	NA	Donor oocytes	Yes
Ozmen et al. (2007) [89]	ICSI	TUNEL	42	Non-significant	2	Grade	Non-significant	Unspecified	No

(continued)

Table 23.2 (continued)

Study	ART	DD test	(*n*)	Fertilization rate	Day of ET	EQ marker	DD vs. EQ	FF inclusion	FF controlled (Y/N)
Payne et al. (2005) [80]	IVF+ICSI	SCSA	95	Significant	2	Development	Non-significant	Unspecified	Yes
Rama Raju et al. (2012) [109]	IVF+ICSI	SCD	247	Non-significant	5	Development	Significant	Female age <40 years, BMI <30	Yes
Sanchez-Martin et al. (2013) [189]	ICSI	SCD	40	NA	NA		NA	Unspecified	No
Seli et al. (2004) [190]	IVF+ICSI	TUNEL	49	NA	2	Development	Significant	Unspecified	No
Sharbatoghli et al. (2012) [57]	ICSI	SCD	120	Non-significant	2 or 3	Grade	Non-significant	Unspecified	No
	ICSI	TUNEL	120	Non-significant	2 or 3	Grade	Non-significant	Unspecified	No
Simon et al. (2010) [119]	IVF	Comet	219	Significant	2 or 3	Grade	Significant	Unspecified	No
	ICSI	Comet	116	Non-significant	2 or 3	Grade	Non-significant	Unspecified	No
Simon et al. (2011a) [115]	IVF	Comet	70	Significant	2 or 3	Grade	Significant	Normal female	Yes
	IVF	Comet	73	Significant	2 or 3	Grade	Significant	Unspecified	No
Simon et al. (2011b) [19]	ICSI	Comet	22	Non-significant	2 or 3	Grade	Non-significant	Unspecified	No
Simon et al. (2014a) [75]	IVF+ICSI	Comet	238	Significant	5	Grade and development	Significant	Unspecified	No
	IVF+ICSI	TUNEL	238	Significant	5	Grade and development	Non-significant	Unspecified	No
	IVF+ICSI	SCSA	102	Non-significant	5	Grade and development	Non-significant	Unspecified	No

Study	ART	DD test	(*n*)	Fertilization rate	Day of ET	EQ marker	DD vs. EQ	FF inclusion	FF controlled (Y/N)
Smit et al. (2010) [191]	IVF+ICSI	SCSA	27	NA	NA	NA	NA	Unspecified	No
Speyer et al. (2010) [126]	IVF	SCSA	192	Non-significant	3 or 5	Development	Non-significant	Female age <45	No
	ICSI	SCSA	155	Non-significant	3 or 5	Development	Non-significant	Female age <45	No
Stevanato et al. (2008) [192]	IVF+ICSI	TUNEL	35	NA	NA		NA	Unspecified	No
Sun et al. (1997) [193]	IVF	TUNEL	143	Significant	NA	Cleavage rate	Significant	Unspecified	No
Tarozzi et al. (2009) [130]	IVF	TUNEL	82	NA		NA	NA	Unspecified	No
	ICSI	TUNEL	50	NA		NA	NA	Unspecified	No
Tavalaee et al. (2009) [194]	IVF+ICSI	SCD	92	Non-significant	3	Development	Non-significant	Unspecified	No
Tomsu et al. (2002) [195]	IVF	Comet	40	NA	3	Grade	Significant	Female age <40 years	Yes
Velez de la Calle et al. (2008) [129]	IVF+ICSI	SCD	622	Significant	2	Grade	Significant	Unspecified	No
Virro et al. (2004) [86]	IVF+ICSI	SCSA	249	Non-significant	2–3	Development	Significant	Unspecified	No
Yang et al. (2013) [196]	ICSI	SCSA	62	NA	NA		NA	Unspecified	No
Zini et al. (2005) [91]	ICSI	SCSA	60	Non-significant	3	Multinucleation	Significant	Female age <40	Yes

TUNEL terminal deoxyuridine nick-end labeling assay, *SCD* sperm chromatin dispersion assay, *SCSA* sperm chromatin structure assay, *FSH* follicle-stimulating hormone, *BMI* body mass index, *IVF* in vitro fertilization, *ICSI* intracytoplasmic sperm injection

[a]Breznik et al. [175]–IVF and ICSI cycles of treatment were not specified

mentation on IVF and ICSI fertilization may be due to the fact that conventional IVF occurs "naturally" as a result of sperm-oocyte interaction, whereas during ICSI treatment this natural selection process is bypassed [49]. With ICSI, the embryologist manually selects morphologically normal and motile sperm [50], which may increase the probability of selecting sperm with low DNA fragmentation [51], as negative correlations between these parameters have been reported [33, 40–42, 52–57]. The differential effect of sperm DNA fragmentation on IVF and ICSI fertilization may also be influenced by the atypical (delayed) sperm nuclear decondensation that occurs after ICSI [58]. These results presented here are also in agreement with the meta-analysis [59], showing that ICSI fertilization rates are higher than IVF rates in patients with unexplained infertility and in normozoospermic men presented with increased sperm DNA fragmentation [45, 60, 61]. In conclusion, sperm DNA fragmentation may be associated with IVF rate but not with ICSI fertilization rates.

23.2.4 Does Sperm DNA Fragmentation Decrease Embryo Quality?

We identified 67 eligible articles that analyzed sperm DNA fragmentation with ART outcomes, of which 22 articles did not have data associating embryo quality with sperm DNA fragmentation. The 45 eligible articles included 62 studies (22 IVF, 24 ICSI, and 16 mixed IVF+ICSI studies) and involved 9055 treatment cycles (3957 IVF, 2409 ICSI, and 2689 mixed IVF+ICSI cycles). Embryo markers such as embryo grade (33 studies), embryo development (20 studies), fragmentation (3 studies), combined embryo grade and development (4 studies), multinucleation (1 study), and embryo cleavage rate (1 study) were used to determine embryo quality in these studies. In 34% (21/62) of the studies (5 TUNEL, 4 SCSA, 7 SCD, and 7 comet), a significant inverse relationship between sperm DNA fragmentation and embryo quality was reported, whereas the remaining 41 studies (18 TUNEL, 14 SCSA, 7 SCD, and 2 comet) showed no significant relationship between these parameters.

Embryo quality was assessed on day 2 or 3 in 48 studies (15 TUNEL, 16 SCSA, 9 SCD, and 8 comet) and on day 5 in 13 studies (5 TUNEL, 5 SCSA, 2 SCD, and 1 comet). Of the 62 studies, 36% of IVF studies (8/22), 21% of ICSI studies (5/24), and 50% of mixed IVF+ICSI studies (8/16) reported a significant correlation between sperm DNA damage and embryo quality (Table 23.3). When the studies were analyzed for embryo markers, delayed embryo development was associated with sperm DNA fragmentation in 37.5% of the studies (9/24), whereas an association between sperm DNA fragmentation and embryo grade was reported in 27.0% of studies (10/37). Studies involving the alkaline comet assay (78%) reported an adverse effect, whereas 22% of TUNEL, 22% of SCSA, and 42% of SCD reported adverse effect of sperm DNA fragmentation on embryo quality. A complete description of studies associating sperm DNA fragmentation with embryo quality is presented in Table 23.2.

Table 23.3 Summary of studies associating sperm DNA fragmentation with embryo quality

	IVF		ICSI		IVF+ICSI	
Embryo quality	Studies (*n*)	Cycles (*n*)	Studies (*n*)	Cycles (*n*)	Studies (*n*)	Cycles (*n*)
Studies reporting no effect	14	3171	19	1925	8	1000
TUNEL	6	708	9	671	3	529
SCSA	5	965	5	574	4	379
SCD	3	1498	3	542	1	92
Comet	0	0	2	138	0	0
Studies reporting adverse effect	8	846	5	424	8	1689
TUNEL	2	318	2	254	1	49
SCSA	1	60	2	142	1	249
SCD	1	66	0	0	4	1093
Comet	4	402	1	28	2	298

These results presented here are consistent with an earlier systematic review, reporting no clear relationship between sperm DNA damage and embryo quality [62]. Although experimental models (where there is diffuse and uniform sperm DNA fragmentation) show that sperm DNA fragmentation can have a profound effect on the developing IVF embryo [63, 64], this cannot be translated to human studies, where a wide spectrum of sperm DNA fragmentation is observed within an ejaculate [5, 65] and the quality of the sperm fertilizing the oocyte is unknown. This analysis reported a slightly higher proportion of the IVF studies (36%) and reported an association between sperm DNA damage and embryo quality than the ICSI studies (21%), although a statistical comparison is not possible due to the heterogeneity of these studies.

A higher proportion of the evaluable studies reported an association between sperm DNA fragmentation and embryo development (37.5%) than between sperm DNA fragmentation and embryo quality (27%). Embryos with a faster cleavage rate are more likely to develop into a blastocyst [66–69] and result in a successful pregnancy following transfer [70]. It is possible that extensive sperm DNA fragmentation could affect normal embryonic development [71, 72] by interfering with a variety of cellular processes, including DNA repair mechanisms, transcription, and cell cycle control [73, 74].

We observed a differential association between sperm DNA fragmentation and embryo quality, when the studies were segregated into groups based on the type of DNA fragmentation measurement assays. Sperm DNA fragmentation detected by the alkaline comet assay was associated with poor embryo quality in 78% of the studies compared to other assays. This association may be due to the increased sensitivity of the comet assays, where both single- and double-strand breaks are measured [75] and the intensity of broken DNA in the comet tail is directly proportional to the level of actual damage [76]. Although the TUNEL assay estimates DNA fragmentation directly, the unique organization of the sperm DNA [2] and the lack of a decondensation step to remove the protamines during the TUNEL protocol may result in the measurement of peripheral DNA damage rather than complete DNA fragmentation, thereby reducing the sensitivity of the assay. In conclusion, there is no consistent relationship between sperm DNA fragmentation and embryo quality (including embryo development); however the relationship between the two parameters may be associated with the ability of the assay to determine both single- and double-strand breaks.

23.2.5 Can Sperm DNA Fragmentation Predict ART Success?

An extensive review of the existing literature and meta-analysis of studies testing the effect of DNA fragmentation on ART treatment was recently published by Simon et al. ([12], published online, ahead of print). In this meta-analysis (56 studies), clinical pregnancy was analyzed in 3734 IVF treatment cycles from 16 studies, 2282 ICSI treatment cycles from 24 studies, and 2052 mixed IVF+ICSI treatment cycles from 16 studies. An overall relationship between sperm DNA fragmentation and clinical pregnancy outcome from 56 studies (including 8068 ART cycles) supported a strong and significant association between the two parameters (odds ratio (OR) = 1.68; 95% CI, 1.49–1.89; $P < 0.0001$) [12].

The relationship between sperm DNA fragmentation and clinical pregnancy outcome were analyzed based on the type of treatment. A significant association between sperm DNA fragmentation and clinical pregnancy was observed for IVF treatment (OR = 1.65; 95% CI, 1.34–2.04; $P < 0.0001$), ICSI treatment (OR = 1.31; 95% CI, 1.08–1.59; $P = 0.0068$), and combined IVF+ICSI treatment (OR = 2.37; 95% CI, 1.89–2.97; $P < 0.0001$) [12]. The association between sperm DNA fragmentation and clinical pregnancy outcome was analyzed by assay type. The analysis with TUNEL assay studies ($n = 2098$ cycles from 18 studies; OR = 2.22; 95% CI, 1.61–3.05; $P < 0.0001$), SCD assay studies ($n = 2359$ cycles from 8 studies; OR = 1.98; 95% CI, 1.19–3.3; $P = 0.0086$), and alkaline comet assay studies ($n = 798$ cycles from 7 studies; OR = 3.56; 95% CI, 1.78–7.09; $P = 0.0003$) all showed a strong association between the two parameters. However, this was not the case with SCSA studies ($n = 2813$ cycles from 23 studies; OR = 1.22; 95% CI: 0.93–1.61; $P = 0.1522$) [12]. The meta-analysis was performed using the fixed and random effect models (Table 23.4).

Previous published meta-analysis [38, 77–79] has concluded that there is very little data to show a relationship between sperm DNA fragmentation and clinical pregnancy outcomes. However, the recent meta-analysis drawn across 56 eligible studies [12] reported a strong and a significant association between the two parameters. Overall, irrespective to the type of treatment or the method of analysis, the sensitivity and specificity of sperm DNA testing to predict clinical pregnancies were 32.6% and 76.4%, respectively, while the positive and negative predictive values to predict a clinical pregnancy were 71.2% and 38.8%, respectively. Although, we observe an increase in the positive and negative predictive values using the alkaline comet assay (81.7% and 46.8%, respectively), the overall predictive value suggests a moderate but significant association between sperm DNA fragmentation and clinical pregnancy.

Table 23.4 Odds ratio of sperm DNA fragmentation and clinical pregnancy outcome

			Fixed effects model		Random effects model			
Effect	No. of studies	No. of cycles	OR (95% CI)	*P* value	OR (95% CI)	*P* value	% of variation across studies I2	Test of heterogeneity (Q2) *p*-value
Overall effect	56	8,068	1.68 [1.49; 1.89]	0.0000	1.84 [1.5; 2.27]	<0.0001	60.9%	< 0.0001
Sperm DNA damage assays								
SCSA	23	2,813	1.18 [0.96; 1.44]	0.1115	1.22 [0.93; 1.61]	0.1522	38.1%	0.0338
TUNEL	18	2,098	2.18 [1.75; 2.72]	0.0000	2.22 [1.61; 3.05]	<0.0001	43.8%	0.0247
COMET	7	798	3.34 [2.32; 4.82]	0.0000	3.56 [1.78; 7.09]	0.0003	65.5%	0.0079
SCD	8	2,359	1.51 [1.18; 1.92]	0.0011	1.98 [1.19; 3.3]	0.0086	72.9%	0.0005
Types of assisted treatment								
IVF	16	3,734	1.65 [1.34; 2.04]	0.0000	1.92 [1.33; 2.77]	0.0005	60.7%	0.0008
ICSI	24	2,282	1.31 [1.08; 1.59]	0.0068	1.49 [1.11; 2.01]	0.0075	48.7%	0.0042
Mixed	16	2,052	2.37 [1.89; 2.97]	0.0000	2.32 [1.54; 3.5]	0.0001	64.4%	0.0002

Significance at 95%

Significance at 95%

Meta-analysis data was obtained from Simon et al. [12]

In conclusion, the updated meta-analysis [12] reported a modest but significant association between sperm DNA damage and clinical pregnancy rate in all three ART treatment groups (IVF, ICSI, and mixed IVF+ICSI studies) with a variable effect according to the type of sperm DNA assay. One explanation for a moderate relationship between the two parameters may be due to patient inclusion factors. Most of the studies have included couples with female factors, and therefore the effect of sperm DNA damage on pregnancy outcome is compromised by female infertility factors [19]. Specifically, in the studies [56, 80–82] more than half of the couples had been diagnosed with female infertility. Whereas, in studies where patients with female infertile factor were eliminated, the odds to predicting a successful pregnancy have significantly increased irrespective to the type of DNA fragmentation testing method [19, 83]. In conclusion, the adverse effect of sperm DNA fragmentation on clinical pregnancies is observed in both IVF and ICSI treatments; however, the odds to predict a clinical pregnancy may vary according to the type of assay used to measure sperm DNA fragmentation.

23.2.6 Is Sperm DNA Fragmentation Associated with Pregnancy Loss?

The existing data associating sperm DNA fragmentation with spontaneous pregnancy loss is limited, yet a negative impact of DNA fragmentation on miscarriage following ARTs is observed in most studies. A meta-analysis [84] analyzed the association of these two parameters by identified 16 articles which included seven articles involving SCSA [14, 30, 34, 55, 85–87], six articles involving TUNEL assay [40, 41, 81, 88–90], two articles involving comet assay [61, 65], and one article involving acridine orange slide-based staining method [91]. These articles included 14 ICSI studies and 11 IVF studies comprising 2969 couples undergoing ART treatment resulting in 1252 pregnancies and 225 spontaneous pregnancy losses [84].

The results of the meta-analysis [84] suggested a significant increase in miscarriage in patients with high DNA damage compared with those with low DNA damage (Relative risk (RR), 2.16; 95% CI, 1.54–3.03; $P < 0.0001$). The meta-analysis also reported a strong association of DNA fragmentation measured by SCSA and TUNEL assays with miscarriages, while that of comet and acridine orange assays did not reach a statistical significance. The impact of DNA fragmentation on miscarriages was observed when DNA fragmentation was measured in the raw semen (RR, 1.65; 95% CI, 1.66–2.33; $P < 0.0001$) as well as the density gradient prepared subpopulation (RR, 3.47; 95% CI, 2.13–5.63; $P < 0.0001$; [84]). Earlier meta-analysis [92] also reported a positive impact of sperm DNA fragmentation on spontaneous pregnancy loss.

Aspects involving spontaneous pregnancy loss are not well understood. However, both maternal and paternal factors are known to be associated with pregnancy loss [93]. The negative impact of sperm DNA fragmentation is more pronounced in animal models where this leads to abnormal embryo development, reduced implantation rate, and frequent pregnancy loss [63, 64, 94]. Such prolonged effect of sperm DNA fragmentation, also known as the late paternal effect [95], may be in part due to the inability of the oocyte to repair the damaged sperm chromatin when it exceeds the threshold value [72]. In conclusion, the findings of the recent meta-analysis suggest that sperm DNA fragmentation is positively associated with pregnancy loss after IVF and ICSI treatments [84].

23.3 Clinical Value of Tests of Sperm DNA Fragmentation

The evidence based on the current literature search supports the fact that there is an influence of sperm DNA fragmentation on male reproductive health, and sperm DNA testing could be incorporated into routine clinical use [96], although some clinical reviews and meta-analyses do not support the clinical use of sperm DNA fragmentation [78, 97]. Despite controversies, in recent years there has been a marked increase in the commercial sperm DNA testing for clinical use. In the following sections, we will discuss some of the evidence in support of the use of sperm DNA testing in infertile men.

23.3.1 Sperm DNA Fragmentation as a Biomarker

DNA fragmentation is a common property of the sperm. Once the damage occurs, the sperm lacks any mechanism to fix it, and therefore the fragmentation occurring to sperm chromatin is a permanent change. Sperm DNA fragmentations is showed to be higher in patients with infertility issues [13–21] and associated with abnormal semen parameters [33, 40–42, 44, 52, 55, 56, 86]. Studies on time to pregnancy have suggested that sperm DNA fragmentation is an excellent predictor of natural conception [14, 28]. Sperm DNA fragmentation is associated with advanced male age [34], exposure to environmental toxins [98, 99], in cancer patients and treatments [65, 100–102], and infertility conditions such as varicocele [18, 103–105]. Sperm DNA fragmentation is also a useful biomarker for various end points during ARTs, such as fertilization rate [41, 43, 106, 107], embryo quality [44, 87, 108], embryo development [41, 65, 109], clinical pregnancy [81, 82, 106, 107], miscarriage [41, 55, 81], and live birth [61, 81, 110]. In conclusion, sperm DNA fragmentation can be used as a biomarker independent of semen parameters.

23.3.2 Diagnosis of Male Infertility

Male factor infertility is the primary cause of infertility in approximately 20–30% of infertile couples. Male factor infertility is contributing factor in another 30–40% of infertile couples in addition to female factors [111, 112]. Thus, male factor infertility is present in half of all couples with infertility issues. To date, the routine method of male factor infertility diagnosis is based on traditional semen analysis [113]. Recently, it is estimated that approximately 15–20% of men with infertility issues have a normal semen analysis profile [114], and therefore a definitive diagnosis of male infertility cannot be performed only on the basis of semen analysis. A number of studies comparing sperm DNA fragmentation status between fertile and infertile men [13–18, 20, 21, 115] have suggested that DNA fragmentation could be a useful biomarker for male infertility diagnosis. Although, sperm DNA fragmentation is correlated with abnormal semen parameters such as sperm concentration, motility, and morphology [33, 40, 41, 44, 52, 55, 56, 86, 116], this is not a consistent finding in all studies [65, 81, 88, 91, 117–119]. Therefore, sperm DNA fragmentation can be considered an independent factor of male infertility and should be used together with the semen analysis as an added parameter to diagnose the status of male reproductive health.

23.3.3 Counseling Infertile Couples Prior to Initiating Infertility Treatment

As discussed earlier, the structure and stability of the sperm chromatin are important for male fertility and normal in vitro fertilization. In a study by Evenson et al. [14], using the sperm chromatin structure assay, DNA fragmentation above the threshold value of 30% is associated with a significant reduction in male infertility potential, and the time to pregnancy in vivo is longer in patients with DNA fragmentation >30% compared to <20%. The likelihood of achieving a natural pregnancy is significantly lower when DNA fragmentation is greater than 30% [120]. Another study examining the effect of DNA fragmentation among first-pregnancy planners with no previous knowledge of their fertility capability suggested that fecundability declined with an increase in sperm DNA fragmentation [28]. These reports summarize that when DNA fragmentation exceeds the threshold value, then male fertility is significantly reduced [14, 28]. Therefore, in couples who are planning for first pregnancy, the DNA fragmentation assay is a good predictor of male fertility potential and negative pregnancy outcomes. In couples where the male partner has extensive DNA fragmentation, counseling to improve their reproductive health and strategies to reduce the level of sperm DNA fragmentation should be provided (Grade B recommendation).

Sperm DNA testing can also be useful in another area of pretreatment counseling involving IUI treatment. A meta-analysis performed in this chapter (unpublished data) involving all the available studies using SCSA [18, 30–32, 34] reported a positive predictive value of 96% when DNA fragmentation is above the threshold (30%), while the sensitivity of the assay was 16%. In couples with high sperm DNA fragmentation, assisted reproduction (IVF or ICSI) should be considered.

23.3.4 Counseling Infertile Couples Planning to Choose Assisted Treatment

The question still remains whether ICSI would be a beneficial treatment of choice if the male partner presents with an increased level of sperm DNA fragmentation. An increase in success rate following ICSI [121, 122] may be attributed to a lower proportion of female factor infertility, where improved oocyte quality would be associated with a better DNA repair capability of the oocytes when fertilized with DNA fragmented sperm [123]. It can also be postulated that selection of physiologically motile and morphologically normal sperm for ICSI insemination [50] by the embryologists increases the probability of choosing sperm with low DNA fragmentation. In such conditions, the probability of selecting sperm with relatively low DNA fragmentation is higher compared to the overall sperm population as these factors (normal morphology and progressive motility) are inversely correlated with sperm DNA fragmentation [19, 33, 40–42, 44, 52–54, 124].

We performed a literature search to identify studies that simultaneously performed sperm DNA fragmentation assays (SCSA, TUNEL, SCD, and comet assays) on patients undergoing IVF and ICSI inseminations. We identified 23 studies that fit this criterion, following elimination of studies using mixed (IVF and ICSI combined) patient group. Of the 23 studies, 18 studies compared the effect of sperm DNA fragmentation with clinical pregnancy outcome following IVF and ICSI treatments. The relationship between sperm DNA fragmentation (above and below the threshold value) and clinical pregnancies (after IVF vs. ICSI insemination) was analyzed by two-by-two table obtained from 15 studies [19, 30, 31, 34, 40, 41, 54, 55, 61, 85, 105, 119, 125–127], while data was not available for three studies [128–130]. This analysis included 5564 treatment cycles from 3853 IVF cycles and 1711 ICSI cycles (unpublished data). Pregnancy rates were comparable between IVF and ICSI treatment when DNA fragmentation was below the threshold value, 34.19% for IVF and 37.15% for ICSI treatment (Chi Sq. = 2.847; df = 1; $p = 0.0915$). However, when the clinical pregnancies were analyzed when sperm DNA fragmentation was above the threshold value, then ICSI had a higher clinical pregnancy rate (32.14%) compared to IVF (16.41%) treatment (Chi Sq. = 20.815; df = 1; $p < 0.0001$). As expected the clinical pregnancy rates were higher in both IVF and ICSI treatments when sperm DNA fragmentation is below the threshold value (unpublished data).

A comprehensive large study by Simon et al. [72], comparing the quality of 2210 embryos (observed on day 2, 3, and 5) obtained from IVF and ICSI insemination at different levels of sperm DNA fragmentation, reported that the quality of ICSI embryos are significantly higher than IVF embryos when patients are presented with high sperm DNA fragmentation (Table 23.5). The literature presented above provides sufficient evidence to show that ICSI treatment is not affected by the level of sperm DNA fragmentation. In fact, the ICSI treatment resulted in twice the amount of pregnancies compared to IVF treatment when the DNA fragmentation was above the threshold value. A meta-analysis reported no difference in miscarriage rates following IVF or ICSI treatments when sperm DNA fragmentation is above the threshold value

Table 23.5 Comparison of embryo quality between IVF and ICSI insemination methods at three levels of sperm DNA fragmentation

Embryo quality		Level of sperm DNA fragmentation		
Observation day	Quality	Low (<30%)	Intermediate (31–70%)	High (>71%)
Two	Good	IVF = ICSI	IVF ↓ + ICSI ↑	IVF ↓ + ICSI ↑
	Poor	IVF ↑ + ICSI ↓	IVF ↑ + ICSI ↓	IVF ↑ + ICSI ↓
Three	Good	IVF = ICSI	IVF ↓ + ICSI ↑	IVF = ICSI
	Poor	IVF ↑ + ICSI ↓	IVF ↑ + ICSI ↓	IVF = ICSI
Five	Good	IVF = ICSI	IVF ↓ + ICSI ↑	IVF = ICSI
	Poor	IVF ↑ + ICSI ↓	IVF ↑ + ICSI ↓	IVF = ICSI

[84]. It can be argued that the outcomes following ICSI treatment may depend on the oocyte quality, where the negative impact of high DNA fragmentation on ART outcomes can be overcome by good quality oocytes that are able to repair the fragmented sperm DNA [131]. Since the success of ARTs has great emotional, financial, and age-related consequences for the couple, the selection of an appropriate treatment (IVF or ICSI) may favor the patient's success.

Based on the results of our meta-analysis [12], the data suggest that tests of sperm DNA damage may provide some predictive value in the context of IVF, ICSI, and mixed IVF + ICSI. An analysis of the 16 IVF studies (with a median pregnancy rate of 32%) revealed a median PPV of 79% and median NPV of 35%. This means that in populations with an overall IVF pregnancy rate of 32%, sperm DNA tests can discriminate between IVF pregnancy rates of 21% (positive test) and 35% (negative test), which represent a clinically important difference in pregnancy rate. An analysis of the 24 ICSI studies (with a median pregnancy rate of 36%) revealed a median PPV of 64% and median NPV of 40%. In the context of ICSI, sperm DNA tests can discriminate between ICSI pregnancy rates of 36% (positive test) and 40% (negative test), which is a small difference of modest clinical value. With the 16 mixed (IVF + ICSI) studies, we observed a median PPV of 70% and median NPV of 50%, suggesting that in populations with an overall mixed (IVF + ICSI) pregnancy rate of 44%, sperm DNA damage assessment can discriminate between mixed (IVF + ICSI) pregnancy rates of 30% (positive test) and 50% (negative test), a notable difference in pregnancy rate of important clinical value. Therefore, couples with high sperm DNA fragmentation and enrolled in an IVF treatment cycle should proceed to ICSI rather than IVF (Grade C recommendation).

23.3.5 As a Biomarker for Reproductive Toxicological Studies

Sperm are particularly vulnerable to xenobiotic action which can result in DNA damage [132]. The exposure to xenobiotics can be classified into three major types such as occupational exposure, environmental exposure, and pharmacological exposure. Studies have shown that sperm DNA fragmentation is higher among coke oven workers in contact with polycyclic aromatic hydrocarbon exposure [133]. Oh et al. [134] had shown that there are elevated levels of DNA fragmentation among the waste incineration workers when compared with men from similar origin. Men working in the factories in contact with organic molecules such as styrene show a significant amount of increase in sperm DNA fragmentation [135]. Similarly, men working in the insecticide and pesticide industries have been proven to show increases in sperm DNA fragmentation [136, 137]. Other occupational exposure such as farmers exposed to insecticides is also known to significantly stimulate sperm DNA fragmentation [136, 137]. Workers exposed to organic chemicals are also reported to exhibit high levels of sperm DNA fragmentation [135].

Today, pharmacological exposure has become very common due to advances in molecular medicine, especially in the field of cancer. Pharmacological intervention for the treatment of diseases results in genotoxicity to sperm and male germ cells. Such exposures are genotoxic to the male germ cells and cannot be avoided. A well-known example for such intervention is cyclophosphamide, which is used as chemotherapeutic agents to treat cancer [138]. Environmental exposure to xenobiotics cannot be avoided in the present-day life because these pollutants are present along with food or water or air. Environmental estrogens and similar compounds are known for their effect on male infertility and sperm DNA fragmentation [139]. Some of the other environmental pollutions that have the ability to induce DNA fragmentation are organo-chlorides [140], smog [98]. Aitken et al. [141] suggested that paternal exposure to xenobiotics not only results in genetic or epigenetic changes to the sperm but also causes adverse consequences for the offspring. Exposure to xenobiotics can result in high levels of sperm DNA fragmentation beyond the capacity of the oocyte to repair and can result in preimplantation failure [132]. Number of studies support the concept that exposure to xenobiotics can have a powerful impact on sperm DNA and its function. Therefore, sperm DNA testing may not only be useful to identify male reproductive health status but also is a method commonly used for toxicological studies (Grade C recommendation).

23.3.6 Unexplained Infertility

We know that 25–30% of couples undergoing ARTs are diagnosed with unexplained infertility [142]. In these cases, men have no obvious history of fertility problems and physical conditions or endocrine issues, and the semen analysis results are normal [143]. The prevalence of high DNA fragmentation is showed in men with unexplained infertility [60, 144, 145]. In a study, when 147 unexplained infertile men were screened for sperm DNA fragmentation, 84% of these patients had DNA fragmentation above the 25% cutoff value used to determine fertile from infertile men [61]. Further analysis of the study [61] reported that approximately 41% of men categorized with unexplained infertility issues have sperm DNA fragmentation above the threshold (52%) to obtain a clinical pregnancy following IVF treatment [61]. Similarly, another study using the SCSA reported that 26% of men diagnosed with unexplained infertility had high DNA fragmentation index [60]. Feijo et al. [145] reported that men with unexplained infertility have high level of sperm DNA fragmentation measured by SCD and TUNEL assays. More than 60% of men with unexplained infertility are showed to have abnormal protamine profile [19], which could be a causative agent for increased sperm DNA fragmentation [20]. These results suggest that to some extent sperm DNA fragmentation assays may help to identify men with fertility problems even when they are presented with normal semen analysis, as reported in unexplained infertility cases. Therefore, in men with unexplained infertility sperm, DNA testing can be used as additional marker of sperm quality to help in the counseling of these couples (Grade C recommendation).

23.4 Why Sperm DNA Testing Is Not Routinely Used Clinically? "Sperm DNA Testing: Pro" Point of View

Sperm DNA test has been performed for more than 30 years. However, vast majority of the data associating the effect of sperm DNA fragmentation on clinical outcomes is published in the last 20 years. A recent literature search using terms related to "sperm DNA damage," "sperm DNA fragmentation," and "sperm DNA integrity," along with "male infertility," "ART," "IVF," and "ICSI" yielded more than 1300 related articles. Despite a well-studied area of research, controversies do exist as to the effect of sperm DNA fragmentation on male infertility and assisted reproductive outcomes. The controversy is largely due to the fair quality of the available studies. In this section, we highlight few facts that would help the readers understand the discrepancies regarding the use of sperm DNA fragmentation for clinical use.

23.4.1 Sperm DNA Testing Is a Broad Term Used to Refer to a Number of Assay Methods

There are four widely used methods to access sperm DNA fragmentation: the comet assay [13], TUNEL assay [146], SCSA [14], and SCD assay [147]. The comet and TUNEL assays are the detect methods to measure DNA strand breaks, while the SCSA and SCD indirectly measure chromatin integrity by measuring the susceptibility of DNA to denaturation [97]. These assays are known to measure different aspects of sperm DNA fragmentation [148, 149], while the ability of these assays to accurately measure the level of DNA fragmentation depends on the technical and biological aspects of each test [150]. A recent meta-analysis [12] associating the four DNA fragmentation assays with ART outcomes suggests that the prognostic value of these assays is different [12]. The odds ratio (OR, 2.35; 95% CI, 1.99–2.78; $P < 0.001$) and relative risk (RR, 1.35; 95% CI, 1.28–1.43; $P < 0.001$) to predict a clinical pregnancy by the direct methods (TUNEL and comet assays including 2897

ART cycles) were higher than the indirect methods (SCSA and SCD assays including 5172 ART cycles) odds ratio (OR, 1.12; 95% CI, 0.98–1.28; $P = 0.096$) and relative risk (RR, 1.04; 95% CI, 0.99–1.09; $P = 0.089$). Although, DNA fragmentation measured by the indirect methods were not significantly associated with clinical pregnancy following ARTs ($P > 0.05$), the overall predictive value (obtained by combining all four sperm DNA tests) was significant [12]. The fact that prior meta-analyses [38, 77–79, 92] have reported an uncertain effect of sperm DNA fragmentation on ART outcome is likely due to the heterogeneity of the studies (combining studies using direct and indirect methods). We believe that future meta-analysis should be performed with independent analyses based on assay type.

23.4.2 The Structural Organization of the Sperm Chromatin Is an "Achilles Heel"

As discussed earlier, each assay measures different aspects of sperm DNA fragmentation. The available literature suggests that there is a wide difference in the threshold values between the assays, not referring to the variations in threshold values observed within the assays. A study comparing three different assays on the same patient population suggests a difference in threshold value, the comet assay (82%), TUNEL (10%), and SCSA (27%; 75), while the threshold for SCD assay may vary between 30% and 35% [44, 105]. These threshold values are primarily based on the range of sperm presented with DNA fragmentation measured by each assays. For example, the ability of an assay to determine the level or percentage of sperm with DNA fragmentation within an individual is variable: TUNEL (0–66%), SCSA (0–44%), SCD assay (0–50%), and the alkaline comet assay (0–100%) [37, 55, 75, 125, 126, 151].

Are the observed differences between assays related to the ability of these assays to access the sperm chromatin? In other words, how much sperm chromatin is accessible within the sperm head by these DNA fragmentation assays? To answer this question, we first have to understand the structural organization of sperm chromatin [152, 153]. The sperm head consists of one half of the genome and tightly packed with the help of protamines [2]. It is reported that the sperm chromatin is six times more compact than that of somatic cells and it is almost crystalline in nature [154]. Recently, Simon et al. [5] demonstrated that the volume of sperm nuclei (28.2 ± 0.2 μ[mu]m^3, [155]) is almost doubled (~63 μ[mu]m^3) by the process of decondensation within the intact sperm (without breaking the cell wall), and the process of lysis and decondensation results in 34-fold increase in volume (~1018 μ[mu]m^3) of the sperm chromatin (after breaking the cell wall). Another experiment [156] reported that decondensation of sperm nucleus increases the ability of TUNEL to detect increased levels of DNA fragmentation in sperm. Similarly, during the alkaline comet assay, the reduction of disulfide bonds connecting protamines using DTT [157] and removal of protamines under alkali conditions [158] help to relax the sperm chromatin [5] and access the complete level of DNA fragmentation within the sperm. In conclusion, due to the condensed nature of the sperm chromatin, the sperm DNA assays should consider decondensation of sperm chromatin prior to DNA fragmentation analysis.

23.4.3 Infertility Is a Multifactorial Issue, While Testing Sperm DNA Testing Is One Part of an Equation

For the past 30 years, several studies have identified factors that could influence the success of an assisted treatment. These factors can be broadly classified into female-derived factors, male-derived factors, and embryonic factors (prior to transfer). In a meta-analysis involving commonly reported factors that are known to influence ART success was reported by van Loendersloot et al. [159]. This meta-analysis reported that some factors (female age, duration of subfertility, basal FSH level) were negatively associated with ART success, and the number of oocytes retrieved was positively associated with ART success, while other factors (parity, indication for subfertility, method of fertilization, and number of embryos transferred and embryo development) was not significantly associated with ART success [159]. It is reasonably known that transfer of good quality blastocysts has increased chances of pregnancy than lower-quality embryos, early-stage blastocysts, or cavitating morula [160, 161]. Among the male-derived factors, male age and functional quality of sperm had no influence on ART success [162]. Based on the recent meta-analysis [12], we now know that there is an association between sperm DNA fragmentation and ART outcome. Despite a significant association between the two parameters, the predictive value of sperm DNA fragmentation to achieve a successful pregnancy is low [19, 75]. One explanation for the low predictive value of sperm DNA fragmentation on ART success can be attributed to the involvement of female-derived factors, where in couples with female factors, the effect of sperm DNA fragmentation on pregnancy outcome is compromised. In support of this theory, a study by Simon et al. [19] concluded that sperm DNA fragmentation can be an independent factor to predict a successful pregnancy (OR, 76.00; 95% CI, 8.69–1714.44; $P < 0.001$) following elimination of couples with known female factors and cases with unexplained causes of infertility. In conclusion, the effect of sperm DNA fragmentation on ART success is likely diminished by the presence of female factors. Therefore, future studies associating these two parameters (sperm DNA fragmentation on ART success) should control for female factors to accurately determine the clinical value of sperm DNA fragmentation [83].

23.4.4 Reliable Testing and Reporting of Sperm DNA Fragmentation

Four assays are commonly used to determine the level of DNA fragmentation in sperm. The current literature reports a wide range of variations within each assay in terms of assay protocol, software used for analysis, the type of sample used (fresh or frozen), study population and control, and reporting of results. These variations observed within the studies question the reliability of DNA fragmentation testing. Assays having standardized protocol along with automated software for analysis such as the SCSA [14] have a strict threshold value ranging from 27% to 30% [86, 163, 117]. When the specified software [14] for SCSA is not used, the ability of the assay to predict ART success at the specified threshold (27–30%) value is not observed [55, 80, 127, 164], and such discrepancies are understandable, while some research groups using alternative software for SCSA have established their own threshold value outside the specified range 27–30%. These studies report a significant association between SCSA and ART outcomes at a lower threshold value [32, 165]. When all the studies using SCSA are summarized using a meta-analysis, the association between DNA fragmentation and ART success is reduced [12].

The slide-based TUNEL assay has a standard protocol (using the commercial kit) but does not use a software to compute the results (the reporting of results is solely based on the technician's observation). In this case, a wide range of threshold value has been reported, 4% [54, 125], 10% [40, 75], 15% [41, 90], 17.6% [108], 20% [52, 88], 35% [81], 36.5% [53], and 48% [118]. Here we see the authors have established the threshold values according to their laboratory conditions, which means the suggested threshold value may not work at another laboratory setting or a different technician. Despite such wide range of threshold values established for TUNEL assay (4–48%), the meta-analysis suggests a strong correlation between DNA fragmentation and ART success [12]. In conclusion, we rely on assays that have been validated with testing of control-fertile populations and with well-established thresholds. Variation in the threshold values may raise concerns, but in cases when there is no standard software to compute the results, threshold values should be established according to the specific laboratory settings.

23.4.5 *Association Between Sperm DNA Fragmentation and ART Outcomes Is a Subject of Experimental Bias*

It is well-known that sperm DNA fragmentation may vary with time. Within an ejaculate, the level of DNA fragmentation is not consistent in all the sperm; some sperm are vulnerable to DNA fragmentation and some don't. In a recent study using the comet assay, it is showed that the level of DNA fragmentation in the sperm population may vary and could be potentially classified into three types [5]. Therefore, under natural conception the sperm fertilizing an oocyte is a random event (in terms of DNA fragmentation) as motile sperm are known to carry fragmented DNA [61, 119]. In accordance with the random selection effect, we see that in all studies conducted on DNA fragmentation and time to pregnancy with first-pregnancy planners, the time for conception increases with an increase in sperm DNA fragmentation [14, 28, 166]. A meta-analysis (presented in Sect. 2.2) consisting of 1135 IUI cycles suggested that sperm DNA fragmentation is strongly associated with IUI outcome, although selection of a motile sperm population by density gradient centrifugation (DGC) is subjected to experimental bias unless DNA fragmentation analysis is performed in the prepared sperm population. Under natural conception as well as IUI treatment, the sperm fertilizing an oocyte is selected randomly in terms of sperm DNA fragmentation. This is not surprising because we know that randomization reduces selection bias and allows us to determine any effects of the treatment efficiently.

Let's consider the scenario of studies that associate sperm DNA fragmentation with IVF or ICSI outcomes. Experimentally, the first line of bias arises from the sperm selection process. Most often in assisted reproduction, DGC is the standard procedure to select the prepared sperm population. Studies comparing DNA fragmentation before and after DGC have reported that the level of DNA fragmentation is reduced in the prepared sperm population [5, 119]. In conventional IVF treatment, the sperm fertilizing an oocyte is random (although prepared sperm population is used), while during ICSI treatment, the embryologists further select for physiologically motile and morphologically normal sperm. Since DNA fragmentation is negatively associated with progressive motility and normal morphology [19, 40, 42, 54, 124], the second sperm selection process may facilitate an additional selection of sperm with absent or low of DNA fragmentation. This is in support of the results presented in the meta-analysis (presented in Sect. 3.4), where the clinical pregnancy rates are twice higher after ICSI treatment compared to IVF treatment when DNA fragmentation is above the threshold value.

The second line of experimental bias arises at the embryo transfer stage. It is well documented that a successful pregnancy is favored by the transfer of high-quality embryos [70]. Irrespective to IVF or ICSI treatments, the best quality blastocysts (generally two) are selected for transfer from the pool of available embryos. Using animal model [63] and in human subjects [72, 167], sperm DNA fragmentation is reported to influence the quality of the embryo. Therefore, in both IVF and ICSI treatments, the good quality embryo used for transfer is presumably fertilized by reasonably good quality sperm, and such sperm does not represent the initial level of DNA fragmentation measured in the ejaculate. Here we see the process of randomization is absent, and during the process of assisted treatment, randomization is impossible.

In studies that associate sperm DNA fragmentation with clinical pregnancy outcome, we assume that the sperm used to fertilize the embryos that were subsequently transferred represents the population of sperm in the ejaculate (in terms of DNA fragmentation). However, this is subjected to experimental bias as these sperm were not randomly selected but in fact selected at two stages. Despite a biased experimental design, several studies and meta-analyses have demonstrated significant association between sperm DNA fragmentation and pregnancy outcome is simply astonishing [12]. We suspect that the effect of sperm DNA fragmentation on ART outcome would be greater if each step during the process of ART was randomized, but such a scenario is not possible under the current clinical setting.

The third line of experimental bias arises in assisted reproduction when the couple undergoing assisted treatment is presented with female factor infertility. Very few studies in the available literature have controlled for female infertility factors and those who did reported a highly significant association between sperm DNA fragmentation and ART outcome [12]. As discussed in Sect. 4.3, despite absence of DNA fragmentation, the presence of female infertility factors may reduce the chances of a successful pregnancy. In a clinical setting of couples where half of them are presented with female infertility factor, the probability of a pregnancy is affected by 50%, even if the sperm have normal DNA. In conclusion, we need to recognize that assisted reproduction is heavily biased. Despite such bias, the current literature [12] still shows a significant negative association between sperm DNA fragmentation and ART outcome supporting a true relationship between the two parameters.

23.5 Conclusion

A clinically useful test for sperm function should have the following characteristics: reliability, cost-efficiency, ability to predict outcomes in vitro and in vivo, and ability to assist clinicians in decision-making [168, 169]. Conventional semen analysis is the only test currently available for men with infertility issues. Although sperm DNA fragmentation shows a correlation with sperm parameters (especially sperm motility, viability, and morphology), these correlations are generally weak. Comparative studies of infertile men and fertile controls report a strong association between sperm DNA fragmentation and infertility. Therefore, sperm DNA fragmentation is associated with male infertility independent of semen parameters. Studies associating semen parameters and fertility in populations of first-pregnancy planners report a weak or no association between the two parameters [170–172]. In contrast, a strong association is observed between sperm DNA fragmentation and time to pregnancy [14, 28] suggesting the importance of sperm DNA integrity testing for male reproductive health.

The primary function of the sperm is to deliver the haploid genetic material to the oocyte. During the process of assisted reproduction, sperm is delivered near the oocyte (IVF) or delivered into the oocyte (ICSI). In such case, it is not reasonable to expect any of the semen parameters to predict ART success [119]. Presumably, sperm DNA fragmentation should be more closely associated with ART outcomes. The meta-analyses and systematic reviews presented here demonstrate that sperm DNA fragmentation is a good predictor of IUI failure and is associated with IVF pregnancy but less so with ICSI outcomes. Sperm DNA fragmentation is also negatively associated with embryo development and implantation and positively associated with miscarriage rates [12].

Another clinical utility of sperm DNA fragmentation is to assist clinicians and infertile couples to help choose the type of assisted treatment. The meta-analysis review presented here on IUI cycles suggests that a sperm DNA fragmentation above the threshold value results in a 96% IUI failure rate. The meta-analysis on IVF and ICSI cycles demonstrates that in couples with DNA fragmentation above the threshold value, clinical pregnancies following ICSI (32.14%) are double than following IVF (16.41%) treatment.

Overall, the evidence presented here (both in vivo and in vitro) and elsewhere favors sperm DNA fragmentation testing as a potential and clinically useful biomarker to predict male infertility and ART outcome [173, 174]. We support the view that sperm DNA testing should be done in addition to the conventional semen analysis for a complete diagnosis of male reproductive health.

References

1. Aitken RJ, de Iuliis GN. On the possible origins of DNA damage in human spermatozoa. Mol Hum Reprod. 2010;16:3–13.
2. Oliva R. Protamines and male infertility. Hum Reprod Update. 2006;12:417–35.
3. Aitken RJ, Baker MA. Oxidative stress and male reproductive biology. Reprod Fertil Dev. 2004;16:581–8.
4. Agarwal A, Prabakaran SA. Oxidative stress and antioxidants in male infertility: a difficult balance. Iran J Reprod Med. 2005;3:1–8.
5. Simon L, Aston KI, Emery BR, Hotaling J, Carrell DT. Sperm DNA damage output parameters measured by the alkaline comet assay and their importance. Andrologia; 2017; 49:e12608.
6. Agarwal A, Guptaa S, Sikka S. The role of free radicals and antioxidants in reproduction. Curr Opin Obstet Gynecol. 2006;18:325–32.
7. Aitken RJ, Koppers AJ. Apoptosis and DNA damage in human spermatozoa. Asian J Androl. 2011;13:36–42.
8. Banks S, King SA, Irvine DS, Saunders PT. Impact of a mild scrotal heat stress on DNA integrity in murine spermatozoa. Reproduction. 2005;129:505–14.
9. Erogul O, Oztas E, Yildirim I, Kir T, Aydur E, Komesli G, Irkilata HC, Irmak MK, Peker AF. Effects of electromagnetic radiation from a cellular phone on human sperm motility: an in vitro study. Arch Med Res. 2006;37:840–3.
10. Kumar D, Salian SR, Kalthur G, Uppangala S, Kumari S, Challapalli S, Chandraguthi SG, Krishnamurthy H, Jain N, Kumar P, Adiga SA. Semen abnormalities, sperm DNA damage and global hypermethylation in health workers occupationally exposed to ionizing radiation. PLoS One. 2013;8:e69927.
11. Durairajanayagam D, Agarwal A, Ong C. Causes, effects and molecular mechanisms of testicular heat stress. Reprod BioMed Online. 2015;30:14–27.
12. Simon L, Zini A, Ciampi A, Dyachenko A, Carrell DT. A systematic review and meta-analysis to determine the effect of sperm DNA damage measured by different assays on IVF and ICSI outcomes. Asian J Androl. 2016b;18:1–11.
13. Hughes CM, Lewis SEM, McKelvey-Martin VJ, Thompson W. A comparison of baseline and induced DNA damage in human spermatozoa from fertile and infertile men, using a modified comet assay. Mol Hum Reprod. 1996;2:613–9.
14. Evenson DP, Jost LK, Marshall D, Zinaman MJ, Clegg E, Purvis K, de Angelis P, Claussen OP. Utility of the sperm chromatin structure assay as a diagnostic and prognostic tool in the human fertility clinic. Hum Reprod. 1999;14:1039–49.
15. Host E, Lindenberg S, Kahn JA, Christensen F. DNA strand breaks in human sperm cells: a comparison between men with normal and oligozoospermic sperm samples. Acta Obstet Gynecol Scand. 1999a;78:336–9.
16. Zini A, Bielcki R, Phang D, Zenzes MT. Correlations between two markers of sperm DNA integrity, DNA denaturation and DNA fragmentation, in fertile and infertile men. Fertil Steril. 2001;75:674–7.
17. Zini A, Fischer MA, Sharir S, Shayegan B, Phang D, Jarvi K. Prevalence of abnormal sperm DNA denaturation in fertile and infertile men. Urology. 2002;60:1069–72.
18. Saleh RA, Agarwal A, Sharma RK, Said TM, Sikka SC, Thomas AJ. Evaluation of nuclear DNA damage in spermatozoa from infertile men with varicocele. Fertil Steril. 2003;80:1431–6.

19. Simon L, Lutton D, McManus J, Lewis SEM. Sperm DNA damage measured by the alkaline Comet assay as an independent predictor of male infertility and IVF success. Fertil Steril. 2011b;95:652–7.
20. Castillo J, Simon L, de Mateo S, Ballesca JL, Lewis SEM, Oliva R. Protamine/DNA ratios and DNA damage in native and density gradient centrifugated sperm from infertile patients. J Androl. 2011;32:324–32.
21. Ji G, Yan L, Wu S, Liu J, Wang L, Zhang S, Shi L, Gu A. Bulky DNA adducts in human sperm associated with semen parameters and sperm DNA fragmentation in infertile men: a cross-sectional study. Environ Health. 2013;12:82.
22. Kayed HF, Mansour RT, Aboulghar MA, Serour GI, Amer AE, Abdrazik A. Screening for chromosomal abnormalities in 2650 infertile couples undergoing ICSI. Reprod BioMed Online. 2006;12:359–70.
23. Brahem S, Mehdi M, Elghezal H, Saad A. The effects of male aging on semen quality, sperm DNA fragmentation and chromosomal abnormalities in an infertile population. J Assist Reprod Genet. 2011;28:425–32.
24. Zhang X, Gabriel MS, Zini A. Sperm nuclear histone to protamine ratio in fertile and infertile men: evidence of heterogeneous subpopulations of spermatozoa in the ejaculate. J Androl. 2006;27:414–20.
25. Aoki VW, Emery BR, Liu L, Carrell DT. Protamine levels vary between individual sperm cells of infertile human male and correlate with viability and DNA integrity. J Androl. 2006;27:890–8.
26. Zini A, Garrels K, Phang D. Antioxidant activity in the semen of fertile and infertile men. Urology. 2000;55:922–6.
27. Koca Y, Ozdal OL, Celik M, Unal S, Balaban N. Antioxidant activity of seminal plasma in fertile and infertile men. Arch Androl. 2003;49:355–9.
28. Spano M, Bonde JP, Hjollund HI, Kolstad HA, Cordelli E, Leter G. Sperm chromatin damage impairs human fertility. The Danish first pregnancy planner study team. Fertil Steril. 2000;73:43–50.
29. Bungum M, Humaidan P, Spano M, Jepson K, Bungum L, Giwercman A. The predictive value of sperm chromatin structure assay (SCSA) parameters for the outcome of intrauterine insemination, IVF and ICSI. Hum Reprod. 2004;19:1401–8.
30. Bungum M, Humaidan P, Axmon A, Spano M, Bungum L, Erenpreiss J, Giwercman A. Sperm DNA integrity assessment in prediction of assisted reproduction technology outcome. Hum Reprod. 2007;22:174–9.
31. Bungum M, Spano M, Humaidan P, Eleuteri P, Rescia M, Giwercman A. Sperm chromatin structure assay parameters measured after density gradient centrifugation are not predictive for the outcome of ART. Hum Reprod. 2008;23:4–10.
32. Yang XY, Zhang Y, Sun XP, Cui YQ, Qian XQ, Mao YD, Liu JY. Sperm chromatin structure assay predicts the outcome of intrauterine insemination. Nat J Androl. 2011;17:977–83.
33. Duran EH, Morshedi M, Taylor S, Oehninger S. Sperm DNA quality predicts intrauterine insemination outcome: a prospective cohort study. Hum Reprod. 2002;17:3122–8.
34. Boe-Hansen GB, Fedder J, Ersboll AK, Christensen P. The sperm chromatin structure assay as a diagnostic tool in the human fertility clinic. Hum Reprod. 2006;21:1576–82.
35. Alkhayal A, San Gabriel M, Zeidan K, Alrabeeah k, Noel D, McGraw R, Bissonnette F, Kadoch IJ, Zini A. Sperm DNA and chromatin integrity in semen samples used for intrauterine insemination. J Assist Reprod Genet. 2013;30:1519–24.
36. Thomson LK, Zieschang JA, Clark AM. Oxidative deoxyribonucleic acid damage in sperm has a negative impact on clinical pregnancy rate in intrauterine insemination but not intracytoplasmic sperm injection cycles. Fertil Steril. 2011;96:843–7.
37. Muriel L, Meseguer M, Fernández JL, Alvarez J, Remohí J, Pellicer A, Garrido N. Value of the sperm chromatin dispersion test in predicting pregnancy outcome in intrauterine insemination: a blind prospective study. Hum Reprod. 2006;21:738–44.
38. The Practice Committee of the American Society for Reproductive Medicine. The clinical utility of sperm DNA integrity testing: a guideline. Fertil Steril. 2013;99:673–7.

39. Simon L, Lewis SEM. Effects of progressive motility and sperm DNA damage on fertilization rates in vitro: is one better than the other? Syst Biol Reprod Med. 2011;57:133–8.
40. Borini A, Tarozzi N, Bizzaro D, Bonu MA, Fava L, Flamigni C, Coticchio G. Sperm DNA fragmentation: paternal effect on early post-implantation embryo development in ART. Hum Reprod. 2006;21:2876–81.
41. Benchaib M, Lornage J, Mazoyer C, Lejeune H, Salle B, Guerin JF. Sperm deoxyribonucleic acid fragmentation as a prognostic indicator of assisted reproductive technology outcome. Fertil Steril. 2007;87:93–101.
42. Caglar GS, Koster F, Schopper B, Asimakopoulos B, Nehls B, Nikolettos N, Diedrich K, Al-Hasani S. Semen DNA fragmentation index, evaluated with both TUNEL and Comet assay, and the ICSI outcome. In Vivo. 2007;21:1075–80.
43. Fang L, Lou LJ, Ye YH, Jin F, Zhou J. A study on correlation between sperm DNA fragmentation index and age of male various parameters of sperm and in vitro fertilization outcome. Chin J Med Genet. 2011;28:432–5.
44. Anifandis G, Bounartzi T, Messini CI, Dafopoulos K, Markandona R, Sotiriou S, Tzavella A, Messinis IE. Sperm DNA fragmentation measured by Halosperm does not impact on embryo quality and ongoing pregnancy rates in IVF/ICSI treatments. Andrologia. 2015;47:295–302.
45. Belloc S, Benkhalifa M, Cohen-Bacrie M, Dalleac A, Amar E, Zini A. Sperm deoxyribonucleic acid damage in normozoospermic men is related to age and sperm progressive motility. Fertil Steril. 2014;101:1588–93.
46. Sakkas D, Urner F, Bianchi P, Bizzaro D, Wagner I, Jaquenoud N, Manicardi C, Campana A. Sperm chromatin anomalies can influence decondensation after intracytoplasmic sperm injection. Hum Reprod. 1996;11:837–43.
47. Lopes S, Sun JG, Jurisicova A, Meriano J, Casper RF. Sperm deoxyribonucleic acid fragmentation is increased in poor quality semen samples and correlates with failed fertilization in intracytoplasmic sperm injection. Fertil Steril. 1998a;69:528–32.
48. Lopes S, Jurisicova A, Casper RF. Gamete-specific DNA fragmentation in unfertilized human oocytes after intracytoplasmic sperm injection. Hum Reprod. 1998b;13:703–8.
49. Ola B, Afnan M, Sharif K, Papaioannou S, Hammadieh N, Barratt CLR. Should ICSI be the treatment of choice for all cases of in-vitro conception? Hum Reprod. 2001;16:2485–90.
50. Sakkas D. Novel technologies for selecting the best sperm for in vitro fertilization and intracytoplasmic sperm injection. Fertil Steril. 2013;99:1023–9.
51. Aziz N, Said T, Paasch U, Agarwal A. The relationship between human sperm apoptosis, morphology and the sperm deformity index. Hum Reprod. 2007;22:1413–9.
52. Benchaib M, Braun V, Lornage J, Hadj S, Salle B, Lejeune H, Guearin JF. Sperm DNA fragmentation decreases the pregnancy rate in an assisted reproductive technique. Hum Reprod. 2003;18:1023–8.
53. Henkel R, Kierspel E, Hajimohammad M, Stalf T, Hoogendijk C, Mehnert C, Menkveld R, Schill WB, Kruger TF. DNA fragmentation of spermatozoa and assisted reproduction technology. Reprod BioMed Online. 2003;7:477–84.
54. Huang CC, Lin DPC, Tsao HM, Cheng TC, Liu CH, Lee MS. Sperm DNA fragmentation negatively correlates with velocity and fertilization rates but might not affect pregnancy rates. Fertil Steril. 2005;84:130–40.
55. Lin HH, Lee RK, Li SH, Lu CH, Sun FJ, Hwu YM. Sperm chromatin structure assay parameters are not related to fertilization rates, embryo quality, and pregnancy rates in in vitro fertilization and intracytoplasmic sperm injection, but might be related to spontaneous abortion rates. Fertil Steril. 2008;90:352–9.
56. Nijs M, Creemers E, Cox A, Franssen K, Janssen M, Vanheusden E, de Jonge C, Ombelet W. Chromomycin A3 staining, sperm chromatin structure assay and hyaluronic acid binding assay as predictors for assisted reproductive outcome. Reprod BioMed Online. 2009;19:671–84.
57. Sharbatoghli M, Valojerdi MR, Amanlou M, Khosravi F, Jafar-abadi MA. Relationship of sperm DNA fragmentation, apoptosis and dysfunction of mitochondrial membrane potential with semen parameters and ART outcome after intracytoplasmic sperm injection. Arch Gynecol Obstet. 2012;286:1315–22.

58. Terada Y, Luetjens CM, Sutovsky P, Schatten G. Atypical decondensation of the sperm nucleus, delayed replication of the male genome, and sex chromosome positioning following intracytoplasmic human sperm injection (ICSI) into golden hamster eggs: does ICSI itself introduce chromosomal anomalies? Fertil Steril. 2000;74:454–60.
59. Johnson LNC, Sasson IE, Sammel MD, Dokras A. Does intracytoplasmic sperm injection improve the fertilization rate and decrease the total fertilization failure rate in couples with well-defined unexplained infertility? A systematic review and meta-analysis. Fertil Steril. 2013;100:704–11.
60. Oleszczuk K, Augustinsson L, Bayat N, Giwercman A, Bungum M. Prevalence of high DNA fragmentation index in male partners of unexplained infertile couples. Andrology. 2013;1:357–60.
61. Simon L, Proutski I, Stevenson M, Jennings D, McManus J, Lutton D, Lewis SEM. Sperm DNA damage has negative association with live birth rates after IVF. Reprod BioMed Online. 2013;26:68–78.
62. Zini A, Jamal W, Cowan L, Al-Hathal N. Is sperm DNA damage associated with IVF embryo quality? A systematic review. J Assist Reprod Genet. 2011;28:391–7.
63. Ahmadi A, Ng SC. Fertilizing ability of DNA-damaged spermatozoa. J Exp Zool. 1999;284:696–704.
64. Fatehi AN, Bevers MM, Schoevers E, Roelen BA, Colenbrander B, Gadella BM. DNA damage in bovine sperm does not block fertilization and early embryonic development but induces apoptosis after the first cleavages. J Androl. 2006;27:176–88.
65. Morris ID, Iiott S, Dixon L, Brison DR. The spectrum of DNA damage in human sperm assessed by single cell gel electrophoresis (Comet assay) and its relationship to fertilization and embryo development. Hum Reprod. 2002;17:990–8.
66. McKiernan S, Bavister B. Timing of development is a critical parameter for predicting successful embryogenesis. Hum Reprod. 1994;9:2123–9.
67. Lonergan P, Khatir H, Piumi F. Effect of time interval from insemination to first cleavage on the developmental characteristics, sex and pregnancy rates following transfer of bovine preimplantation embryos. J Reprod Fertil. 1999;117:159–67.
68. Lee MJ, Lee RKK, Lin MH, Hwu YM. Cleavage speed and implantation potential of early-cleavage embryos in IVF or ICSI cycles. J Assist Reprod Genet. 2012;29:745–50.
69. Knez K, Tomazevic T, Vrtacnik-Bokal E, Virant-Klun I. Developmental dynamics of IMSI-derived embryos: a time-lapse prospective study. Reprod BioMed Online. 2013;27:161–71.
70. van Montfoort A, Dumoulin J, Kester A, Evers J. Early cleavage is a valuable addition to existing embryo selection parameters: a study using single embryo transfers. Hum Reprod. 2004;19:2103–8.
71. Bordignon V, Smith LC. Ultraviolet-irradiated spermatozoa activate oocytes but arrest preimplantation development after fertilization and nuclear transplantation in cattle. Biol Reprod. 1999;61:1513–20.
72. Simon L, Murphy K, Shamsi MB, Liu L, Emery B, Aston KI, Hotaling J, Carrell DT. Paternal influence of sperm DNA integrity on early embryonic development. Hum Reprod. 2014b;29:2402–12.
73. Jackson SP, Bartek J. The DNA-damage response in human biology and disease. Nature. 2009;461:1071–8.
74. Bazrgar M, Gourabi H, Yazdi PE, Vazirinasab H, Fakhri M, Hassani F, Valojerdi MR. DNA repair signalling pathway genes are overexpressed in poor-quality pre-implantation human embryos with complex aneuploidy. Eur J Obstet Gynecol Reprod Biol. 2014;175:152–6.
75. Simon L, Liu L, Murphy K, Ge S, Hotaling J, Aston KI, Emery B, Carrell DT. Comparative analysis of three sperm DNA damage assays and sperm nuclear protein content in couples undergoing assisted reproduction treatment. Hum Reprod. 2014a;29:904–17.
76. Martins CF, Dode MN, Bao SN, Rumpf R. The use of the acridine orange test and the TUNEL assay to assess the integrity of freeze-dried bovine spermatozoa DNA. Genet Mol Res. 2007;6:94–104.
77. Li L, Wang L, Cai J, Huang H. Correlation of sperm DNA damage with IVF and ICSI outcomes: a systematic review and meta-analysis. J Assist Reprod Genet. 2006;23:367–76.

78. Collins JA, Barnhart KT, Schlegel PN. Do sperm DNA integrity tests predict pregnancy with in vitro fertilization? Fertil Steril. 2008;89:823–31.
79. Zhao J, Zhang Q, Wang Y, Li Y. Whether sperm deoxyribonucleic acid fragmentation has an effect on pregnancy and miscarriage after in vitro fertilization/intracytoplasmic sperm injection: a systematic review and meta-analysis. Fertil Steril. 2014;102:998–1005.
80. Payne JF, Raburn DJ, Couchman GM, Price TM, Jamison MG, Walmer DK. Redefining the relationship between sperm deoxyribonucleic acid fragmentation as measured by the sperm chromatin structure assay and outcomes of assisted reproductive techniques. Fertil Steril. 2005;84:356–64.
81. Frydman N, Prisant N, Hesters L, Frydman R, Tachdjian G, Cohen-Bacrie P, Fanchin R. Adequate ovarian follicular status does not prevent the decrease in pregnancy rates associated with high sperm DNA fragmentation. Fertil Steril. 2008;89:93–8.
82. Meseguer M, Santiso R, Garrido N, García-Herrero S, Remohí J, Fernandez JL. Effect of sperm DNA fragmentation on pregnancy outcome depends on oocyte quality. Fertil Steril. 2011;95:124–8.
83. Giwercman A, Lindstedt L, Larsson M, Bungum M, Spano M, Levine RJ, Rylander L. Sperm chromatin structure assay as an independent predictor of fertility in vivo: a case–control study. Int J Androl. 2010;32:221–7.
84. Robinson L, Gallos JD, Conner SJ, Rajkhowa M, Miller D, Lewis SEM, Kirkman-Brown J, Coomarasamy A. The effect of sperm DNA fragmentation on miscarriage rates: a systematic review and meta-analysis. Hum Reprod. 2012;27:2908–17.
85. Gandini L, Lombardo F, Paoli D, Caruso F, Eleuteri P, Leter G, Ciriminna R, Culasso F, Dondero F, Lenzi A, Spano M. Full-term pregnancies achieved with ICSI despite high levels of sperm chromatin damage. Hum Reprod. 2004;19:1409–17.
86. Virro MR, Larson-Cook KL, Evenson DP. Sperm chromatin structure assay (SCSA) parameters are related to fertilization, blastocyst development, and ongoing pregnancy in in vitro fertilization and intracytoplasmic sperm injection cycles. Fertil Steril. 2004;81:1289–95.
87. Check JH, Graziano V, Cohen R, Krotec J, Check ML. Effect of an abnormal sperm chromatin structural assay (SCSA) on pregnancy outcome following (IVF) with ICSI in previous IVF failures. Arch Androl. 2005;51:121–4.
88. Greco E, Scarselli F, Iacobelli M, Rienzi L, Ubaldi F, Ferrero S, Franco G, Anniballo N, Mendoza C, Tesarik J. Efficient treatment of infertility due to sperm DNA damage by ICSI with testicular spermatozoa. Hum Reprod. 2005;20:226–30.
89. Ozmen B, Caglar GS, Koster F, Schopper B, Diedrich K, Al-Hasani S. Relationship between sperm DNA damage, induced acrosome reaction and viability in ICSI patients. Reprod BioMed Online. 2007;15:208–14.
90. Esbert M, Pacheco A, Vidal F, Florensa M, Riqueros M, Ballesteros A, Garrido N, Calderon G. Impact of sperm DNA fragmentation on the outcome of IVF with own or donated oocytes. Reprod BioMed Online. 2011;23:704–10.
91. Zini A, Meriano J, Kader K, Jarvi K, Laskin CA, Cadesky K. Potential adverse effect of sperm DNA damage on embryo quality after ICSI. Hum Reprod. 2005;20:3476–80.
92. Zini A, Boman JM, Belzile E, Ciampi A. Sperm DNA damage is associated with an increased risk of pregnancy loss after IVF and ICSI: systematic review and meta-analysis. Hum Reprod. 2008;23:2663–8.
93. Ford HB, Schust DJ. Recurrent pregnancy loss: etiology, diagnosis, and therapy. Rev Obstet Gynecol. 2009;2:76–83.
94. Perez-Crespo M, Moreira P, Pintado B, Gutierrez-Adan A. Factors from damaged sperm affect its DNA integrity and its ability to promote embryo implantation in mice. J Androl. 2008;29:47–54.
95. Tesarik J, Greco E, Mendoza C. Late, but not early, paternal effect on human embryo development is related to sperm DNA fragmentation. Hum Reprod. 2004;19:611–5.
96. Barratt CLR, De Jonge CJ. Clinical relevance of sperm DNA assessment: an update. Fertil Steril. 2010;94:1958–9.
97. Zini A, Sigman M. Are tests of sperm DNA damage clinically useful? Pros and cons. J Androl. 2009;30:219–29.

98. Evenson DP, Wixon R. Environmental toxicants cause sperm DNA fragmentation as detected by the sperm chromatin structure assay (SCSA(R)). Toxicol Appl Pharmacol. 2005;207:532–7.
99. Speit G, Vasquez M, Hartmann A. The comet assay as an indicator test for germ cell genotoxicity. Mutat Res. 2009;681:3–12.
100. Stahl O, Eberhard J, Jepson K, Spano K, Cwikiel M, Cavallin-Stahl E, Giwercman A. Sperm DNA integrity in testicular cancer patients. Hum Reprod. 2006;21:3199–205.
101. O'Flaherty C, Hales BF, Chan P, Robaire B. Impact of chemotherapeutics and advanced testicular cancer or Hodgkin lymphoma on sperm deoxyribonucleic acid integrity. Fertil Steril. 2009;94:1374–9.
102. Maselli J, Hales BF, Robaire B. Paternal exposure to testis cancer chemotherapeutics alters sperm fertilizing capacity and affects gene expression in the eight-cell stage rat embryo. Andrology. 2014;2:259–66.
103. Smith R, Kaune H, Parodi D, Madariaga M, Rios R, Morales I, Castro A. Increased sperm DNA damage in patients with varicocele: relationship with seminal oxidative stress. Hum Reprod. 2006;21:986–93.
104. Agarwal A, Sharma RK, Desai NR, Prabakaran S, Tavares A, Sabanegh E. Role of oxidative stress in pathogenesis of varicocele and infertility. Urology. 2009;73:461–9.
105. Ni K, Steger K, Yang H, Wang H, Hu K, Chen B. Sperm protamine mRNA ratio and DNA fragmentation index represent reliable clinical biomarkers for men with varicocele after microsurgical varicocele ligation. J Urol. 2014;192:170–6.
106. Gu LJ, Chen ZW, Chen ZJ, Xu JF, Li M. Sperm chromatin anomalies have an adverse effect on the outcome of conventional in vitro fertilization: a study with strictly controlled external factors. Fertil Steril. 2009;92:1344–6.
107. Gu LJ, Lu WH, Chen ZW. Effects of fertilization and pregnancy after embryo transfer—sperm DNA damage in vitro fertilization. Chin J Birth Health Hered. 2011;19:111–2.
108. Avendano C, Franchi A, Duran H, Oehninger S. DNA fragmentation of normal spermatozoa negatively impacts embryo quality and intracytoplasmic sperm injection outcome. Fertil Steril. 2010;94:549–57.
109. Rama Raju GA, Prakash GJ, Krishna KM, Madan K, Narayana TS, Krishna CHR. Noninsulin-dependent diabetes mellitus: effects on sperm morphological and functional characteristics, nuclear DNA integrity and outcome of assisted reproductive technique. Andrologia. 2012;44:490–8.
110. Wang WB, Zhao LW, Xiang ZQ, Zhou XZ, Gui YL, He CH. Correlation analysis of the results of double fluorescence (AO/PI) staining and clinical outcomes. J Reprod Contracept. 2012;23:111–8.
111. Mosher WD, Pratt WF. Fecundity and infertility in the United States: incidence and trends. Fertil Steril. 1991;56:192–3.
112. Thonneau P, Marchand S, Tallec A, Ferial ML, Ducot B, Lansac J, Lopes P, Tabaste JM, Spira A. Incidence and main causes of infertility in a resident population (1, 850, 000) of three French regions (1988–1989). Hum Reprod. 1991;6:811–6.
113. World Health Organization. WHO laboratory manual for the examination of human semen and sperm-cervical mucus interaction. Cambridge: Cambridge University Press; 2010.
114. Agarwal A, Allamaneni SS. Sperm DNA damage assessment: a test whose time has come. Fertil Steril. 2005;84:850–3.
115. Simon L, Castillo J, Oliva R, Lewis S. The relationship between human sperm protamines, DNA damage and assisted reproductive outcomes. Reprod BioMed Online. 2011a;23:724–34.
116. Tomlinson MJ, Moffatt O, Manicardi GC, Bizzaro D, Afnan M, Sakkas D. Interrelationships between seminal parameters and sperm nuclear DNA damage before and after density gradient centrifugation: implications for assisted conception. Hum Reprod. 2001;16:2160–5.
117. Larson-Cook KL, Brannian JD, Hansen KA, Kasperson KM, Aamold ET, Evenson DP. Relationship between the outcomes of assisted reproductive techniques and sperm DNA fragmentation as measured by the sperm chromatin structure assay. Fertil Steril. 2003;80:895–902.

118. Bakos HW, Thompson JG, Feil D, Lane M. Sperm DNA damage is associated with assisted reproductive technology pregnancy. Int J Androl. 2007;31:518–26.
119. Simon L, Brunborg G, Stevenson M, Lutton D, McManus J, Lewis SEM. Clinical significance of sperm DNA damage in assisted reproductive outcome. Hum Reprod. 2010;25:1594–608.
120. Evenson DP, Wixon R. Data analysis of two in vivo fertility studies using sperm chromatin structure assay—derived DNA fragmentation index vs. pregnancy outcome. Fertil Steril. 2008;90:1229–31.
121. Fishel S, Aslam I, Lisi F, Rinaldi L, Timson J, Jacobson M, Gobetz L, Green S, Campbell A, Lisi R. Should ICSI be the treatment of choice for all cases if in-vitro conception? Hum Reprod. 2000;15:1278–83.
122. Oehninger S, Gosden RG. Should ICSI be the treatment of choice for all cases of in-vitro conception? No, not in light of the scientific data. Hum Reprod. 2002;17:2237–42.
123. Lewis SEM. The place of sperm DNA fragmentation testing in current day fertility management. Middle East Fertil Soc J. 2013;18:78–82.
124. Said TM, Agarwal A, Sharma RK, Thomas AJ, Sikka SC. Impact of sperm morphology on DNA damage caused by oxidative stress induced by beta-nicotinamide adenine dinucleotide phosphate. Fertil Steril. 2005;83:95–103.
125. Host E, Lindenberg S, Smidt-Jensen S. The role of DNA strand breaks in human spermatozoa used for IVF and ICSI. Acta Obstet Gynecol Scand. 2000;79:559–63.
126. Speyer BE, Pizzey AR, Ranieri M, Joshi R, Delhanty JD, Serhal P. Fall in implantation rates following ICSI with sperm with high DNA fragmentation. Hum Reprod. 2010;25:1609–18.
127. Jiang HH, He XJ, Song B, Cao YX. Sperm chromatin integrity test for predicting the outcomes of IVF and ICSI. Nat J Androl. 2011;17:1083–6.
128. Hammadeh ME, Al Hasani S, Rosenbaum P, Schmidt W, Hammadeh CF. Reactive oxygen species, total antioxidant concentration of seminal plasma and their effect on sperm parameters and outcome of IVF/ICSI patients. Arch Gynecol Obstet. 2008;277:515–26.
129. Velez de la Calle JFV, Muller A, Walschaerts M, Clavere JL, Jimenez C, Wittemer C, Thonneau P. Sperm deoxyribonucleic acid fragmentation as assessed by the sperm chromatin dispersion test in assisted reproductive technology programs: results of a large prospective multicenter study. Fertil Steril. 2008;90:1792–9.
130. Tarozzi N, Nadalini M, Stronati A, Prato LD, Coticchio G, Borini A. Anomalies in sperm chromatin packing: impactions for assisted reproductive treatment. Reprod BioMed Online. 2009;18:486–95.
131. Meseguer M, Martınez-Conejero JA, O'Connor JE, Pellicer A, Remoh J, Garrido N. The significance of sperm DNA oxidation in embryo development and reproductive outcome in an oocyte donation program: a new model to study a male infertility prognostic factor. Fertil Steril. 2008;89:1191–9.
132. Aitken RJ, de Iuliis GN. Origins and consequences of DNA damage in male germ cells. Reprod BioMed Online. 2007;14:727–33.
133. Hsu PC, Chen IY, Pan CH, Wu KY, Pan MH, Chen JR, Chen CJ, Chien GP, Hsu CH, Liu CS, Wu MT. Sperm DNA damage correlates with polycyclic aromatic hydrocarbons biomarker in coke oven workers. Int Arch Occup Environ Health. 2006;79:349–56.
134. Oh E, Lee E, Im H, Kang HS, Jung WW, Nam HW, Kim EM, Sul D. Evaluation of immuno and reproductive toxicities and association between immunotoxicological and genotoxicological parameters in waste incineration workers. Toxicology. 2005;210:65–80.
135. Migliore L, Nacearali A, Zanello A, Scarpato R, Bramanti L, Mariani M. Assessment of sperm DNA integrity in workers exposed to styrene. Hum Reprod. 2002;17:2912–8.
136. Bian Q, Xu LC, Wang SL, Xu L, Collins MD, Chang HC, Song L, Liu J, Wang S, Wang X. Study on the relation between occupational fenvalerate exposure and spermatozoa DNA damage of pesticide factory workers. Occup Environ Med. 2004;61:999–1005.
137. Xia Y, Cheng S, Bian Q, Xu L, Collins MD, Chang HC, Song L, Liu J, Wang S, Wang X. Genotoxic effects on spermatozoa of carbaryl-exposed workers. Toxicol Sci. 2005;85:615–23.

138. Hales BF, Barlon TS, Robaire B. Impact of paternal exposure to chemotherapy on offspring in the rat. J Natl Cancer Inst Monogr. 2005;34:28–31.
139. Anderson D, Schmid TE, Batimgartner A, Cemeli-Carratala E, Brinkworth MH, Wood JM. Oestrogenic compounds and oxidative stress (in human sperm and lymphocytes in the Comet assay). Mutat Res. 2003;544:173–8.
140. Spano M, Toft G, Hagmar L, Eleuteri P, Rescia M, Rignell-Hydbom A, Tyrkiel E, Zvyezday V, Bonde JP, INUENDO. Exposure to PCB and p.p′-DDE in European and Inuit populations: impact on human sperm chromatin integrity. Hum Reprod. 2005;20:3488–99.
141. Aitken RJ, Koopman P, Lewis SEM. Seeds of concern. Nature. 2004;432:48–52.
142. Gleicher N, Barad D. Unexplained infertility: does it really exist? Hum Reprod. 2006;21:1951–5.
143. Hamada A, Esteves SC, Nizza M, Agarwal A. Unexplained male infertility: diagnosis and management. Int Braz J Urol. 2012;38:576–94.
144. Host E, Lindenberg S, Ernst E, Christensen F. DNA strand breaks in human spermatozoa: a possible factor, to be considered in couples suffering from unexplained infertility. Acta Obstet Gynecol Scand. 1999b;78:622–5.
145. Feijo CM, Esteves SC. Diagnostic accuracy of sperm chromatin dispersion test to evaluate sperm deoxyribonucleic acid damage in men with unexplained infertility. Fertil Steril. 2014;101:58–63.
146. Gorczyca W, Gong J, Drazynkiewicz Z. Detection of DNA strand breaks in individual apoptotic cells by the in situ terminal deoxynucleotidyl transferase and nick translation assay. Cancer Res. 1993;53:1945–51.
147. Fernandez JL, Muriel L, Goyanes V, Segrelles E, Gosálvez J, Enciso M, LaFromboise M, De Jonge C. Simple determination of human sperm DNA fragmentation with an improved sperm chromatin dispersion test. Fertil Steril. 2005;84:833–42.
148. Henkel R, Hoogendijk CF, Bouic PJ, Kruger TF. TUNEL assay and SCSA determine different aspects of sperm DNA damage. Andrologia. 2010;42:305–13.
149. Schulte RT, Ohl DA, Sigman M, Smith GD. Sperm DNA damage in male infertility: etiologies, assays, and outcomes. J Assist Reprod Genet. 2010;27:3–12.
150. Tavukcuoglu IS, Al-Azawi T, Khaki AA, Khaki A, Khalil A, Al-Hasani S. Clinical value of DNA fragmentation evaluation tests under ART treatments. J Turk Ger Gynecol Assoc. 2012;13:270–4.
151. Lopez G, Lafuente R, Checa MA, Carreras R, Brassesco M. Diagnostic value of sperm DNA fragmentation and sperm high-magnification for predicting outcome of assisted reproduction treatment. Asian J Androl. 2013;15:790–4.
152. Ward WS, Zalensky AO. The unique, complex organization of the transcriptionally silent sperm chromatin. Crit Rev Eukaryot Gene Expr. 1996;6:139–47.
153. Wykes SM, Krawetz SA. The structural organization of sperm chromatin. J Biol Chem. 2003;278:29471–7.
154. Fuentes-Mascorro G, Serrano H, Rosado A. Sperm chromatin. Arch Androl. 2000;45:215–25.
155. Gilmore JA, McGann LE, Liu J, Gao DY, Peter AT, Kleinhans FW, Critser JK. Effect of cryoprotectant solutes on water permeability of human spermatozoa. Biol Reprod. 1995;53:985–95.
156. Mitchell LA, De Iuliis GN, Aitken RJ. The TUNEL assay consistently underestimates DNA damage in human spermatozoa and is influenced by DNA compaction and cell vitality: development of an improved methodology. Int J Androl. 2011;34:2–13.
157. Liu L, Aston KI, Carrell DT. Protamine extraction and analysis of human sperm protamine 1/protamine 2 ratio using Acid gel electrophoresis. Methods Mol Biol. 2013;927:445–50.
158. Gosalvez J, Rodriguez-Predreira M, Mosquera A, Lopez-Fernandez C, Esteves SC, Agarwal A, Fernandez JL. Characterisation of a subpopulation of sperm with massive nuclear damage, as recognised with the sperm chromatin dispersion test. Andrologia. 2014;46:602–9.
159. van Loendersloot LL, van Wely M, Limpens J, Bossuyt PM, Repping S, van der Veen F. Predictive factors in in vitro fertilization (IVF): a systematic review and meta-analysis. Hum Reprod Update. 2010;16:577–89.

160. Goto S, Kadowaki T, Tanaka S, Hashimoto H, Kokeguchi S, Shiotani M. Prediction of pregnancy rate by blastocyst morphological score and age, based on 1,488 single frozen-thawed blastocyst transfer cycles. Fertil Steril. 2011;95:948–52.
161. van den Abbeel E, Balaban B, Ziebe S, Lundin K, Cuesta MJG, Klein BM, Helmgaard L, Arce JC. Association between blastocyst morphology and outcome of single-blastocyst transfer. Reprod BioMed Online. 2013;27:353–61.
162. Papathanasiou A, Bhattacharya S. Prognostic factors for IVF success: diagnostic testing and evidence-based interventions. Semin Reprod Med. 2015;33:65–76.
163. Larson KL, de Jonge CJ, Barnes AM, Jost LK, Evenson DP. Sperm chromatin structure assay parameters as predicted of failed pregnancy following assisted reproductive techniques. Hum Reprod. 2000;15:1717–22.
164. Dar S, Grover SA, Moskovtsev SI, Swanson S, Baratz A, Librach CL. In vitro fertilization–intracytoplasmic sperm injection outcome in patients with a markedly high DNA fragmentation index (>50%). Fertil Steril. 2013;100:75–80.
165. Micinski P, Pawlicki K, Wielgus E, Bochenek M, TworkowskaI I. The sperm chromatin structure assay (SCSA) as prognostic factor in IVF/ICSI program. Reprod Biol. 2009;9:65–70.
166. Loft S, Kold-Jensen T, Hjollund NH, Giwercman A, Gyllemborg J, Ernst E, Olsen J, Scheike T, Poulsen HE, Bonde JP. Oxidative DNA damage in human sperm influences time to pregnancy. Hum Reprod. 2003;18:1265–72.
167. Shoukir Y, Chardonnens D, Campana A, Sakkas D. Blastocyst development from supernumerary embryos after intracytoplasmic sperm injection: a paternal influence? Hum Reprod. 1998;13:1632–7.
168. Sigman M. Refining the measurement of sperm DNA fragmentation. Fertil Steril. 2012;98: 1123.
169. Oehninger S, Franken DR, Ombelet W. Sperm functional tests. Fertil Steril. 2014;102:1528–33.
170. Bonde JP, Ernst E, Jensen TK, Hjollund NH, Kolstad H, Henriksen TB, Scheike T, Giwercman A, Olsen J, Skakkebaek NE. Relation between semen quality and fertility: a population-based study of 430 first-pregnancy planners. Lancet. 1998;352:1172–7.
171. Andersen AG, Ziebe S, Jorgensen N, Petersen JH, Skakkebaek NE, Andersen AN. Time to pregnancy in relation to semen quality assessed by CASA before and after sperm separation. Hum Reprod. 2002;17:173–7.
172. Buck Louis GM, Sundaram R, Schisterman EF, Sweeney A, Lynch CD, Kim S, Maisog JM, Gore-Langton R, Eisenberg ML, Chen Z. Semen quality and time-to-pregnancy, the LIFE study. Fertil Steril. 2014;101:453–62.
173. Bungum M. Sperm DNA integrity assessment: a new tool in diagnosis and treatment of fertility. Obstet Gynecol Int. 2012;2012:531042.
174. Palermo GD, Neri QV, Cozzubbo T, Rosenwaks Z. Perspectives on the assessment of human sperm chromatin integrity. Fertil Steril. 2014;102:1508–17.
175. Breznik BP, Kovacic B, Vlaisavljevic V. Are sperm DNA fragmentation, hyperactivation, and hyaluronan-binding ability predictive for fertilization and embryo development in in vitro fertilization and intracytoplasmic sperm injection? Fertil Steril. 2013;99:1233–41.
176. Daris B, Goropevnek A, Hojnik N, Vlaisavljevi V. Sperm morphological abnormalities as indicators of DNA fragmentation and fertilization in ICSI. Arch Gynecol Obstet. 2010;281:363–7.
177. Gosalvez J, Caballero P, Lopez-Fernandez C, Ortega L, Guijarro JA, Fernandez JL, Johnston SD, Nunez-Calonge R. Can DNA fragmentation of neat or swim-up spermatozoa be used to predict pregnancy following ICSI of fertile oocyte donors? Asian J Androl. 2013;15:812–8.
178. Guerin P, Matillon C, Bleau G, Levy R, Menezo Y. Impact of sperm DNA fragmentation on ART outcome. Gynecol Obstet Fertil. 2005;33:665–8.
179. Hammadeh ME, Radwan M, Al-Hasani S, Micu R, Rosenbaum P, Lorenz M, Schmidt W. Comparison of reactive oxygen species concentration in seminal plasma and semen parameters in partners of pregnant and nonpregnant patients after IVF/ICSI. Reprod BioMed Online. 2006;13:696–706.

180. Kennedy C, Ahlering P, Rodriguez H, Levy S, Sutovsky P. Sperm chromatin structure correlates with spontaneous abortion and multiple pregnancy rates in assisted reproduction. Reprod BioMed Online. 2011;22:272–6.
181. Lazaros L, Vartholomatos G, Pamporaki C, Kosmas I, Takenaka A, Makrydimas G, Sofikitis N, Stefos T, Zikopoulos K, Hatzi E, Georgiou I. Sperm flow cytometric parameters are associated with ICSI outcome. Reprod BioMed Online. 2013;26:611–8.
182. Lewis SEM, O'Connell M, Stevenson M, Thompson-Cree L, McClure N. An algorithm to predict pregnancy in assisted reproduction. Hum Reprod. 2004;19:1385–94.
183. Marchetti C, Obert G, Deffosez A, Formstecher P, Marchetti P. Study of mitochondrial membrane potential, reactive oxygen species, DNA fragmentation and cell viability by flow cytometry in human sperm. Hum Reprod. 2002;17:1257–65.
184. Na L, Li L. Effect of sperm DNA damage on the outcome of in vitro fertilization-embryo transfer. Guangxi Med J. 2011;33:257–60.
185. Nasr-Esfahani MH, Salehi M, Razavi S, Anjlmshoa M, Rozahani S, Moulavi F, Mardani M. Effect of sperm DNA damage and sperm protamine deficiency on fertilization and embryo development post-ICSI. Reprod BioMed Online. 2005;11:198–205.
186. Nicopoullos JDM, Gilling-Smith C, Almeida PA, Homa S, Norman-Taylor JQ, Ramsay JWA. Sperm DNA fragmentation in subfertile men: the effect on the outcome of intracytoplasmic sperm injection and correlation with sperm variables. Br J Urol Int. 2008;101:1553–60.
187. Nijs M, De Jonge C, Cox A, Janssen M, Bosmans E, Ombelet W. Correlation between male age, WHO sperm parameters, DNA fragmentation, chromatin packaging and outcome in assisted reproduction technology. Andrologia. 2011;43:174–9.
188. Nunez-Calonge R, Caballero P, Lopez-Fernandez C, Guijarro JA, Fernandez JL, Johnston S, Gosalvez J. An improved experimental model for understanding the impact of sperm DNA fragmentation on human pregnancy following ICSI. Reprod Sci. 2012;19:1163–8.
189. Sanchez-Martin P, Sanchez-Martín F, Gonzalez-Martinez M, Gosalvez J. Increased pregnancy after reduced male abstinence. Syst Biol Reprod Med. 2013;59:256–60.
190. Seli E, Gardner DK, Schoolcraft WB, Moffatt O, Sakkas D. Extent of nuclear DNA damage in ejaculated spermatozoa impacts on blastocyst development after in vitro fertilization. Fertil Steril. 2004;82:378–83.
191. Smit M, Romijn JC, Wildhagen MF, Veldhoven JLM, Weber RFA, Dohle GR. Decreased sperm DNA fragmentation after surgical varicocelectomy is associated with increased pregnancy rate. J Urol. 2010;183:270–4.
192. Stevanato J, Bertolla RP, Barradas V, Spaine DM, Cedenho AP, Ortiz V. Semen processing by density gradient centrifugation does not improve sperm apoptotic deoxyribonucleic acid fragmentation rates. Fertil Steril. 2008;90:889–90.
193. Sun JG, Jurisicova A, Casper RF. Detection of deoxyribonucleic acid fragmentation in human sperm: correlation with fertilization in vitro. Biol Reprod. 1997;56:602–7.
194. Tavalaee M, Razavi S, Nasr-Esfahani MH. Influence of sperm chromatin anomalies on assisted reproductive technology outcome. Fertil Steril. 2009;91:1119–26.
195. Tomsu M, Sharma V, Miller D. Embryo quality and IVF treatment outcome may correlate with different sperm comet parameters. Hum Reprod. 2002;17:1856–62.
196. Yang XY, Wang LL, Chen P, Zhang Y, Zhang W, Cui YG, Zhang W, Liu JY. Impact of sperm DNA fragmentation index and sperm malformation rate on the clinical outcome of ICSI. Nat J Androl. 2013;19:1082–7.

Chapter 24
Sperm DNA Tests Are Clinically Useful: CON

Katherine Rotker and Mark Sigman

24.1 Introduction

The diagnostic semen analysis remains the mainstay laboratory test in the evaluation of the infertile man. However, conventional semen parameters have limited diagnostic value for male fertility and are poor predictors of reproductive outcomes. There is significant overlap between semen parameters in groups of fertile and infertile men [1]. Therefore, substantial efforts have been made to identify improved diagnostic tests to provide a more accurate infertility diagnosis than by evaluation of standard semen parameters alone. Sperm DNA integrity assays have gained interest as a potential test to discriminate infertile from fertile men. Despite a growing body of literature, controversy still exists regarding the ability of these assays to provide clinically useful data in the evaluation of the infertile man. The Practice Committee of the American Society for Reproductive Medicine (ASRM), the American Urological Association (AUA) practice guidelines, and the European Society for Human Reproduction and Embryology (ESHRE) have concluded that current data doesn't support the use of sperm DNA testing on a routine basis [2–4]. In this chapter we will discuss the reasons that, despite future promise, sperm DNA damage testing in its current state is not a routinely clinically useful test.

K. Rotker (✉)
Department of Urology, UMASS Medical School & Memorial Healthcare System, Worcester, MA, USA
e-mail: katherine.rotker@umassmemorial.org

M. Sigman
Department of Surgery (Urology), Warren Alpert School of Medicine of Brown University, Rhode Island Hospital and The Miriam Hospital, Providence, RI, USA

A. Zini, A. Agarwal (eds.), *A Clinician's Guide to Sperm DNA and Chromatin Damage*, https://doi.org/10.1007/978-3-319-71815-6_24

24.2 Inherent Issues

In its most basic form, a diagnostic test should provide information that affects patient management. A successful test should ideally direct management or at least provide valuable information on prognosis. In this case, a sperm DNA test should reliably differentiate a fertile from an infertile man or provide a reliable, clinically relevant prognosis for intercourse or ART success. Not all DNA fragmentation is pathologic. Some DNA nicking occurs as part of the normal process of winding and unwinding DNA, and a certain amount of single-stranded DNA breaks may be repaired by the oocyte [5]. Current assays do not selectively differentiate clinically important DNA fragmentation from clinically insignificant fragmentation. Perhaps for this reason, although DNA damage has been associated with male infertility, fertile men also possess detectable levels of DNA damage [6]. Therefore, upper threshold levels are set, but a portion of fertile men fall over the threshold, and a portion of infertile men fall under the threshold.

The task of proving the clinical usefulness of sperm DNA testing is made more difficult by the significant heterogeneity present in the tests and thresholds. As discussed further in other chapters of this book, several assays exist to measure sperm DNA and chromatin damage. Each assay measures different aspects of sperm DNA and chromatin integrity, and some have undergone more rigorous testing than others. Furthermore, even using the same assay, sample preparation, handling, and conditions can significantly impact the final test results. Finally, not all assays have standardized and clinically relevant threshold values for the upper normal level. For these reasons, it is difficult to combine studies and make broad conclusions. Additionally, most of the evaluable studies on sperm DNA tests have poorly controlled clinical parameters including female factors, female age, and number of embryos transferred, making the ability to draw clinical conclusions difficult.

Sperm DNA integrity testing determines the percentage of cells with DNA fragmentation or chromatin defects. As this implies, not all sperm within a sample have high levels of fragmentation. Animal models have provided strong evidence that sperm DNA fragmentation is highly correlated with fertility potential and even pregnancy loss [7]. However, these experiments may or may not translate to equivalent clinical effects because unlike sperm DNA damage in humans, DNA damage in animal models is induced experimentally and is present in all spermatozoa [7]. Most assays to evaluate sperm DNA integrity involve treatment of the sample (e.g., DNA-binding dye) which makes the individual sperm unusable for advanced reproductive techniques (ART). This necessitates that the sample used for testing is different than the one utilized for ART. Put another way, current tests do not provide information on the DNA status of individual sperm used to fertilize ova.

Although to what degree is debated, some intraindividual variability exists in these tests over time. Therefore, it can be difficult to extrapolate results from a single test to future attempts at intercourse or ART. A study examined a group of couples undergoing IUI, IVF, or ICSI for more than one cycle. In those couples with an initial normal DNA fragmentation, tests in subsequent cycles showed DNA fragmentation above the threshold in 15%. Additionally, for those with initially high DNA fragmentation scores, 37% were found to have normal scores on subsequent testing [8]. A more recent analysis in 2011 again found a high intraindividual coefficient of variation for DNA fragmentation index utilizing a sperm chromatin structure assay. In this study 11% of patients identified as being in the normal category were reassigned to the high fragmentation category in subsequent testing. Additionally, 4.4% of those identified as high DNA fragmentation initially were subsequently categorized as normal [9]. This alone would make it difficult to counsel a couple to make a significant management decision, for example, not attempting intercourse and moving straight to advanced reproductive techniques, based on an initial positive result.

The test is also limited by the fact that no proven treatment exists. Sperm DNA fragmentation has been associated with numerous environmental toxins and exposures. However, testing fails to differentiate different exposures or provide clinical information beyond what is known without testing, i.e., that one should try to avoid these exposures if possible. For example, although the DNA fragmentation percentage may be higher in a patient who smokes, one hardly needs a test to recommend that a patient stop smoking [10]. Although limited studies suggest oral antioxidant treatment decreases sperm DNA fragmentation, no convincing data exists for any treatment to improve pregnancy rates related to DNA fragmentation. Therefore, diagnosing a patient with high DNA fragmentation at this time doesn't allow for a proven treatment or intervention.

Finally, in the current healthcare environment, more attention is drawn to efficient use of resources and containment of costs. New diagnostic tests need not only to meet the burdens of sensitivity, specificity, and clinical relevance, but they must also be cost-effective.

24.3 Evidence-Based Utility

24.3.1 Intercourse

One possible arena for sperm DNA testing is in the couple planning for first-time pregnancy. A 2008 meta-analysis showed a strong association between sperm DNA damage and failure to achieve a natural pregnancy with a combined odds ratio of 7.15 [11]. In the two included studies with a median pregnancy rate of 64%, the median positive predictive value of the assay was 73%, and the median negative predictive value was 68% [12, 13]. An odds ratio of 7.15 sounds great, and this indication is often stated to be an area of greatest value for sperm DNA testing. However, when one considers the prevalence of infertility in the study populations, the clinical value is more questionable. In one of the most commonly quoted studies included, 25.6% of patients failed to achieve pregnancy. Of those patients, the sperm DNA test was abnormal in only 6.2% [12]. The sensitivity of the assay was only

19%, meaning that the test failed to identify infertility in four out of five infertile patients. Also notable was that out of the 132 patients tested, only 6 (3.7%) were found to have high DNA fragmentation and did not achieve pregnancy. This means that 96.3% paid for a test that didn't provide any benefit or guidance. Most worrisome, out of all the patients with an abnormal test, 40% still achieved pregnancy. Therefore, it would be difficult to counsel even those patients who did have an abnormal test not to try pregnancy by intercourse since they would still have a 40% success rate. A test that proves diagnostic to very few patients and provides limited prognostic ability at best to those for whom it is positive would be unlikely to change management and be clinically useful.

An additional study published in 2010 compared sperm parameters and DFI values between fertile and infertile men and found that a higher DNA fragmentation index was more common in the group of infertile men than in the fertile group. Thus, the odds ratio of being in the infertile group increased as the DFI increased. Of note, 49% of infertile men and 10% of fertile men had DFI values of >20%. As a diagnostic test, the sensitivity was only 51% with a specificity of 89%, indicating again that while there is an association between higher DFI and infertility, it falls far short of being a good diagnostic test that should be routinely used for couples trying to conceive. Moving the threshold to 30% increased the specificity (fewer false-positive results) to 96%, but sensitivity dropped to 21% [14].

Finally, the sperm DNA test is most accurate when used during the month of attempted conception. In both the studies of pregnancy by intercourse, predictive ability was best if the test was done close to the time of intercourse and performed more poorly when it was performed further ahead of time. This makes the assay impractical for couples attempting conception by intercourse each month. Take, for example, a couple newly considering pregnancy. If diagnosed with high levels of fragmentation, the sample could differ the following month, and they would still have a reasonable chance of conception. Therefore, the couple should continue to attempt conception by intercourse for 12 months just as they would if they had never had the test performed rendering the test clinically useless in this scenario.

24.3.2 *Intrauterine Insemination*

Another possible indication for sperm DNA testing would be in the infertile couple who has failed intercourse and is determining the utility of IUI versus advancing to IVF or ICSI. A number of studies have found an association between sperm DNA damage [15, 16] and lower IUI pregnancy rates, but in only one study was an odds ratio able to be calculated [17]. In this study, an odds ratio of 9.9 was derived, and a PPV of 97% and a NPV of 24% were calculated. However, the sensitivity of the assay was only 20.7%, meaning that the test again failed to identify four out of five couples that did not conceive by IUI. Out of all samples tested, abnormal results were obtained in only 17%, but 80% of patients didn't go on to conceive with IUI. The test would have to be performed on 83.4% of people for whom it would have no diagnostic or prognostic value in order to benefit only 16.6% of people. In this study, the sample used for IUI was the same sample utilized for testing raising concern about the accuracy of testing performed remotely. In clinical practice, there would need to be time after the test resulted in order for it to affect management decisions. Additionally, this is based on a single study. More studies are needed for a proper statistical evaluation and would certainly be necessary before adding sperm DNA testing to routine clinical practice.

24.3.3 IVF and ICSI

The literature regarding sperm DNA damage and its effect on IVF/ICSI outcome is controversial at best, and numerous studies and a number of recent meta-analyses have been performed. Each meta-analysis reaches slightly different conclusions suggesting that if any difference does exist in IVF/ICSI outcomes between men with high and normal levels of DNA damage, it is likely slight and very unlikely to be clinically significant enough to warrant the additional cost of testing.

In one of the earliest meta-analyses, Li et al. concluded that the SCSA assay had no significant effect on the chance of clinical pregnancy after IVF or ICSI treatment and that the TUNEL assay was associated with significant decreases in the chance of IVF clinical pregnancy but was not associated with changes in IVF fertilization, ICSI fertilization, or ICSI clinical pregnancy [18]. A total of eight articles met inclusion/exclusion criteria at that time (five utilizing TUNEL assay and three utilizing SCSA), and for the only significant finding, the clinical pregnancy rate using IVF was 27.75% for those with positive sperm DNA testing and 43.11% for those with a negative test (RR 0.68, 95% CI 0.54–0.85, $p = 0.0006$). A meta analysis published in 2008 included 13 studies in analysis and found a small but statistically significant association between sperm DNA integrity test results and pregnancy in IVF and ICSI cycles but concluded the difference was "not strong enough to provide a clinical indication for routine use of these tests in infertility evaluation of men" [19]. The studies included varied widely, and the sensitivity of the tests ranged from 6% to 71%, and the specificity ranged from 38% to 98%. The American Society for Reproductive Medicine performed a meta-analysis in 2013 and concluded that "existing data do not support a consistent relationship between abnormal DNA integrity and reproductive outcomes" [2]. Another meta-analysis of 21 articles in 2014 found no association between DFI and clinical pregnancy by IVF or ICSI [20].

In contrast, Zhao et al. performed a meta-analysis in 2014 where 16 studies met inclusion criteria. They found a significant decrease in pregnancy rates in patients with high DNA damage using all techniques combined (IUI/IVF/ICSI) with a small odds ratio of 0.81 (95% CI 0.70–0.95; $p = 0.008$). When stratified by a type of procedure, an association was found with IVF but not ICSI [21]. A meta-analysis in 2016 also concluded that "there is sufficient evidence in the existing literature suggesting that sperm DNA damage has a negative effect on clinical pregnancy following IVF and/or ICSI treatment" [22]. This included 41 studies in the analysis and found a combined odds ratio of all studies (IVF, ICSI, and IVF/ICSI combined) utilizing a random effects model to be 1.84 (95% CI 15–2.27, $p = 0.0001$). Notably, this robust effect was only noted for studies utilizing the TUNEL, comet, and SCD assays. No effect was noted in the studies utilizing the SCSA assay. The inclusion of the SCD and comet assays differentiates this analysis from the ASRM evaluation which primarily included studies utilizing SCSA and TUNEL assays. This points out that the prognostic significance may very well depend on the type of assay utilized. This issue needs to be clarified since assays such as the SCSA are the most commonly employed ones in clinical practice. Until more data is accumulated, the value of these tests for IVF and ICSI remains questionable. In addition, even if the assays are used to predict lower ART success, management is not affected since couples will still proceed with ICSI as the test does not predict inability to conceive but a slightly lower pregnancy rate by ART in those with high DNA fragmentation.

24.3.4 Pregnancy Loss

A theoretical risk exists that successful fertilization with DNA-damaged sperm may cause de novo mutations in the offspring, despite the ability of the oocyte and embryo to repair this DNA damage [5]. No relationship has been found between level of sperm DNA fragmentation and characteristics of children born after ART [23]. In addition, current testing does not allow for evaluation of the DNA integrity in the individual sperm that is utilized for ART.

However, the relationship between sperm DNA fragmentation and recurrent pregnancy loss has been examined. An early meta-analysis looked at the association between high DNA fragmentation and pregnancy loss and included 11 studies. It found that sperm DNA damage was statistically significantly associated with pregnancy loss when IVF/ICSI studies were combined with an odds ratio of 2.48 (95% CI 1.52–4.04, $p = <0.0001$). With an overall pregnancy loss rate of 18%, the median positive predictive value was 37%, and the median negative predictive value was 90% [24]. A more recent meta-analysis included 14 publications and found a significant association between DNA damage and miscarriage rate with a slightly lower combined OR of 2.28 (95% CI 1.55–3.35, $p = <0.001$) for IVF/ICSI studies combined [21].

The major issue is what clinically one would do with these results, other than cause anxiety, which in itself has been implicated in poor pregnancy outcomes [25]. Take, for example, a couple considering IVF/ICSI. Using current data, those with a negative test would still have a pregnancy loss rate of 10% but would be reassured. In fact, 60% of all pregnancy loss cases would have a negative test (sensitivity 40%). However, those with a positive test would have a 37% chance of pregnancy loss. This means that 63% of couples with a positive test would still go on to have a viable, term pregnancy with IVF/ICSI. One can hardly tell a couple not to proceed to IVF/ICSI because they have high DNA fragmentation if they have a two-thirds chance that any pregnancy will go to term. If data on effective treatments for DNA fragmentation accumulate and clearly show a positive effect, this may be the one area where the test could be useful in this very selected population. However, testing in its current state is not clinically useful for this concern.

24.4 Conclusion

As a routine test in the infertile couple, sperm DNA testing adds expense to the healthcare system and does not provide a clinical benefit for most couples. The techniques and thresholds are not standardized, and the results are variable over time. With suboptimal sensitivity and specificity, the tests do not differentiate clinically significant from insignificant fragmentation and cannot evaluate individual sperm used for ART. Finally, with no proven treatment, the test fails to change management. Despite the potential, at this point, DNA fragmentation testing does not meet the criteria of a clinically useful diagnostic test in the evaluation of the infertile male.

References

1. Guzick DS, et al. Sperm morphology, motility, and concentration in fertile and infertile men. N Engl J Med. 2001;345(19):1388–93.
2. Practice Committee of the American Society for Reproductive Medicine. The clinical utility of sperm DNA integrity testing: a guideline. Fertil Steril. 2013;99(3):673–7.
3. Barratt CL, et al. Sperm DNA: organization, protection and vulnerability: from basic science to clinical applications—a position report. Hum Reprod. 2010;25(4):824–38.
4. American Urological Association. The optimal evaluation of the infertile male: best practice statement reviewed and validity confirmed; 2011. Accessed 1 Aug 2016. Available from: http://www.auanet.org/education/guidelines/male-infertility-d.cfm
5. Ahmadi A, Ng SC. Fertilizing ability of DNA-damaged spermatozoa. J Exp Zool. 1999;284(6):696–704.
6. Zini A, et al. Correlations between two markers of sperm DNA integrity, DNA denaturation and DNA fragmentation, in fertile and infertile men. Fertil Steril. 2001;75(4):674–7.
7. Fernandez-Gonzalez R, et al. Long-term effects of mouse intracytoplasmic sperm injection with DNA-fragmented sperm on health and behavior of adult offspring. Biol Reprod. 2008;78(4):761–72.
8. Erenpreiss J, et al. Intra-individual variation in sperm chromatin structure assay parameters in men from infertile couples: clinical implications. Hum Reprod. 2006;21(8):2061–4.
9. Oleszczuk K, Giwercman A, Bungum M. Intra-individual variation of the sperm chromatin structure assay DNA fragmentation index in men from infertile couples. Hum Reprod. 2011;26(12):3244–8.
10. Potts RJ, et al. Sperm chromatin damage associated with male smoking. Mutat Res. 1999;423(1–2):103–11.
11. Evenson DP, Wixon R. Data analysis of two in vivo fertility studies using sperm chromatin structure assay-derived DNA fragmentation index vs. pregnancy outcome. Fertil Steril. 2008;90(4):1229–31.
12. Evenson DP, et al. Utility of the sperm chromatin structure assay as a diagnostic and prognostic tool in the human fertility clinic. Hum Reprod. 1999;14(4):1039–49.

13. Spano M, et al. Sperm chromatin damage impairs human fertility. The Danish first pregnancy planner study team. Fertil Steril. 2000;73(1):43–50.
14. Giwercman A, et al. Sperm chromatin structure assay as an independent predictor of fertility in vivo: a case-control study. Int J Androl. 2010;33(1):e221–7.
15. Duran EH, et al. Sperm DNA quality predicts intrauterine insemination outcome: a prospective cohort study. Hum Reprod. 2002;17(12):3122–8.
16. Muriel L, et al. Value of the sperm chromatin dispersion test in predicting pregnancy outcome in intrauterine insemination: a blind prospective study. Hum Reprod. 2006;21(3):738–44.
17. Bungum M, et al. Sperm DNA integrity assessment in prediction of assisted reproduction technology outcome. Hum Reprod. 2007;22(1):174–9.
18. Li Z, et al. Correlation of sperm DNA damage with IVF and ICSI outcomes: a systematic review and meta-analysis. J Assist Reprod Genet. 2006;23(9–10):367–76.
19. Collins JA, Barnhart KT, Schlegel PN. Do sperm DNA integrity tests predict pregnancy with in vitro fertilization? Fertil Steril. 2008;89(4):823–31.
20. Zhang Z, et al. Sperm DNA fragmentation index and pregnancy outcome after IVF or ICSI: a meta-analysis. J Assist Reprod Genet. 2015;32(1):17–26.
21. Zhao J, et al. Whether sperm deoxyribonucleic acid fragmentation has an effect on pregnancy and miscarriage after in vitro fertilization/intracytoplasmic sperm injection: a systematic review and meta-analysis. Fertil Steril. 2014;102(4):998–1005 e8.
22. Simon L, et al. A systematic review and meta-analysis to determine the effect of sperm DNA damage on in vitro fertilization and intracytoplasmic sperm injection outcome. Asian J Androl. 2017;19(1):80–90.
23. Bungum M, et al. Spermatozoa DNA damage measured by sperm chromatin structure assay (SCSA) and birth characteristics in children conceived by IVF and ICSI. Int J Androl. 2012;35(4):485–90.
24. Zini A, et al. Sperm DNA damage is associated with an increased risk of pregnancy loss after IVF and ICSI: systematic review and meta-analysis. Hum Reprod. 2008;23(12):2663–8.
25. Terzioglu F, et al. The effect of anxiety and depression scores of couples who underwent assisted reproductive techniques on the pregnancy outcomes. Afr Health Sci. 2016;16(2):441–50.

Part V
Treatment Options for Men with Sperm DNA Damage

Chapter 25
Antioxidant Therapy

Ahmad Majzoub and Ashok Agarwal

25.1 Introduction

Infertility, defined as the inability to conceive after at least 12 months of regular, unprotected intercourse, is caused by male-related factors in almost half of the reported cases [1–3]. While several causes for male factor infertility have been recognized, the etiology remains unknown in the majority of the cases [2]. In search of molecular causes of infertility, oxidative stress, a condition caused either by too high levels of oxidants or too low amounts of antioxidants in the body, has been suggested as a significant contributor to idiopathic male infertility.

Reactive oxygen species (ROS) are molecules derived from oxygen metabolism that play an important role in cell signaling and homeostasis. Normally, small amounts of ROS are produced by sperm cells to exhibit beneficial sperm functions such as promotion of sperm capacitation, regulation of sperm maturation, and enhancement of cellular signaling pathways [4]. On the other hand, abnormally high ROS levels can cause harmful effects such as sperm DNA damage, lipid peroxidation (LPO), and deactivation of several enzymes necessary for spermatogenesis [5]. In the reproductive tract, ROS are kept in equilibrium with the antioxidant defense mechanisms that exist in the body [6].

Antioxidants are molecules that are capable of neutralizing or eliminating free radicals, thereby preventing their damaging cellular effects. Two antioxidant systems exist: (i) the enzymatic system comprised by superoxide dismutase, catalase, and glutathione peroxidase and (ii) the nonenzymatic antioxidant system which

A. Majzoub
Department of Urology, Hamad Medical Corporation, Doha, Qatar

A. Agarwal (✉)
American Center for Reproductive Medicine, Glickman Urological and Kidney Institute, Cleveland Clinic, Cleveland, OH, USA
e-mail: Agarwaa@ccf.org

A. Zini, A. Agarwal (eds.), *A Clinician's Guide to Sperm DNA and Chromatin Damage*, https://doi.org/10.1007/978-3-319-71815-6_25

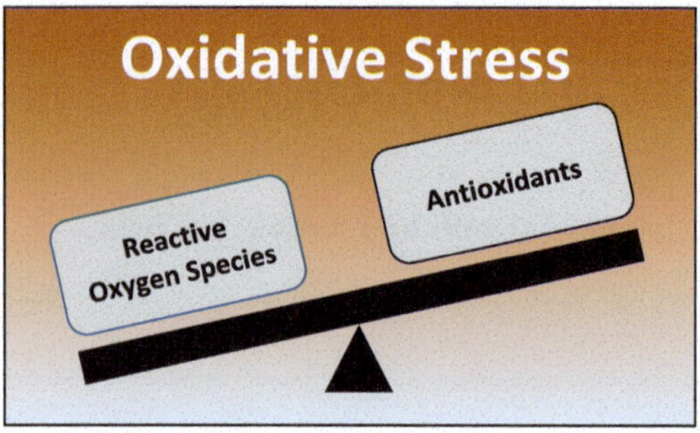

Fig. 25.1 Oxidative stress

includes ascorbic acid (vitamin C), urate, tocopherol (vitamin E), pyruvate, glutathione, lycopene, β[beta]-carotene, taurine, and hypotaurine [7]. When excessive amounts of ROS are produced, or when antioxidant activity fails, the equilibrium state between oxidation and reduction is disrupted, resulting in oxidative stress (Fig. 25.1). The sperm cells' characteristic sparse cytoplasm renders them exceptionally vulnerable to oxidative stress as they lack the cytoplasmic enzyme repair systems necessary for antioxidant activity. Moreover, spermatozoa also contain an extraordinary high amount of polyunsaturated fatty acids in their plasma membrane making them susceptible to ROS-induced LPO.

Studies have shown that up to 25% of infertile men have significantly higher levels of ROS in their semen when compared with fertile men [8]. Moreover, significant negative correlations have been detected between oxidative stress and semen parameters, fertilization rate, embryonic development, and pregnancy rate [9, 10]. Thus, identifying and treating increased ROS production and/or low levels of antioxidants should be an integral step in infertility management. While antioxidant supplementation has been proposed as a favorable approach to increase the scavenging capacity of seminal plasma [11], controversy still surrounds its actual clinical utility. This is mainly because studies examining different antioxidant forms revealed considerable variations in the dosage or combinations used as well as the outcome.

25.2 Antioxidants

Antioxidants are readily available biologic or chemical compounds present either in normal diet or taken as oral supplements. Among all available antioxidants, the most frequently utilized compounds include vitamins C and E, carnitine, N-acetyl cysteine, selenium, and zinc (Table 25.1). Although the number of studies demonstrating a positive influence for antioxidant therapy is increasing, additional comprehensive placebo-controlled trials are required to establish a clearer role of antioxidants in the prevention of oxidative stress [12, 13]. Moreover, the uncontrolled or exaggerated use of antioxidants should be disfavored. In this context, one has to consider the concept of the so-called antioxidant paradox, which highlights the potential of antioxidants to cause both positive and serious negative effects on

Table 25.1 Mechanism of action of endogenous antioxidants and commonly utilized nonenzymatic antioxidants

Antioxidants	Mechanism of action
Enzymatic	
Superoxide dismutase	Neutralizes superoxide anions
Catalase	Breaks H_2O_2 into H_2O and O_2
Glutathione peroxidase	Scavenges free radicals
Nonenzymatic antioxidants	
Tocopherol (vitamin E)	Neutralizes free radicals
Ascorbic acid (vitamin C)	Neutralizes free radicals
Carnitine	Neutralizes free radicals and acts as an energy source
Coenzyme Q10	In its reduced form, scavenges free radicals intermediate in mitochondrial electron transport system
N-acetyl cysteine	Enhances enzymatic antioxidant activity
Folic acid	Scavenges free radicals
Selenium	Enhancement of enzymatic antioxidant activity
Zinc	Inhibition of NADPH oxidase

male fertility and well-being. It is believed that an overdose of antioxidants may disrupt the fine bodily balance between oxidation and reduction causing "reductive stress," which is as dangerous for cells as oxidative stress [14–17]. An increase in sperm DNA decondensation is one example that has been reported to occur as a consequence of higher doses of vitamin C [18, 19]. It may induce chromosomal abnormalities, leading to cytoplasmic fragments in the embryo and can be deleterious for early embryo development. Menezo et al. [18] assessed the effect of 90 days' treatment with oral antioxidants consisting of vitamin C (400 mg), vitamin E (400 mg), β[beta]-carotene (18 mg), zinc (500 μmol), and selenium (1 μmol) on sperm DNA fragmentation and DNA decondensation. Despite reporting a significant decrease in sperm DNA fragmentation from 32.4% to 26.2% (using sperm chromatin structure assay, $P < 0.001$), a significant increase in sperm DNA decondensation was observed from 17.5% to 21.5% ($P < 0.001$). The authors attributed this increase to vitamin C influenced reduction in disulfide bonds and opening of disulfide bridges [18].

As stated previously, antioxidants exist in two forms: enzymatic or naturally occurring antioxidants and nonenzymatic antioxidants which are principally obtained from food supplements.

25.2.1 *Enzymatic Antioxidants*

The glutathione peroxidase/reductase system provides the main endogenous antioxidant protection against lipid peroxidation in the epididymis and testes [20]. Through scavenging lipid peroxides and hydrogen peroxide (H_2O_2), these enzymes confer protection for lipid constituents, thus preserving sperm viability and motility [21]. In vitro, studies have confirmed the protective effect of glutathione reductase on tail-beat frequency, LPO, and sperm membrane characteristics [22]. Superoxide dismutase scavenges both extracellular and intracellular superoxide anions through catalyzing the conversion of superoxide into oxygen and H_2O_2, thus preventing lipid peroxidation of the plasma membrane [23]. Additionally, it aids in the decomposition of H_2O_2, after conjugating with catalase or glutathione peroxidase [23]. Superoxide dismutase also optimizes sperm functional capabilities before fertilization through preventing premature sperm hyperactivation and capacitation induced by superoxide radicals before ejaculation [24]. On the other hand, catalase activates nitric oxide (NO)-induced sperm capacitation, which is a complex mechanism involving H_2O_2 [25]. It is believed that low levels of H_2O_2, which is principally under the control of catalase, are required for optimal sperm capacitation [26].

25.2.2 Nonenzymatic Antioxidants

25.2.2.1 Vitamin E (Dose 200–600 IU/Day)

Vitamin E (α[alpha]-tocopherol), an organic fat-soluble compound located mainly in cell membranes, is a powerful antioxidant capable of quenching free hydroxyl radicals and superoxide anions. Such activity is favored because it reduces lipid peroxidation initiated by ROS at the level of plasma membranes. Vitamin E is available in food such as nuts, vegetable and olive oils, leafy vegetables (spinach), fortified cereals, and meat.

In Vivo Studies

Vitamin E has been investigated in many studies, the majority of which conveyed a significant benefit on semen parameters. In a placebo-controlled study, 300 mg of daily vitamin E resulted in significant improvement in sperm motility, reduction of oxidative stress measures, and a resultant 21% spontaneous pregnancy rate in the treatment group compared to 0% in the placebo group [27]. Studies investigating vitamin E in combination with other vitamins have specifically revealed a significant improvement in sperm concentration [28, 29] together with a decrease in SDF [28] and seminal ROS [29]. ElSheikh et al. investigated the combination of vitamin E with clomiphene citrate and demonstrated a significant improvement in sperm concentration ($p = 0.001$) and sperm motility ($p < 0.001$) [30].

In Vitro Studies

The in vitro antioxidant activity of vitamin E was investigated on 122 semen samples, where at a dose of 10 mmol/1, significant suppression of lipid peroxidation was detected, leading to preservation of sperm motility [31]. The in vitro use of vitamins E and C also had favorable effects on sperm function tests, where a reduction in the levels of ROS and SDF was observed in both normozoospermic and asthenozoospermic samples [32].

25.2.2.2 Vitamin C (500–1000 mg/Day)

Vitamin C (ascorbic acid) is a water-soluble compound found in seminal plasma at concentrations about ten times higher than that in blood serum [33]. Vitamin C provides protection for human spermatozoa against endogenous oxidative damage through its ability to neutralize hydroxyl, superoxide, and hydrogen peroxide radicals [34]. Studies have confirmed the presence of lower vitamin C levels and higher ROS levels in the seminal plasma of asthenozoospermic men [35]. Additionally, a dose-dependent positive correlation between vitamin C levels and sperm motility [36] and percentage of normal sperm morphology [37] was detected. Vitamin C is mainly obtained through the intake of fruits (citrus fruits) and vegetables (tomatoes and potatoes).

In Vivo Studies

Vitamin C has been mainly investigated in combination with other vitamins and minerals [38, 39]. Patients treated with vitamins C and E had a significant reduction in the percentage of sperm DNA fragmentation (SDF) and a significant improvement in clinical pregnancy and implantation rates following intracytoplasmic sperm injection (ICSI) [39]. Similarly, combination therapy with zinc, vitamin E, and vitamin C resulted in a significant increase in sperm motility and decrease in SDF [40]. A randomized double-blind, placebo-controlled trial investigated a combined antioxidant regimen, including vitamin C, using Menevit (lycopene 6 mg, vitamin E 400 IU, vitamin C 100 mg, zinc 25 mg, selenium 26 mcg, folate 0.5 mg, garlic 1 g) in couples undergoing ICSI. The authors reported a significant improvement in viable pregnancy rate in the treatment group, where 38.5% of transferred embryos resulted in a viable fetus compared to 16% in the placebo group [41]. On the contrary, another randomized, controlled double-blind study by Rolf et al. failed to show improvement in semen parameters, sperm survival, or pregnancy rates in couples with male factor infertility after the administration of high-dose oral vitamin C and E for 56 days [42].

In Vitro Studies

Vitamin C, at higher doses (>1000 mmol/1), has been found to paradoxically increase ROS levels causing worsening of sperm motility in vitro [43]. However, at therapeutic doses, a dose-dependent effect was observed, with optimal motility achieved after incubation in 800 mmol/1 for 6 h [43]. As previously stated, the in vitro combination of vitamins C and E significantly reduced the levels of ROS and SDF in both normozoospermic and asthenozoospermic samples [32].

25.2.2.3 Carnitine (500–2000 mg/Day)

Carnitine is a water-soluble antioxidant that may be considered as a fuel source as it is actively involved in sperm motility. It assists in free fatty acid utilization and prevents lipid oxidation [44]. Carnitines are readily obtained from red meat and dairy products. The main forms used in the treatment of male subfertility are L-carnitine (LC) and L-acetyl carnitine (LAC).

In Vivo Studies

Most studies involving carnitines have demonstrated a significant influence particularly on sperm motility [45–47]. Lenzi et al. demonstrated significant improvement in sperm motility and pregnancy rate in patients with oligoasthenoteratozoospermia (OAT) receiving a combination of LC and LAC [45]. Similarly, Balercia et al. confirmed such response to therapy specifically among patients with lower baseline values of motility [47]. Cavallini et al. investigated patients with low-grade varicocele and idiopathic infertility and demonstrated significant improvement in all semen parameters in addition to higher spontaneous pregnancy rates among patients treated with LC and LAC in comparison to placebo (21.8% versus 1.7%, respectively) [46].

In Vitro Studies

Aliabadi et al. compared the effect LC and LAC to pentoxifylline (PF) on testicular sperm motility and chromatin integrity in mice. While sperm motility was significantly improved with LC, LAC, and PF, sperm chromatin quality only improved significantly following the administration of LC and LAC [48]. Human studies have also conveyed similar results. Al-Dujaily et al. [49] investigated semen from 100 infertile men dividing their samples into four groups: control, PF only, LC only, and a combination of PF and LC groups. Results revealed a statistically significant increase in the percentage of progressive motility, the highest of which occurred among the combination group (LC + PF) [49]. Furthermore, a favorable response to LC on sperm motility was also detected after incubation and centrifugation.

25.2.2.4 Coenzyme Q10 (100–600 mg/Day)

Coenzyme Q10 (CoQ10) is an essential antioxidant that is ubiquitous to almost all body tissues. It is highly concentrated in the sperm mitochondria where it plays an integral role in energy production [50]. Dietary sources of CoQ10 include fish, meat, whole grains, and certain vegetables such as parsley and cabbage.

In Vivo Studies

CoQ10 has been shown to significantly improve sperm concentration and motility in comparison to placebo [51]. Safarinejad randomly assigned 212 infertile men with idiopathic OAT to receive either a 300 mg CoQ10 or a placebo orally for a period of 26 weeks. He demonstrated a significant increase in sperm density and motility with CoQ10 therapy ($P = 0.01$) [51]. In another study, the same author reported a beneficial effect on spontaneous pregnancy rates in men receiving CoQ10 [52]. Moreover, improvement in fertilization rate after ICSI treatment has also been reported in patients receiving 60 mg/day of oral CoQ10 [50]. Gvozdjáková et al. investigated the effect of CoQ10 in combination with L-carnitine, vitamin E, and vitamin C (Carni-Q-Nol) demonstrating improvement in sperm function with a pregnancy rate of 45% after 6 months of treatment [53].

In Vitro Studies

The beneficial effect of CoQ10 on sperm motility was also observed in vitro. In one study, semen samples from 38 asthenozoospermic men were incubated for 24 h in HAM's medium alone, HAMs with 1% dimethyl sulfide, and HAMs with 5 μ[mu]M or 50 μ[mu]M CoQ10, respectively. A significant increase in motility was observed in the 50 μ[mu]M CoQ10 subgroup ($P < 0.05$) [50].

25.2.2.5 N-Acetyl Cysteine (300–600 mg/Day)

N-acetyl cysteine (NAC) is an amino acid that is converted in the body to cysteine, a precursor to glutathione, thereby exhibiting its antioxidant properties. Glutathione is an intracellular sulfhydryl or thiol group-containing compound that is capable of replacing the protein (–SH) groups eliminated during oxidative stress. Deficiency of glutathione was found to be associated with sperm mid-piece instability and abnormal motility [54]. While NAC is not available in food, cysteine is highly present in proteins such as meat and eggs and in vegetables (broccoli, red peppers, and onions).

In Vivo Studies

Treatment with NAC (600 mg daily) resulted in a significant improvement in sperm motility in comparison to placebo in 120 patients with idiopathic infertility [55]. Moreover, authors reported higher serum total antioxidant capacity and lower total peroxide and oxidative stress index in the NAC-treated group compared with the control group. The combination of 600 mg NAC and 200 μ[mu]g selenium (Se) resulted in a significant improvement in all semen parameters with a dose-dependent positive correlations between the sum of Se and NAC concentrations, mean sperm concentration, motility, and percent of normal morphology [55].

In Vitro Studies

A direct dose- and time-dependent reduction of seminal ROS after exposure of human spermatozoa to NAC was reported by Oeda et al. [56]. The authors concluded that the treatment of patients with NAC might be a useful option in reducing oxidative stress. Prolonged in vitro incubation of human spermatozoa is associated with the activation of mitochondrial ROS and loss of protein (–SH) groups. Aitken et al. [57] demonstrated that the addition of nucleophilic (–SH)-containing proteins to semen samples generated a protective effect against ROS-induced motility reduction. NAC was also found to exhibit an inhibitory effect on germ cell apoptosis in the human seminiferous tubules in vitro [58].

25.2.2.6 Folic Acid (0.25–5 mg/Day)

Folic acid is a B vitamin carrying free radical scavenging abilities. It plays a vital role in nucleic acid synthesis and amino acid metabolism. It can be supplied by foods such as vegetables (mainly dark-green leafy vegetables), fruits, nuts, beans, dairy products, meats, eggs, and grains.

In Vivo Studies

In a double-blind, placebo-controlled interventional study, 108 fertile men and 103 subfertile men were randomized into four groups: (i) folic acid only, (ii) zinc only, (iii) a combination of both folic acid and zinc, and (iv) placebo. After 26 weeks of treatment, a statistically significant 74% increase in total normal sperm concentration was noted among subfertile men receiving combination therapy [59]. Another double-blind, placebo-controlled study evaluated endocrine and semen parameters of 47 fertile and 40 subfertile males before and after treatment with folic acid and zinc sulfate. After 26 weeks of treatment, a significant improvement in sperm concentration of subfertile males was detected with no documented effect on other semen and endocrine parameters [60]. Using a branded mixture of antioxidants containing 0.5 mg of folic acid, Tremellen et al. reported significant improvement in pregnancy rates following assisted reproductive techniques [41]. On the other hand, high doses of folic acid may result in methylation of promoter regions in several genes involved in cancer and neurobehavioral disorders [61]. Thus, folic acid supplementation must be carefully prescribed in order to avoid placing patients in unnecessary health risks.

In Vitro Studies

One study evaluating the effects of several antioxidants on seminal plasma of patients undergoing ART reported an inverse correlation between seminal plasma folate and sperm DNA fragmentation index (DFI) [62].

25.2.2.7 Selenium (50–200 mcg/Day)

Selenium (Se) is an essential trace element mainly involved in normal testicular development and spermatogenesis, protecting sperm DNA against oxidative stress damage. The precise mechanism by which Se eliminates oxidative stress is not well-established. It is believed to exert its biochemical and cellular effects through the activity of glutathione peroxidases and thioredoxin reductases, thus playing an integral role in the function of biologic glutathione. Morphologic sperm mid-piece abnormalities and impairment of sperm motility were associated with Se deficiency [63]. As for any other antioxidant and micronutrient, the daily selenium intake has to be balanced because both high and low intake may cause numerous sperm abnormalities and can thus affect male fertility [64]. Dietary Se can be found in seafood, nuts, cereals, meat, and dairy products.

In Vivo Studies

Few studies have documented a beneficial effect for Se on semen parameters in subfertile men. As previously noted, Safarinejad et al. [65] reported a statistically significant improvement in all semen parameters in men receiving 200 μ[mu]g of Se either alone or in combination with NAC for 26 weeks [65]. The combination of Se with vitamin E resulted in an increase in sperm motility [66, 67]. However, these changes in sperm parameters did not exert a significant influence on the overall pregnancy rates [66]. In a recent literature review, Se was found to have a favorable influence on the viability of spermatozoa by providing a protective effect against ROS [64].

In Vitro Studies

Most in vitro studies examined the effects of Se on cryopreservation techniques. Early reports on the in vitro use of Se as a semen extender revealed a protective effect against freezing injury [68]. The addition of 1 and 2 μ[mu]g/ml of Se to the semen before freezing significantly increased the post-thaw motility compared to non-treated specimens. Animal studies also conveyed similar results, where the addition of similar concentrations of Se to semen extenders significantly improved post-thaw sperm motility, viability, membrane integrity, and semen total antioxidant capacity and reduced DFI in water buffalo sperm [69].

25.2.2.8 Zinc (50–250 mg/Day)

Zinc is another essential trace mineral involved in DNA and RNA metabolism and has anti-apoptotic and antioxidant properties. Its effect on spermatogenesis appears to be protective through prevention of premature oxidation of sulfhydryl groups during epididymal maturation [70–72]. Although the antioxidant properties of zinc were first utilized in antiaging supplements and immune boosters, studies have shown an inverse association between the seminal concentration of zinc and male fertility potential [73]. Dietary zinc deficiency causes increased oxidative stress [74] and poor sperm morphology [75].

In Vivo Studies

Omu et al. compared zinc therapy to no therapy in men with asthenozoospermia for a period of 3 months revealing a significant improvement in sperm count ($P < 0.02$), progressive motility ($P < 0.05$), fertilizing capacity ($P < 0.01$), and a reduction in the incidence of antisperm antibodies ($P < 0.01$) among the treatment group [40]. Additionally, oral zinc supplementation successfully restored seminal catalase-like activity and improved sperm concentration and progressive motility in a group of asthenozoospermic men [76]. As noted earlier, several randomized controlled trials have demonstrated a beneficial effect of oral intake of zinc + folate on semen parameters [59, 60].

In Vitro Studies

Similar to the reported animal study on Se, Dorostkar et al. investigated the in vitro use of zinc sulfate as a semen extender demonstrating a protective effect of low doses of zinc (0.288 mg/L) against freezing-thawing oxidative damage [77].

25.3 Systematic Reviews of Antioxidants

Several systematic reviews investigated the available evidence on antioxidant use in male subfertility yielding variable conclusions. A Cochrane review of 48 randomized controlled clinical trials including 4179 subfertile men was recently performed [78]. Live birth and pregnancy rates were reported in four and seven trials, respectively. Despite a considerable variability in the reported antioxidant effect on semen parameters, a statistically significant improvement in live birth rate (OR 4.21, 95% CI 2.08–8.51, $P < 0.0001$) and clinical pregnancy rate (OR 3.43, 95% CI 1.92–6.11, $P < 0.0001$) were detected [78]. Different selection criteria were utilized in other literature reviews. Ross et al. [79] analyzed 17 randomized trials, including a total of 1665 infertile men in whom oral antioxidants were compared to placebo or no treatment. Semen parameters and reported pregnancy rates were the outcome measures analyzed. Despite the methodological and clinical heterogeneity, an improvement in sperm after antioxidant therapy was reported in 14 out of 17 trials. Pregnancy rates were measured in seven trials, six of which showed a significant improvement after antioxidant therapy. The authors concluded that the use of oral antioxidants in infertile men may have beneficial effects on sperm quality and pregnancy rates. In an attempt to evaluate the impact of oral antioxidants on measures of sperm oxidative stress and DNA damage, Gharagozloo and Aitken selected 20 trials that assessed

Table 25.2 Available evidence on the effect of antioxidants in the treatment of male infertility

Antioxidant supplementation has been shown to:	
Improve semen parameters (concentration, motility, and morphology)	[12, 28, 29, 40, 45–47, 51, 52, 55, 65, 79]
Reduce seminal oxidative stress	[12, 13, 27, 28, 64]
Reduce sperm DNA fragmentation	[13, 29, 39, 40]
Improve clinical pregnancy rate	[27, 39, 41, 46, 52, 78, 79]
Improve live birth rate	[78]
Provide protection for sperm in vitro against the detrimental effects of incubation time and freezing-thawing	[13, 32, 43, 49, 50, 57, 58, 62, 69, 77]

such an association [12]. The analysis showed that 19 out of the 20 studies reported a significant reduction in oxidative stress or DNA damage after treatments with antioxidants. Moreover, a significant improvement in sperm motility was observed in seven out of the seven studies particularly performed on asthenozoospermic patients [12]. In addition to addressing the effect of oral antioxidants on sperm dysfunction and DNA damage, Zini and Al-Hathal also investigated the in vitro use of antioxidants prior to assisted reproduction revealing a protective effect for antioxidants against exogenous ROS, sperm cryopreservation, and thawing [13].

Although many reviews generally demonstrate a favorable influence of antioxidants on male fertility (Table 25.2), the optimum regimen of antioxidants is still unknown. Many experts suggest an individualized treatment approach, whereby the dose and type of antioxidant given to a particular patient should be adjusted according to the clinical presentation and/or the level of seminal oxidative stress.

25.4 Conclusion

The use of antioxidant therapy for the treatment of male subfertility has been investigated with several undersized studies. Despite the presence of considerable evidence confirming their beneficial effects in reversing oxidative stress-induced sperm dysfunction and in improving pregnancy rates, the heterogeneous nature of the study designs hampers our ability to implement an ideal treatment modality and calls for the conduct of large-scale randomized controlled trials. Furthermore, the optimum safe management of oxidative stress is critical and only possible with antioxidants that work in synergy with some selectivity for the male reproductive tract. The uncontrolled use of antioxidant formulations with random ingredients and dosages may have negative influences on male fertility adding to the plight of couples who are desperate to have a healthy child. The in vitro use of antioxidants is undoubtedly relevant in the era of ART but must also be applied carefully as improper dosage or combination with unfavorable media compounds could lead to unexpected adverse effects. Finally, additional studies are needed to determine the optimal antioxidant preparation to be used in vivo and in vitro.

References

1. Irvine DS. Epidemiology and aetiology of male infertility. Hum Reprod. 1998;13(Suppl 1): 33–44.
2. Sharlip ID, et al. Best practice policies for male infertility. Fertil Steril. 2002;77(5):873–82.
3. Nieschlag E, Behre HM. Andrology. Male reproductive health and dysfunction. Berlin: Springer; 2000.
4. Ford CE, et al. The chromosomes in a patient showing both mongolism and the Klinefelter syndrome. Lancet. 1959;1(7075):709–10.
5. Brooker RJ. Genetics: analysis and principles. 4th ed. Ohio: McGraw-Hill Higher Education; 2011.
6. Aitken RJ, Clarkson JS, Fishel S. Generation of reactive oxygen species, lipid peroxidation, and human sperm function. Biol Reprod. 1989;41(1):183–97.
7. Sies H. Strategies of antioxidant defense. Eur J Biochem. 1993;215(2):213–9.
8. Agarwal A, et al. Reactive oxygen species as an independent marker of male factor infertility. Fertil Steril. 2006;86(4):878–85.
9. Tremellen K. Oxidative stress and male infertility—a clinical perspective. Hum Reprod Update. 2008;14(3):243–58.
10. Agarwal A, Saleh RA, Bedaiwy MA. Role of reactive oxygen species in the pathophysiology of human reproduction. Fertil Steril. 2003;79(4):829–43.
11. Gharagozloo P, et al. A novel antioxidant formulation designed to treat male infertility associated with oxidative stress: promising preclinical evidence from animal models. Hum Reprod. 2016;31(2):252–62.
12. Gharagozloo P, Aitken RJ. The role of sperm oxidative stress in male infertility and the significance of oral antioxidant therapy. Hum Reprod. 2011;26(7):1628–40.
13. Zini A, Al-Hathal N. Antioxidant therapy in male infertility: fact or fiction? Asian J Androl. 2011;13(3):374–81.
14. Ufer C, et al. Redox control in mammalian embryo development. Antioxid Redox Signal. 2010;13(6):833–75.
15. Henkel RR. Leukocytes and oxidative stress: dilemma for sperm function and male fertility. Asian J Androl. 2011;13(1):43–52.
16. Naviaux RK. Oxidative shielding or oxidative stress? J Pharmacol Exp Ther. 2012; 342(3):608–18.
17. Chen SJ, et al. Influence of reactive oxygen species on human sperm functions and fertilizing capacity including therapeutical approaches. Arch Gynecol Obstet. 2013;288(1):191–9.
18. Menezo YJ, et al. Antioxidants to reduce sperm DNA fragmentation: an unexpected adverse effect. Reprod BioMed Online. 2007;14(4):418–21.
19. Giustarini D, et al. Is ascorbate able to reduce disulfide bridges? A cautionary note. Nitric Oxide. 2008;19(3):252–8.
20. Mora-Esteves C, Shin D. Nutrient supplementation: improving male fertility fourfold. Semin Reprod Med. 2013;31(4):293–300.
21. Lanzafame FM, et al. Oxidative stress and medical antioxidant treatment in male infertility. Reprod BioMed Online. 2009;19(5):638–59.
22. Griveau JF, Le Lannou D. Effects of antioxidants on human sperm preparation techniques. Int J Androl. 1994;17(5):225–31.
23. Agarwal A, et al. Role of antioxidants in treatment of male infertility: an overview of the literature. Reprod BioMed Online. 2004;8(6):616–27.
24. de Lamirande E, Gagnon C. Capacitation-associated production of superoxide anion by human spermatozoa. Free Radic Biol Med. 1995;18(3):487–95.
25. de Lamirande E, Leclerc P, Gagnon C. Capacitation as a regulatory event that primes spermatozoa for the acrosome reaction and fertilization. Mol Hum Reprod. 1997;3(3):175–94.
26. Bize I, et al. Hydrogen peroxide is involved in hamster sperm capacitation in vitro. Biol Reprod. 1991;44(3):398–403.

27. Suleiman SA, et al. Lipid peroxidation and human sperm motility: protective role of vitamin E. J Androl. 1996;17(5):530–7.
28. Kodama H, et al. Increased oxidative deoxyribonucleic acid damage in the spermatozoa of infertile male patients. Fertil Steril. 1997;68(3):519–24.
29. Comhaire FH, et al. The effects of combined conventional treatment, oral antioxidants and essential fatty acids on sperm biology in subfertile men. Prostaglandins Leukot Essent Fat Acids. 2000;63(3):159–65.
30. ElSheikh MG, et al. Combination of vitamin E and clomiphene citrate in treating patients with idiopathic oligoasthenozoospermia: a prospective, randomized trial. Andrology. 2015;3(5):864–7.
31. Aitken RJ, Clarkson JS. Significance of reactive oxygen species and antioxidants in defining the efficacy of sperm preparation techniques. J Androl. 1988;9(6):367–76.
32. Sierens J, et al. In vitro isoflavone supplementation reduces hydrogen peroxide-induced DNA damage in sperm. Teratog Carcinog Mutagen. 2002;22(3):227–34.
33. Jacob RA, Pianalto FS, Agee RE. Cellular ascorbate depletion in healthy men. J Nutr. 1992;122(5):1111–8.
34. Fraga CG, et al. Ascorbic acid protects against endogenous oxidative DNA damage in human sperm. Proc Natl Acad Sci U S A. 1991;88(24):11003–6.
35. Lewis SE, et al. The impact of sperm DNA damage in assisted conception and beyond: recent advances in diagnosis and treatment. Reprod BioMed Online. 2013;27(4):325–37.
36. Dawson EB, et al. Effect of ascorbic acid supplementation on the sperm quality of smokers. Fertil Steril. 1992;58(5):1034–9.
37. Thiele JJ, et al. Ascorbic acid and urate in human seminal plasma: determination and interrelationships with chemiluminescence in washed semen. Hum Reprod. 1995;10(1):110–5.
38. Baker HW, et al. Protective effect of antioxidants on the impairment of sperm motility by activated polymorphonuclear leukocytes. Fertil Steril. 1996;65(2):411–9.
39. Greco E, et al. Reduction of the incidence of sperm DNA fragmentation by oral antioxidant treatment. J Androl. 2005;26(3):349–53.
40. Omu AE, et al. Indications of the mechanisms involved in improved sperm parameters by zinc therapy. Med Princ Pract. 2008;17(2):108–16.
41. Tremellen K, et al. A randomised control trial examining the effect of an antioxidant (Menevit) on pregnancy outcome during IVF-ICSI treatment. Aust N Z J Obstet Gynaecol. 2007;47(3):216–21.
42. Rolf C, et al. Antioxidant treatment of patients with asthenozoospermia or moderate oligoasthenozoospermia with high-dose vitamin C and vitamin E: a randomized, placebo-controlled, double-blind study. Hum Reprod. 1999;14(4):1028–33.
43. Verma A, Kanwar KC. Human sperm motility and lipid peroxidation in different ascorbic acid concentrations: an in vitro analysis. Andrologia. 1998;30(6):325–9.
44. Mongioi L, et al. The role of carnitine in male infertility. Andrology. 2016;4:800–7.
45. Lenzi A, et al. A placebo-controlled double-blind randomized trial of the use of combined l-carnitine and l-acetyl-carnitine treatment in men with asthenozoospermia. Fertil Steril. 2004;81(6):1578–84.
46. Cavallini G, et al. Cinnoxicam and L-carnitine/acetyl-L-carnitine treatment for idiopathic and varicocele-associated oligoasthenospermia. J Androl. 2004;25(5):761–70; discussion 771–2.
47. Balercia G, et al. Placebo-controlled double-blind randomized trial on the use of L-carnitine, L-acetylcarnitine, or combined L-carnitine and L-acetylcarnitine in men with idiopathic asthenozoospermia. Fertil Steril. 2005;84(3):662–71.
48. Aliabadi E, et al. Effects of L-carnitine and L-acetyl-carnitine on testicular sperm motility and chromatin quality. Iran J Reprod Med. 2012;10(2):77–82.
49. Al-Dujaily S, Al-Sultani YK, Shams Alddin NN. DNA normality following in vitro sperm preparation with pentoxifylline and L-carnitine for asthenozoospermic infertile men. Glob J Med Res. 2013;13(7):25–30.
50. Lewin A, Lavon H. The effect of coenzyme Q10 on sperm motility and function. Mol Asp Med. 1997;18(Suppl):S213–9.

51. Safarinejad MR. Efficacy of coenzyme Q10 on semen parameters, sperm function and reproductive hormones in infertile men. J Urol. 2009;182(1):237–48.
52. Safarinejad MR. The effect of coenzyme Q(1)(0) supplementation on partner pregnancy rate in infertile men with idiopathic oligoasthenoteratozoospermia: an open-label prospective study. Int Urol Nephrol. 2012;44(3):689–700.
53. Gvozdjakova A, et al. Coenzyme Q(1)(0), alpha-tocopherol, and oxidative stress could be important metabolic biomarkers of male infertility. Dis Markers. 2015;2015:827941.
54. Lenzi A, et al. Glutathione treatment of dyspermia: effect on the lipoperoxidation process. Hum Reprod. 1994;9(11):2044–50.
55. Ciftci H, et al. Effects of N-acetylcysteine on semen parameters and oxidative/antioxidant status. Urology. 2009;74(1):73–6.
56. Oeda T, et al. Scavenging effect of N-acetyl-L-cysteine against reactive oxygen species in human semen: a possible therapeutic modality for male factor infertility? Andrologia. 1997;29(3):125–31.
57. Aitken RJ, et al. Sperm motility is lost in vitro as a consequence of mitochondrial free radical production and the generation of electrophilic aldehydes but can be significantly rescued by the presence of nucleophilic thiols. Biol Reprod. 2012;87(5):110.
58. Erkkila K, et al. N-acetyl-L-cysteine inhibits apoptosis in human male germ cells in vitro. J Clin Endocrinol Metab. 1998;83(7):2523–31.
59. Wong WY, et al. Effects of folic acid and zinc sulfate on male factor subfertility: a double-blind, randomized, placebo-controlled trial. Fertil Steril. 2002;77(3):491–8.
60. Ebisch IM, et al. Does folic acid and zinc sulphate intervention affect endocrine parameters and sperm characteristics in men? Int J Androl. 2006;29(2):339–45.
61. Aarabi M, et al. High-dose folic acid supplementation alters the human sperm methylome and is influenced by the MTHFR C677T polymorphism. Hum Mol Genet. 2015;24(22):6301–13.
62. Boxmeer JC, et al. Low folate in seminal plasma is associated with increased sperm DNA damage. Fertil Steril. 2009;92(2):548–56.
63. Noack-Fuller G, De Beer C, Seibert H. Cadmium, lead, selenium, and zinc in semen of occupationally unexposed men. Andrologia. 1993;25(1):7–12.
64. Ahsan U, et al. Role of selenium in male reproduction—a review. Anim Reprod Sci. 2014;146(1–2):55–62.
65. Safarinejad MR, Safarinejad S. Efficacy of selenium and/or N-acetyl-cysteine for improving semen parameters in infertile men: a double-blind, placebo controlled, randomized study. J Urol. 2009;181(2):741–51.
66. Vezina D, et al. Selenium-vitamin E supplementation in infertile men. Effects on semen parameters and micronutrient levels and distribution. Biol Trace Elem Res. 1996;53(1–3):65–83.
67. Keskes-Ammar L, et al. Sperm oxidative stress and the effect of an oral vitamin E and selenium supplement on semen quality in infertile men. Arch Androl. 2003;49(2):83–94.
68. Siegel RB, et al. Effect of in vitro selenium supplementation on bovine sperm motility. Theriogenology. 1980;13(5):357–67.
69. Dorostkar K, Alavi-Shoushtari SM, Mokarizadeh A. Effects of in vitro selenium addition to the semen extender on the spermatozoa characteristics before and after freezing in water buffaloes (Bubalus bubalis). Vet Res Forum. 2012;3(4):263–8.
70. Henkel R, et al. Elimination of zinc from the flagella of spermatozoa during epididymal transit is important for motility. Reprod Technol. 2001;10:280–5.
71. Henkel R, Baldauf C, Schill WB. Resorption of the element zinc from spermatozoa by the epididymal epithelium. Reprod Domest Anim. 2003;38(2):97–101.
72. Bjorndahl L, Kvist U. Human sperm chromatin stabilization: a proposed model including zinc bridges. Mol Hum Reprod. 2010;16(1):23–9.
73. Chia SE, et al. Comparison of zinc concentrations in blood and seminal plasma and the various sperm parameters between fertile and infertile men. J Androl. 2000;21(1):53–7.
74. Nair N, et al. Short-term zinc deficiency in diet induces increased oxidative stress in testes and epididymis of rats. Indian J Exp Biol. 2005;43(9):786–94.

75. Hunt CD, et al. Effects of dietary zinc depletion on seminal volume and zinc loss, serum testosterone concentrations, and sperm morphology in young men. Am J Clin Nutr. 1992;56(1):148–57.
76. Hadwan MH, Almashhedy LA, Alsalman AR. Oral zinc supplementation restores superoxide radical scavengers to normal levels in spermatozoa of Iraqi asthenospermic patients. Int J Vitam Nutr Res. 2015;85(3–4):65–73.
77. Dorostkar K, Alavi Shoushtari SM, Khaki A. Effects of in vitro zinc sulphate additive to the semen extender on water buffalo (Bubalusbubalis) spermatozoa before and after freezing. Int J Fertil Steril. 2014;8(3):325–32.
78. Showell MG, et al. Antioxidants for male subfertility. Cochrane Database Syst Rev. 2014;(12):CD007411.
79. Ross C, et al. A systematic review of the effect of oral antioxidants on male infertility. Reprod BioMed Online. 2010;20(6):711–23.

Chapter 26
Varicocelectomy

Matheus Roque and Sandro C. Esteves

26.1 Introduction

Varicocele is defined as a dilatation of the pampiniform plexus veins. It is a common condition found both in men with normal spermatogenesis and in men with abnormal semen parameters. Varicocele has been considered the most common cause of male infertility, affecting about 15–20% of the general population, 35–40% of men presenting with primary infertility [1–3], and up to 80% of men with secondary infertility [3]. Despite being more common on the left side, varicoceles are found bilaterally in up to 50% of the patients [3, 4]. On the contrary, isolated right side varicocele is a rare condition that may be associated with situs inversus, retroperitoneal tumors, and insertion of the spermatic vein into the right renal vein [4, 5].

The diagnosis of varicocele is primarily based on physical examination. However, imaging studies have been indicated when the physical examination is inconclusive or in cases of recurrence after previous repair. Only clinically palpable varicocele has been clearly associated with infertility [6]. The most widely used classification is the Dubin grading system, which classifies the varicocele on a scale of 1–3, with grade 3 being present on visual inspection of the scrotum, grade 2 being palpable, and grade 1 only being palpable with the aid of Valsalva maneuver [7].

M. Roque
ORIGEN - Center for Reproductive Medicine, Rio de Janeiro, Brazil
e-mail: matheusroque@origen.com.br

S.C. Esteves (✉)
Andrology and Human Reproduction Clinic, ANDROFERT, Campinas, Brazil
e-mail: s.esteves@androfert.com.br

A. Zini, A. Agarwal (eds.), *A Clinician's Guide to Sperm DNA and Chromatin Damage*, https://doi.org/10.1007/978-3-319-71815-6_26

Varicocele can impair spermatogenesis through several distinct pathophysiological mechanisms, namely, scrotal hyperthermia, hormonal disturbances, testicular hypoperfusion, hypoxia, and backflow of toxic metabolites (Fig. 26.1). Recent studies, however, indicate that oxidative stress is a central element in the pathophysiology of varicocele-related infertility. As a matter of fact, both reactive oxygen species (ROS) and apoptosis markers are elevated in the semen of infertile men with varicocele [8–11]. Despite having an important physiological role in fertility [12], ROS in excess may overcome the body's antioxidant protection and result in oxidative stress (OS). As human spermatozoa contain high concentrations of unsaturated fatty acids, lipid peroxidation ensues in the presence of excessive ROS [13]. As a result, damage to sperm membrane occurs, affecting both sperm motility and sperm-oocyte fusion. Furthermore, OS may negatively affect the sperm chromatin by inducing breaks in the DNA strands [5, 14, 15]. Notwithstanding, the reasons why some patients with varicocele are infertile, whereas the majority of patients are not, remain unclear [16].

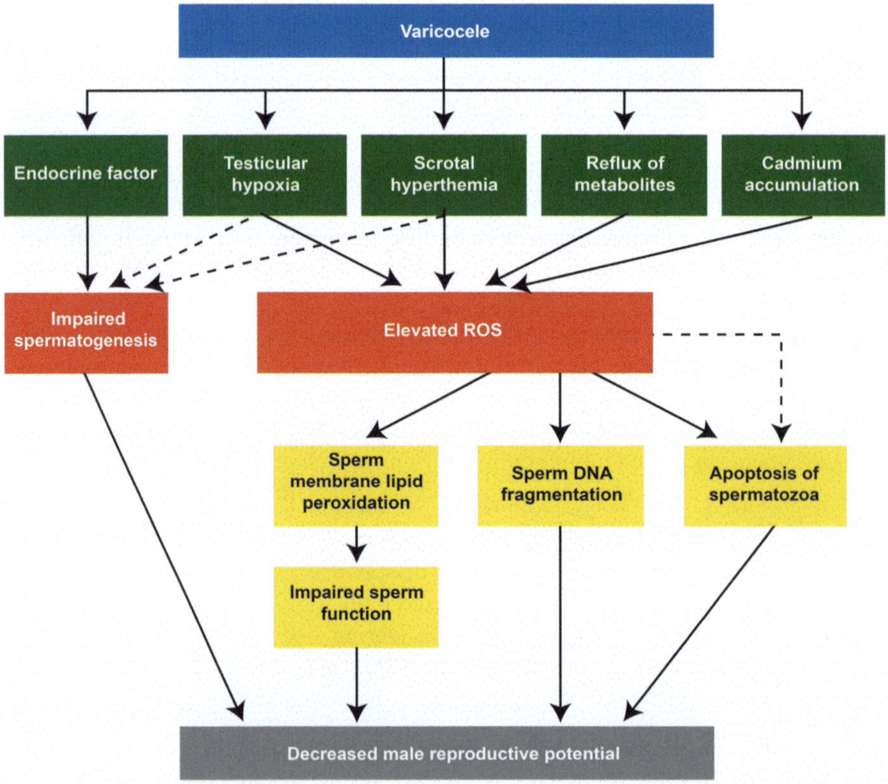

Fig. 26.1 The detrimental effect of varicocele on male reproduction (Reprinted from: Cho et al. [10] (This figure is available under the terms of the Creative Commons Attribution-NonCommercial-ShareAlike License (CC BY-NC-SA), which permits noncommercial use, distribution, and reproduction in any medium))

Although sperm with fragmented DNA are able to fertilize oocytes with an apparent similar efficiency as sperm without DNA fragmentation [16, 17], it has been found that sperm DNA fragmentation (SDF) may negatively impact embryo development through its effects on the integrity of the embryonic genome [18, 19]. In fact, SDF has been associated not only with infertility but also with poor outcomes in assisted reproduction treatments, including miscarriages [20–22].

Whereas the routine use of OS markers, including SDF, has been debated [23], the assessment of SDF in men with varicocele may provide valuable information to guide therapeutic interventions [11, 24, 25]. For instance, determining which patients are affected by SDF could enable clinicians to better select varicocele candidates for early surgical interventions [26]. Moreover, oxidative stress markers can be used to monitor the effectiveness of interventions [16]. In fact, varicocele repair may alleviate OS and reduce SDF, thus leading to improved fertility, both natural and assisted [27–31].

In this chapter, we summarize (1) the current evidence concerning the association between varicocele and sperm DNA fragmentation and (2) the benefit of varicocele repair in infertile men with elevated SDF.

26.2 Varicocele and Oxidative Stress

Although small quantities of ROS play important roles in sperm function, a disproportionate increase in ROS usually leads to OS that may cause damage to both nuclear and mitochondrial sperm DNA, including base modifications, strand breaks, and chromatin cross-links [11]. OS has also been implicated in apoptosis-like processes affecting sperm maturation and nuclear protamination [10].

Several studies comparing fertile men with and without varicocele have found that the former exhibit increased levels of seminal OS markers. However, it is still unknown by which mechanisms fertility is maintained in these men [15, 32–34]. Likewise, OS markers are also elevated in infertile men with varicocele. Elevated levels of ROS, nitric oxide, and lipid peroxidation products are common findings [35–37], thus indicating that the presence of varicocele exacerbates the generation of oxidative stress [16]. Furthermore, an association between varicocele grade and OS seems to exist, as the larger the varicocele, the higher the levels of OS [38–42]. Others have demonstrated that men with varicocele had diminished seminal antioxidant capacity when compared to fertile counterparts [9, 32, 33, 37, 42–45].

Added to this, ROS generation has been associated with scrotal hyperthermia, testicular hypoxia, reflux of adrenal and renal metabolites, cadmium accumulation, and epididymal dysfunction [5, 10]. However, it is likely that intrinsic factors either protecting or exacerbating the harmful effects of oxidation on germ cells exist, thus modulating the fertility status of men with varicocele [5]. In this scenario, sperm DNA fragmentation is probably the manifestation of these aforementioned factors on spermatogenesis [9].

26.3 Varicocele and Sperm DNA Fragmentation

As depicted in Fig. 26.1, there are several distinct mechanisms, namely, scrotal hyperthermia, hormonal disturbances, testicular hypoperfusion, hypoxia, and backflow of toxic metabolites related to the pathophysiology of varicocele. All of them are associated with ROS generation and ROS-mediated oxidative stress, including lipid peroxidation, which damages not only the sperm membrane but also the DNA contents [5]. As a consequence, DNA fragmentation ensues both in mitochondrial and nuclear DNA. Although mitochondrial DNA is more susceptible to ROS, sperm nuclear damage has a greater clinical significance [10]. It is therefore prime to discuss how the distinct pathophysiological mechanisms involved in varicocele are associated with oxidative stress and sperm DNA fragmentation, as we will see in the sections below.

26.3.1 Heat Stress

Spermatogenesis is optimal at temperatures 2.50 °C lower than the body's temperature. However, due to the reflux of abdominal blood through incompetent valves of the internal spermatic and cremasteric veins into the pampiniform plexus, scrotal temperature increases in patients with varicocele. Scrotal hyperthermia is the most widely accepted hypothesis to explain oxidative stress in varicocele [46]. ROS production from mitochondria, plasma membrane, cytoplasm, and peroxisome increase in the presence of heat stress. The cell damage due to hyperthermia occurs in different grades in the various cell compartments [10]. In the testes, spermatogonia B and developing spermatozoa are highly vulnerable to heat stress. On the contrary, spermatogonia A, Leydig and Sertoli cells are thermo-resistant [5]. Figure 26.2 depicts the association between heat stress and ROS production in varicocele.

26.3.2 Testicular Hypoxia

Studies evaluating venographic pressure and testis histopathology showed that tissue ischemia occurs if venous hydrostatic pressure of internal testicular vein exceeds the testicular arteriolar pressure [47, 48]. Ischemia signs, including arteriolar occlusion by microthrombi, germ cell degeneration, Leydig cell atrophy, and fibrotic

Fig. 26.2 (continued) that is mediated through a variety of mechanisms and targets lipids, proteins, sugars, and nucleic acids. Excessive ROS overwhelm primary sperm defenses against oxidative stress—the tight packing of sperm DNA and seminal antioxidants. The harmful effects of oxidative stress are caused by lipid peroxidation of sperm plasma membrane and nuclear as well as mitochondrial sperm DNA damage (Adapted by permission from Macmillan Publishers Ltd.: Nature Reviews Urology. Agarwal et al. [5])

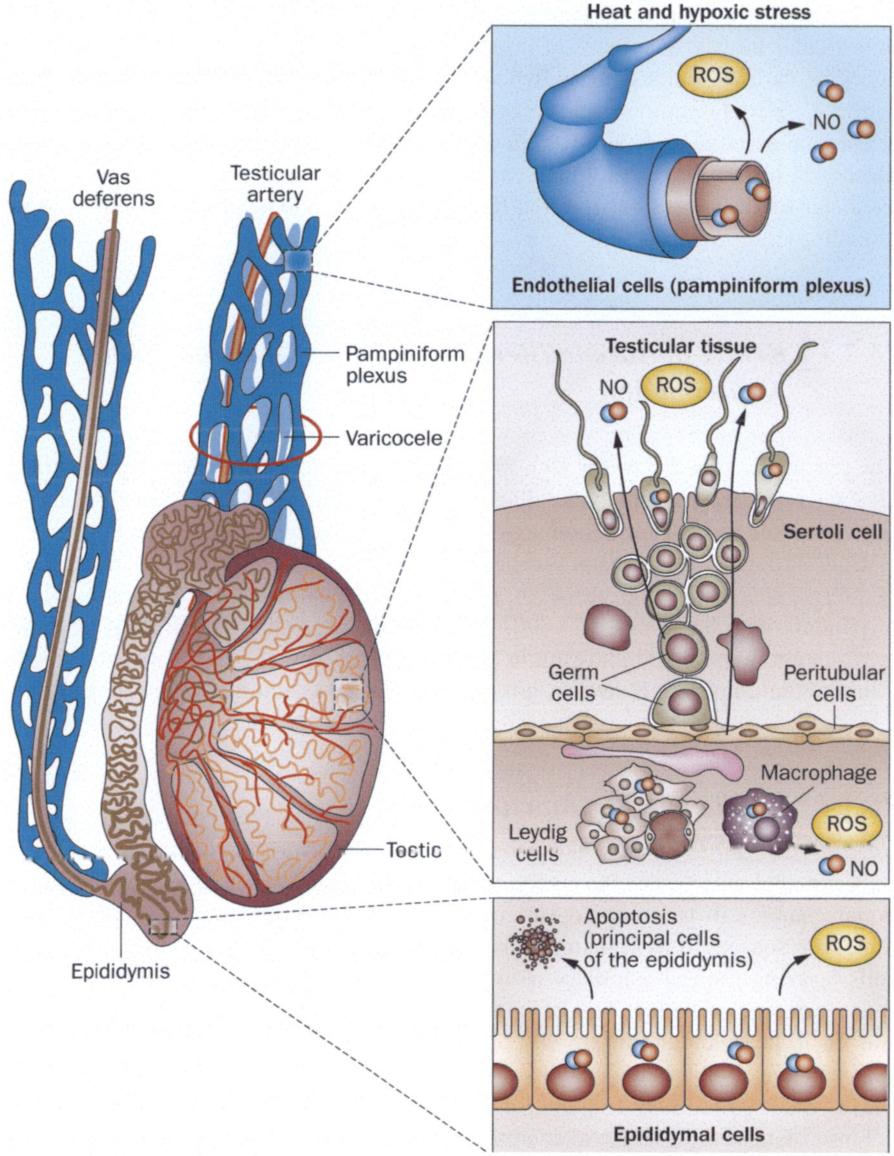

Fig. 26.2 Oxidative stress is the central and common pathogenic mediator of testicular damage in varicocele, while exposure to heat, hypoxia, and toxic adrenal and renal metabolites are stimulators of reactive oxygen and nitrogen species generation. ROS encompass a broad category of highly reactive substances formed as byproducts of oxidative and reductive metabolic reactions. Reactive nitrogen species constitute a subset of ROS that contains nitrogen atoms. Three components can release ROS in men with varicocele under heat and hypoxic stress: the principal cells in the epididymis, the endothelial cells in the dilated pampiniform plexus, and the testicular cells (developing germ cells, Leydig cells, macrophages, and peritubular cells). An imbalance between seminal ROS and their neutralizing antioxidants in men with varicocele results in oxidative stress

thickening of the basement membranes of seminiferous tubules have been observed in testicular biopsy specimens of infertile men with varicocele [47]. ROS are produced by various sources during hypoxia, including activation of hypoxia inducible factor 1 (HIF-1), mitochondrial dysfunction, xanthine dehydrogenase/oxidase, membrane-associated NAPDH oxidase 5 (NOX5), and phospholipase A2 [5]. Moreover, hypoxia can lead to increase in the expression of leptin and cytokines in testicular tissue, including IL-1 and IL-6, which can induce the generation of ROS [40, 49–51].

26.3.3 Reflux of Adrenal/Renal Metabolites and Cadmium Accumulation

The retrograde blood flow through the left testicular vein with adrenal prostaglandins and renal and adrenal metabolites can induce cellular OS [52]. Norepinephrine can contribute to vasospasm and aggravate hypoxia, generating more ROS [5].

Cadmium is a natural metal that has been identified in elevated levels in the wall of internal spermatic veins, testicular tissue biopsy specimens, and the seminal fluid of patients with varicocele [53–55]. It is hypothesized that increased hydrostatic pressure and hypoxia might result in a porous blood-testis barrier that enables cadmium to build up [55]. However, it is still unclear how cadmium affects fertility.

26.3.4 Epididymis Dysfunction

Experimental varicoceles have been used to study epididymal structural and functional changes in response to varicocele [5]. In the epididymis, there are three important sources of ROS, namely, the luminal fluid from the testis, the endothelial cells layering the rich capillary network around the caput, and the metabolically active principal cells [5]. The initial epididymal segment seems to be the primary site for ROS accumulation. In all epididymal segments, there also seems to exist cells capable of generating enzymatic and nonenzymatic antioxidants. Hypoxia and heat stress are the likely triggers for the imbalance between ROS and antioxidant defenses. Under these stressful conditions, the principal cells can generate excessive ROS that when combined with impaired production of antioxidants result in oxidative damage to the maturing sperm and epididymal cells [10].

26.3.5 Clinical Data

A meta-analysis of seven studies assessed SDF rates in men with varicocele. Higher sperm DNA damage was found in patients with varicocele than controls. The overall estimate showed a mean difference of 9.84% (95% CI 9.19–10.49; $P < 0.00001$)

in SDF rates between patients and controls [56]. In another review article, the authors identified 16 case-control studies that measured SDF in fertile and infertile men with varicocele [9]. The control groups were formed by sperm donors, fertile men, or infertile men without varicocele. Nine studies investigated the association between varicocele and SDF in infertile men; SDF rates were higher in infertile men with varicocele than infertile men without varicocele in four studies. The remaining seven studies specifically included fertile men with varicocele. In six of them, SDF rates were higher in men with varicocele (and no history of infertility) than fertile men or sperm donors without varicocele [9].

In a multicenter study, we evaluated SDF by sperm chromatin dispersion (SCD) test in 593 men with various etiologies attending infertility clinics. A total of 98 men with varicocele and 80 fertile controls were included [46]. Both men with varicocele and those with leukocytospermia exhibited the highest SDF rates among the studied men, with 35.7% (±18.3%) and 41.7% (±17.6%) damaged sperm, respectively. The SDF rates were also higher in testicular cancer patients and in couples with repeated in vitro fertilization (IVF)/ICSI failure than controls ($P < 0.05$) [46]. Importantly, we identified two distinctive sperm subpopulations within fragmented DNA in the varicocele subgroup, namely, standard fragmented sperm and degraded sperm (DDS), similarly than previously reported [57–59]. Spermatozoa with standard fragmented DNA exhibited either the absence or the presence of a small halo of chromatin dispersion around a compact nucleoid. On the contrary, spermatozoa with degraded DNA exhibited a ghost-like morphology owing to massive single- and double-strand DNA breaks as well as nuclear protein damage [59]. The rates of degraded sperm (DDSi), determined by the proportion of degraded sperm in the whole population of spermatozoa with fragmented DNA, were eightfold higher in varicocele than donors. Although DDS is not pathognomonic of varicocele, it was possible to identify varicocele based solely on SCD results with 94% accuracy, thus making it an attractive marker for the presence of varicocele [46] (Fig. 26.3).

26.4 Varicocelectomy and Sperm DNA Fragmentation

Varicocele treatment is generally recommended when the following criteria are met: (1) presence of clinical varicoceles on physical examination regardless of its grade, (2) presence of infertility, (3) female partner with normal fertility or with a potentially treatable cause of infertility and time to pregnancy is not a major concern, and (4) male partner has abnormal semen parameters [6]. However, the identification and treatment of the underlying pathology is one of the main objectives when managing infertile men [1]. Given that abnormalities in sperm chromatin may be present even in men with semen analysis within normal ranges [60], it seems sound to offer SDF testing to all infertile men undergoing fertility evaluation, including those with varicocele. Testing for SDF has been proposed not only to identify those patients in whom SDF is contributory to infertility but also to offer interventions to alleviating SDF and potentially improve pregnancy outcome, both naturally and with assisted reproductive technology (ART) [61].

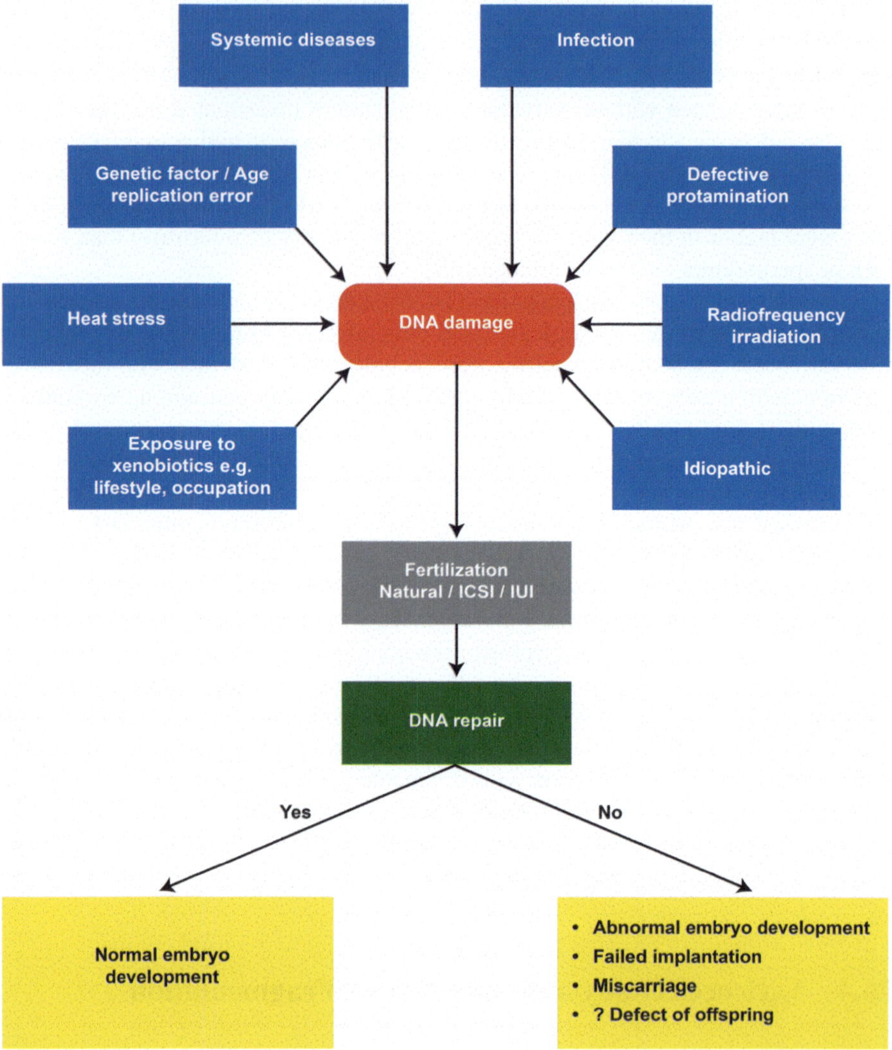

Fig. 26.3 The possible etiologies and consequences of sperm DNA damage (Reprinted from: Cho et al. [10]. (This figure is available under the terms of the Creative Commons Attribution-NonCommercial-ShareAlike License (CC BY-NC-SA), which permits noncommercial use, distribution, and reproduction in any medium))

As aforementioned, varicocele is associated with OS and is one of the major causes of SDF. Therefore, it seems logical that varicocele repair may result in improvements in overall semen quality, including SDF [9, 11, 62]. In fact, the levels of oxidative-stress markers, including 4977-bp mitochondrial DNA deletion, 8-OHdG, TBARS, and nitrate plus nitrite content are decreased or normalized after varicocelectomy [15, 37, 42, 63]. Furthermore, varicocele repair has been shown to improve or normalize TAC levels both in the seminal plasma and peripheral blood, as well as retinol, selenium, and zinc levels [63–65]. These studies indicate that varicocelectomy is beneficial not only for alleviating OS and its negative effect on fertility but also for preventing and protecting against the progressive nature of varicocele and its consequent upregulation of systemic OS [30]. On the contrary, some studies have failed to demonstrate reduction of OS markers after varicocelectomy [66–68], making it unclear why not all men improve after varicocelectomy [69].

As far as SDF is concerned, a meta-analysis including six studies evaluated the effect of varicocelectomy. The authors found that SDF rates were overall reduced, with a mean difference of −3.37% (95% CI −4.09–2.65; $P < 0.00001$) [56]. Subsequently, others have corroborated these aforementioned findings. Kadioglu et al. retrospectively analyzed 92 consecutive infertile men presenting with clinical varicocele and who were subjected to subinguinal microsurgical varicocele repair. Sperm DNA fragmentation was evaluated using the terminal deoxynucleotidyl transferase dUTP nick end labeling (TUNEL) assay. In addition to the improvements in conventional semen parameters, there was a significant decrease in DNA fragmentation index (DFI) from a preoperative mean of 42.6% to a postoperative mean of 20.5% ($P < 0.001$) [70]. Ni et al. evaluated 42 subfertile patients with clinical varicocele and altered seminal parameters subjected to microsurgical varicocelectomy. SDF was measured by sperm chromatin structure assay (SCSA), and the protamine-1/2 mRNA ratio was also assessed. The preoperative results were compared to a control group of semen donors. The protamine-1/2 ratio and SDF indexes were significantly higher preoperatively in the patient group than in the control group. After varicocelectomy, the mean P1/P2 ratio was significantly improved after a mean time of 3–6 months in men who were able to impregnate their wives, and postoperative results did not differ from the control group. Overall, SDF was also significantly lower 3–6 months after surgery when compared to the preoperative levels, although still higher than in controls. However, in the group of patients unable to impregnate their wives naturally after a follow-up of 6 months, postoperative P1/P2 mRNA and SDF rates were not different compared to the preoperative levels [71]. Lastly, Smit et al. prospectively evaluated 49 men with clinical varicocele, oligozoospermia, and at least 1 year of infertility subjected to varicocelectomy. These authors also observed postoperative improvements in sperm parameters and decreases in SDF indexes. Lower postoperative SDF results were associated with a higher chance of pregnancy, both naturally and with ART [72]. Notwithstanding, the repair of subclinical varicoceles is not warranted. In a recent study, Garcia-Peiró et al. evaluated 60 infertile patients with varicocele using several SDF methods (TUNEL, SCD, and SCSA). While SDF rates decreased after repairing clinical varicoceles, there were no improvements in SDF rates in infertile patients with subclinical varicocele subjected to surgery [79]. In conclusion, fair evidence indicates that (1) SDF is reduced after varicocelectomy in infertile men with clinical varicocele, and (2) a decrease in SDF is associated with a higher chance of pregnancy. Table 26.1 summarizes the main results of the studies examining the role of varicocelectomy on SDF.

Table 26.1 Studies examining the effects of varicocelectomy on sperm DNA fragmentation

Study	Design	Patients	Main results	Conclusions
Zini et al. [27]	Retrospective	37 men subjected to varicocelectomy[a]	Mean (±SE) SDF rates before and after microsurgical varicocelectomy (6 months interval) were 27.7 ± 2.9 vs. 24.6 ± 2.7% ($P = 0.04$)	Varicocelectomy improves sperm DNA integrity in infertile men with clinical varicocele
Sakamoto et al. [37]	Retrospective	28 azoospermic, 30 oligozoospermic (15 with and 15 without varicocele) and 30 patients with normal semen characteristics (15 with and 15 without varicocele). Varicocele repair was performed in all men with varicocele	SDF assessed by TUNEL was lower postoperatively (post: 27.5 ± 19.4%; pre: 79.6 ± 13.6%; $P < 0.001$	Men with varicocele, regardless of presenting with normal or abnormal semen analyses, have higher seminal oxidative stress. Varicocelectomy reduces sperm DNA damage
Werthman et al. [73]	Retrospective	11 patients with varicocele subjected to varicocelectomy[a]	90% of the patients showed a significant decrease in the rates of SDF 3–6 months after varicocelectomy	Men with high levels of sperm DNA fragmentation and varicoceles should be counseled to undergo varicocele repair before proceeding to other fertility treatments
Moskovtsev et al. [74]	Retrospective	9 men subjected to varicocelectomy[a]	Improvements in SDF were observed in 78% of the treated patients (pre: 44.7% ± 12.8; post: 28.4 ± 9.5% ($P < 0.03$)	The cause-specific treatment of SDF led to a significant decrease in sperm DNA damage
Smit et al. [75]	Prospective	49 men subjected to varicocelectomy[a]	Improvements in SDF were observed in the treated subjects (pre: 35.2%; post: 30.2%; $P = 0.019$)	Varicocelectomy significantly decreased DNA fragmentation and should be considered in infertile men with palpable varicocele, abnormal semen analysis, and no major female factors
Lacerda et al. [68]	Prospective	27 adolescents between 15 and 19 years old with grades 2 or 3 varicocele subjected to varicocelectomy[a]	A higher proportion of sperm with intact nuclear DNA, as assessed by the comet assay, was observed after varicocelectomy	Varicocelectomy in adolescents was associated with an increase in sperm DNA integrity

Zini et al. [9]	Prospective	25 men subjected to varicocelectomy[a]	Improvements in SDF were observed in the treated subjects (pre: 18 ± 11%; post (4 months): 10 ± 5%; post (6 months): 7 ± 3%	Varicocele repair was associated with improvements in sperm DNA integrity and chromatin compaction
La Vignera et al. [76]	Not stated	30 men with oligoastheno-teratozoospermia and grade 3 left varicocele subjected to varicocelectomy[a]	SDF rates significantly decreased after surgery from 5.0 ± 3.0% to 2.1 ± 0.4% ($P < 0.05$), and these postoperative results were similar to that of healthy controls (2.0 ± 1.0%)	Varicocelectomy was associated with reduction in sperm DNA fragmentation. Postoperative SDF of treated men similar to healthy fertile men without varicocele
Li et al. [77]	Not stated	19 infertile men subjected to varicocelectomy and 19 normozoospermic men serving as controls	DFI decreased from 28.4 ± 15.6% before surgery to 22.4 ± 12.9% 3 months postoperatively	Microsurgical varicocele repair can be considered a treatment option in infertile men with palpable varicocele
Baker et al. [78]	Retrospective	22 men with clinical varicocele subjected to varicocelectomy[a]	DFI decreased from a preoperative mean of 40.8% to a postoperative mean of 24.5% ($P = 0.001$)	Varicocele ligation resulted in DFI decrease. Patients considering varicocelectomy with the intent of improving semen parameters should be encouraged
Smit et al. [72]	Prospective	49 infertile men with a palpable varicocele and oligozoospermia who underwent varicocelectomy[a]	The DFI decreased from 35.2% before to 30.2% after surgery ($P = 0.033$)	After varicocelectomy sperm parameters significantly improved and sperm DNa fragmentation was significantly decreased. Low DFI values are associated with a higher chance of pregnancy

(continued)

Table 26.1 (continued)

Study	Design	Patients	Main results	Conclusions
García-Peiró et al. [79]	Not stated	60 infertile patients with varicocele (15 with untreated clinical varicoceles, 19 with clinical varicoceles subjected to varicocele repair, 16 with untreated subclinical varicocele, and 10 with subclinical varicocele subjected to varicocele repair)	SDF assessed by different methods (TUNEL, SCD, and SCSA) were elevated (and not statistically different) in men with both clinical and subclinical varicocele	Although both infertile patients with clinical and subclinical varicocele have impaired sperm DNA quality, varicocelectomy was shown to improve SDF only in those with clinical varicocele
			SDF was reduced after varicocele repair in men with clinical varicocele but not in those with subclinical varicocele	
Kadioglu et al. [70]	Retrospective	92 infertile men subjected to varicocelectomy[a]	Mean DFI decreased after varicocele repair (pre: 42.6%; post: 20.5% ($P < 0.001$)	Varicocelectomy improve semen parameters and sperm DNA integrity in infertile men with varicocele
Ni et al. [71]	Prospective	42 infertile men subjected to varicocelectomy and 10 normozoospermic healthy donors	SDF decreased from a preoperative of 27.45 ± 6.35% (preoperative) to a postoperative mean ± SD of 20.65 ± 3.56% (3 months postoperative) and 19.03 ± 4.26% (6 months postoperative) in couples that achieved pregnancy	Decrease in DFI after varicocele repair was associated with a higher chance of achieving pregnancy

DFI DNA fragmentation index, *TUNEL* terminal deoxynucleotidyl transferase dUTP nick end labeling, *SCD* sperm chromatin dispersion, *SCSA* sperm chromatin structure assay

[a]The study compared preoperative and postoperative sperm DNA fragmentation (SDF) in the same patient

26.5 Future Research

A variety of tests has been developed to measure SDF in sperm, as discussed in detail elsewhere in this book. Nowadays, the most commonly used tests are sperm chromatin structure assay (SCSA), terminal deoxynucleotidyl transferase-mediated fluorescein-dUTP nick-end labeling (TUNEL), COMET, and sperm chromatin dispersion (SCD) test. However, it is still unknown which test would be optimal to detect DNA damage in men with varicocele. And further research is needed to determine which SDF thresholds would better discriminate infertile from fertile men with varicocele.

Recently, a clinical guideline on the use of SDF testing based on clinical scenarios shed some light on the role of SDF testing in men with varicocele [80]. In their paper, Agarwal et al. reviewed the existing literature and recommended SDF testing for (i) infertile men with large varicocele (grades 2 and 3) and normal conventional semen analysis (WHO criteria) and (ii) infertile men with small varicocele (grade 1) and borderline or normal semen analysis. The rationale is to aid the clinical decision of recommending varicocelectomy to these patients. The authors advocate surgery to the aforementioned subjects with high SDF rates (grade C recommendation). They argued that SDF testing could identify men with already compromised sperm function and otherwise "normal" conventional parameters. Given that the authors' recommendation was mainly based on retrospective studies, more data is needed to elucidate the role of SDF testing to both diagnosis and management of varicocele.

The development of genomics, epigenomics, proteomics, and metabolomics biomarkers may also help to understand the pathophysiology of varicocele and why some men are infertile whereas others are not. Proteomic studies have suggested that varicocele leads to a deviation from homeostasis toward a dynamic equilibrium in an altered state [81, 82]. In adolescents, a general dysfunction is observed in the seminal plasma proteome whereas functions critical for fertilization are underrepresented in adults [81]. It seems that the proteomic signature differs when men with varicocele are compared to controls without varicocele [82]. New studies identifying molecular markers related to oxidative stress and SDF in men with varicoceles are very much anticipated, as molecular markers seem to hold promise as a better means of selecting patients that require treatment [83].

26.6 Conclusions

Significant advancements have been obtained in biomolecular techniques, enabling us to better understand the mechanisms involved in testicular damage caused by varicocele. Fair evidence indicates that varicocele exacerbates the generation of reactive oxygen species (ROS), which is associated with oxidative stress. Although small quantities of ROS have important roles in sperm function, a disproportionate increase in ROS may lead to OS that can cause damage to nuclear and mitochondrial sperm DNA. Therefore, both OS and SDF play an important role in the pathophysiology of varicocele-related infertility. Sperm DNA fragmentation has been associated with infertility and poorer reproductive outcomes, both natural and assisted. It has been suggested that SDF testing should be included during male infertility workup as infertile men with so-called "normal" semen analysis may present with elevated rates of SDF. Furthermore, assessment of OS markers, including SDF, may allow the identification of men with abnormal markers who may be the best candidates for surgery. Varicocele repair may alleviate oxidative stress and as a consequence decrease the proportion of spermatozoa exhibiting SDF. As a result, fertility can be either restored or improved, and better outcomes are expected if assisted reproduction is required.

References

1. Esteves SC, Miyaoka R, Agarwal A. An update on the clinical assessment of the infertile male. [corrected]. Clinics (Sao Paulo). 2011;66:691–700.
2. Shiraishi K, Matsuyama H, Takihara H. Pathophysiology of varicocele in male infertility in the era of assisted reproductive technology. Int J Urol. 2012;19:538–50.
3. Gorelick JI, Goldstein M. Loss of fertility in men with varicocele. Fertil Steril. 1993;59:613–6.
4. Alsaikhan B, Alrabeeah K, Delouya G, Zini A. Epidemiology of varicocele. Asian J Androl. 2016;18:179–81.
5. Agarwal A, Hamada A, Esteves SC. Insight into oxidative stress in varicocele-associated male infertility: part 1. Nat Rev Urol. 2012;9:678–90.
6. Practice Committee of the American Society for Reproductive Medicine, Society for Male Reproduction and Urology. Report on varicocele and infertility: a committee opinion. Fertil Steril. 2014;102:1556–60.
7. Miyaoka R, Esteves SC. A critical appraisal on the role of varicocele in male infertility. Adv Urol. 2012;2012:597495.
8. Agarwal A, Sharma RK, Desai NR, Prabakaran S, Tavares A, Sabanegh E. Role of oxidative stress in pathogenesis of varicocele and infertility. Urology. 2009;73:461–9.
9. Zini A, Dohle G. Are varicoceles associated with increased deoxyribonucleic acid fragmentation? Fertil Steril. 2011;96:1283–7.
10. Cho CL, Esteves SC, Agarwal A. Novel insights into the pathophysiology of varicocele and its association with reactive oxygen species and sperm DNA fragmentation. Asian J Androl. 2016;18:186–93.
11. Esteves SC. Novel concepts in male factor infertility: clinical and laboratory perspectives. J Assist Reprod Genet. 2016;33:1319–35.
12. Griveau JF, Le Lannou D. Reactive oxygen species and human spermatozoa: physiology and pathology. Int J Androl. 1997;20:61–9.
13. Ni K, Steger K, Yang H, Wang H, Hu K, Zhang T, Chen B. A comprehensive investigation of sperm DNA damage and oxidative stress injury in infertile patients with subclinical, normozoospermic and astheno/oligozoospermic clinical varicocele. Andrology. 2016;4:816–24.
14. Tremellen K. Oxidative stress and male infertility—a clinical perspective. Hum Reprod Update. 2008;14:243–58.
15. Blumer CG, Restelli AE, Giudice PT, Soler TB, Fraietta R, Nichi M, Bertolla RP, Cedenho AP. Effect of varicocele on sperm function and semen oxidative stress. BJU Int. 2012;109:259–65.
16. Hamada A, Esteves SC, Agarwal A. Insight into oxidative stress in varicocele-associated male infertility: part 2. Nat Rev Urol. 2012;10:26–37.

17. Sakkas D, Alvarez JG. Sperm DNA fragmentation: mechanisms of origin, impact on reproductive outcome, and analysis. Fertil Steril. 2010;93:1027–36.
18. Aitken RJ, Krausz C. Oxidative stress, DNA damage and the Y chromosome. Reproduction. 2001;122:497–506.
19. Seli E, Gardner DK, Schoolcraft WB, Moffatt O, Sakkas D. Extent of nuclear DNA damage in ejaculated spermatozoa impacts on blastocyst development after in vitro fertilization. Fertil Steril. 2004;82:378–83.
20. Avendaño C, Franchi A, Duran H, Oehninger S. DNA fragmentation of normal spermatozoa negatively impacts embryo quality and intracytoplasmic sperm injection outcome. Fertil Steril. 2010;94:549–57.
21. Robinson L, Gallos ID, Conner SJ, Rajkhowa M, Miller D, Lewis S, Kirkman O, Brown J, Coomarasamy A. The effect of sperm DNA fragmentation on miscarriage rates: a systematic review and meta-analysis. Hum Reprod. 2012;27:2908–17.
22. Zini A, Boman JM, Belzile E, Ciampi A. Sperm DNA damage is associated with an increased risk of pregnancy loss after IVF and ICSI: systematic review and meta-analysis. Hum Reprod. 2008;23:2663–8.
23. Practice Committee of the American Society for Reproductive Medicine. The clinical utility of sperm DNA integrity testing: a guideline. Fertil Steril. 2013;99:673–7.
24. Esteves SC. Clinical relevance of routine semen analysis and controversies surrounding the 2010 World Health Organization criteria for semen examination. Int Braz J Urol. 2014;40:443–53.
25. Esteves SC, Sharma RK, Gosálvez J, Agarwal A. A translational medicine appraisal of specialized andrology testing in unexplained male infertility. Int Urol Nephrol. 2014;46:1037–52.
26. Majzoub A, Esteves SC, Gonsálvez J, Agarwal A. Specialized sperm function tests in varicocele and the future of andrology laboratory. Asian J Androl. 2016;18:205–12.
27. Zini A, Blumenfeld A, Libman J, et al. Beneficial effect of microsurgical subinguinal varicocelectomy on human sperm DNA integrity. Hum Reprod. 2005;20:1018–21.
28. Marmar JL, Agarwal A, Prabaskan S, Agarwal R, Short RA, et al. Reassessing the value of varicocelectomy as a treatment for male subfertility with a new meta-analysis. Fertil Steril. 2007;88:639–48.
29. Kroese AC, de Lange NM, Collins J, Evers JL. Surgery or embolization for varicoceles in subfertile men. Cochrane Database Syst Rev. 2012;10:CD000479.
30. Tiseo BC, Esteves SC, Cocuzza MS. Summary evidence on the effects of varicocele treatment to improve natural fertility in subfertile men. Asian J Androl. 2016;18:239–45.
31. Esteves SC, Roque M, Agarwal A. Outcome of assisted reproductive technology in men with treated and untreated varicocele: systematic review and meta-analysis. Asian J Androl. 2016;18:254–8.
32. Pasqualotto FF, Sundaram A, Sharma RK, Borges E Jr, Pasqualotto EB, Agarwal A. Semen quality and oxidative stress scores in fertile and infertile patients with varicocele. Fertil Steril. 2008;89:602–7.
33. Mostafa T, Anis T, Imam H, El-Nashar AR, Osman IA. Seminal reactive oxygen species—antioxidant relationship in fertile males with and without varicocele. Andrologia. 2009;41:125–9.
34. Zylbersztejn DS, Andreoni C, Del Giudice PT, Spaine DM, Borsari L, Souza GH, Bertolla RP, Fraietta R. Proteomic analysis of seminal plasma in adolescents with and without varicocele. Fertil Steril. 2013;99:92–8.
35. Saleh RA, Agarwal A, Sharma RK, Said TM, Sikka SC, Thomas AJ Jr. Evaluation of nuclear DNA damage in spermatozoa from infertile men with varicocele. Fertil Steril. 2003;80:1431–6.
36. Mehraban D, Ansari M, Keyhan H, Sedighi Gilani M, Naderi G, Esfehani F. Comparison of nitric oxide concentration in seminal fluid between infertile patients with and without varicocele and normal fertile men. Urol J. 2005;2:106–10.
37. Sakamoto Y, Ishikawa T, Kondo Y, Yamaguchi K, Fujisawa M. The assessment of oxidative stress in infertile patients with and without varicocele. BJU Int. 2008;101:1547–52.
38. Köksal IT, Tefekli A, Usta M, Erol H, Abbasoglu S, Kadioglu A. The role of reactive oxygen species in testicular dysfunction associated with varicocele. BJU Int. 2000;86:549–52.

39. Allamaneni SS, Naughton CK, Sharma RK, Thomas AJ Jr, Agarwal A. Increased seminal reactive oxygen species levels in patients with varicoceles correlate with varicocele grade but not with testicular size. Fertil Steril. 2004;82:1684–6.
40. Ishikawa T, Fujioka H, Ishimura T, Takenaka A, Fujisawa M. Increased testicular 8-hydroxy-2′-deoxyguanosine in patients with varicocele. BJU Int. 2007;100:863–6.
41. Abd-Elmoaty MA, Saleh R, Sharma R, Agarwal A. Increased levels of oxidants and reduced antioxidants in semen of infertile men with varicocele. Fertil Steril. 2010;94:1531–4.
42. Mostafa T, Anis TH, El-Nashar A, Imam H, Othman IA. Varicocelectomy reduces reactive oxygen species levels and increases antioxidant activity of seminal plasma from infertile men with varicocele. Int J Androl. 2001;24:261–5.
43. Pasqualotto FF, Sharma RK, Nelson DR, Thomas AJ Jr, Agarwal A. Relationship between oxidative stress, semen characteristics, and clinical diagnosis in men undergoing infertility investigation. Fertil Steril. 2000;73:459–64.
44. Sharma RK, Pasqualotto FF, Nelson DR, Thomas AJ Jr, Agarwal A. The reactive oxygen species-total antioxidant capacity score is a new measure of oxidative stress to predict male infertility. Hum Reprod. 1999;14:2801–7.
45. Hendin BN, Kolettis PN, Sharma RK, Thomas AJ Jr, Agarwal A. Varicocele is associated with elevated spermatozoal reactive oxygen species production and diminished seminal plasma antioxidant capacity. J Urol. 1999;161:1831–4.
46. Esteves SC, Gosálvez J, López-Fernández C, Núñez-Calonge R, Caballero P, Agarwal A, Fernández J. Diagnostic accuracy of sperm DNA degradation index (DDSi) as a potential noninvasive biomarker to identify men with varicocele-associated infertility. Int Urol Nephrol. 2015;47:1471–7.
47. Gat Y, Zukerman Z, Chakraborty J, Gornish M. Varicocele, hypoxia and male infertility. Fluid mechanics analysis of the impaired testicular venous drainage system. Hum Reprod. 2005;20:2614–9.
48. Gat Y, Gornish M, Navon U, Chakraborty J, Bachar GN, Ben-Shlomo I. Right varicocele and hypoxia, crucial factors in male infertility: fluid mechanics analysis in male infertility: fluid mechanics analysis of the impaired testicular drainage system. Reprod BioMed Online. 2006;13:510–5.
49. Ambrosini G, Nath AK, Sierra-Honigmann MR, Flores-Riveros J. Transcriptional activation of the human leptin gene in response to hypoxia. Involvement of hypoxia inducible factor 1. J Biol Chem. 2002;277:34601–9.
50. Nallella KP, Allamaneni SS, Pasqualotto FF, Sharma RK, Thomas AJ Jr, Agarwal A. Relationship of interleukin-6 with semen characteristics and oxidative stress in patients with varicocele. Urology. 2004;64:1010–3.
51. Sahin Z, Celik-Ozenci C, Akkoyunlu G, Korgun ET, Acar N, Erdogru T, Demir R, Ustunel I. Increased expression of interleukin-1α and interleukin-1β is associated with experimental varicocele. Fertil Steril. 2006;85(Suppl 1):1265–75.
52. Ito H, Fuse H, Minagawa H, Kawamura K, Murakami M, Shimazaki J. Internal spermatic vein prostaglandins in varicocele patients. Fertil Steril. 1982;37:218–22.
53. Benoff S, Hurley IR, Barcia M, Mandel FS, Cooper GW, Hershlag A. A potential role for cadmium in the etiology of varicocele-associated infertility. Fertil Steril. 1997;67:336–47.
54. Benoff SH, Millan C, Hurley IR, Napolitano B, Marmar JL. Bilateral increased apoptosis and bilateral accumulation of cadmium in infertile men with left varicocele. Hum Reprod. 2004;19:616–27.
55. Jeng SY, Wu SM, Lee JD. Cadmium accumulation and metallothionein overexpression in internal spermatic vein of patients with varicocele. Urology. 2009;73:1231–5.
56. Wang YJ, Zhang RQ, Lin YJ, Zhang RG, Zhang WL. Relationship between varicocele and sperm DNA damage and the effect of varicocele repair: a meta-analysis. Reprod BioMed Online. 2012;25:307–14.
57. Fernández JL, Muriel L, Goyanes V, Segrelles E, Gosálvez J, Enciso M, LaFromboise M, De Jonge C. Simple determination of human sperm DNA fragmentation with an improved sperm chromatin dispersion (SCD) test. Fertil Steril. 84:833–42.

58. Enciso M, Muriel L, Fernández JL, Goyanes V, Segrelles E, Marcos M, Montejo JM, Ardoy M, Pacheco A, Gosálvez J. Infertile men with varicocele show a high relative proportion of sperm cells with intense nuclear damage level, evidenced by the sperm chromatin dispersion (SCD) test. J Androl. 2006;27:106–11.
59. Gosálvez J, Rodríguez-Predreira M, Mosquera A, López-Fernández C, Esteves SC, Agarwal A. Characterization of a subpopulation with massive nuclear damage, as recognized with the sperm chromatin dispersion (SCD) test. Andrologia. 2014;46:602–9.
60. Feijó CM, Esteves SC. Diagnostic accuracy of sperm chromatin dispersion test to evaluate sperm deoxyribonucleic acid damage in men with unexplained infertility. Fertil Steril. 2014;101:58–63.
61. Agarwal A, Cho CL, Esteves SC. Should we evaluate and treat sperm DNA fragmentation? Curr Opin Obstet Gynecol. 2016;28:164–71.
62. Esteves SC, Oliveira FV, Bertolla RP. Clinical outcome of intracytoplasmic sperm injection in infertile men with treated and untreated clinical varicocele. J Urol. 2010;184:1442–6.
63. Chen SS, Huang WJ, Chang LS, Wei YH. Attenuation of oxidative stress after varicocelectomy in subfertile patients with varicocele. J Urol. 2008;179:639–42.
64. Cervellione RM, Cervato G, Zampieri N, Corroppolo M, Camoglio F, Cestaro B, Ottolenghi A. Effect of varicocelectomy on the plasma oxidative stress parameters. J Pediatr Surg. 2006;41:403–6.
65. Hurtado de Catalfo GE, Ranieri-Casilla A, Marra FA, de Alaniz MJ, Marra CA. Oxidative stress biomarkers and hormonal profile in human patients undergoing varicocelectomy. Int J Androl. 2007;30:519–30.
66. Yesilli C, Mungan G, Seçkiner I, Akduman B, Açikgöz S, Altan K, Mungan A. Effect of varicocelectomy on sperm creatine kinase, HspA2 chaperone protein (creatine kinase-M type), LDH, LDH-X, and lipid peroxidation product levels in infertile men with varicocele. Urology. 2005;66:610–5.
67. Rodriguez Peña M, Alescio L, Russell A, Lourenco da Cunha J, Alzu G, Bardoneschi E. Predictors of improved seminal parameters and fertility after varicocele repair in young adults. Andrologia. 2009;41:277–81.
68. Lacerda JI, Del Giudice PT, da Silva BF, Nichi M, Fariello RM, Fraietta R, Restelli AE, Blumer CG, Bertolla RP, Cedenho AP. Adolescent varicocele: improved sperm function after varicocelectomy. Fertil Steril. 2011;95:994–9.
69. Redmon JB, Carey P, Pryor JL. Varicocele—the most common cause of male factor infertility? Hum Reprod Update. 2002;8:53–8.
70. Kadioglu TC, Aliyev E, Celtik M. Microscopic varicocelectomy significantly decreases the sperm DNA fragmentation index in patients with infertility. Biomed Res Int. 2014;2014:695713.
71. Ni K, Steger K, Yang H, Wang H, Hu K, Chen B. Sperm protramine mRNA ratio and DNA fragmentation index represent reliable clinical biomarkers for men with varicocele after microsurgical varicocele ligation. J Urol. 2014;192:170–6.
72. Smit M, Romijn JC, Wildhagen MF, Veldhoven JLM, Webert RFA, Dohle GR. Decreased sperm DNA fragmentation after surgical varicocelectomy is associated with increased pregnancy rate. J Urol. 2013;189(1 Suppl):S146–50.
73. Werthman P, Wixon R, Kasperson K, Evenson DP. Significant decrease in sperm deoxyribonucleic acid fragmentation after varicocelectomy. Fertil Steril. 2008;90:1800–4.
74. Moskovtsev SI, Lecker I, Mullen JB, Jarvi K, Willis J, White J, Lo KC. Cause-specific treatment in patients with high sperm DNA damage resulted in significant DNA improvement. Syst Biol Reprod Med. 2009;55:109–15.
75. Smit M, Romijn JC, Wildhagen MF, Veldhoven JL, Weber RF, Dohle GR. Decreased sperm DNA fragmentation after surgical varicocelectomy is associated with increased pregnancy rate. J Urol. 2010;183:270–4.
76. Vignera L, Condorelli R, Vicari E, D'Agata R, Calogero AE. Effects of varicocelectomy on sperm DNA fragmentation, mitochondrial function, chromatin condensation, and apoptosis. J Androl. 2012;33:389–96.

77. Li F, Yamaguchi K, Okada K, Matsushita K, Ando M, Chiba K, Yue H, Fujisawa M. Significant improvement of sperm DNA quality after microsurgical repair of varicocele. Syst Biol Reprod Med. 2012;58:274–7.
78. Baker K, McGill J, Sharma R, Agarwal A, Sabanegh E Jr. Pregnancy after varicocelectomy: impact of postoperative motility and DFI. Urology. 2013;81:760–6.
79. García-Peiró A, Ribas-Maynou J, Oliver-Bonet M, Navarro J, Checa MA, Nikolaou A, Amengual MJ, Abad C, Benet J. Multiple determinations of sperm DNA fragmentation show that varicocelectomy is not indicated for infertile patients with subclinical varicocele. Biomed Res Int. 2014;2014:181396.
80. Agarwal A, Majzoub A, Esteves SC, Ko E, Ramasamy R, Zini A. Clinical utility of sperm DNA fragmentation testing: practice recommendations based on clinical scenarios. Transl Androl Urol. 2016;5:935–50.
81. Camargo M, Intasqui P, Bertolla RP. Proteomic profile of seminal plasma in adolescents and adults with treated and untreated varicocele. Asian J Androl. 2016;18:194–201.
82. Agarwal A, Sharma R, Samanta L, Durairajanayagam D, Sabanegh E. Proteomic signatures of infertile men with clinical varicocele and their validation studies reveal mitochondrial dysfunction leading to infertility. Asian J Androl. 2016;18:282–91.
83. Esteves SC, Agarwal A. Afterword to varicocele and male infertility: current concepts and future perspectives. Asian J Androl. 2016;18:319–22.

Chapter 27
Physiological Intracytoplasmic Sperm Insemination Based on Hyaluronic Acid-Binding Ability

Mohammad Hossein Nasr-Esfahani, Shaghayegh Foroozan-Boroojeni, and Marziyeh Tavalaee

27.1 Introduction

Among millions of sperm entering the female reproductive tract naturally, only a few gain the opportunity to meet the oocyte. Therefore, it appears that nature uses firm and decisive barriers to select the most qualified spermatozoa [1]. Despite the presence of numerous physiological barriers, some of these barriers are known, like those present in cervical mucus, but the type and exact mechanisms of most of these barriers remain to be explored. It is assumed that the sperm which reach the oviduct are highly prolific and may have passed most, if not all, the required strict criteria for successful fertilization and development. Yet, one might believe the process of fertilization is a purely random event. This notion, however, remains vetoed by the fact that the overwhelming majority of motile sperm in subfertile men are incapable of fertilization even in vitro and numerous evidence showing a negative correlation between DNA fragmentation and semen parameters [2–4]. Notwithstanding these natural barriers in vivo, assisted reproductive techniques (ARTs), especially intracytoplasmic sperm injection (ICSI), bypass them all, to accomplish fertilization and development [5].

Ejaculated sperm population is highly heterogeneous and may contain apoptotic sperm with high degree of DNA fragmentation along with abnormal DNA packaging [6, 7]. In addition, traditional sperm processing like density gradient centrifuga-

M.H. Nasr-Esfahani (✉)
Department of Reproductive Biotechnology, Reproductive Biomedicine Research Center, Royan Institute for Biotechnology, ACECR, Isfahan, Iran

Isfahan Fertility and Infertility Center, Isfahan, Iran
e-mail: mh.nasr-esfahani@royaninstitute.org

S. Foroozan-Boroojeni • M. Tavalaee
Department of Reproductive Biotechnology, Reproductive Biomedicine Research Center, Royan Institute for Biotechnology, ACECR, Isfahan, Iran
e-mail: shaqayeqforoozan@gmail.com; tavalaee.m@royaninstitute.org

A. Zini, A. Agarwal (eds.), *A Clinician's Guide to Sperm DNA and Chromatin Damage*, https://doi.org/10.1007/978-3-319-71815-6_27

tion (DGC) and swim up, in certain cases, may further aggravate the severity of this phenomenon as result of production of reactive oxygen species due to exposure of sperm to shearing forces during processing and/or also ROS produced by somatic cells present in semen [1]. Indeed in this regard, Avendaño et al. [8] revealed higher percentage of spermatozoa with normal morphology showing DNA damage in infertile and subfertile population compared to fertile individuals [8], and Ramos et al. [9] believe that around 50% of injected sperm during ICSI contain damaged DNA [9], and therefore, one out of every two oocytes is wasted due to improper selection of sperm during ICSI [8]. Considering the negative correlation between sperm DNA fragmentation and semen parameters [2–4], the number of oocyte lost due to insemination of sperm with damaged DNA during ICSI is increased in couples with severe male infertility. These effects are all due to the fact that sperm lack DNA repair mechanisms and cannot repair DNA breaks post-spermiogenesis, and repair of these breaks is carried out by oocyte which highly depends on the severity of DNA damage, age, and quality of inseminated oocyte. Consequently, these situations are further intensified in aged couples [10, 11].

Nowadays, ARTs contribute to over five million births all over the world and the amount is increasing day by day [1]. Despite this momentous achievement, which has had and will have ongoing emotional, social, and economic impacts, some experts believe that there is a price to pay for passing on the subfertility or infertility phenotypes, namely, increased abortion rate, obstetric complication, fetal anomalies, and possible increase in risk of cancer [12, 13]. In addition, these procedures remain sub-efficient and are far from being perfect and effective [1]. Therefore, it is believed that these dearths might be reduced by selecting more fecund sperm in the ejaculate rather than mere selection of sperm based on viability and morphology, and neglecting other important aspect of sperm, such as DNA integrity [14–16]. In regard to this, researchers have used different approaches to imitate the natural barriers [17–19]. Some of these approaches are completely independent of routine sperm processing procedures like swim up and DGC, while other approaches are carried out along with these procedures. In addition, some procedures isolate a subpopulation of sperm with high DNA integrity, while other procedures select "a single physiological sperm" with intact DNA rather than a subpopulation. Therefore, a procedure which can recover an adequate number of sperm with high degree of intact DNA may have the greatest advantage [17]. In this regard, one of the approaches to imitate natural sperm selection is based on the ability of sperm to bind to hyaluronic acid [20, 21]. This procedure selects "a physiological sperm" and is commonly used along with DGC or swim-up procedure.

27.2 Hyaluronic Acid

Hyaluronic acid (HA) belongs to glycosaminoglycans (GAGs) and has a polysaccharide chain of proteoglycans (PGs), a class of molecules that have essential roles as a component of the extracellular matrix (ECM). HA is unique and dissimilar to other GAGs, since this molecule does not bind to core proteins and is non-sulfated [22]. HA is ubiquitous in all of connective tissues and ECM in mammals and is evolutionarily conserved, indicating the functional and structural importance of this molecule [23]. Despite its simple structure, hyaluronan functions in most cell biological mechanisms such as survival, differentiation, proliferation, migration, adhesion, motility, and intracellular signal transduction. HA exists in two forms: high molecular weight (HMW) and low molecular weight (LMW) [22, 24, 25].

27.3 HA Receptors and Their Functional Role in Sperm Physiology

HA receptors such as CD44 and sperm adhesion molecule 1 (SPAM1) also known as PH-20 are expressed on plasma membrane of spermatozoa in many species including humans. Various roles related to sperm maturation, motility, and fertilization have been envisaged for these receptors [26, 27].

CD44 is the most well-known receptor of HA with high specificity for this GAG which is present in all cells. Despite its ubiquitous presence, all cells do not bind to HA [23]. Structurally, CD44 is a transmembrane glycoprotein with an extracellular domain for binding to hyaluronan, a hydrophobic domain, and an intracellular domain which is believed to be involved in initiating several signal transduction pathways. HA binds to CD44 in a multivalent manner occurring mostly in lipid rafts and so leading to stabilization of CD44-containing complexes on the cell surface [28]. Several studies have shown that the dynamic of interaction between CD44 and hyaluronan is regulated by these lipid rafts and many functions are envisioned for interaction of HA-CD44 such as increasing human sperm motility mediated through intracellular Ca2+ concentration, preventing apoptosis, and protecting sperm from immune system [22, 29–31] (Fig. 27.1).

SPAM1 is the most widely conserved mammalian sperm antigen and considered as a functional hyaluronidase present in sperm, so this molecule is a "hyase." Structurally, SPAM1 is a single-chain glycoprotein which has four functional domains (Fig. 27.2):

- Neutral hyase domain (NHD): This domain is in charge of flagellar activity and breakage of HA present in cumulus—oocyte complex ECM.
- HA-binding domain (HABD): SPAM1 is able to bind to HA via this domain and this interaction leads to Ca^{2+} signaling required for acrosome reaction.
- Zona pellucida (ZP) binding domain (ZPBD): Sperm, after passing the cumulus-oocyte complex, is confronted with ZP and to traverse this structure and reach the oocyte, this task is achieved by this domain.
- Acidic hyase domain (AHD): This domain helps sperm to breakdown HA in ZP and perivitelline space and allows it to reach its destination.

SPAM1 is produced and secreted in male and female reproductive tracts and is translocated to spermatozoa to increase their fertilization potential. In humans, to attain successful in vitro fertilization (IVF), certain level of hyases should be present

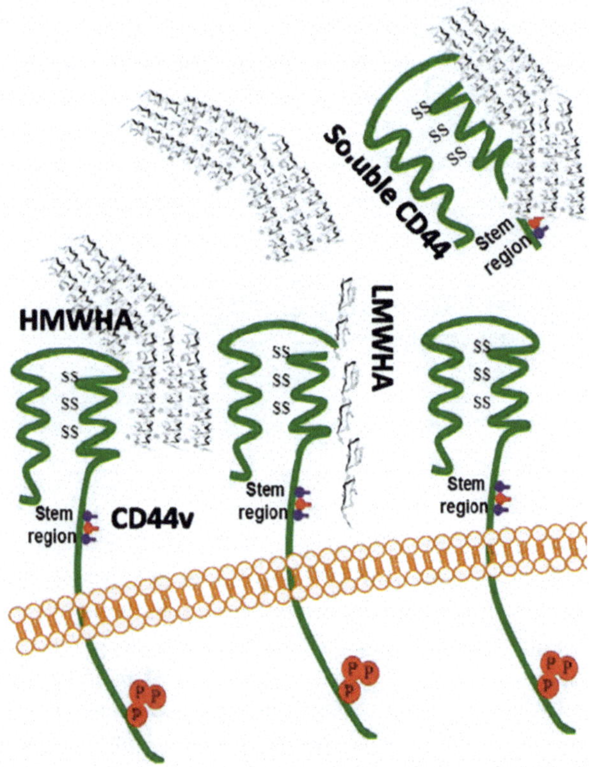

Fig. 27.1 Interaction between CD44 and hyaluronan (Modified figure from Murai [29])

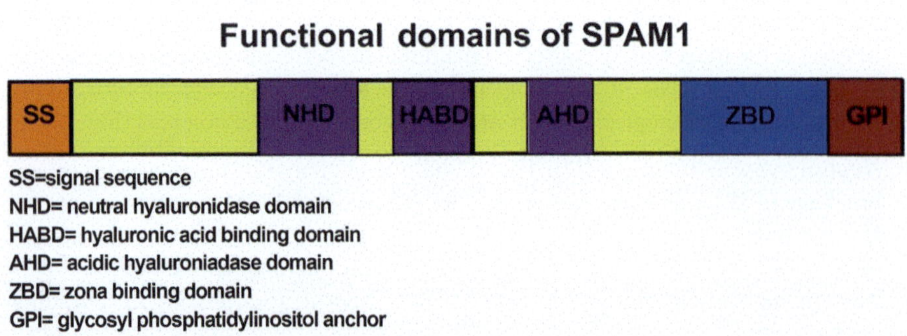

Fig. 27.2 Four functional domains of SPAM

[32–34]. There are also other types of HA receptors (e.g., RHAMM) which have functions in sperm [22, 35]. However, it is not well established which of these receptors play the main role in sperm binding to HA.

27.4 Hyaluronic Acid-Binding Assay and Sperm Selection

At the end of the twentieth century and the beginning of the twenty-first century, Huszar and his colleagues were working on specific sperm maturation markers in fresh ejaculated and cryopreserved-thaw spermatozoa and showed that the presence of HA in the medium could improve human sperm motility and viability [36]. Based on these findings, further studies showed the existence of HA receptors on head region of sperm membrane with intact acrosome [37]. These authors verified that only viable mature sperm have the ability to bind to solid HA [38]. In addition, the proportion of sperm presenting DNA fragmentation and active caspase-3 showed reduced ability to bind to HA compared to unselected sperm. Therefore, mature sperm with intact chromatin can be selected through solid HA for clinical application, especially for ICSI [38, 39]. In one study, these authors categorized individuals according to percentage of sperm bound to HA (≥80%, between 60–80% and ≤60–65%), and they suggested that the first group are fertile and there is no need of intervention, the second group could be treated by intrauterine insemination (IUI), and the third group are candidates for ICSI [38]. The results of another experiment revealed that in vitro sperm selection by using coated dishes with HA for ICSI could improve the outcome of ICSI procedure and reduce chromosomal aneuploidy [40]. After that, many laboratories and researchers tried to evaluate HA-binding assay or used HA-coated dishes to evaluate semen quality [40–49] (Table 27.1). Technically, performing a HA-binding assay in a laboratory is easy and cost-effective. Besides commercially available systems, a "homemade" HA sperm selection dish can be prepared with little effort in any laboratory [21, 41, 43]. Currently, two ready-to-use kits are available for researchers or infertility clinics: (1) a dish with microdots of HA hydrogel attached to the surface of the dish known as PICSI (physiologic ICSI) and (2) a viscous medium containing HA (SpermSlow). In both procedures (see section below), the sperm is prepared via sperm washing or centrifugation [50].

27.5 PICSI or Physiologic ICSI

To perform the PICSI procedure, semen samples are processed by swim up or DGC. Then, hyaluronan microdots are directly covered by processed sperm suspension or covered by suitable sperm diluent, and then processed semen samples are introduced into these droplets at a later stage. Concomitantly with preparation of these droplets, PVP (polyvinylpyrrolidone) or other required droplets for micromanipulation are prepared and the dish is covered with oil. Then, adequate time is provided for

Table 27.1 Comparison and correlation analysis for sperm chromatin maturity [aniline blue (AB) and chromomycin A3 (CMA3)], DNA integrity [acridine orange (AO), terminal deoxynucleotidyl transferase dUTP nick end labeling (TUNEL), and sperm chromatin dispersion (SCD)], apoptosis (caspase-3), and chromosomal aneuploidy [fluorescence in situ hybridization (FISH)] in sperm population selected based on HA-binding ability

Author, year	Analysis approach	HA-binding method	Assessed parameters	
Huszar et al. (2003) [37]	Comparison	Homemade	AB staining	↓
Cayli et al. (2004) [39]	Comparison	PICSI	Immunostaining of caspase-3	↓
Jakab et al. (2005) [40]	Comparison	Homemade	Chromosomal aneuploidy	↓
Nasr-Esfahani et al. (2008) [41]	Correlation	Homemade	CMA3 staining	↓
			SCD	↓
Tarozzi et al. (2009) [42]	Comparison	PICSI	TUNEL	↓
Razavi et al. (2009) [43]	Comparison	Homemade	CMA3 staining	↓
			SCD	–
Parmegiani et al. (2010) [44]	Comparison	SpermSlow	SCD	↓
Yagci et al. (2010) [45]	Comparison	PICSI	AO staining	↓
Vozdova et al. (2012) [46]	Comparison	PICSI	Chromosomal aneuploidy	↓
Mongkolchaipak et al. (2013) [47]	Comparison	PICSI	TUNEL	↓
			Chromosomal aneuploidy	↓
Molnar et al. (2014) [48]	Correlation	PICSI	AB staining	↓
Huang et al. (2015) [49]	Comparison	PICSI	AO staining	↓

↓: A significant difference was observed between control (semen) and HA-selected sperm (comparison) or a significant correlation was observed between % HA-bound sperm with the assessed parameters (correlation)
–: No statistical significant difference was observed

hyaluronan microdots to hydrate and sperm to bind to HA. Afterwards, hyaluronan-bound sperm are identified based on vigorous tail beating but without progressive movement. The selected sperm are collected by the aid of an ICSI needle and introduced to the PVP drop. Among the selected sperm, viable sperm with the best morphology are selected for insemination of oocytes [41, 51].

27.6 SpermSlow

For ICSI using SpermSlow, a small droplet of DGC or swim-up prepared sperm is placed in the vicinity of a larger droplet containing viscous medium (SpermSlow medium). The droplets are connected together with help of a pipette tip. Alongside with preparation of these droplets, other required droplets for micromanipulation

Table 27.2 Sperm selection procedure based on hyaluronic acid-binding ability and ICSI outcomes

Author, year	HA-binding method	Control group	No. of patients in control group / No. of patients in treatment group	% Fertilization	% High quality embryo	% Chemical pregnancy	% Implantation	% Clinical pregnancy	% Ongoing pregnancy	Live birth	Pregnancy loss
Nasr-Esfahani et al. (2008) [41]	Homemade	C-ICSI	50 / 50	↑	–	D.N.A	–	–	D.N.A	D.N.A	D.N.A
Ciray et al. (2008) [52]	PICSI	Unbound sperm	10[a] / 10	–	–	D.N.A	D.N.A	D.N.A	D.N.A	D.N.A	D.N.A
Van den bergh et al. (2009) [53]	SpermSlow	Unbound sperm	44[a] / 44	–	D.N.A	D.N.A	D.N.A	D.N.A	D.N.A	D.N.A	D.N.A
Parmegiani et al. (2010) [54]	SpermSlow	C-ICSI	112 / 94	–	↑	D.N.A	–	–	D.N.A	–	–
Parmegiani et al. (2010) [54]	SpermSlow	C–ICSI	293 / 86	–	↑	D.N.A	↑	–	D.N.A	D.N.A	–
Choe et al. (2012) [55]	SpermSlow	C-ICSI	18[a] / 18	–	–	D.N.A	D.N.A	D.N.A	D.N.A	D.N.A	D.N.A
Majumdar and Majumdar (2013) [56]	PICSI	C-ICSI	71 / 80	–	–	–	–	–	D.N.A	–	–

(continued)

Table 27.2 (continued)

Author, year	HA-binding method	Control group	No. of patients in control group / No. of patients in treatment group	% Fertilization	% High quality embryo	% Chemical pregnancy	% Implantation	% Clinical pregnancy	% Ongoing pregnancy	Live birth	Pregnancy loss
Worrilow et al. (2013) [57]	PICSI	C-ICSI	237 245	–	D.N.A	D.N.A	–	–	D.N.A	D.N.A	↓[b]
Mokanszki et al. (2014) [58]	PICSI	C-ICSI	140 110	↑[b]	D.N.A	D.N.A	↑[b]	↑	D.N.A	↑b	↓

↑: Statistical significant increase, ↓: Statistical significant decrease, , –: No statistical significant change was observed
C-ICSI conventional ICSI, *DNA* data not available
[a]Sibling oocytes
[b]Significant when patients were divided base on hyaluronic acid-binding score

are prepared and the dish is covered with oil. After passage of adequate time, a single viable hyaluronan-bound sperm with normal morphology is collected with aid of a micromanipulation or injection needle from the interface of the two droplets. The selected sperm are used for insemination of oocytes [41, 51].

We carried out a literature search in PubMed and found 13 clinical trials using HA-binding assay as bases for sperm selection procedure [41, 44, 52–58]. A brief summary of these clinical trials is provided below and in Table 27.2.

27.7 Sperm Selection Based on Hyaluronic Acid-Binding and ART

In the literature, the HA trials can be divided into two groups based on control group. Seven out of nine studies used conventional ICSI procedure as a control group and two studies used HA-unbound sperm. It is important to note that in control of the former group, in insemination samples, both bound and unbound sperm were present, while in the control of the latter group, only unbound sperm were used for insemination. As shown in Table 27.2, only one study observed significant increase in fertilization rate using homemade dishes [41]. Two studies by one group observed increase in embryo quality compared to control group [44, 54]. Two out of nine studies observed significant improvement: one for implantation rate [54], while the other for clinical pregnancy rate [58]. The latter also observed a reduction in pregnancy loss [58] (Table 27.2).

To evaluate the heterogeneity observed between the outcomes of these trials, two studies further evaluated the role of HA-binding score on clinical outcomes of ICSI. Worrilow et al. [57] used a cutoff value of 65% HA binding: patients with ≤65% score were divided into control and HA-binding (HAB) selection groups and those with >65% were divided to non-participatory (NP), control, or HAB groups. Although they did not observe any significant differences in clinical outcomes overall, when they divided their participants according to HA-binding score, they observed a significant decrease in pregnancy loss in patients with ≤65% score in favor of HAB group [57]. In addition, Mokanszki et al. [58] categorized patients into two groups according to hyaluronan binding score >50% and ≤50% and observed significant increase in fertilization, implantation, and clinical pregnancy rates and a significant decrease in pregnancy loss in group with HBA score <50% compared to control group with less than <50% HBA, which did not use the PICSI procedure [58]. These two latter studies suggest that sperm selection based on HA-binding ability should be implemented for couples with severe male infertility with low binding score. In other words, implementation of HA-binding assay for couples with high HBA score has no beneficial effects, since the person performing the ICSI procedure is also selecting a viable sperm with best morphology, which is very likely to have a high HA-binding potential. Therefore, this procedure has beneficial effects in the group of patients with low binding ability, and selection based on viability and morphology alone cannot select sperm with high HA-binding ability, specially in severe male factor infertility.

In contrast, Huang et al. [49] compared the percentage of intact DNA between population of microscopic sperm selection and HA-binding selection and reported a lack of statistical difference between these two sperm selection methods based on acridine orange staining. Moreover they stated "A well-trained embryologist will have the same ability to choose sperm with intact DNA by conventional microscopic selection as with HA-binding sperm selection." However, they did not conduct a clinical evaluation of the two procedures to see whether the two methods would affect ICSI clinical outcomes [49]. Parmegiani et al. [51] also compared two commercial systems, PICSI and SpermSlow, and concluded no significant difference between these two procedures for clinical purposes [51].

Assisted reproductive procedure used in all of the aforementioned studies was ICSI. Searching PubMed database revealed other studies that investigated the usage of HA-binding assay for other techniques. Ye et al. [59] showed that HA-binding assay has a significant correlation with fertilization rate when IVF was performed [59]. In contrast, Tarozzi et al. [42] found no significant correlation between HA-binding ability and clinical outcomes of IVF [42]. In another study by Kovacs et al. [60], they tried to predict fertilization potential of semen sample in couples with unexplained infertility undergoing IVF treatment via HA-binding assay, but they concluded that this procedure did not foretell spontaneous fertilization potential in these couples. Therefore, they suggested that HA-binding screening does not help with the selection of an artificial reproductive technique [60]. Furthermore, Yildirim et al. [61] tried to assess prognostic ability of HBA in IUI. They observed that "HBA does not predict IUI outcome in couples with unexplained infertility or mild male factor infertility, but it can be used together with semen parameters to verify sperm quality" [61].

HA binds to its receptors on the surface of sperm. These receptors are lost during the process of capacitation [62]. Considering the fact that sperm processing media contain albumin, it is very likely that capacitation is initiated or may be completed [63] by the time that HA-binding assay is implemented. Therefore, good sperm which have the ability to undergo capacitation may have lost their ability to bind to HA, and they might become part of unbound sperm population. Whether such a discrepancy may account for variations reported between studies remains to be explored. Indeed, Parmegiani et al. [51] suggested that the ability of sperm to bind to HA decreases after a certain period of time and binding ability is regulated by sperm hyaluronidase activity, the PH-20. They believe that hyaluronidase activity reduces HA binding since it digests the HA and allows sperm to detach themselves from the binding site and restore their motility, until they find the chance to bind to new HA in another area [51]. However, to our knowledge, we have seen no study which has focused on this concept, i.e., loss of HA activity as sperm become capacitated.

In conclusion, based on the clinical studies reported thus far, sperm selection by HA binding may improve the ICSI outcomes of couples with low HA-binding capacity. The rate of pregnancy loss may also be decreased. However, to make solid conclusions, further multicenter clinical trials are needed, so that further meta-analysis can be carried out. Nevertheless, in these studies, factors such as time after processing should be also considered as a variable factor. It is important to note that a meta-analysis already exists in this field. In the meta-analysis by Beck-Fruchter et al. [14], seven studies with 1437 cycles were included. They concluded that the use of the hyaluronic acid-binding sperm selection technique yielded no improvement in fertilization and pregnancy rates." A meta-analysis of all available studies showed an improvement in embryo quality and implantation rate; an analysis of prospective studies only showed an improvement in embryo quality. Evidence does not support routine use of hyaluronic acid-binding assays in all ICSI cycles. Identification of patients that might benefit from this technique needs further study" [14].

27.8 Comparison of Sperm Selection Based on Hyaluronic Acid-Binding with Other Novel Sperm Selection Procedures

ICSI has gained tremendous popularity in ARTs and accounts for a considerable number of birth per annum, especially in developed countries due to late marriage and increase rate of male infertility. Therefore, selection of the "best sperm" through novel sperm selection procedures is opening its way to ART laboratories [17, 19]. Selection of the best procedure can be achieved through comparison of these techniques. There is only one study so far comparing HA binding with Zeta sperm selection procedure based on surface electrical charge and showed that Zeta procedure has a higher ability to select sperm with intact chromatin using sperm chromatin dispersion assay and chromomycin A3 (CMA3) staining for assessing DNA integrity and protamine deficiency, respectively. These authors stated that in Zeta procedure, sperm are selected based on their surface electric charge (Zeta potential) and only one of sialylated glycoproteins involved in production of the electric is PH-20 or CD44, the receptor for HA. However, it is important to note that in this study, homemade dishes were used, and to solidify such a conclusion, further studies are required to compare with PICSI dishes [43].

27.9 HA Sperm Selection and Patient Management

Today, HA sperm selection procedure is advised for couples with low HA-binding score. Considering the fact that beyond the semen analysis, sperm chromatin integrity tests (especially those directly assessing DNA fragmentation) are gaining their place in infertility management, carrying out HA-ICSI selection based on DNA fragmentation may have important role in patient management. In addition, variations observed between studies might be related to the time and medium used to carry out HA sperm selection, since both duration and exposure to medium containing different serum concentration increase the chance of capacitation and increase loss of PH-20 involved in HA binding. Therefore, future studies should take these points into consideration for research to conclude on the efficiency of this procedure in ART management.

27.10 Conclusion

HA sperm selection has been inspired from innate physiological processes and selected sperm through this procedure have higher quality in terms of chromatin integrity, chromosomal euploidy, maturity, and morphology. However, the data derived from randomized clinical studies suggest that not all couples undergoing ICSI will gain from this procedure. To date, it appears that couples with severe male infertility with low HA-binding score may benefit from it in that they will experience lower rates of early pregnancy loss.

References

1. Rappa KL, Rodriguez HF, Hakkarainen GC, Anchan RM, Mutter GL, Asghar W. Sperm processing for advanced reproductive technologies: where are we today? Biotechnol Adv. 2016;34(5):578–87. https://doi.org/10.1016/j.biotechadv.2016.01.007. Epub 2016 Feb 1.2
2. Tavalaee M, Kiani-Esfahani A, Nasr-Esfahani MH. Relationship between phospholipase C-zeta, semen parameters, and chromatin status. Syst Biol Reprod Med. 2017;63:259–68.
3. Boushaba S, Belaaloui G. Sperm DNA fragmentation and standard semen parameters in algerian infertile male partners. World J Mens Health. 2015;33(1):1–7. https://doi.org/10.5534/wjmh.2015.33.1.1. Epub 2015 Apr 23
4. Evgeni E, Charalabopoulos K, Asimakopoulos B. Human sperm DNA fragmentation and its correlation with conventional semen parameters. J Reprod Infertil. 2014;15(1):2–14.
5. Sakkas D, Ramalingam M, Garrido N, Barratt CL. Sperm selection in natural conception: what can we learn from mother nature to improve assisted reproduction outcomes? Hum Reprod Update. 2015;21(6):711–26. https://doi.org/10.1093/humupd/dmv042. Review
6. Aitken RJ, Smith TB, Jobling MS, Baker MA, De Iuliis GN. Oxidative stress and male reproductive health. Asian J Androl. 2014;16(1):31–8. https://doi.org/10.4103/1008–682X.122203. Review
7. Aitken RJ, Baker MA. Causes and consequences of apoptosis in spermatozoa; contributions to infertility and impacts on development. Int J Dev Biol. 2013;57(2–4):265–72. https://doi.org/10.1387/ijdb.130146ja. Review
8. Avendaño C, Franchi A, Taylor S, Morshedi M, Bocca S, Oehninger S. Fragmentation of DNA in morphologically normal human spermatozoa. Fertil Steril. 2009;91(4):1077–84. https://doi.org/10.1016/j.fertnstert.2008.01.015.
9. Ramos L, De Boer P, Meuleman EJ, Braat DD, Wetzels AM. Evaluation of ICSI-selected epididymal sperm samples of obstructive azoospermic males by the CKIA system. J Androl. 2004;25(3):406–11.
10. Gunes S, Al-Sadaan M, Agarwal A. Spermatogenesis, DNA damage and DNA repair mechanisms in male infertility. Reprod Biomed Online. 2015;31(3):309–19. https://doi.org/10.1016/j.rbm0.2015.06.010. Epub 2015 Jun 19
11. González-Marín C, Gosálvez J, Roy R. Types, causes, detection and repair of DNA fragmentation in animal and human sperm cells. Int J Mol Sci. 2012;13(11):14026–52. https://doi.org/10.3390/ijms131114026.
12. Hansen M, Kurinczuk JJ, Milne E, de Klerk N, Bower C. Assisted reproductive technology and birth defects: a systematic review and meta-analysis. Hum Reprod Update. 2013;19(4):330–53. https://doi.org/10.1093/humupd/dmt006. Review
13. Rimm AA, Katayama AC, Diaz M, Katayama KP. A meta-analysis of controlled studies comparing major malformation rates in IVF and ICSI infants with naturally conceived children. J Assist Reprod Genet. 2004;21(12):437–43.

14. Beck-Fruchter R, Shalev E, Weiss A. Clinical benefit using sperm hyaluronic acid binding technique in ICSI cycles: a systematic review and meta-analysis. Reprod Biomed Online. 2016;32(3):286–98. https://doi.org/10.1016/j.rbm0.2015.12.001. Review
15. Lewis SE, Kumar K. The paternal genome and the health of the assisted reproductive technology child. Asian J Androl. 2015;17(4):616–22. https://doi.org/10.4103/1008–682X.153301. Review
16. de Wagenaar B, Berendsen JT, Bomer JG, Olthuis W, van den Berg A, Segerink LI. Microfluidic single sperm entrapment and analysis. Lab Chip. 2015;15(5):1294–301. https://doi.org/10.1039/c41c01425a.
17. Nasr-Esfahani MH, Deemeh MR, Tavalaee M. New era in sperm selection for ICSI. Int J Androl. 2012;35(4):475–84. https://doi.org/10.1111/j.1365–2605.2011.01227.x. Review
18. Bassiri F, Tavalaee M, Shiravi AH, Mansouri S, Nasr-Esfahani MH. Is there an association between HOST grades and sperm quality? Hum Reprod. 2012;27(8):2277–84. https://doi.org/10.1093/humrep/des155.
19. Said TM, Land JA. Effects of advanced selection methods on sperm quality and ART outcome: a systematic review. Hum Reprod Update. 2011;17(6):719–33. https://doi.org/10.1093/humupd/dmr032. Review
20. Oehninger S, Franken DR, Ombelet W. Sperm functional tests. Fertil Steril. 2014;102(6):1528–33. https://doi.org/10.1016/j.fertnstert.2014.09.044. Review
21. Nasr-Esfahani MH, Marziyeh T. Sperm selection for ICSI using the hyaluronic acid binding assay. Methods Mol Biol. 2013;927:263–8.
22. Karousou E, D'Angelo ML, Kouvidi K, Vigetti D, Viola M, Nikitovic D, De Luca G, Passi A. Collagen VI and hyaluronan: the common role in breast cancer. Biomed Res Int. 2014;2014:606458. https://doi.org/10.1155/2014/606458. Review
23. Rodriguez-Martinez H, Tienthai P, Atikuzzaman M, Vicente-Carrillo A, Rubér M, Alvarez-Rodriguez M. The ubiquitous hyaluronan: functionally implicated in the oviduct? Theriogenology. 2016;86(1):182–6. https://doi.org/10.1016/j.theriogenology.2015.11.025. Review
24. Zhao G, Yan G, Cheng J, Zhou X, Fang T, Sun H, Hou Y, Hu Y. Hyaluronic acid prevents immunosuppressive drug-induced ovarian damage via up-regulating PGRMC1 expression. Sci Rep. 2015;5:7647. https://doi.org/10.1038/srep07647.
25. Darzynkiewicz Z, Balazs EA. Genome integrity, stem cells and hyaluronan. Aging (Albany NY). 2012;4(2):78–88. Review
26. Bains R, Adeghe J, Carson RJ. Human sperm cells express CD44. Fertil Steril. 2002;78(2):307–12.
27. Hardy CM, Clydesdale G, Mobbs KJ, Pekin J, Lloyd ML, Sweet C, Shellam GR, Lawson MA. Assessment of contraceptive vaccines based on recombinant mouse sperm protein PH20. Reproduction. 2004;127(3):325–34.
28. Grass GD, Dai L, Qin Z, Parsons C, Toole BP. CD147: regulator of hyaluronan signaling I invasiveness and chemoresistance. Adv Cancer Res. 2014;123:351–73. https://doi.org/10.1016/B978–0-12–800092–2.00013–7. Review
29. Murai T. Lipid raft-mediated regulation of Hyaluronan-CD44 interactions in inflammation and cancer. Front Immunol. 2015;6:420. https://doi.org/10.3389/fimmu.2015.00420. Review
30. Peach RJ, Hollenbaugh D, Stamenkovic I, Aruffo A. Identification of hyaluronic acid binding sites in the extracellular domain of CD44. J Cell Biol. 1993;122(1):257–64.
31. Misra S, Hascall VC, Markwald RR, Ghatak S. Interactions between Hyaluronan and its receptors (CD44, RHAMM) regulate the activities of inflammation and cancer. Front Immunol. 2015;6:201. https://doi.org/10.3389/fimmu.2015.00201. Review
32. Gmachl M, Sagan S, Ketter S, Kreil G. The human sperm protein PH-20 has hyaluronidase activity. FEBS Lett. 1993;336(3):545–8.
33. Martin-Deleon PA. Germ-cell hyaluronidases: their roles in sperm function. Int J Androl. 2011;34(5 Pt 2):e306–18. https://doi.org/10.1111/j.1365–2605.2010.01138.x. Review
34. Modelski MJ, Menlah G, Wang Y, Dash S, Wu K, Galileo DS, Martin-DeLeon PA. Hyaluronidase 2: a novel germ cell hyaluronidase with epididymal expression and functional roles in mammalian sperm. Biol Reprod. 2014;91(5):109. https://doi.org/10.1095/biolreprod.113.115857.

35. Kornovski BS, McCoshen J, Kredentser J, Turley E. The regulation of sperm motility by a novel hyaluronan receptor. Fertil Steril. 1994;61(5):935–40.
36. Cayli S, Jakab A, Ovari L, Delpiano E, Celik-Ozenci C, Sakkas D, Ward D, Huszar G. Biochemical markers of sperm function: male fertility and sperm selection for ICSI. Reprod Biomed Online. 2003;7(4):462–8. Review
37. Huszar G, Ozenci CC, Cayli S, Zavaczki Z, Hansch E, Vigue L. Hyaluronic acid binding by human sperm indicates cellular maturity, viability, and unreacted acrosomal status. Fertil Steril. 2003;79(Suppl 3):1616–24.
38. Huszar G, Jakab A, Sakkas D, Ozenci CC, Cayli S, Delpiano E, Ozkavukcu S. Fertility testing and ICSI sperm selection by hyaluronic acid binding: clinical and genetic aspects. Reprod Biomed Online. 2007;14(5):650–63. Review
39. Cayli S, Sakkas D, Vigue L, Demir R, Huszar G. Cellular maturity and apoptosis in human sperm: creatine kinase, caspase-3 and Bcl-XL levels in mature and diminished maturity sperm. Mol Hum Reprod. 2004;10(5):365–72.
40. Jakab A, Sakkas D, Delpiano E, Cayli S, Kovanci E, Ward D, Revelli A, Huszar G. Intracytoplasmic sperm injection: a novel selection method for sperm with normal frequency of chromosomal aneuploidies. Fertil Steril. 2005;84(6):1665–73. Erratum in: Fertil Steril. 2006 Aug;86(2):498
41. Nasr-Esfahani MH, Razavi S, Vahdati AA, Fathi F, Tavalaee M. Evaluation of sperm selection procedure based on hyaluronic acid binding ability on ICSI outcome. J Assist Reprod Genet. 2008;25(5):197–203. https://doi.org/10.1007/s10815–008–9223–4.
42. Tarozzi N, Nadalini M, Bizzaro D, Serrao L, Fava L, Scaravelli G, Borini A. Sperm-hyaluronan-binding assay: clinical value in conventional IVF under Italian law. Reprod Biomed Online. 2009;19(Suppl 3):35–43.
43. Razavi SH, Nasr-Esfahani MH, Deemeh MR, Shayesteh M, Tavalaee M. Evaluation of zeta and HA-binding methods for selection of spermatozoa with normal morphology, protamine content and DNA integrity. Andrologia. 2010;42(1):13–9. https://doi.org/10.1111/j.1439–0272.2009.00948.x.
44. Parmegiani L, Cognigni GE, Bernardi S, Troilo E, Ciampaglia W, Filicori M. "Physiologic ICSI": hyaluronic acid (HA) favors selection of spermatozoa without DNA fragmentation and with normal nucleus, resulting in improvement of embryo quality. Fertil Steril. 2010;93(2):598–604. https://doi.org/10.1016/j.fertnstert.2009.03.033.
45. Yagci A, Murk W, Stronk J, Huszar G. Spermatozoa bound to solid state hyaluronic acid show chromatin structure with high DNA chain integrity: an acridine orange fluorescence study. J Androl. 2010;31(6):566–72. https://doi.org/10.2164/jandr01.109.008912.
46. Vozdova M, Kasikova K, Oracova E, Prinosilova P, Rybar R, Horinova V, Gaillyova R, Rubes J. The effect of the swim-up and hyaluronan-binding methods on the frequency of abnormal spermatozoa detected by FISH and SCSA in carriers of balanced chromosomal translocations. Hum Reprod. 2012;27(3):930–7. https://doi.org/10.1093/humrep/der445.
47. Mongkolchaipak S, Vutyavanich T. No difference in high-magnification morphology and hyaluronic acid binding in the selection of euploid spermatozoa with intact DNA. Asian J Androl. 2013;15(3):421–4. https://doi.org/10.1038/aja.2012.163.
48. Molnar Z, Mokanszki A, Kassai Bazsane Z, Bhattoa HP, Benyo M, Olah E, Jakab A. Sperm concentration, hyaluronic acid-binding capacity, aneuploidy and persistent histones in testicular cancer. Hum Reprod. 2014;29(9):1866–74. https://doi.org/10.1093/humrep/deu179.
49. Huang MT, Kuo-Kuang Lee R, Lu CH, Chen YJ, Li SH, Hwu YM. The efficiency of conventional microscopic selection is comparable to the hyaluronic acid binding method in selecting spermatozoa for male infertility patients. Taiwan J Obstet Gynecol. 2015;54(1):48–53. https://doi.org/10.1016/j.tjog.2014.11.006.
50. Ebner T, Filicori M, Tews G, Parmegiani L. A plea for a more physiological ICSI. Andrologia. 2012;44(Suppl 1):2–19. https://doi.org/10.1111/j.1439–0272.2011.01266.x. Review
51. Parmegiani L, Cognigni GE, Bernardi S, Troilo E, Taraborrelli S, Arnone A, Maccarini AM, Filicori M. Comparison of two ready-to-use systems designed for sperm-hyaluronic acid binding selection before intracytoplasmic sperm injection: PICSI vs. sperm slow: a prospective, randomized trial. Fertil Steril. 2012;98(3):632–7. https://doi.org/10.1016/j.fertnstert.2012.05.043.

52. Ciray HN, Coban O, Bayram A, Kizilkanat A, Bahçeci M. Preliminary study of embryo development following assessment of male and female gametes. Reprod Biomed Online. 2008;16(6):875–80.
53. Van Den Bergh MJ, Fahy-Deshe M, Hohl MK. Pronuclear zygote score following intracytoplasmic injection of hyaluronan-bound spermatozoa: a prospective randomized study. Reprod Biomed Online. 2009;19(6):796–801.
54. Parmegiani L, Cognigni GE, Ciampaglia W, Pocognoli P, Marchi F, Filicori M. Efficiency of hyaluronic acid (HA) sperm selection. J Assist Reprod Genet. 2010;27(1):13–6. https://doi.org/10.1007/s10815-009-9380-0.
55. Choe SA, Tae JC, Shin MY, Kim HJ, Kim CH, Lee JY, Hwang D, Kim KC, Suh CS, Jee BC. Application of sperm selection using hyaluronic acid binding in intracytoplasmic sperm injection cycles: a sibling oocyte study. J Korean Med Sci. 2012;27(12):1569–73. https://doi.org/10.3346/jkms.2012.27.12.1569.
56. Majumdar G, Majumdar A. A prospective randomized study to evaluate the effect of hyaluronic acid sperm selection on the intracytoplasmic sperm injection outcome of patients with unexplained infertility having normal semen parameters. J Assist Reprod Genet. 2013;30(11):1471–5. https://doi.org/10.1007/s10815-013-0108-9.
57. Worrilow KC, Eid S, Woodhouse D, Perloe M, Smith S, Witmyer J, Ivani K, Khoury C, Ball GD, Elliot T, Lieberman J. Use of hyaluronan in the selection of sperm for intracytoplasmic sperm injection (ICSI): significant improvement in clinical outcomes—multicenter, double-blinded and randomized controlled trial. Hum Reprod. 2013;28(2):306–14. https://doi.org/10.1093/humrep/des417.
58. Mokánszki A, Tóthné EV, Bodnár B, Tándor Z, Molnár Z, Jakab A, Ujfalusi A, Oláh É. Is sperm hyaluronic acid binding ability predictive for clinical success of intracytoplasmic sperm injection: PICSI vs. ICSI? Syst Biol Reprod Med. 2014;60(6):348–54. https://doi.org/10.3109/19396368.2014.948102.
59. Ye H, Huang GN, Gao Y, Liu DY. Relationship between human sperm-hyaluronan binding assay and fertilization rate in conventional in vitro fertilization. Hum Reprod. 2006;21(6):1545–50.
60. Kovacs P, Kovats T, Sajgo A, Szollosi J, Matyas S, Kaali SG. The role of hyaluronic acid binding assay in choosing the fertilization method for patients undergoing IVF for unexplained infertility. J Assist Reprod Genet. 2011;28(1):49–54. https://doi.org/10.1007/s10815-010-9479-3.
61. Yildirim M, Duvan CI, Pekel A, Ayrim A, Kafali H. Can hyaluronan binding assay predict the outcome of intrauterine insemination in couples with unexplained or mild male factor infertility? J Reprod Infertil. 2015;16(1):18–23.
62. Redgrove KA, Nixon B, Baker MA, Hetherington L, Baker G, Liu DY, Aitken RJ. The molecular chaperone HSPA2 plays a key role in regulating the expression of sperm surface receptors that mediate sperm-egg recognition. PLoS One. 2012;7(11):e50851. https://doi.org/10.1371/journal.pone.0050851.
63. De Jonge C. Biological basis for human capacitation. Hum Reprod Update. 2005;11(3):205–14. Review

Chapter 28
Advanced Sperm Processing/Selection Techniques

Ashok Agarwal and Manesh Kumar Panner Selvam

28.1 Introduction

A total of five million births all over the world and around 2–4% of births in developed countries are the result of ART [1, 2]. Half of the DNA contributed to the offspring is by the sperm. Numerous techniques were developed to isolate superior-quality spermatozoa with intact chromatin condensation and without chromosomal abnormalities for use in ART. Currently available conventional techniques such as density gradient centrifugation (DGC), the swim-up and the glass wool filtration techniques select sperm based on their motility and morphology. However, the important factors that affect the fertility such as oxidative stress and DNA integrity cannot be assessed by any of these conventional techniques [3, 4].

In many laboratories, DNA integrity-based testing is done prior to the use in ART. This allows to select spermatozoa with high DNA integrity to achieve high fertilization rates, whereas the use of sperm with poor DNA integrity in the ART procedure is associated with decreased implantation and pregnancy rates [5–7]. In a prospective study, our group has also demonstrated that increased DNA damage to spermatozoa is associated with poor ART outcome [8]. Similarly, another meta-analysis reported that reduced fertilization rates by natural conception are associated with poor DNA integrity of spermatozoa [9].

An increase in the incidence of infertility coupled with progress in the field of biotechnology has led researchers to develop advanced techniques beyond the conventional selection methods in order to reduce the oxidative and physiological damage caused by the sperm selection process. Hence, several advanced sperm selection techniques were introduced to select spermatozoa with high DNA integrity to increase the success rate of ART.

A. Agarwal (✉) • M.K. Panner Selvam
American Center for Reproductive Medicine, Glickman Urological and Kidney Institute, Cleveland Clinic, Cleveland, OH, USA
e-mail: agarwaa@ccf.org; manesh.balu@gmail.com

A. Zini, A. Agarwal (eds.), *A Clinician's Guide to Sperm DNA and Chromatin Damage*, https://doi.org/10.1007/978-3-319-71815-6_28

28.2 Selection Based on Net Electric Charge

28.2.1 Electrophoresis

Morphologically normal and mature spermatozoa have a high concentration of sialic acid residues in the sperm membrane and therefore possess a higher negative charge compared to immature and abnormal spermatozoa. Based on the size and surface charge differences, electrophoresis is used to separate functionally active normal spermatozoa from immature, abnormal sperm and leukocytes present in the semen sample.

28.2.1.1 Microflow Cell

The microflow cell consists of outer and inner chambers. Outer chambers are connected with platinum-coated titanium electrodes, and the inner chamber is divided into two compartments, the inoculation chamber to load 400 μL of semen and the collection compartment filled with buffer to collect the separated spermatozoa. A polycarbonate membrane (5 μm) present between the two chambers filters out the sperm from the leukocytes and epithelial germ cells present in the semen (Fig. 28.1). Briefly, the sample and the buffer are equilibrated in loading and collecting compartments, respectively, for 5 min before electrophoresis at 23 °C with a constant current of 75 mA and variable voltage of 18–21 mV [10]. The sorted spermatozoa are recovered from the collection chamber and can be used for ART.

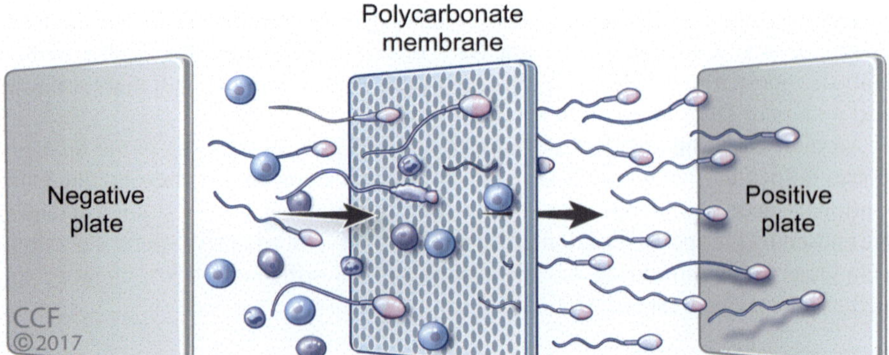

Fig. 28.1 Microflow cell separation of spermatozoa from leukocytes using polycarbonate separation membranes and sorting based on the movement in the applied electric field (Reprinted with permission, Cleveland Clinic Center for Medical Art & Photography ©2011–2017. All Rights Reserved)

28.2.1.2 Microelectrophoresis

Similarly, a microelectrophoresis technique to isolate the negatively charged spermatozoa (NCS) from neat semen sample as well as from the double density gradient-prepared sperm was developed by Simon et al. [11]. The sterile microelectrophoresis unit consists of electrophoresis, egg inoculation, and bubble restriction chambers. Basically, microelectrophoresis of sperm is carried out under the ICSI stage. 10–15 μL of semen are electrophoresed in the buffer with increasing current (6–14 mA) and variable voltage (30–100 V). During electrophoresis, the sperm are monitored with an inverted microscope under 200X magnification, and based on the movement of the sperm under the influence of electric current, sperm are picked up using the ICSI pipette [11].

ART Outcome

The microflow cell was able to separate the viable and morphologically normal motile sperm with high DNA integrity from the semen samples of infertile men [10]. Similarly, NCS isolated using microelectrophoresis had significantly lower DNA fragmentation [11]. Sperm sorted by electrophoresis were also free of oxidative DNA damage and exhibited normal zona pellucida binding [12, 13]. Ainsworth et al. effectively used the sperm selected with high DNA integrity, to establish pregnancy from the semen sample with high DNA fragmentation by ICSI [14]. This method can be a handy and convenient tool for the isolation of spermatozoa for ART.

28.2.2 Zeta Potential

Mature spermatozoa possess a negative electric surface charge ranging from −16 mV to −20 mV across the plasma membrane [15]. This negative electric charge is known as zeta potential or electrokinetic potential which is used for sorting the high-quality spermatozoa from the low-graded sperm using positively charged centrifuge tube.

In this technique, 100 μL of the washed sperm are suspended in 5 mL of serum-free HEPES-HTF medium. After rapidly pulling the tube after rotating it two to three times in a latex glove, the negatively charged mature sperm stick to the walls of the positively charged (2–4 mV) plastic centrifuge tube (Fig. 28.2). After keeping the tube still at room temperature for 1 min, it is centrifuged at 300 × g for 5 min, and the fluid is subsequently discarded. Finally, sperm holding negative zeta potential attached to the walls are recovered in the 0.2 mL of serum-supplemented HEPES-HTF medium, which neutralizes the charge on the test-tube wall [16].

ART Outcome

Sperm samples processed by means of the zeta potential technique contained highly motile, hyperactive, mature spermatozoa with normal morphology and intact DNA [17]. Protamine-deficient spermatozoa were eliminated by this technique, and high-quality sperm with less DNA fragmentation are retained [18]. Negative zeta potential sperm in IVF had a higher fertilization rate (65.79%) compared with sperm isolated with double density gradient centrifugation.

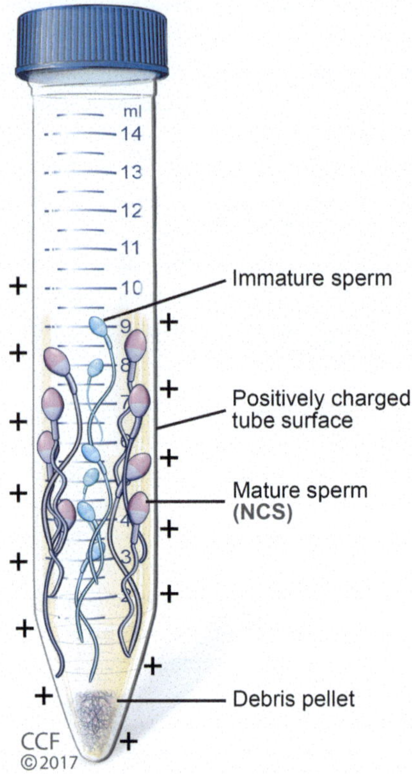

Fig. 28.2 Selection of spermatozoa using zeta potential principle. The negatively charged mature sperm sticks to the walls of the positively charged centrifuge tube, while non-mature sperm in the suspension are discarded (Reprinted with permission, Cleveland Clinic Center for Medical Art & Photography ©2011–2017. All Rights Reserved)

28.3 Annexin V Affinity-Based Separation

In normal healthy spermatozoa, phospholipids and phosphatidylserine (PS) present on the plasma membrane are directed toward the protoplasm of viable spermatozoa. However, when a cell undergoes apoptosis, PS translocates from the inner leaflet of the plasma membrane to the outer leaflet and is then exposed on the outer surface of the sperm plasma membrane [19]. Annexin V, a 35 kDa protein, has high affinity to bind to PS and can thus serve as biomarker for apoptotic cells.

28.3.1 Magnetic-Activated Cell Sorting (MACS)

In this method, apoptotic sperm cells are separated from normal matured cells with high DNA integrity. Micromagnetic beads (0.5 μm) coated with annexin V are incubated with liquefied semen. 100 μL of sperm sample are mixed with 100 μL of homogenized magnetic microbeads and incubated at room temperature for 15 min. Then, the suspension is passed through a specially designed MACS column placed in the activated magnetic field on either side of the column (Fig. 28.3a, b). Apoptotic spermatozoa bind to the magnetic beads and are retained in the column by the external magnetic field (Fig. 28.3c). When rinsing the column with buffer, the unbound healthy sperm cells flow through the selection column, and a fraction of spermatozoa with normal morphology and minimum DNA damage is collected.

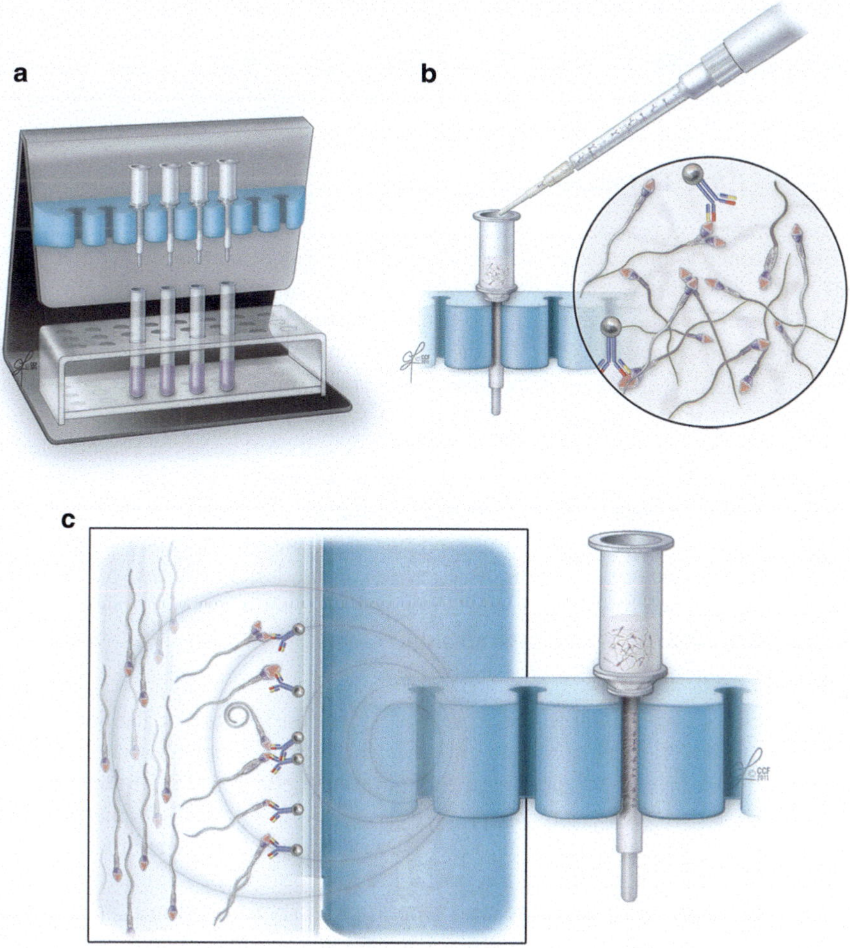

Fig. 28.3 (**a**) Magnetic-activated cell sorting and collection device. The MACS columns are placed on the stand surrounded by magnetic field. (**b**) Loading the MACS columns with liquefied semen (apoptotic and non-apoptotic sperm) labeled with annexin V-coated micromagnetic beads. (**c**) Activated magnetic field retains the apoptotic sperm bound to micromagnetic beads coated with annexin V in the column and allows the non-apoptotic healthy sperm cells to flow through the selection column (Reprinted with permission, Cleveland Clinic Center for Medical Art & Photography ©2011–2017. All Rights Reserved)

28.3.2 Annexin V-Based Glass Wool Filtration

By modifying the conventional glass wool filtration technique, Paasch et al. introduced this technique to sort out non-apoptotic spermatozoa. Here, the solid phase containing glass wool fibers is linked with annexin V molecules. When the sample is passed through the column, apoptotic spermatozoa bind to the solid phase and are thus filtered out, separating them from healthy sperm passing through the filtration system [20]. This is a promising technique which can select the spermatozoa of high motility and normal mitochondrial potential with superior fertilizing ability.

28.3.3 Flow Cytometry

Flow cytometry analyzes cells based on their physical and fluorescence properties. Flow cytometry sorters were initially used for sex sorting of spermatozoa and also employed to identify DNA fragmentation in spermatozoa using fluorescent apoptotic markers [21]. Later, this technique was also used to separate DNA-damaged (annexin V-positive) sperm from non-apoptotic (annexin V-negative) spermatozoa. 10 × 106 sperm were washed and suspended in the 195 μL of binding buffer. To this, 5 μL of FITC-labeled annexin V are added and incubated in the dark for 15 min at room temperature. Finally, the volume is made to 1 mL by adding 800 μL of binding buffer [22]. Spermatozoa are passed through the flow channel and sorted out based on the fluorescence signals generated by the stained cells. Spermatozoa are examined at a flow rate of <100 cells/sec. Fractions containing annexin V-positive and annexin V-negative cells are collected separately in the wash medium.

ART Outcome

MACS-selected sperm subjected to cryopreservation for further use in ART have shown high levels of normal mitochondrial membrane potential with high DNA integrity and decreased percentage of apoptotic cells [23–27]. In addition, the sperm-oocyte penetration capacity was high in MACS-selected spermatozoa. Also, in comparison with the zeta method, it was found that MACS is able to isolate a higher proportion of sperm with a normal acrosome and protamine content [28]. Embryo cleavage and pregnancy rates were high in sperm used in ICSI selected by MACS compared with DGC in oligo-, astheno-, and teratozoospermic men [29–31]. Use of bioluminescent magnetic nanoparticles was in initial stages of development to isolate high-quality sperm for use in ART [32] and found to be safe and reliable for use in an assisted reproduction program.

Even though flow cytometry and annexin V-based glass wool filtration can efficiently isolate annexin V-positive spermatozoa and allow for recovery of non-apoptotic sperm cells, there is a lack of clinical studies using these sperm in IVF and ICSI procedures.

28.4 Microfluidics

Microfluidics is a novel technique for separating spermatozoa based on their morphology and motility using a microchannel. These channels are made of polydimethylsiloxane (PDMS) silicon polymers that are nontoxic and transparent [33]. Different microfluidic devices were developed to separate sperm such as the passively driven microfluidic device [34, 35], the chemoattractant microfluidic device [36], chemotaxis device [37], microfluidic fertilization device [38], macro-microfluidic sperm sorter [39], Zech selector [40], circular microfluidic device [41], microgroove and channel device [42], and boundary-following behavior-based passive microfluidic device [43].

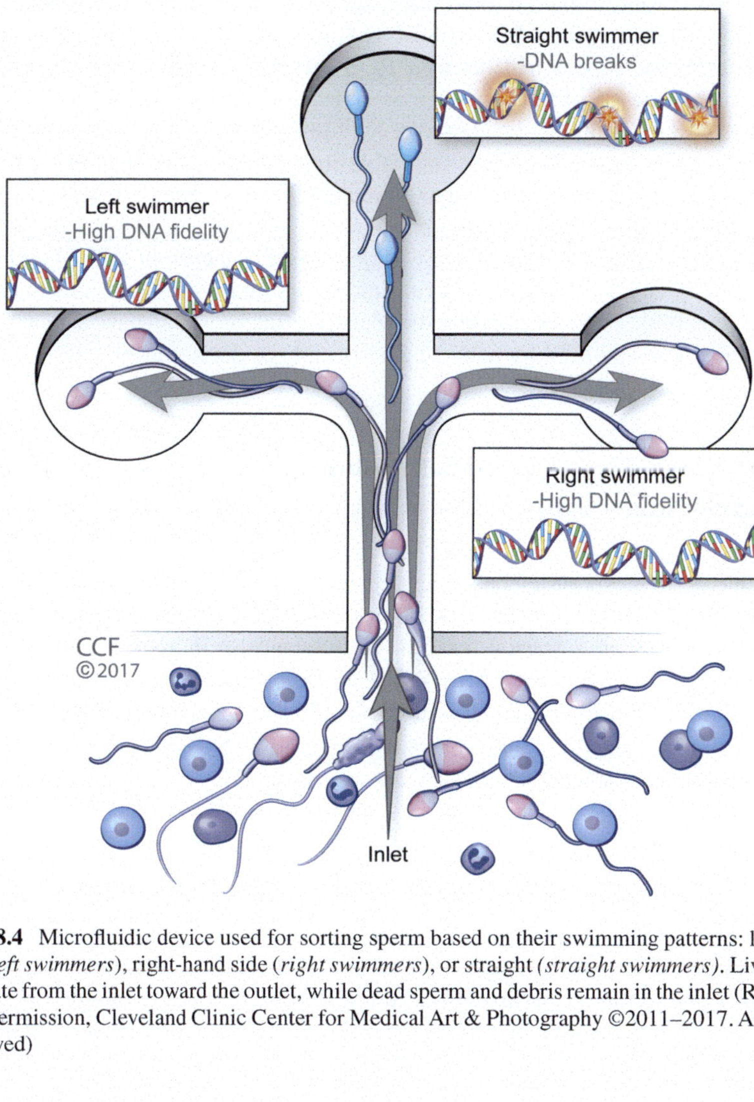

Fig. 28.4 Microfluidic device used for sorting sperm based on their swimming patterns: left-hand side (*left swimmers*), right-hand side (*right swimmers*), or straight *(straight swimmers)*. Live sperm navigate from the inlet toward the outlet, while dead sperm and debris remain in the inlet (Reprinted with permission, Cleveland Clinic Center for Medical Art & Photography ©2011–2017. All Rights Reserved)

The recently developed passive microfluidic device separates sperm with high DNA integrity based on their boundary-following behavior. The device contains a radial network of 52 μ channels which enables the sorting of sperm as left, right, and straight swimmers through the channel (Fig. 28.4). Initially, a 200 μL aliquot of raw semen is loaded into the inlet ring using a plastic syringe and kept undisturbed for 15 min. The temperature of the device and the media is maintained at 37 °C. Motile sperm move and flow through the microchannel in the medium mimicking the viscosity of female reproductive tract fluid. Whereas dead and non-motile sperm are retained in the inlet, motile sperm are collected in a micropipette from the outlets of the microchannel [43].

ART Outcome

Sperm sorted using the microfluidic technology are motile with normal morphology, reduced chromosomal abnormalities, increased chromatin condensation, and high sperm DNA integrity of up to 80% [34, 40, 41, 44]. Also, sperm recovered using microfluidic sorters had reduced ROS levels compared with conventional swim-up technique [39, 45].

The use of a microfluidic device shortened the time in the ICSI treatment of porcine sperm and increased the number of viable embryos without reducing the in vitro production efficiency. An application in human ART is suggested [46, 47]. The technique requires only a low concentration of sperm in a murine IVF model [48]. A robotic-assisted reproduction platform was developed to carry out IVF on a chip by fertilizing the preloaded ova with superior-quality spermatozoa selected by microfluidic technique [49]. Thus, the microfluidic sperm sorting proved to have a great potential in clinical IVF and ICSI for achieving early embryo development.

28.5 Morphology and High-Resolution Microscopy-Based Selection

Abnormal sperm morphology has a major impact on the fertilization and male fertility [50, 51]. Therefore, selection of high-quality spermatozoa based on the morphology is a necessary criterion for their subsequent use in assisted reproduction. Conventional selection of sperm by using a 400× magnification microscope for ICSI does not reveal important structural abnormalities such as nuclear vacuoles. Hence, high magnification microscopes with magnifications up to 6300 × are used to analyze these morphological defects.

28.5.1 Motile Sperm Organelle Morphology Examination

This technique assesses the morphology of the sperm head components (acrosome, post-acrosomal lamina), the mid-piece, the tail region, the mitochondria, and the nucleus chromatin content and also for the presence and size of vacuoles in real time of live spermatozoa. Sperm are generally examined under the digitally enhanced light microscope using Nomarski optics that increases magnification by 6300× [52].

In brief, 1 μL of sperm suspension is mixed with 5 μL droplet of modified HTF medium containing 7% polyvinylpyrrolidone solution (PVP medium; Irvine Scientific). The microdroplets containing motile sperm are placed in a sterile glass petri dish and observed under high magnification. Images of the spermatozoa are captured, and the morphological evaluation is carried out on the monitor [53]. Based on the nuclear vacuoles, spermatozoa are graded and selected. Increased levels of DNA fragmentation are associated with large vacuoles [52].

28.5.2 Birefringence

Sperm birefringence is noticed in the mature sperm nucleus and associated with the nucleoproteins. Due to the presence of subacrosomal protein filaments oriented in longitudinal fashion, birefringence (double refraction) is exhibited by spermatozoa when light passes through the protoplasm. Spermatozoa exhibit either partial or total birefringence based on the composition of the protoplasm. In live sperm cells, birefringence is evaluated under an inverted microscope using Hoffman contrast, polarizing and analyzing lens [54]. This technique distinguishes acrosome-reacted from non-reacted spermatozoa [54].

Birefringence is directly associated with DNA integrity [55]. Partial and total birefringence spermatozoa differ in their DNA fragmentation by 7.3% and 19.5%, respectively [55].

ART Outcome

Spermatozoa with more than 50% vacuolated nuclei are associated with DNA fragmentation [56]. MSOME-selected sperm further used for intracytoplasmic morphologically selected sperm injection (IMSI) are significantly and positively associated with fertilization and pregnancy rates as well as pregnancy outcome compared with standard ICSI [57, 58]. Moreover, this technique also presented low rates of chromosomal aneuploidy and miscarriage [57, 59]. Additionally, Garolla et al. successfully demonstrated the selection of sperm with low DNA damage by using a combination of MSOME and birefringence [60].

In cases of oligoasthenoteratozoospermia, the use of IMSI is preferred over ICSI as it increased implantation and pregnancy rate with decreased miscarriage [61]. Even though IMSI in combination with MSOME has beneficial effects on the improvement in the embryo quality compared with ICSI [62, 63], certain studies indicate no significant advantage of either of these two techniques over the other [64]. This was also pointed out in a meta-analysis implicating that the outcomes of IMSI and ICSI do not differ significantly [65]. Accordingly, MSOME-based selection remains a potential method for the selection of high-quality sperm. However, more clinical studies have to be conducted to demonstrate its efficacy in ART.

28.6 Possible Future of Sperm Selection Methods

Confocal light absorption and scattering spectroscopic (CLASS) microscopy works on the combination of the two principles, the light scattering spectroscopy and confocal microscopy, to visualize subcellular structures of the sperm including the chromatin [66, 67]. The sperm are selected based on the high chromatin integrity without damaging the structure of the spermatozoa.

Interferometric phase microscopy (IPM) is a live cell imaging system used for label-free morphological evaluation and selection of spermatozoa [68]. IPM tracks the sub-nanometric changes in the cells by capturing the two-dimensional optical path delay or optical cell thickness [68]. Under low-power illumination at different sperm spatial points, the cell optical thickness is quantified and presented as a holographic image. Holographic imaging is done in a single exposure without scanning the spermatozoa [69]. This technique was able to identify sperm abnormalities with high accuracy and makes it a suitable tool for selection of sperm in ART use [68, 69].

Raman spectrometry is used to evaluate the integrity of the sperm nuclear DNA and protamine content based on the light scattered when a specific wavelength of light is focused on the sperm head [70]. It provides complete information about the chromatin packing in the spermatozoa and can be used to select the superior-quality sperm with minimal damage for further use in the ICSI procedure [70].

A synthetic oligopeptide (DWI) labeled with the dye terminal rhodamine B was designed against the p53 protein to evaluate DNA breaks in human spermatozoa (Fig. 28.5) [71]. In this technique, the plasma membrane is permeabilized to stain the spermatozoa. However, more research is needed to optimize the permeabilization process and allow this technique for selection of live spermatozoa with intact DNA for further use in ICSI, IVF, and IMSI.

28.7 Limitations of Advanced Sperm Selection Techniques

For an overview of the limitations of advanced sperm selection techniques, see Table 28.1.

28.8 Conclusion

It is an established fact that the presence of damaged DNA in spermatozoa leads to poor fertilization, pregnancy failure, and birth defects. Various advanced sperm selection techniques discussed in this chapter are currently available for ART as a treatment to overcome the male infertility. Most of these techniques are sophisticated and expensive and lack clinical data to document their efficacy.

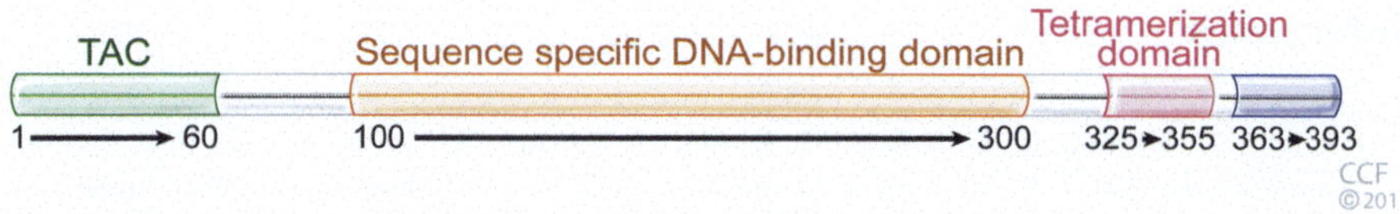

Fig. 28.5 Multi-domain organization of p53 protein. It contains N-terminal transcription-activation domain (TAD) (1–60), a central sequence-specific DNA-binding core domain (100–300), and a multifunctional C-terminal domain (300–393) that contains the tetramerization domain (325–355) and, at the extreme carboxyl terminus, a stretch of 30 amino acids that is rich in basic residues (363–393) (Reprinted with permission, Cleveland Clinic Center for Medical Art & Photography ©2011–2017. All Rights Reserved)

Table 28.1 Limitations of advanced sperm selection techniques

Technique	Limitations
Microflow cell	Complexity of apparatus
	Restricted for daily routine use
Microelectrophoresis	Low yield due to limited volume that can be analyzed
	Not suitable for IUI
Zeta potential	Low sperm recovery rate
	Cannot be used for oligozoospermic samples
	Cannot be used on sperm extracted from testicular/epididymal region or in a humid environment as the surface charges are neutralized
	Samples need to be processed immediately after collection as the sperm lose their negative charge when they undergo capacitation
MACS	MACS cannot remove the leukocytes, immature germ cells, and epithelial cells; it has to be subjected to DGC
	Sperm can be used for IVF and IUI, not much benefit in ICSI
	High cost of the equipment restricted its use in small centers
Annexin V-based glass wool filtration	Debris are noticed in sample after filtration
Microfluidics	Cannot sort high volumes of sperm and hence it is not suitable for IUI
MSOME	Due to prolonged incubation at 37 °C, sperm exhibit decreased motility and vitality
	Highly skilled and technical person is required to carry out the technique

Therefore, further evaluation of these techniques is required by carrying out sound clinical studies. Success rates can be increased by complete andrological examination of the men and choosing the most suitable sperm selection method for establishing pregnancy in the female partner. Therefore, it is most important to improve the efficacy of these techniques and maintain their safety.

References

1. Poenicke K, Grunewald S, Glander H, Paasch U. Sperm selection in assisted reproductive techniques. In: Rao KA, Agarwal A, Srinivas MS, editors. Andrology laboratory manual. 1st ed. India: Jaypee Brothers Pvt Ltd; 2010. p. 173–87.
2. Centers for Disease Control and Prevention ASfRM, Society for Assisted Reproductive Technology. Assisted reproductive technology fertility clinic success rates report. In: Services UDoHaH, (Atlanta, GA 2014); 2012.
3. Henkel R. Sperm preparation: state-of-the-art–physiological aspects and application of advanced sperm preparation methods. Asian J Androl. 2012;14(2):260–9.
4. Said TM, Land JA. Effects of advanced selection methods on sperm quality and ART outcome: a systematic review. Hum Reprod Update. 2011;17(6):719–33.
5. Sharma R, Said T, Agarwal A. Sperm DNA damage and its clinical relevance in assessing reproductive outcome. Asian J Androl. 2004;6(2):139–48.
6. Lopes S, Sun J-G, Jurisicova A, Meriano J, Casper RF. Sperm deoxyribonucleic acid fragmentation is increased in poor-quality semen samples and correlates with failed fertilization in intracytoplasmic sperm injection. Fertil Steril. 1998;69(3):528–32.
7. Sun J-G, Jurisicova A, Casper RF. Detection of deoxyribonucleic acid fragmentation in human sperm: correlation with fertilization in vitro. Biol Reprod. 1997;56(3):602–7.
8. Saleh RA, Agarwal A, Nada EA, El-Tonsy MH, Sharma RK, Meyer A, et al. Negative effects of increased sperm DNA damage in relation to seminal oxidative stress in men with idiopathic and male factor infertility. Fertil Steril. 2003;79:1597–605.
9. Medicine PCotASfR. The clinical utility of sperm DNA integrity testing: a guideline. Fertil Steril. 2013;99(3):673–7.
10. Ainsworth C, Nixon B, Aitken R. Development of a novel electrophoretic system for the isolation of human spermatozoa. Hum Reprod. 2005;20(8):2261–70.
11. Simon L, Murphy K, Aston KI, Emery BR, Hotaling JM, Carrell DT. Optimization of microelectrophoresis to select highly negatively charged sperm. J Assist Reprod Genet. 2016;33(6):679–88.
12. Aitken RJ, Hanson AR, Kuczera L. Electrophoretic sperm isolation: optimization of electrophoresis conditions and impact on oxidative stress. Hum Reprod. 2011;26(8):1955–65.
13. Fleming S, Ilad R, Griffin AG, Wu Y, Ong K, Smith H, et al. Prospective controlled trial of an electrophoretic method of sperm preparation for assisted reproduction: comparison with density gradient centrifugation. Hum Reprod. 2008;23(12):2646–51.
14. Ainsworth C, Nixon B, Jansen R, Aitken R. First recorded pregnancy and normal birth after ICSI using electrophoretically isolated spermatozoa. Hum Reprod. 2007;22(1):197–200.
15. Ishijima S, Okuno M, Mohri H. Zeta potential of human X-and Y-bearing sperm. Int J Androl. 1991;14(5):340–7.
16. Chan PJ, Jacobson JD, Corselli JU, Patton WC. A simple zeta method for sperm selection based on membrane charge. Fertil Steril. 2006;85(2):481–6.
17. Razavi S, Nasr-Esfahani M, Deemeh M, Shayesteh M, Tavalaee M. Evaluation of zeta and HA-binding methods for selection of spermatozoa with normal morphology, protamine content and DNA integrity. Andrologia. 2010;42(1):13–9.
18. Zarei-Kheirabadi M, Tavalaee M, Deemeh M, Arabi M, Forouzanfar M, Javadi GR, et al. Evaluation of ubiquitin and annexin V in sperm population selected based on density gradient centrifugation and zeta potential (DGC-Zeta). J Assist Reprod Genet. 2012;29(4):365–71.
19. Vermes I, Haanen C, Steffens-Nakken H, Reutellingsperger C. A novel assay for apoptosis flow cytometric detection of phosphatidylserine expression on early apoptotic cells using fluorescein labelled annexin V. J Immunol Methods. 1995;184(1):39–51.
20. Paasch U, Grunewald S, Glander H. Sperm selection in assisted reproductive techniques. Soc Reprod Fertil Suppl. 2007;65:515–25.
21. Garner DL, Evans KM, Seidel GE. Sex-sorting sperm using flow cytometry/cell sorting. Spermatogenesis: Methods Protoc. 2013:279–95.

22. Hoogendijk CF, Kruger TF, Bouic PJ, Henkel RR. A novel approach for the selection of human sperm using annexin V-binding and flow cytometry. Fertil Steril. 2009;91(4):1285–92.
23. Grunewald S, Paasch U, Said TM, Rasch M, Agarwal A, Glander H-J. Magnetic-activated cell sorting before cryopreservation preserves mitochondrial integrity in human spermatozoa. Cell Tissue Bank. 2006;7(2):99–104.
24. Makker K, Agarwal A, Sharma RK. Magnetic activated cell sorting (MACS): utility in assisted reproduction. Indian J Exp Biol. 2008;46:491–7.
25. Gil M, Sar-Shalom V, Sivira YM, Carreras R, Checa MA. Sperm selection using magnetic activated cell sorting (MACS) in assisted reproduction: a systematic review and meta-analysis. J Assist Reprod Genet. 2013;30(4):479–85.
26. Lee T-H, Liu C-H, Shih Y-T, Tsao H-M, Huang C-C, Chen H-H, et al. Magnetic-activated cell sorting for sperm preparation reduces spermatozoa with apoptotic markers and improves the acrosome reaction in couples with unexplained infertility. Hum Reprod. 2010;25(4):839–46.
27. Said TM, Agarwal A, Zborowski M, Grunewald S, Glander HJ, Paasch U. ANDROLOGY LAB CORNER*: utility of magnetic cell separation as a molecular sperm preparation technique. J Androl. 2008;29(2):134–42.
28. Zahedi A, Tavalaee M, Deemeh M, Azadi L, Fazilati M, Nasr-Esfahani M. Zeta potential vs apoptotic marker: which is more suitable for ICSI sperm selection? J Assist Reprod Genet. 2013;30(9):1181–6.
29. Dirican EK, Özgün OD, Akarsu S, Akın KO, Ercan Ö, Uğurlu M, et al. Clinical outcome of magnetic activated cell sorting of non-apoptotic spermatozoa before density gradient centrifugation for assisted reproduction. J Assist Reprod Genet. 2008;25(8):375–81.
30. de Fried EP, Denaday F. Single and twin ongoing pregnancies in two cases of previous ART failure after ICSI performed with sperm sorted using annexin V microbeads. Fertil Steril. 2010;94(1):351. e15-. e18
31. Rawe VY, Boudri HU, Sedó CA, Carro M, Papier S, Nodar F. Healthy baby born after reduction of sperm DNA fragmentation using cell sorting before ICSI. Reprod Biomed Online. 2010;20(3):320–3.
32. Vasquez ES, Feugang JM, Willard ST, Ryan PL, Walters KB. Bioluminescent magnetic nanoparticles as potential imaging agents for mammalian spermatozoa. J Nanobiotechnol. 2016;14(1):20.
33. Xia Y, Whitesides GM. Soft lithography. Annu Rev Mater Sci. 1998;28(1):153–84.
34. Cho BS, Schuster TG, Zhu X, Chang D, Smith GD, Takayama S. Passively driven integrated microfluidic system for separation of motile sperm. Anal Chem. 2003;75(7):1671–5.
35. Chung Y, Zhu X, Gu W, Smith GD, Takayama S. Microscale integrated sperm sorter. Microfluid Tech: Rev Protoc. 2006:227–44.
36. Cheng S-Y, Heilman S, Wasserman M, Archer S, Shuler ML, Wu M. A hydrogel-based microfluidic device for the studies of directed cell migration. Lab Chip. 2007;7(6):763–9.
37. Xie L, Ma R, Han C, Su K, Zhang Q, Qiu T, et al. Integration of sperm motility and chemotaxis screening with a microchannel-based device. Clin Chem. 2010;56(8):1270–8.
38. Lopez-Garcia MC, Monson R, Haubert K, Wheeler M, Beebe D. Sperm motion in a microfluidic fertilization device. Biomed Microdevices. 2008;10(5):709–18.
39. Asghar W, Velasco V, Kingsley JL, Shoukat MS, Shafiee H, Anchan RM, et al. Selection of functional human sperm with higher DNA integrity and fewer reactive oxygen species. Adv Healthc Mater. 2014;3(10):1671–9.
40. Ebner T, Shebl O, Moser M, Mayer R, Arzt W, Tews G. Easy sperm processing technique allowing exclusive accumulation and later usage of DNA-strandbreak-free spermatozoa. Reprod Biomed Online. 2011;22(1):37–43.
41. Nosrati R, Vollmer M, Eamer L, San Gabriel MC, Zeidan K, Zini A, et al. Rapid selection of sperm with high DNA integrity. Lab Chip. 2014;14(6):1142–50.
42. Tung C-k, Ardon F, Fiore AG, Suarez SS, Wu M. Cooperative roles of biological flow and surface topography in guiding sperm migration revealed by a microfluidic model. Lab Chip. 2014;14(7):1348–56.

43. Eamer L, Vollmer M, Nosrati R, San Gabriel MC, Zeidan K, Zini A, et al. Turning the corner in fertility: high DNA integrity of boundary-following sperm. Lab Chip. 2016;16(13):2418–22.
44. Seiringer M, Maurer M, Shebl O, Dreier K, Tews G, Ziehr S, et al. Efficacy of a sperm-selection chamber in terms of morphology, aneuploidy and DNA packaging. Reprod Biomed Online. 2013;27(1):81–8.
45. Zhang QC, Wang W, Li WX, Zhang Q, Liang GT, Yan W, Zhou XM. Sperm sorting based on the imitation of the physiological process on the microfluidic chip. Zhonghuanankexue= Natl J Androl. 2012;18(9):803–6.
46. Matsuura K, Uozumi T, Furuichi T, Sugimoto I, Kodama M, Funahashi H. A microfluidic device to reduce treatment time of intracytoplasmic sperm injection. Fertil Steril. 2013;99(2):400–7.
47. Clark SG, Haubert K, Beebe DJ, Ferguson CE, Wheeler MB. Reduction of polyspermic penetration using biomimetic microfluidic technology during in vitro fertilization. Lab Chip. 2005;5(11):1229–32.
48. Suh RS, Zhu X, Phadke N, Ohl DA, Takayama S, Smith GD. IVF within microfluidic channels requires lower total numbers and lower concentrations of sperm. Hum Reprod. 2006;21(2):477–83.
49. Tsai VF, Chang HC, Hsieh JT, Wo AM. Application of microfluidic technologies to the quantification and manipulation of sperm. Urol Sci. 2016;27(2):56–9.
50. Kruger T, Coetzee K. The role of sperm morphology in assisted reproduction. Hum Reprod Update. 1999;5(2):172–8.
51. Van der Merwe F, Kruger T, Oehninger S, Lombard C. The use of semen parameters to identify the subfertile male in the general population. Gynecol Obstet Investig. 2005;59(2):86–91.
52. Bartoov B, Berkovitz A, Eltes F, Kogosowski A, Menezo Y, Barak Y. Real-time fine morphology of motile human sperm cells is associated with IVF-ICSI outcome. J Androl. 2002;23(1):1–8.
53. Franco JG Jr. Motile sperm organelle morphology examination (MSOME). In non-invasive sperm selection for in vitro fertilization. New York: Springer; 2015. p. 81–90.
54. Gianaroli L, Magli MC, Collodel G, Moretti E, Ferraretti AP, Baccetti B. Sperm head's birefringence: a new criterion for sperm selection. Fertil Steril. 2008;90(1):104–12.
55. Rappa KL, Rodriguez HF, Hakkarainen GC, Anchan RM, Mutter GL, Asghar W. Sperm processing for advanced reproductive technologies: where are we today? Biotechnol Adv. 2016;34(5):578–87.
56. Oliveira JBA, Massaro FC, Baruffi RLR, Mauri AL, Petersen CG, Silva LF, et al. Correlation between semen analysis by motile sperm organelle morphology examination and sperm DNA damage. Fertil Steril. 2010;94(5):1937–40.
57. Antinori M, Licata E, Dani G, Cerusico F, Versaci C, d'Angelo D, et al. Intracytoplasmic morphologically selected sperm injection: a prospective randomized trial. Reprod Biomed Online. 2008;16(6):835–41.
58. Balaban B, Yakin K, Alatas C, Oktem O, Isiklar A, Urman B. Clinical outcome of intracytoplasmic injection of spermatozoa morphologically selected under high magnification: a prospective randomized study. Reprod Biomed Online. 2011;22(5):472–6.
59. Figueira RCS, Braga DPAF, Pasqualotto EB, Pasqualotto FF, Iaconelli A, Borges E. The role of morphological nuclear integrity of the sperm cells in preimplantation genetic aneuploidy screening cycles outcome. J fur Reproduktionsmedizin und Endokrinologie. 2010;7:250–1.
60. Garolla A, Cosci I, Menegazzo M, De Palo R, Ambrosini G, Sartini B, et al. Sperm selected by both birefringence and motile sperm organelle morphology examination have reduced deoxyribonucleic acid fragmentation. Fertil Steril. 2014;101(3):647–52.
61. Setti AS, Ferreira RC. Braga DPdAF, FigueiraRdCS, Iaconelli A, Borges E. Intracytoplasmic sperm injection outcome versus intracytoplasmic morphologically selected sperm injection outcome: a meta-analysis. Reprod Biomed Online. 2010;21(4):450–5.
62. De Vos A, Van de Velde H, Bocken G, Eylenbosch G, Franceus N, Meersdom G, et al. Does intracytoplasmic morphologically selected sperm injection improve embryo development? A randomized sibling-oocyte study. Hum Reprod. 2013;28(3):617–26.

63. Klement AH, Koren-Morag N, Itsykson P, Berkovitz A. Intracytoplasmic morphologically selected sperm injection versus intracytoplasmic sperm injection: a step toward a clinical algorithm. Fertil Steril. 2013;99(5):1290–3.
64. Knez K, Tomazevic T, Zorn B, Vrtacnik-Bokal E, Virant-Klun I. Intracytoplasmic morphologically selected sperm injection improves development and quality of preimplantation embryos in teratozoospermia patients. Reprod Biomed Online. 2012;25(2):168–79.
65. Teixeira DM, Barbosa MA, Ferriani RA, Navarro PA, Raine-Fenning N, Nastri CO, et al. Regular (ICSI) versus ultra-high magnification (IMSI) sperm selection for assisted reproduction. Cochrane Libr. 2013;
66. Itzkan I, Qiu L, Fang H, Zaman MM, Vitkin E, Ghiran IC, et al. Confocal light absorption and scattering spectroscopic microscopy monitors organelles in live cells with no exogenous labels. Proc Natl Acad Sci. 2007;104(44):17255–60.
67. Yetunde I, Vasiliki M. Effects of advanced selection methods on sperm quality and ART outcome. Minerva Ginecol. 2013;65(5):487–96.
68. Girshovitz P, Shaked NT. Compact and portable low-coherence interferometer with off-axis geometry for quantitative phase microscopy and nanoscopy. Opt Express. 2013;21(5):5701–14.
69. Haifler M, Girshovitz P, Band G, Dardikman G, Madjar I, Shaked NT. Interferometric phase microscopy for label-free morphological evaluation of sperm cells. Fertil Steril. 2015;104(1):43–7. e2
70. Huser T, Orme CA, Hollars CW, Corzett MH, Balhorn R. Raman spectroscopy of DNA packaging in individual human sperm cells distinguishes normal from abnormal cells. J Biophotonics. 2009;2(5):322–32.
71. Enciso M, Pieczenik G, Cohen J, Wells D. Development of a novel synthetic oligopeptide for the detection of DNA damage in human spermatozoa. Hum Reprod. 2012;27(8):2254–66.

Chapter 29
Use of Testicular Sperm for ICSI: Pro

Sandro C. Esteves and Matheus Roque

29.1 Introduction

Infertility, defined by the inability of a sexually active and non-contracepting couple to achieve pregnancy in 1 year, affects approximately 8–15% of couples. Of these, the male factor is solely responsible in ~20% and contributory in another 30–40% of couples. Although male infertility is usually associated with the presence of abnormal semen parameters, it may be present even when the conventional semen analysis is normal [1, 2], which occurs in approximately 15% of the cases [3]. Despite its multifactorial nature, male factor infertility is not yet fully understood, and approximately half of the cases are deemed unexplained or idiopathic [4–6].

Increasing evidence indicates that sperm DNA damage is more common in infertile patients than in fertile counterparts and that DNA integrity is important for normal embryo development [7, 8]. Sperm DNA damage is also important because genetic information passed on to the next generation depends on sperm DNA integrity [9, 10]. As a consequence, sperm DNA fragmentation (SDF) testing has emerged as an important tool for assessing male fertility potential [11, 12]. The test has been proposed as complementary to but different from the information provided by routine semen analysis [7, 13, 14]. Some authors advocate its use as a routine testing in the clinical evaluation of male factor infertility [10, 13–16].

Furthermore, the literature is rich in studies claiming an association between elevated sperm DNA damage and poor assisted reproductive outcomes (revised by Agarwal et al. 2016) [13]. It has been found that although sperm with fragmented DNA are able to fertilize an egg with apparently the same efficiency as sperm

S.C. Esteves (✉)
Andrology and Human Reproduction Clinic, ANDROFERT, Campinas, Brazil
e-mail: s.esteves@androfert.com.br

M. Roque
ORIGEN - Center for Reproductive Medicine, Rio de Janeiro, RJ, Brazil
e-mail: matheusroque@origen.com.br

A. Zini, A. Agarwal (eds.), *A Clinician's Guide to Sperm DNA and Chromatin Damage*, https://doi.org/10.1007/978-3-319-71815-6_29

without DNA fragmentation, SDF negatively impacts embryo quality by compromising integrity of the embryonic genome [17–19]. These alterations may jeopardize in vitro fertilization (IVF)/intracytoplasmic sperm injection (ICSI) outcomes [20–22], including by increasing the rates of miscarriage [22, 23], but also be associated with a higher risk of birth defects in the offspring [7]. The use of the term "late paternal effect" has been suggested for the developmental disadvantage conferred to embryos by spermatozoa carrying damaged DNA [24].

Notwithstanding, the impact of sperm DNA damage on reproductive outcomes may be modulated by the cytoplasmic and genomic quality of the oocyte, which is closely related to the women's age. Moreover, the quality of sperm DNA is also related to the paternal age, and this may further exacerbate the negative effects of SDF seen in assisted reproductive techniques (ART) cycles performed in women of advanced age [25–27]. Along the same lines, SDF has also a greater impact on the outcomes of IVF/ICSI cycles among women with reduced ovarian reserve [28].

Since several etiological factors have been implicated in the impairment of sperm DNA content, including environmental lifestyle factors, varicocele, male accessory gland infections, advanced paternal age, and systemic diseases, assessment of sperm DNA fragmentation (SDF) offers an opportunity to better understand and treat such sperm dysfunctions [9, 12, 13]. Thus, several strategies have been attempted to overcome SDF in couples subjected to ART. In addition to varicocele repair [29], oral antioxidant intake [30, 31], and use of short ejaculatory abstinence periods [32] and recurrent ejaculations before fertilization [33, 34], sperm selection techniques such as magnetic cell sorting [35, 36], physiological ICSI [37], and intracytoplasmic morphologically selected sperm injection [38–40] have been proposed. However, none of these interventions, alone or in combination, have been unequivocally proven to be of clinical value to bypass the potential detrimental effect of abnormal SDF on ART outcomes [2]. Among the sperm selection techniques, it has been advocated that the use of testicular sperm for ICSI instead of ejaculated sperm in men with high SDF would be of benefit [14]. In this chapter, we discuss the available evidence regarding the use of testicular sperm to overcome high levels of SDF in ejaculated sperm using a SWOT (strengths, weaknesses, opportunities, and threats) analysis.

29.2 Strengths

The post-testicular induced DNA fragmentation occurs mainly by reactive oxygen species (ROS) during sperm transport through the seminiferous tubules and the epididymis. This potential damage could be avoided or at least decreased by bypassing the epididymis and using testicular sperm [27]. Previous studies observed that sperm DNA damage is significantly higher both in ejaculated sperm [41] and sperm from the cauda epididymis [42, 43] than testicular sperm.

The epithelial cells of the epididymis may be involved in ROS-induced DNA damage through hydroxyl 1 radical or nitric oxide [44, 45] or through the activation of sperm caspases and endonucleases by physicochemical factors such as high temperature [45, 46] and environmental factors [47]. In infertile men with varicocele, for instance, who usually have higher SDF than counterparts without varicocele, reactive oxygen and nitrogen species are released not only by the endothelial cells in the dilated pampiniform plexus and the testicular cells (developing germ cells, Leydig cells, macrophages, and peritubular cells) but also by the principal cells in the epididymis [48, 49]. Thus, the use of testicular sperm obtained by testicular sperm aspiration (TESA) or extraction (TESE) would be of clinical interest in cases of high levels of DNA fragmentation in the semen and repeated implantation failure [27], as the probability of selecting spermatozoa free of DNA damage for ICSI will increase [50]. Likewise, the fertilization of an oocyte by genomically intact testicular spermatozoa will increase the chances of creating a normal embryonic genome that will ultimately increase the likelihood of pregnancy and live birth [50].

The first study to propose the use of testicular sperm as an alternative to ejaculated sperm in men with fertility compromised by sperm DNA damage was published in 2005 [41]. The authors evaluated 18 couples who had at least two previous unsuccessful ICSI with ejaculated sperm and whose seminal evaluation showed ≥15% of SDF assessed by the terminal deoxyribonucleotidyl transferase-mediated dUTP nick-end labeling (TUNEL) assay. Testicular sperm were obtained by testis biopsy, and SDF was evaluated on prepared smears containing minced testicular tissue in a similar manner as for ejaculated sperm smears. Two hundred spermatozoa per sample were analyzed in both ejaculated and the testicular specimens collected on the same day. But in the second ICSI attempt, all sperm injections were performed with testicular sperm. The mean ± SD SDF rates in testicular sperm and ejaculated sperm were 4.8 ± 3.6% and 23.6 ± 5.1%, respectively ($P < 0.001$). There were no significant differences in fertilization and cleavage rates and also in the proportion of embryos with good morphology when the first and second ICSI attempts were compared. However, whereas only one pregnancy – that spontaneously aborted – was obtained in the cycles with ejaculated sperm, eight clinical pregnancies (four singletons and four twins) were obtained in the cycles carried out with testicular sperm. No miscarriages were recorded.

In 2010, two studies [27, 51] compared DNA damage in ejaculated and testicular spermatozoa. Moskovtsev et al. evaluated 12 men with persistently high DNA damage despite taking oral antioxidants for 3 months. They compared the levels of DNA fragmentation by TUNEL in testicular sperm obtained by TESE with that of ejaculated sperm collected on the day of ICSI. The rates of SDF in ejaculated sperm were threefold higher than testicular sperm (39.7 ± 14.8 vs. 13.3 ± 7.3, $P < 0.001$) [51]. In another study, Sakkas and Alvarez showed that pregnancy outcomes were improved using testicular sperm rather than ejaculated sperm in patients with high levels of sperm DNA fragmentation. These authors studied 72 patients with DNA fragmentation by TUNEL >20% and found statistically higher implantation

($P = 0.0021$) and clinical pregnancy rates ($P = 0.035$) and lower miscarriage rates in ICSI cycles with testicular sperm [27]. Subsequently, Mehta et al. evaluated a small cohort of 24 men with oligozoospermia (<5 million/mL), SDF by TUNEL >7%, and previous failed ICSI attempts [52]. Patients were subjected to microdissection testicular sperm extraction (micro-TESE), and the retrieved sperm were used for ICSI. Clinical pregnancy was achieved in 50% of 24 couples in the first cycle, and all pregnancies resulted in deliveries of healthy babies. The mean TUNEL-positive level was 24.5% for ejaculated sperm and 4.6% for testicular sperm.

In a recent prospective comparative study evaluating a larger cohort of 172 infertile men with elevated SDF subjected to ICSI for the first time, Esteves et al. [50] compared treatment outcomes between ejaculated and testicular sperm. In this aforementioned study, the authors enrolled infertile men with idiopathic mild to moderate oligozoospermia (5–15 million spermatozoa/ml) presenting with persistent high SDF (>30%) despite oral antioxidant therapy with a combination of vitamins C and E, folic acid, selenium, and zinc for 3 months. On the day of oocyte retrieval, SDF was assessed in all patients after 2–3 days of ejaculatory abstinence using the sperm chromatin dispersion (SCD) test. In the group of patients undergoing sperm retrieval, performed either by testicular sperm extraction (TESE) or testicular sperm aspiration (TESA), SDF was also assessed in testicular specimens using the SCD method combining a dual fluorescent probe to target both the DNA and proteins. This method allowed for discrimination between spermatozoa and other cell elements in testicular suspensions. The rates of SDF in these aforementioned men were fivefold higher in the semen (40.7 ± 9.9%) than in the testis (8.3 ± 5.3%; $P < 0.001$; Fig. 29.1); all sperm injections were performed with testicular sperm. On the contrary, SDF rates were 40.9 ± 10.2% in the group of patients subjected to ICSI with ejaculated sperm. The comparison groups were similar with regard to male and female demographic characteristics. However, the miscarriage rates were lower, whereas the live birth rates were higher in the couples subjected to sperm injections with testicular sperm (Fig. 29.2). The adjusted relative risk for miscarriage and live birth between testicular and ejaculated groups were 0.29 (95% CI, 0.10–0.82; $P = 0.019$) and 1.76 (95% CI, 1,15–2.70, P-0.008), respectively. The number needed to treat by testicular compared to ejaculated samples to obtain an additional live birth per fresh transfer cycles was 4.9 (95% CI, 2.8–16.8). To our knowledge, this is the largest and best-designed study published to date comparing ICSI outcomes using ejaculated and testicular sperm in couples with elevated SDF.

29.3 Weaknesses

The available evidence favoring the use of testicular sperm for ICSI in cases with high SDF is still limited. Most studies have evaluated a small cohort of men [27, 41, 51, 52]. Only one prospective comparative study, albeit not randomized, was powered to detect differences in live birth rates [50]. Given the lack of

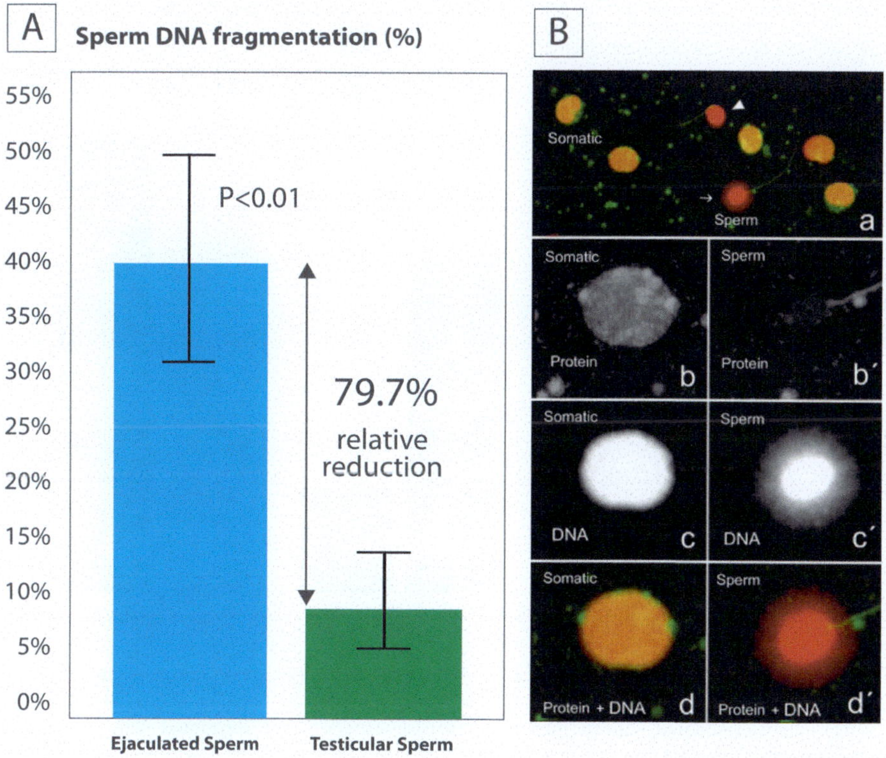

Fig. 29.1 (**a**) Comparison of sperm DNA fragmentation rates in ejaculated and testicular sperm of 81 infertile men undergoing ICSI. Use of testicular sperm for ICSI resulted in a fivefold reduction in SDF (absolute reduction, 32.6%, relative reduction, 79.7%). (**b**) Sperm chromatin dispersion (SCD) for assessment of SDF in testicular sperm. A variant of the Halosperm test (Halotech DNA, Spain) that combines a dual fluorescent cocktail probe to discriminate somatic cells from spermatozoa was used. Spermatozoa and somatic cells exhibit differences in the wavelength emission associated with each fluorochrome (green for proteins and red for DNA). Spermatozoa exhibit only red fluorescence on the sperm head owing to protamine removal, while nonsperm cells fluoresce yellow as a result of the combined emission of both fluorochromes (**a**). Spermatozoa exhibiting red fluorescence with a green flagellum and no halo of chromatin dispersion represented those with fragmented DNA (arrow cap). In contrast, spermatozoa exhibiting red fluorescence with a green flagellum and haloes of chromatin dispersion represented those with non-fragmented DNA (arrow). A somatic cell with its typical high protein and DNA contents and a spermatozoon with its characteristic low protein remnant and high DNA content are seen in panels "b" and "c," respectively, using a single-channel fluorescence emission. After merging the information provided by protein and DNA selective staining, somatic cells and spermatozoa can be easily distinguished (d and d'). In addition, the sperm tail fluoresces green, and this feature also helps to distinguish spermatozoa from other cell elements (a and d') (Adapted with permission from Elsevier 2015, [50]. Reprinted with permission from Springer 2016 [14])

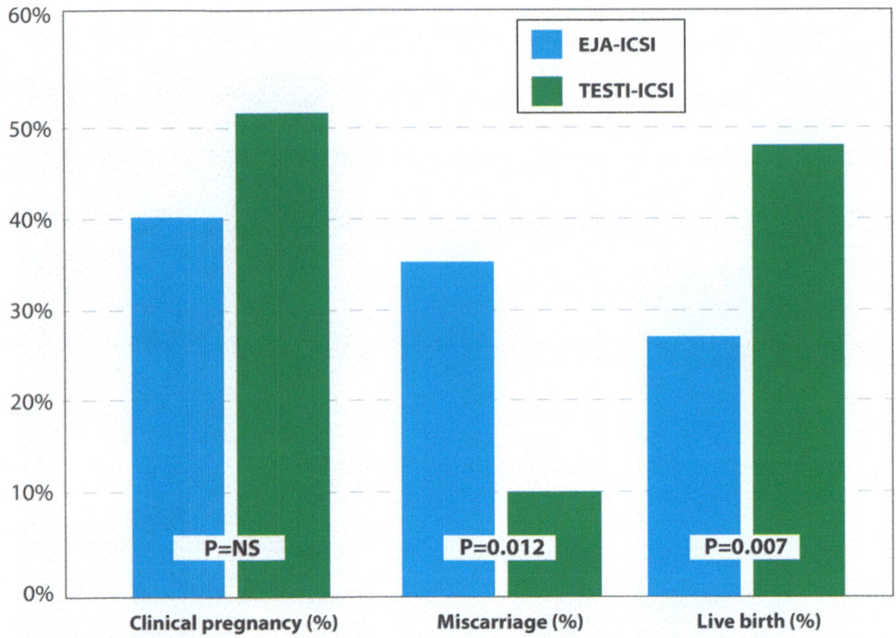

Fig. 29.2 Clinical pregnancy, miscarriage, and live birth rates after sperm injections using either ejaculated sperm (EJA-ICSI; $n = 91$) or testicular sperm retrieved by TESE or TESA (TESTI-ICSI; $n = 81$) cohorts (Adapted with permission from Elsevier 2015,[50]. Reprinted with permission from Springer 2016 [14])

randomized clinical trials supporting the routine use of testicular strategy in cases involving high DNA fragmentation, the current evidence should be interpreted with caution. Furthermore, the cost-effectiveness of implementing this strategy should be determined, as does its efficacy in other subgroups of men, including those with semen parameters within normal limits and in men with severe oligozoospermia. Along the same lines, the usefulness of testicular ICSI in specific etiology categories that has been associated with high SDF, such as varicocele, needs to be determined. Lastly, it is also important to assess the health of offspring generated from fathers with infertility associated with SDF and who have used testicular sperm for obtaining fatherhood.

It is important to recognize that testicular sperm may not always overcome the problem of SDF. It is well known that sperm DNA damage may also occur in the seminiferous tubule epithelium by apoptosis or it can be due to defects in chromatin remodeling during spermiogenesis [27]. Moreover, despite being associated with low rates of complications, sperm retrievals are invasive procedures that may result in postoperative pain, hematoma, and testicular atrophy [53]. Thus, their application should be only justified after a careful examination of the benefits and risks and reserved for selected men who have failed less invasive treatments for known and unknown causes of sperm DNA damage.

29.4 Opportunities

Given the importance of SDF to both natural and medically assisted reproductive outcomes, several strategies have been attempted to alleviate SDF and/or select sperm with higher-quality chromatin content for ART. The intake of oral antioxidants [30, 31], treatment of subclinical genital infections, varicocelectomy (discussed in Chap. 26), and the use of recurrent ejaculations and short abstinence periods before fertilization [32, 54] alone or combined with micromanipulation-based sperm selection techniques (discussed in Chaps. 27 and 28) have been attempted (Fig. 29.3). Yet none of these interventions, alone or combined, have been unequivocally proven to be of clinical value to bypass the potential detrimental effect of abnormal SDF on assisted reproductive technology (ART) outcomes [2].

The use of testicular sperm for ICSI (TESTI-ICSI) has emerged as an attractive alternative to overcome infertility in men with high SDF who are candidates to ART, including those with oligozoospermia and persistent high levels of SDF after antioxidant therapy [41, 50]. On the contrary, the use of testicular sperm for ICSI in cases of cryptozoospermia and repeated implantation failures where SDF can be a contributory cause has been poorly studied [55–57]. To our knowledge, there are few reports assessing ICSI outcomes in men with cryptozoospermia [55, 56].

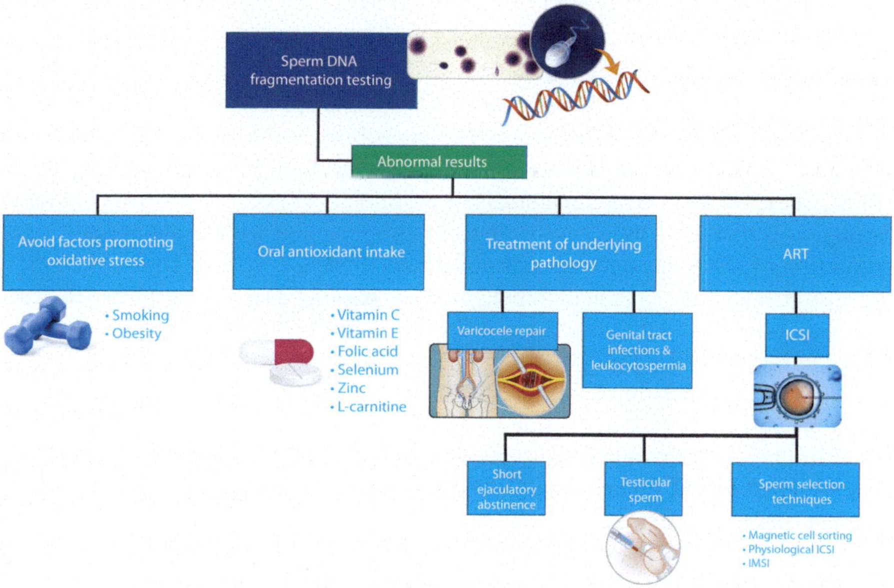

Fig. 29.3 Possible treatment alternatives to overcome high sperm DNA fragmentation. The figure highlights the role of SDF testing to better manage couples facing infertility. Possible treatment strategies to overcome high SDF are indicated. ART, assisted reproductive technology; ICSI, intracytoplasmic sperm injection; IMSI, intracytoplasmic morphologically selected sperm injection or ultrahigh magnification sperm injection (Reprinted with permission from Springer 2016 [14])

Ben-Ami et al. studied 17 cryptozoospermic men who underwent several failed ICSI cycles with ejaculated sperm, followed by cycles using testicular sperm extracted by testicular sperm extraction (TESE) [55]. Despite no significant differences in fertilization rates between the groups, testicular sperm yielded higher implantation rate (20.7% vs. 5.7%; $P = 0.003$), higher pregnancy rate (42.5% vs. 15.1%; $P = 0.004$), and higher delivery rate (27.5% vs. 9.4%; $P = 0.028$). Hauser et al. studied 13 couples whose male partner had virtual azoospermia or cryptozoospermia [56]. The patients were subjected to multiple ICSI cycles with ejaculated and fresh and frozen testicular sperm, and the results indicated that fertilization rates (50.0% vs. 38.2%, $P < 0.05$), high-quality embryo rates (65.3% vs. 53.2%, $P < 0.05$), and implantation rates (18.1% vs. 5.1%; $P = 0.04$) favored fresh testicular sperm compared with ejaculated sperm. In a recent systematic review and meta-analysis including five cohort studies encompassing 272 ICSI cycles and 4596 injected oocytes, Abhyankar et al. evaluated ICSI outcomes in cryptozoospermic patients comparing TESTI-ICSI versus ejaculated sperm for ICSI. The authors didn't find any difference in pregnancy rates (relative risk [RR] 0.53, 95% CI 0.19–1.42, $P = 0.21$) and fertilization rates (RR 0.91, 95% CI 0.78–1.06, $P = 0.21$) between TESTI-ICSI and ejaculated groups. In conclusion, the available literature does not support the use of testicular instead of ejaculated sperm in men with cryptozoospermia submitted to ICSI [57]. And as far as repeated implantation failure is concerned, Weissman et al. reported success with the use of testicular sperm in four couples with multiple failed ICSI attempts [58]. However, all aforementioned studies compared fertility outcomes without assessing SDF, making it difficult to ascertain that SDF was the effect modulator.

Furthermore, it is yet to be determined if testicular sperm could overcome infertility in cases of repeated miscarriage. The plausibility of a role for TESTI-ICSI in such cases relies on the positive association between high SDF and miscarriage in IVF/ICSI cycles. In a recent meta-analysis evaluating 2969 couples, the risk of miscarriage was increased by 2.2-fold when semen specimens with an abnormally high proportion of DNA damage were used for ICSI (95% CI, 1.54–3.03; $P < 0.00001$) (Robinson et al. 2012). In another meta-analysis pooling data of 14 studies, elevated SDF was associated with higher miscarriage rates in ICSI (OR 2.68; 95% CI 1.40–5.14; $P = 0.003$) cycles [59].

Altogether, the existing evidence, albeit limited, indicates that TESTI-ICSI may overcome infertility related to SDF, but more research is needed to confirm these initial findings. Furthermore, there are also opportunities to explore the effectiveness of TESTI-ICSI compared to other laboratory preparation methods used to deselect sperm with damaged DNA, such as magnetic cell sorting (MACS), physiological ICSI (PCSI), and intracytoplasmic morphologically selected sperm injection (IMSI). In a recent study, it has been suggested that live birth rates were higher in couples whose male partners had been subjected to ICSI with testicular sperm (49.8%) than other laboratory selection techniques, such as IMSI (28.7%) and PICSI (38.3%). The worse live birth rates were observed when no intervention had been carried out to deselect sperm with SDF (24.2%) compared with testicular sperm (49.8%; $P = 0.020$) [60].

29.5 Threats

While defective spermatozoa passing the testicular barrier can be eventually deselected via natural apoptotic-like process [61], it is possible that testicular sperm originating from a subpopulation that would be blocked in its ontogeny during the maturation process is selected for ICSI cycles using testicular sperm and carries putative deficiencies [62]. It has been shown that aneuploidy rates were higher in testicular sperm obtained from men with nonobstructive azoospermia compared to epididymal sperm and ejaculated sperm [63–66]. While testicular spermatozoa appear favorable for ICSI in terms of lower DNA damage, this potential advantage could be offset by the higher aneuploidy rates in testicular spermatozoa [66]. In one study, Moskovtsev et al. compared aneuploidy rates at the testicular and post-testicular levels in the same patients with persistently high SDF despite prior 3-month oral antioxidant therapy. Although SDF rates were almost threefold lower in testicular sperm (40.6 ± 14.8% vs. 14.9 ± 5.0%, $P < 0.05$), higher aneuploidy rates for chromosomes 18, 21, X, and Y were observed in testicular spermatozoa [67]. Notwithstanding, these findings are yet to be confirmed in larger series comprising both men with oligozoospermia and normal semen parameters. The limited evidence favoring ICSI outcomes with the use of testicular sperm in men with high SDF calls for continuous monitoring until the safety of this strategy is confirmed. Any genetic and epigenetic effects in the offspring will require a more extensive investigation and long-term follow-up.

29.6 Conclusions

Fair evidence indicates that sperm DNA fragmentation is associated with poorer ART outcomes. There is a rationale for the use of testicular sperm for ICSI owing to the improvement in live birth rates in men with high SDF, defined by the presence of >30% spermatozoa with fragmented DNA in the neat semen. The threshold level of 30% for proceeding to TESTI-ICSI derives from few studies using SCD and TUNEL. The biological plausibility of this favorable effect relates to the fact that post-testicular exposure of spermatozoa to oxidative DNA damage in the epididymis is avoided. Given the limited evidence in favor of TESTI-ICSI and the potential risks associated with sperm retrieval, the method should be reserved for selected men who have failed less invasive treatments for known and unknown causes of sperm DNA damage. Ample opportunities exist to further investigate the role of testicular sperm for ICSI (1) in different subgroups of men with high DNA damage, (2) in comparison with other laboratory methods of sperm selection, and (3) in the health of offspring.

References

1. Esteves SC. Clinical relevance of routine semen analysis and controversies surrounding the 2010 World Health Organization criteria for semen examination. Int Braz J Urol. 2014;40:443–53.
2. Practice Committee of the American Society for Reproductive Medicine. Diagnostic evaluation of the infertile male: a committee opinion. Fertil Steril. 2015;103:18–25.
3. Hamada A, Esteves SC, Nizza M, Agarwal A. Unexplained male infertility: diagnosis and management. Int Braz J Urol. 2012;38:576–94.
4. Brandes M, Hamilton CJ, De Bruin JP, Nelen WL, Kremer JA. The relative contribution of IVF to the total ongoing pregnancy rate in a subfertile cohort. Hum Reprod. 2010;25:118–26.
5. Esteves SC. A clinical appraisal of the genetic basis in unexplained male infertility. J Hum Reprod Sci. 2013;6:176–82.
6. Esteves SC, Chan P. A systematic review of recent clinical practice guidelines and best practice statements for the evaluation of the infertile male. Int Urol Nephrol. 2015;47:1441–56.
7. Lewis SE, John Aitken R, Conner SJ, Iuliis GD, Evenson DP, Henkel R, et al. The impact of sperm DNA damage in assisted conception and beyond: recent advances in diagnosis and treatment. Reprod BioMed Online. 2013;27:325–37.
8. Esteves SC, Gosálvez J, López-Fernández C, Núñez-Calonge R, Caballero P, Agarwal A, Fernández JL. Diagnostic accuracy of sperm DNA degradation index (DDSi) as a potential noninvasive biomarker to identify men with. Int Urol Nephrol. 2015;47:1471–7.
9. Lewis SE. Should sperm DNA fragmentation testing be included in the male infertility work-up? Reprod BioMed Online. 2015;31:134–7.
10. Gosálvez J, Lopez-Fernandez C, Fernandez JL, Esteves SC, Johnston SD. Unpacking the mysteries of sperm DNA fragmentation: ten frequently asked questions. J Reprod Biotechnol Fertil. 2015;4:1–16.
11. Spano M, Bonde JP, Hjollund HI, Kolstad HA, Cordelli E, Leter G. Sperm chromatin damage impairs human fertility. The Danish First Pregnancy Planner Study Team. Fertil Steril. 2000;73:43–50.
12. Esteves SC, Sharma RK, Gosálvez J, Agarwal A. A translational medicine appraisal of specialized andrology testing in unexplained male infertility. Int Urol Nephrol. 2014;46:1037–52.
13. Agarwal A, Cho CL, Esteves SC. Should we evaluate and treat sperm DNA fragmentation? Curr Opin Obstet Gynecol. 2016;28:164–71.
14. Esteves SC. Novel concepts in male factor infertility: clinical and laboratory perspectives. J Assist Reprod Genet. 2016. https://doi.org/10.1007/s10815–016–0763–8.
15. Feijo CM, Esteves SC. Diagnostic accuracy of sperm chromatin dispersion test to evaluate sperm deoxyribonucleic acid damage in men with unexplained infertility. Fertil Steril. 2014;101:58–63.
16. Majzoub A, Esteves SC, Gosálvez J, Agarwal A. Specialized sperm function tests in varicocele and the future of andrology laboratory. Asian J Androl. 2016;18:205–12.
17. Aitken RJ, Krausz C. Oxidative stress, DNA damage and the Y chromosome. Reproduction. 2001;122:497–506.
18. Seli E, Gardner DK, Schoolcraft WB, Moffatt O, Sakkas D. Extent of nuclear DNA damage in ejaculated spermatozoa impacts on blastocyst development after in vitro fertilization. Fertil Steril. 2004;82:378–83.
19. Lewis SE, Aitken RJ. DNA damage to spermatozoa has impacts on fertilization and pregnancy. Cell Tissue Res. 2005;322:33–41.
20. Bungum M, Humaidan P, Axmon A, Spano M, Bungum L, Erenpreiss J, et al. Sperm DNA integrity assessment in prediction of assisted reproduction technology outcome. Hum Reprod. 2007;22:174–9.
21. Avendaño C, Franchi A, Duran H, Oehninger S. DNA fragmentation of normal spermatozoa negatively impacts embryo quality and intracytoplasmic sperm injection outcome. Fertil Steril. 2010;94:549–57.

22. Robinson L, Gallos ID, Conner SJ, Rajkhowa M, Miller D, Lewis S, et al. The effect of sperm DNA fragmentation on miscarriage rates: a systematic review and meta-analysis. Hum Reprod. 2012;27:2908–17.
23. Zini A, Boman JM, Belzile E, Ciampi A. Sperm DNA damage is associated with an increased risk of pregnancy loss after IVF and ICSI: systematic review and meta-analysis. Hum Reprod. 2008;23:2663–8.
24. Tesarik J, Greco E, Mendoza C. Late, but not early, paternal effect on human embryo development is related to sperm DNA fragmentation. Hum Reprod. 2004;19:611–5.
25. Wyrobek AJ, Eskenazi B, Young S, Arnheim N, Tiemann-Boege I, Jabs EW, Glaser RL, Pearson FS, Evenson D. Advancing age has differential effects on DNA damage, chromatin integrity, gene mutations, and aneuploidies in sperm. Proc Natl Acad Sci U S A. 2006;103:9601–6.
26. Belloc S, Cohen-Bacrie P, Benkhalifa M, Cohen-Bacrie M, De MJ, Hazout A, et al. Effect of maternal and paternal age on pregnancy and miscarriage rates after intrauterine insemination. Reprod BioMed Online. 2008;17:392–7.
27. Sakkas D, Alvarez JG. Sperm DNA fragmentation: mechanisms of origin, impact on reproductive outcome, and analysis. Fertil Steril. 2010;93:1027–36.
28. Ji J, Pan C, Fei Q, Ni W, Yang X, Zhang L, et al. Effect of sperm DNA fragmentation on the clinical outcomes for in vitro fertilization and intracytoplasmic sperm injection in women with different ovarian reserve. Fertil Steril. 2015;103:910–6.
29. Wang YJ, Zhang RQ, Lin YJ, Zhang RG, Zhang WL. Relationship between varicocele and sperm DNA damage and the effect of varicocele repair: a meta-analysis. Reprod BioMed Online. 2012;25:307–14.
30. Zini A, San Gabriel M, Baazeem A. Antioxidants and sperm DNA damage: a clinical perspective. J Assist Reprod Genet. 2009;26:427–32.
31. Abad C, Amengual ML, Gosálvez J, Coward K, Hannaoui N, Benet J, et al. Effects of oral antioxidant treatment upon the dynamics of human sperm DNA fragmentation and subpopulations of sperm with highly degraded DNA. Andrologia. 2013;45:211–6.
32. Agarwal A, Gupta S, Du Plessis S, Sharma R, Esteves SC, Cirenza C, Eliwa J, Al-Najjar W, Kumaresan D, Haroun N, Philby S, Sabanegh E. Abstinence time and its impact on basic and advanced semen parameters. Urology. 2016;94:102–10.
33. Raziel A, Friedler S, Schachter M, Kaufman S, Omanski A, Soffer Y, et al. Influence of a short or long abstinence period on semen parameters in the ejaculate of patients with nonobstructive azoospermia. Fertil Steril. 2001;76:485–90.
34. Gosálvez J, González-Martínez M, López-Fernández C, Fernández JL, Sánchez-Martín P. Shorter abstinence decreases sperm deoxyribonucleic acid fragmentation in ejaculate. Fertil Steril. 2011;96:1083–6.
35. Said TM, Grunewald S, Paasch U, Rasch M, Agarwal A, Glander HJ. Advantage of combining magnetic cell separation with sperm preparation techniques. Reprod BioMed Online. 2005;10:740–6.
36. Sharma RK, Kattoor AJ, Ghulmiyyah J, Agarwal A. Effect of sperm storage and selection techniques on sperm parameters. Syst Biol Reprod Med. 2015;61:1–12.
37. Parmegiani L, Cognigni GE, Bernardi S, Troilo E, Taraborrelli S, Arnone A, et al. Comparison of two ready-to-use systems designed for sperm-hyaluronic acid binding selection before intracytoplasmic sperm injection: PICSI vs. sperm slow: a prospective, randomized trial. Fertil Steril. 2012;98:632–7.
38. Antinori M, Licata E, Dani G, Cerusico F, Versaci C, d'Angelo D, et al. Intracytoplasmic morphologically selected sperm injection: a prospective randomized trial. Reprod BioMed Online. 2008;16:835–41.
39. Cassuto NG, Hazout A, Bouret D, Balet R, Larue L, Benifla JL, et al. Low birth defects by deselecting abnormal spermatozoa before ICSI. Reprod BioMed Online. 2014;28:47–53.
40. Gosálvez J, Migueles B, López-Fernández C, Sanchéz-Martín F, Sáchez-Martín P. Single sperm selection and DNA fragmentation analysis: the case of MSOME/IMSI. Nat Sci. 2013;5:7–14.

41. Greco E, Scarselli F, Iacobelli M, Rienzi L, Ubaldi F, Ferrero S, et al. Efficient treatment of infertility due to sperm DNA damage by ICSI with testicular spermatozoa. Hum Reprod. 2005;20:226–30.
42. Steele EK, McClure N, Maxwell RJ, Lewis SE. A comparison of DNA damage in testicular and proximal epididymal spermatozoa in obstructive azoospermia. Mol Hum Reprod. 1999;5:831–5.
43. Suganuma R, Yanagimachi R, Meistrich ML. Decline in fertility of mouse sperm with abnormal chromatin during epididymal passage as revealed by ICSI. Hum Reprod. 2005;20:3101–8.
44. Britan A, Maffre V, Tone S, Drevet JR. Quantitative and spatial differences in the expression of tryptophan-metabolizing enzymes in mouse epididymis. Cell Tissue Res. 2006;324:301–10.
45. Hamada A, Esteves SC, Agarwal A. Insight into oxidative stress in varicocele-associated male infertility: part 2. Nat Rev Urol. 2013;10:26–37.
46. Banks S, King SA, Irvine DS, Saunders PT. Impact of a mild scrotal heat stress on DNA integrity in murine spermatozoa. Reproduction. 2005;129:505–14.
47. Rubes J, Selevan SG, Sram RJ, Evenson DP, Perreault SD. GSTM1 genotype influences the susceptibility of men to sperm DNA damage associated with exposure to air pollution. Mut Res. 2007;625:20–8.
48. Agarwal A, Hamada A, Esteves SC. Insight into oxidative stress in varicocele-associated male infertility: part 1. Nat Rev Urol. 2012;9(12):678–90.
49. Cho CL, Esteves SC, Agarwal A. Novel insights into the pathophysiology of varicocele and its association with reactive oxygen species and sperm DNA fragmentation. Asian J Androl. 2016;18(2):186–93.
50. Esteves SC, Sánchez-Martín F, Sánchez-Martín P, Schneider DT, Gosálvez J. Comparison of reproductive outcome in oligozoospermic men with high sperm DNA fragmentation undergoing intracytoplasmic sperm injection with ejaculated and testicular sperm. Fertil Steril. 2015;104:1398–405.
51. Moskovtsev SI, Jarvi K, Mullen JBM, Cadesky KI, Hannam T, Lo KC. Testicular spermatozoa have statistically significantly lower DNA damage compared with ejaculated spermatozoa in patients with unsuccessful oral antioxidant treatment. Fertil Steril. 2010;93:1142–6.
52. Mehta A, Bolyakov A, Schlegel PN, Paduch DA. Higher pregnancy rates using testicular sperm in men with severe oligospermia. Fertil Steril. 2015;104:1382–7.
53. Esteves SC, Miyaoka R, Agarwal A. Sperm retrieval techniques for assisted reproduction. Int Braz J Urol. 2011;37:570–83.
54. Gosalvez J, Gonzalez-Martínez M, Lopez-Fernandez C, Fernandez JL, Sanchez-Martín P. Shorter abstinence decreases sperm deoxyribonucleic acid fragmentation in ejaculate. Fertil Steril. 2011;96:1083–6.
55. Ben-Ami I, Raziel A, Strassburger D, Komarovsky D, Ron-El R, Friedler S. Intracytoplasmic sperm injection outcome of ejaculated versus extracted testicular spermatozoa in cryptozoospermic men. Fertil Steril. 2013;99:1867–71.
56. Weissman A, Horowitz E, Ravhon A, Nahum H, Golan A, Levran D. Pregnancies and live births following ICSI with testicular spermatozoa after repeated implantation failure using ejaculated spermatozoa. Reprod BioMed Online. 2008;17:605–9.
57. Abhyankar N, Kathrins M, Niederberger C. Use of testicular versus ejaculated sperm for intracytoplasmic sperm injection among men with cryptozoospermia: a meta-analysis. Fertil Steril. 2016;105:1469–75.
58. Hauser R, Bibi G, Yogev L, Carmon A, Azem F, Botchan A, Yavetz H, Klieman SE, Lehavi O, Amit A, Ben-Yosef D. Virtual azoospermia and cryptozoospermia—fresh/frozen testicular or ejaculate sperm for better IVF outcome? J Androl. 2011;32:484–90.
59. Zhao J, Zhang Q, Wang Y, Li Y. Whether sperm deoxyribonucleic acid fragmentation has an effect on pregnancy and miscarriage after in vitro fertilization/intracytoplasmic sperm injection: a systematic review and meta-analysis. Fertil Steril. 2014;102:998–1005.
60. Bradley CK, McArthur SJ, Gee AJ, Weiss KA, Schmidt U, Toogood L. Intervention improves assisted conception intracytoplasmic sperm injection outcomes for patients with high levels of sperm DNA fragmentation: a retrospective analysis. Andrology. 2016;4:903–10.

61. García-Peiró A, Martínez-Heredia J, Oliver-Bonet M, Abad C, Amengual MJ, Navarro J, et al. Protamine 1 to protamine 2 ratio correlates with dynamic aspects of DNA fragmentation in human sperm. Fertil Steril. 2011;95:105–9.
62. Muriel L, Goyanes V, Segrelles E, Gosalvez J, Alvarez JG, Fernandez JL. Increased aneuploidy rate in sperm with fragmented DNA as determined by the sperm chromatin dispersion (SCD) test and FISH analysis. J Androl. 2007;28:38–49.
63. Bernardine L, Gianaroli L, Fortini D, Conte N, Magli C, Cavani S, et al. Frequency of hyper-hypohaploidy and diploidy in ejaculate, epididymal and testicular germ cells of infertile patients. Hum Reprod. 2000;15:2165–72.
64. Mateizel I, Verheyen G, Van Assche E, Tournaye H, Liebaers I, Van Steirteghem A. FISH analysis of chromosome X, Y and 18 abnormalities in testicular sperm from azoospermic patients. Hum Reprod. 2002;17:2249–57.
65. Palermo GD, Colombero LT, Hariprashad JJ, Schlegel PN, Rosenwaks Z. Chromosome analysis of epididymal and testicular sperm in azoospermic patients undergoing ICSI. Hum Reprod. 2002;17:570–5.
66. Egozcue J, Sarrate Z, Codina-Pascual M, Egozcue S, Oliver-Bonet M, Blanco J, et al. Meiotic abnormalities in infertile males. Cytogenet Genome Res. 2005;11:337–42.
67. Moskovtsev SI, Alladin N, Lo KC, Jarvi K, Mullen JBM, Librach CL. A comparison of ejaculated and testicular spermatozoa aneuploidy rates in patients with high sperm DNA damage. Syst Biol Reprod Med. 2012;58:142–8.

Chapter 30
Debate on the Use of Testicular Sperm for ICSI: Con

Peter T.K. Chan

30.1 Introduction

In the previous chapter, Dr. Esteves provided compelling evidence why surgically retrieved testicular sperm can provide superior reproductive outcomes compared to using ejaculated sperm for ICSI in some infertile couples. In reality, the statement that "testicular sperm performs better than ejaculated sperm with ICSI" is at best controversial. The purpose of this chapter is to present alternative interpretations and critiques on the existing data in the current literature and to provide readers different perspectives on this complex and controversial issue of testicular versus ejaculated sperm on ICSI outcomes.

Surgical sperm retrieval procedure from the testis for ICSI generally can be performed percutaneously under local anesthesia without requiring a scrotal incision in an outpatient office setting. However, testicular sperm aspiration (TESA) and extraction (TESE) can be associated with complications [1–5] such as bleeding, hematoma, pain, scrotal swelling, and infection. Men who have baseline impaired spermatogenic function are at higher risks for complications as they may require multiple testicular punctures to obtain adequate amount of sperm. This, along with the cost and added complexity of sperm processing in the embryology laboratory associated with surgically retrieved testicular sperm, is among the reasons why ejaculated sperm is the first choice for ICSI in patients attempting their first trial of ICSI, so long as they are of adequate quantity and quality, as reflected by their motility and morphology, for the number of mature oocyte retrieved in the ICSI

P.T.K. Chan (✉)
Department of Surgery (Urology), McGill University and the McGill Univeristy Health Centre, Montréal, QC, Canada
e-mail: McGillSperminator@yahoo.com

A. Zini, A. Agarwal (eds.), *A Clinician's Guide to Sperm DNA and Chromatin Damage*, https://doi.org/10.1007/978-3-319-71815-6_30

cycle. Indeed, most earlier studies have stated that regardless whether the source of sperm for ICSI is from the testis or ejaculation, ICSI outcomes were similar [6–11], and, in particular, testicular sperm do not necessarily perform better than ejaculated sperm [12]. Thus, despite the strong arguments provided by Dr. Esteves in the previous chapter that testicular sperm perform better than ejaculated sperm, most experts would argue against using testicular sperm upfront for the first ICSI cycle among men with adequate number of usable ejaculated sperm. The same notion holds true even among those with subnormal semen parameters or with repeated failure with IUI or conventional IVF.

30.2 How the Idea of Using Testicular Sperm Instead of Ejaculated Sperm for ICSI Came About

The recommendation of using testicular sperm despite having adequate usable ejaculated sperm for ICSI generally is usually made when the infertile couple has one or more of the following conditions. First, there is previously history of ICSI failure at postfertilization steps including poor embryo quality, failure of implantation, or early pregnancy loss at first trimester. Second, there are anomalies in semen parameters, particularly with regard to the quality of sperm such as severe astheno-teratospermia or impaired sperm chromatin integrity that cannot be corrected or reversed (e.g., by lifestyle modification, medical treatment for underlying infection/inflammation, correction of clinical varicoceles, usage of antioxidants or other empirical therapies). Third, there is absence of significant female infertility factor to account for the ICSI failure.

The idea behind using testicular sperm for ICSI after failure with ejaculated sperm probably originated from the early observations by various investigators [13, 14] that in some men with severe oligo-astheno-teratospermia (OAT) or cryptozoospermia or sperm DNA damage, testicular sperm may have better quality and perform better with ICSI. This idea then somehow gets extrapolated to infer that other men with adequate ejaculated sperm but failed ICSI could also benefit from using testicular sperm to repeat ICSI. What one may not realize is that studies showing testicular sperm performed better than ejaculated sperm in severe OAT or cryptozoospermia may have included, albeit inadvertently, men with partial obstruction of the excurrent ductal system (e.g., incomplete ejaculatory ductal obstruction, postvasectomy reversal, inflammation of the epididymis or other parts of the excurrent ductal system) or ejaculatory dysfunction (neurogenic or situational) who have normal spermatogenic function. Indeed, some reports claiming superior ICSI outcomes with testicular sperm either left out or provided imprecise description of important information on the patient characteristics such as past history, physical examination (physique, testicular volume, etc.), hormonal profile, etc. [13, 15, 16]. To be fair, even experienced clinicians may sometimes have doubt whether a cryptozoospermic man may have partial obstruction of the excurrent ductal system contributing to their poor semen parameters. Even in studies when efforts were made to obtain testicular biopsies to confirm spermatogenic dysfunction, a significant portion of subjects may have incomplete data [13] to completely rule out the inclusion of men with normal spermatogenesis with obstructive causes of infertility. Fresh testicular sperm from men with obstruction and normal spermatogenesis may have better quality [17, 18] than post-testicular sperm. Hence, it is not surprising that testicular sperm could perform better with ICSI than with the aged and degenerated sperm that eventually make it to the semen from a severely obstructed system. Using testicular sperm for ICSI in such a scenario may yield different outcomes than in men with impaired spermatogenic function or other testicular factors contributing to poor ejaculated sperm quantitatively and qualitatively.

30.3 Reasons Why All Parties Willingly Accept Using Testicular Sperm Instead of Ejaculated Sperm for ICSI

With the significant negative factors including risks and cost associated with testicular surgical sperm retrieval and with another cycle of ICSI, why would all the involved parties (reproductive urologists, REIs, embryologists, patients) readily accept and go forward with this treatment plan? The reason perhaps is more than just their beliefs that it would yield better outcome (which as we will see later in this chapter is based on circumstantial evidence at best). The thought processes of how the various parties involved readily come to an agreement to proceed with another ICSI cycle using testicular sperm are worth a discussion.

It is conceivable that part of the reasons of their acceptance is that there are enough gains for all involved parties to repeat ICSI with testicular sperm. First, the REI and the reproductive center would welcome additional treatment cycles for the obvious reason of financial gain. Even for urologists, performing testicular sperm extraction for ICSI represents additional financial gain that would not have been present otherwise if the couples are to use only ejaculated sperm. The relative risks of repeating ICSI with testicular sperm for both treating parties are generally acceptable and outweighed by these gains. Financial gain aside, when counseling these couples, having something potentially promising to offer them is far better than admitting that they do not know what went wrong, that they have reached the limit of their knowledge or ability, and that the couple should seek help from bigger and better centers. Even from the patients, particularly those who are frustrated with repeated ICSI failure and are desperate for success, knowing that there is hope with something as "simple" as using testicular sperm obtained through a relatively minor procedure is indeed comforting. Despite recurrent failure, many of these couples are financially prepared and willing to give it one more trial while accepting the associated risks and burdens, even if it is just for the purpose of having a proper "closure" of their journey. Another very important point: these couples are well prepared for yet another failure. Thus, any success would be a bonus—nothing to lose but all to gain! With these thoughts in mind, it is understandable why the notion of repeating ICSI with testicular sperm would face little resistance or challenge by all involved parties and that any favorable evidence, even when they are circumstantial at best, would be welcomed and inadequately scrutinized to justify their presumptions that testicular sperm is better than ejaculated sperm for ICSI.

30.4 Any Scientific Basis Indicating that Testicular Sperm Are Better than Ejaculated Sperm?

Some studies have speculated on the biological mechanisms that support why sperm surgically retrieved from the testes are better than epididymal [17, 18] and ejaculated sperm [14, 19–22], as Dr. Esteves discussed in the previous chapter. Unfortunately, the citation of these studies serves only to support a view (that testicular sperm is "better" than ejaculated sperm) that the authors have already accepted. Virtually every report claiming better reproductive outcomes with ICSI with testicular sperm has quoted these same studies in their discussion to "support" their reported findings. To have a more balanced perspective, readers should be aware also that there are studies in the literature indicating that testicular sperm is "biologically inferior" to post-testicular and ejaculated sperm for reproduction. The rationales include poor motility, poor fertilizing capacity, and even higher aneuploidy rates associated with testicular sperm [21, 23–30]—all can potentially be linked to adverse reproductive outcomes. It is not difficult to imagine that for investigators reporting inferior reproductive outcomes with testicular sperm than ejaculated sperm, this latter group of studies will be quoted and emphasized in their discussion instead. Thus, a detailed discussion of the underlying biological mechanisms, though extremely important to allow advancement in our understanding on the physiological processes of human reproduction, serves little in settling the debate of whether testicular sperm is superior to ejaculated sperm for ICSI.

30.5 Critiques on the Current Literature Demonstrating Testicular Sperm Is Better than Ejaculated Sperm for ICSI

30.5.1 The Difficulties in Conducting a Proper Study Design

To demonstrate that testicular sperm yields superior results with ICSI to ejaculated sperm, properly designed comparative studies must be conducted and confirmed by other centers with comparable results. Obviously, properly designed randomized controlled trials (RCT) would be ideal. As any investigators would agree, conducting an RCT with enough power to detect a significant improvement in the ICSI outcomes of testicular vs ejaculated sperm is far from being easy. Just to recruit enough subjects or couples that would match with various important variables such as age (particularly female age), reproductive status (ovarian reserve, baseline FSH), lifestyle and comorbidities, semen parameters, and baseline sperm chromatin quality would be extremely difficult. Further, the procedures involved in the processing of ejaculated and testicular sperm in the embryology laboratory are distinctive enough to make proper blinding from the embryologists in the treatment arms complicated in a trial setting. From the perspectives of the infertile couples, under a research trial setting, when presented with the choices of repeating (and thus paying for) the same treatment that previously or repeatedly failed versus another potentially better choice (instead of being presented with two different approaches that may potentially perform better than their past failed cycles), it is understandable that many couples may decline to participate in the trial and request to repeat ICSI using testicular sperm. This would certainly make recruitment and randomization difficult and prone to bias. Thus, the literature on this topic consists mainly of retrospective case series with large variations in the characteristics of the comparison or control groups and in the comparative models used.

30.5.2 The Impact of Publication Bias

Despite the inclusion of some levels of quantitative or statistical analyses in their comparative models, case series in any subject in medical science or clinical research tend to have small number of subjects. More importantly, by nature of them being retrospective, they were not exactly planned out by the investigators but likely observed by chance by the investigators to have favorable outcomes. This means that perhaps the investigators noticed a trend of the outcomes (e.g., a series of ICSI cycles with testicular sperm seemed to have better outcomes than with ejaculated) and then followed on this hunch to carry out data analysis to develop a manuscript. Unfortunately, this research methodology, though seemingly reasonable and logical, would lead to publication bias.

Let us assume that the ultimate truth is that the outcomes of ICSI with testicular sperm are NOT different from those with ejaculated sperm. Then in a small series of patients, simply by chance, the investigators may observe that ICSI with testicular sperm yields BETTER outcomes than with ejaculated sperm, leading to the production of a manuscript supporting a false claim. Of course, sometimes with a small sample size, an observed difference in the outcomes between groups may not pass a proper statistical analysis to demonstrate its significance. This disappointing result often led investigators to perform more complex statistical or analytical maneuvers on the raw data to develop alternative comparative models until they reach one that could demonstrate statistically significant differences in some measured variables between groups for publication. Alternatively, some investigators would choose to highlight a clinical trend between group results despite the absence of a statistically significant difference. In other times, the investigators may simply call off the study.

Moreover, investigators who failed to notice a difference between using testicular or ejaculated sperm for ICSI may simply not have initiated further analyses to avoid wasting time, energy, money, and other resources to generate a manuscript with negative results that may be rejected for publication. As a result, the current literature on the subject may contain preferentially studies from investigators that noticed, perhaps by chance, a difference in a small retrospective series of patients from their centers. Without understanding the impact of this publication bias, when seeing a series of publications from various reputable centers and investigators, using various methodologies and perhaps sophisticated analyses, coming to a similar conclusion, one could easily be misled to believe the face value of these reports. The impact of this publication bias may go even further. Seeing so many existing publications, some from world-renowned groups of investigators and large centers, as listed by Dr. Esteves in the previous chapter, supporting the use of testicular sperm for ICSI for better outcomes, other investigators who do not notice a benefit with testicular sperm for ICSI in their centers would understandably hesitate to report their negative results unless they have, instead of data from yet another whimsy case series, solid and high-quality data from a properly designed RCT to prove otherwise. Thus, few contemporary publications exist on this subject demonstrating no statistically significant differences in ICSI outcomes between using testicular or ejaculated sperm [11, 31, 32].

30.5.3 The Need to Demonstrate Impact on Relevant Clinical Outcomes

But let's take a closer look at the existing studies supporting the use of testicular sperm for a repeat ICSI. What reproductive outcomes should studies include to illustrate superiority when using testicular sperm compared to ejaculated sperm for ICSI? Obviously various outcomes from sperm quality (motility, morphology, chromatin structure integrity, aneuploidy, etc.), fertilization rate, embryo qualities, implantation rate, clinical pregnancy rate, ongoing pregnancy rate, and miscarriage rate are all considered important parameters. For clinicians and particularly for infertile couples, however, it is healthy live-birth rate that matters most. Thus, studies that reported a statistically significant superiority of various reproductive outcomes other than live-birth rate [10, 16, 33] or did not report the rate of healthy live-birth [16, 20, 33, 34] inevitably limit the impact of their studies on modifying the counseling strategies clinicians can use for their patients. In fact, it is puzzlingly rare to see investigators of these studies publishing subsequent reports to include live-birth rates of their series with expanded sample sizes. Theoretically speaking, if using testicular sperm for ICSI yield better outcomes in most parameters but not a significantly higher live-birth rate, this may imply a higher rate of subsequent adverse outcome such as failure of implantation, early or late pregnancy loss, or miscarriage. In other words, while using testicular sperm for ICSI may allow the infertile couples to advance further in their progress on the reproductive journey, they may risk eventual failure at a more advanced stage of pregnancy which can be more devastating and dangerous than an early failure. Thus, demonstration of improvement in healthy live-birth rate is a key for these types of studies.

30.5.4 Improper Comparison and Additional Confounding Factors in the Current Literature

On the methodology and design of the studies, simply demonstrating success with live-births [35, 36] or whatever relevant reproductive outcomes [10, 16, 33] when using testicular sperm with ICSI among couples with previous failure of ICSI with ejaculated sperm cannot be considered convincing evidence. First, these studies were generally conducted in large, reputable reproductive centers with presumably higher overall success rate than the average reproductive centers. Therefore, previous failures of ICSI performed in smaller, less experienced centers and later success in bigger centers with special expertise may simply be a reflection of the higher level of experience of the bigger centers rather than any true benefits of using testicular sperm for ICSI. Further, even when these couples had undergone previous failed ICSI with ejaculated sperm within *the same centers*, the fact that these same couples had subsequent success in ICSI with testicular sperm cannot be fairly attributed to any potential benefits of using testicular sperm. This is simply because all the subjects began with a 0% or very poor success (from previous failed ICSI cycles with ejaculated sperm); the outcomes of a subsequent trial of ICSI (with testicular sperm) can thus only be better. It is important to appreciate that there exists also a series of couples who have success with a repeat ICSI simply using ejaculated sperm again. But this latter group offers little innovation or interest and as a result was not discussed in most of the publications. Indeed, in one of the most recent studies on this subject, Pabuccu et al. [34] reported a clinical pregnancy rate per started ICSI cycles with testicular sperm to be over 40% in couples with repeated ART failure (mean 3.2 trials of previous failed ART). But in couples with a significantly more complex history of recurrent ART failure (mean 4.0 trials of previous failed ART, $p < 0.02$), repeating ICSI with ejaculated sperm once again yielded a clinical pregnancy rate of still 20%. This highlights the importance of having a proper comparison group to allow proper interpretation of study outcomes.

Another important consideration is that the better outcomes observed in repeat ICSI with testicular sperm may be attributed to modifications of other factors in the latest cycle that can allow for higher success rates (e.g., more efficient stimulation protocol, embryo transfer performed more cautiously with more experienced personnel or significantly more embryo transferred per cycle in the subsequent testicular sperm cycle, use of ICSI instead of mainly or only conventional IVF in previously failed cycle, etc.) [15, 36]. The couples may also have changed their lifestyle significantly (weight reduction, use of antioxidant, cessation of smoking, etc.) that led to better fertility status and treatment outcomes.

30.6 Looking Forward

Clearly, we still lack adequate, definitive evidence to conclude that testicular sperm performs better with ICSI than ejaculated sperm. For investigators who truly believe ICSI with testicular is better, in addition to striving to conduct better investigations, it is important to define what subgroups of patients (e.g., based on semen parameters, previous ART outcomes, age or other reproductive status) would benefit, and to what extent would such a benefit be, from repeating ICSI with testicular sperm. Equally valuable is to identify those couples who are UNLIKELY to benefit from a repeat ICSI cycle with testicular sperm. This is a particularly important consideration when there are significant coexisting female infertility factors in the couples, as most studies on this subject have excluded female partners with poor ovarian reserves or responses [13, 15, 16, 20, 34, 37]. Likewise, some men with infertility due to certain well-described, though rare, specific defects identified in the ejaculated sperm such as complete globozoospermia characterized by secondary absence of acrosome [38–44], macrocephalospermia [45, 46], and sperm neck defects with centriole dysfunction [47–54] should not undergo testicular sperm extraction, as their testicular sperm will likely have the same defect and thus would not contribute to an improved success rate.

There are further questions that we must be prepared to answer. As discussed above, several studies [20, 36, 37] on this subject indicated that one of the important reasons why testicular sperm performs better than ejaculated sperm is due to their better sperm chromatin structure, as determined by various molecular assays. Does it mean that the benefits of using testicular sperm are only found in men with better testicular sperm chromatin structure results but not in those with results that are equally bad or worse than those in ejaculated sperm? If so, does that mean before contemplating using testicular sperm for another ICSI cycle, these men should first undergo a testicular sperm extraction and measure sperm chromatin structure from both the testicular and ejaculated sperm and compare? Though the cost and risk of this evaluation are significant, at least this approach is less costly (and perhaps less risky) than a full ICSI cycle. To go one step further, if an infertile couple can only undergo one ICSI cycle (for financial, health, or other personal reasons), should they undergo testicular sperm and ejaculated sperm chromatin evaluation to decide what sperm to use for the one ICSI cycle that they can afford? Then should every couple have this evaluation prior to using ICSI? In other words, should we know what source of sperm to use upfront instead of waiting for ICSI failure with ejaculated sperm?

Finally, one potential benefit of facing this controversy is that the male partners of many of these "idiopathic" ART failure couples would get a referral to see a urologist for fertility evaluation that would otherwise not happen. At least in theory, this would allow significant pathologies and health risks including smoking, obesity, varicoceles, obstruction, inflammation, infection, testicular cancer, erectile dysfunction, and genetic and endocrinological anomalies to be diagnosed and managed. However, if the view that "testicular sperm with ICSI is better" prevails, all parties will persuade these couples to this route rather than offering proper evaluation and treatment to the male partners that may truly benefit their reproductive and general health. While awaiting further evidence, clinicians must recognize the limitations of the quality of current scientific evidence in the literature on the use of surgically retrieved testicular sperm for another cycle of ICSI to infertile couples experiencing unexplained failure of ICSI with ejaculated sperm and provide proper counseling to these frustrated, vulnerable, and often desperate couples, with prudent considerations on the risks, financial and psychosocial burdens, cost-effectiveness, and efficacy of further fertility treatment options.

Disclaimer The contents of this chapter are presented for informational and academic purposes only. It should not be used by patients in isolation without proper clinical counseling with experienced healthcare professionals to make any clinical decisions on their fertility management.

References

1. Friedler S, Raziel A, Strassburger D, Soffer Y, Komarovsky D, Ron-El R. Testicular sperm retrieval by percutaneous fine needle sperm aspiration compared with testicular sperm extraction by open biopsy in men with non-obstructive azoospermia. Hum Reprod. 1997;12(7):1488–93.
2. Schlegel PN, Su LM. Physiological consequences of testicular sperm extraction. Hum Reprod. 1997;12(8):1688–92.
3. Ron-El R, Strauss S, Friedler S, Strassburger D, Komarovsky D, Raziel A. Serial sonography and colour flow Doppler imaging following testicular and epididymal sperm extraction. Hum Reprod. 1998;13(12):3390–3.
4. Okada H, Dobashi M, Yamazaki T, Hara I, Fujisawa M, Arakawa S, Kamidono S. Conventional versus microdissection testicular sperm extraction for nonobstructive azoospermia. J Urol. 2002;168(3):1063–7.
5. Ramasamy R, Yagan N, Schlegel PN. Structural and functional changes to the testis after conventional versus microdissection testicular sperm extraction. Urology. 2005;65(6):1190–4.
6. Ghazzawi IM, Sarraf MG, Taher MR, Khalifa FA. Comparison of the fertilizing capability of spermatozoa from ejaculates, epididymal aspirates and testicular biopsies using intracytoplasmic sperm injection. Hum Reprod. 1998;13(2):348–52.
7. Ubaldi F, Nagy ZP, Rienzi L, Tesarik J, Anniballo R, Franco G, Menchini-Fabris F, Greco E. Reproductive capacity of spermatozoa from men with testicular failure. Hum Reprod. 1999;14(11):2796–800.
8. Bukulmez O, Yucel A, Yarali H, Bildirici I, Gurgan T. The origin of spermatozoa does not affect intracytoplasmic sperm injection outcome. Eur J Obstet Gynecol Reprod Biol. 2001;94(2):250–5.
9. Nicopoullos JD, Gilling-Smith C, Almeida PA, Norman-Taylor J, Grace I, Ramsay JW. Use of surgical sperm retrieval in azoospermic men: a meta-analysis. Fertil Steril. 2004;82(3):691–701.
10. Bendikson KA, Neri QV, Takeuchi T, Toschi M, Schlegel PN, Rosenwaks Z, Palermo GD. The outcome of intracytoplasmic sperm injection using occasional spermatozoa in the ejaculate of men with spermatogenic failure. J Urol. 2008;180(3):1060–4.
11. Amirjannati N, Heidari-Vala H, Akhondi MA, Hosseini Jadda SH, Kamali K, Sadeghi MR. Comparison of intracytoplasmic sperm injection outcomes between spermatozoa retrieved from testicular biopsy and from ejaculation in cryptozoospermic men. Andrologia. 2012;44(Suppl 1):704–9.
12. Nagy Z, Liu J, Cecile J, Silber S, Devroey P, Van Steirteghem A. Using ejaculated, fresh, and frozen-thawed epididymal and testicular spermatozoa gives rise to comparable results after intracytoplasmic sperm injection. Fertil Steril. 1995;63(4):808–15.

13. Hourvitz A, Shulman A, Madjar I, Levron J, Levran D, Mashiach S, Dor J. In vitro fertilization treatment for severe male factor: a comparative study of intracytoplasmic sperm injection with testicular sperm extraction and with spermatozoa from ejaculate. J Assist Reprod Genet. 1998;15(6):386–9.
14. Moskovtsev SI, Alladin N, Lo KC, Jarvi K, Mullen JB, Librach CL. A comparison of ejaculated and testicular spermatozoa aneuploidy rates in patients with high sperm DNA damage. Syst Biol Reprod Med. 2012;58(3):142–8.
15. Ben-Ami I, Raziel A, Strassburger D, Komarovsky D, Ron-El R, Friedler S. Intracytoplasmic sperm injection outcome of ejaculated versus extracted testicular spermatozoa in cryptozoospermic men. Fertil Steril. 2013;99(7):1867–71.
16. Hauser R, Bibi G, Yogev L, Carmon A, Azem F, Botchan A, Yavetz H, Klieman SE, Lehavi O, Amit A, Ben-Yosef D. Virtual azoospermia and cryptozoospermia—fresh/frozen testicular or ejaculate sperm for better IVF outcome? J Androl. 2011;32(5):484–90.
17. Steele EK, McClure N, Maxwell RJ, Lewis SE. A comparison of DNA damage in testicular and proximal epididymal spermatozoa in obstructive azoospermia. Mol Hum Reprod. 1999;5(9):831–5.
18. O'Connell M, McClure N, Lewis SE. A comparison of mitochondrial and nuclear DNA status in testicular sperm from fertile men and those with obstructive azoospermia. Hum Reprod. 2002;17(6):1571–7.
19. Tesarik J, Ubaldi F, Rienzi L, Martinez F, Iacobelli M, Mendoza C, Greco E. Caspase-dependent and -independent DNA fragmentation in Sertoli and germ cells from men with primary testicular failure: relationship with histological diagnosis. Hum Reprod. 2004;19(2):254–61.
20. Greco E, Scarselli F, Iacobelli M, Rienzi L, Ubaldi F, Ferrero S, Franco G, Anniballo N, Mendoza C, Tesarik J. Efficient treatment of infertility due to sperm DNA damage by ICSI with testicular spermatozoa. Hum Reprod. 2005;20(1):226–30.
21. Moskovtsev SI, Jarvi K, Mullen JB, Cadesky KI, Hannam T, Lo KC. Testicular spermatozoa have statistically significantly lower DNA damage compared with ejaculated spermatozoa in patients with unsuccessful oral antioxidant treatment. Fertil Steril. 2010;93(4):1142–6.
22. Sakkas D1, Alvarez JG. Sperm DNA fragmentation: mechanisms of origin, impact on reproductive outcome, and analysis. Fertil Steril. 2010;93(4):1027–36.
23. Bernardini L, Gianaroli L, Fortini D, Conte N, Magli C, Cavani S, Gaggero G, Tindiglia C, Ragni N, Venturini PL. Frequency of hyper-, hypohaploidy and diploidy in ejaculate, epididymal and testicular germ cells of infertile patients. Hum Reprod. 2000;15(10):2165–72.
24. Levron J, Aviram-Goldring A, Madgar I, Raviv G, Barkai G, Dor J. Sperm chromosome abnormalities in men with severe male factor infertility who are undergoing in vitro fertilization with intracytoplasmic sperm injection. Fertil Steril. 2001;76(3):479–84.
25. Burrello N, Calogero AE, De Palma A, Grazioso C, Torrisi C, Barone N, Pafumi C, D'Agata R, Vicari E. Chromosome analysis of epididymal and testicular spermatozoa in patients with azoospermia. Eur J Hum Genet. 2002;10(6):362–6.
26. Mateizel I, Verheyen G, Van Assche E, Tournaye H, Liebaers I, Van Steirteghem A. FISH analysis of chromosome X, Y and 18 abnormalities in testicular sperm from azoospermic patients. Hum Reprod. 2002;17(9):2249–57.
27. Palermo GD, Colombero LT, Hariprashad JJ, Schlegel PN, Rosenwaks Z. Chromosome analysis of epididymal and testicular sperm in azoospermic patients undergoing ICSI. Hum Reprod. 2002;17(3):570–5.
28. Gianaroli L, Magli MC, Cavallini G, Crippa A, Nadalini M, Bernardini L, Menchini Fabris GF, Voliani S, Ferraretti AP. Frequency of aneuploidy in sperm from patients with extremely severe male factor infertility. Hum Reprod. 2005;20(8):2140–52.
29. Rodrigo L, Rubio C, Mateu E, Simón C, Remohí J, Pellicer A, Gil-Salom M. Analysis of chromosomal abnormalities in testicular and epididymal spermatozoa from azoospermic ICSI patients by fluorescence in-situ hybridization. Hum Reprod. 2004;19(1):118–23.
30. Rodrigo L, Rubio C, Peinado V, Villamón R, Al-Asmar N, Remohí J, Pellicer A, Simón C, Gil-Salom M. Testicular sperm from patients with obstructive and nonobstructive azoosper-

mia: aneuploidy risk and reproductive prognosis using testicular sperm from fertile donors as control samples. Fertil Steril. 2011;95(3):1005–12.
31. Gnoth C, Markhinin V, Maxrath B, Skonieczny T, Friol K, Roos J, Rahimi G, Godehardt E. Impact of sperm cell source on the results of intracytoplasmic sperm injection. Arch Gynecol Obstet. 2015;291(3):663–9.
32. Abhyankar N, Kathrins M, Niederberger C. Use of testicular versus ejaculated sperm for intracytoplasmic sperm injection among men with cryptozoospermia: a meta-analysis. Fertil Steril. 2016;105(6):1469–1475.e1. https://doi.org/10.1016/j.fertnstert.2016.02.013. Epub 2016 Feb 28
33. Alrabeeah K, Yafi F, Flageole C, Phillips S, Wachter A, Bissonnette F, Kadoch IJ, Zini A. Testicular sperm aspiration for nonazoospermic men: sperm retrieval and intracytoplasmic sperm injection outcomes. Urology. 2014;84(6):1342–6.
34. Pabuccu EG, Caglar GS, Tangal S, Haliloglu AH, Pabuccu R. Testicular versus ejaculated spermatozoa in ICSI cycles of normozoospermic men with high sperm DNA fragmentation and previous ART failures. Andrologia. 2016. https://doi.org/10.1111/and.12609. [Epub ahead of print]
35. Weissman A, Horowitz E, Ravhon A, Nahum H, Golan A, Levran D. Pregnancies and live births following ICSI with testicular spermatozoa after repeated implantation failure using ejaculated spermatozoa. Reprod BioMed Online. 2008;17(5):605–9.
36. Mehta A, Bolyakov A, Schlegel PN, Paduch DA. Higher pregnancy rates using testicular sperm in men with severe oligospermia. Fertil Steril. 2015;104(6):1382–7.
37. Esteves SC, Sánchez-Martín F, Sánchez-Martín P, Schneider DT, Gosálvez J. Comparison of reproductive outcome in oligozoospermic men with high sperm DNA fragmentation undergoing intracytoplasmic sperm injection with ejaculated and testicular sperm. Fertil Steril. 2015;104(6):1398–405.
38. Dirican EK, Isik A, Vicdan K, Sozen E, Suludere Z. Clinical pregnancies and livebirths achieved by intracytoplasmic injection of round headed acrosomeless spermatozoa with and without oocyte activation in familial globozoospermia: case report. Asian J Androl. 2008;10:332–6.
39. Tejera A, Mollá M, Muriel L, Remohí J, Pellicer A, et al. Successful pregnancy and childbirth after intracytoplasmic sperm injection with calcium ionophore oocyte activation in a globozoospermic patient. Fertil Steril. 2008;90:1202.e1–5.
40. Kyono K, Nakajo Y, Nishinaka C, Hattori H, Kyoya T, et al. A birth from the transfer of a single vitrified-warmed blastocyst using intracytoplasmic sperm injection with calcium ionophore oocyte activation in a globozoospermic patient. Fertil Steril. 2009;91:931.e7–11.
41. Banker MR, Patel PM, Joshi BV, Shah PB, Goyal R. Successful pregnancies and a live birth after intracytoplasmic sperm injection in globozoospermia. J Hum Reprod Sci. 2009;2:81–2.
42. Egashira A, Murakami M, Haigo K, Horiuchi T, Kuramoto T. A successful pregnancy and live birth after intracytoplasmic sperm injection with globozoospermic sperm and electrical oocyte activation. Fertil Steril. 2009;2037(92):e5–9.
43. Taylor SL, Yoon SY, Morshedi MS, Lacey DR, Jellerette T, et al. Complete globozoospermia associated with PLCζ deficiency treated with calcium ionophore and ICSI results in pregnancy. Reprod BioMed Online. 2010;20:559–64.
44. Sermondade N, Hafhouf E, Dupont C, Bechoua S, Palacios C, et al. Successful childbirth after intracytoplasmic morphologically selected sperm injection without assisted oocyte activation in a patient with globozoospermia. Hum Reprod. 2011;26:2944–9.
45. Escalier D. Genetic approach to male meiotic division deficiency: the human macronuclear spermatozoa. Mol Hum Reprod. 2002;8(1):1–7.
46. Achard V, Paulmyer-Lacroix O, Mercier G, Porcu G, Saias-Magnan J, Metzler-Guillemain C, Guichaoua MR. Reproductive failure in patients with various percentages of macronuclear spermatozoa: high level of aneuploid and polyploid spermatozoa. J Androl. 2007;28(4):600–6.
47. Chemes HE, Puigdomenech ET, Carizza C, Brugo Olmedo S, Zanchetti F, et al. Acephalic spermatozoa and abnormal development of the head–neck attachment. A human syndrome of genetic origin. Hum Reprod. 1999;14:1811–8.

48. Saias-Magnan J, Metzler-Guillemain C, Mercier G, Carles-Marcorelles F, Grillo JM, et al. Failure of pregnancy after intracytoplasmic sperm injection with decapitated spermatozoa: case report. Hum Reprod. 1999;14:1989–92.
49. Porcu G, Mercier G, Boyer P, Achard V, Banet J, et al. Pregnancies after ICSI using sperm with abnormal head–tail junction from two brothers: case report. Hum Reprod. 2003;18:562–7.
50. Emery BR, Thorp C, Malo JW, Carrell DT. Pregnancy from intracytoplasmic sperm injection of a sperm head ad detached tail. Fertil Steril. 2004;81:686–8.
51. Rawe VY, Díaz ES, Abdelmassih R, Wójcik C, Morales P, et al. The role of sperm proteasomes during sperm aster formation and early zygote development: implications for fertilization failure in humans. Hum Reprod. 2008;23:573–80.
52. Gambera L, Falcone P, Mencaglia L, Collodel G, Serafini F, et al. Intracytoplasmic sperm injection and pregnancy with decapitated sperm. Fertil Steril. 2010;93:1347.e7–12.
53. Nakamura S, Terada Y, Rawe VY, Uehara S, Morito Y, et al. A trial to restore defective human sperm centrosomal function. Hum Reprod. 2005;20:1933–7.
54. Terada Y, Schatten G, Hasegawa H, Yaegashi N. Essential roles of the sperm centrosome in human fertilization: developing the therapy for fertilization failure due to sperm centrosomal dysfunction. Tohoku J Exp Med. 2010;220:247–58.

Chapter 31
Strategies to Diminish DNA Damage in Sperm Samples Used for ART

Jaime Gosálvez, Ashok Agarwal, and Sandro C. Esteves

31.1 Introduction

31.1.1 Sperm DNA Fragmentation and Reproductive Outcome

In general, individuals presenting high levels of sperm DNA fragmentation (SDF) in their ejaculates have poor semen quality parameters, including reduced sperm count, motility, and morphology [1–3]. Moreover, assisted reproductive outcomes of couples whose male partner has high SDF are poorer than those in whom SDF is not a contributory factor [4]. It has been reported that SDF levels are three times higher in men attending infertility clinics with different etiology categories than those observed in sperm donors [5, 6]. Furthermore, SDF has been shown to accurately discriminate populations of infertile from normal men. At a cutoff level of 16%, SDF assessed by the sperm chromatin dispersion test (SCD) discriminate both populations with sensitivity of 85% and specificity of 75% [6, 7]. This means that SDF results in a net ejaculate provide useful information that is complementary to but more distinct than those of conventional semen analysis. Overall, the actual role of SDF testing has been undervalued. We believe that there are at least two crucial aspects requiring further research, namely, (1) quantitative SDF, which accounts for

J. Gosálvez (✉)
University Autonoma Madrid, Madrid, Spain
e-mail: jaime.gosalvez@uam.es

A. Agarwal
American Center for Reproductive Medicine, Glickman Urological and Kidney Institute, Cleveland Clinic, Cleveland, OH, USA
e-mail: agarwaa@ccf.org

S.C. Esteves
Andrology and Human Reproduction Clinic, ANDROFERT, Campinas, Brazil
e-mail: s.esteves@androfert.com.br

A. Zini, A. Agarwal (eds.), *A Clinician's Guide to Sperm DNA and Chromatin Damage*, https://doi.org/10.1007/978-3-319-71815-6_31

the relative amount of sperm affected in the neat ejaculate and/or post-processing, and (2) qualitative SDF, which accounts for the presence of single- or double-strand breaks or alternative DNA configurations to a Watson-Crick and the respective association to the capacity of the oocyte for DNA repair.

In general, a direct relationship between a discrete value of SDF and the reproductive outcome cannot be clearly demonstrated [8]. This is partially due to the fact that ART has been refined and is able to decrease the probability of selecting defective sperm for fertilization. Additionally, there are confounding factors that may account for the conflicting results concerning the predictive value of SDF on pregnancy outcomes. For instance, it is important to estimate the amount of iatrogenic sperm DNA damage generated during sperm handling in vitro before fertilization. Secondly, it is

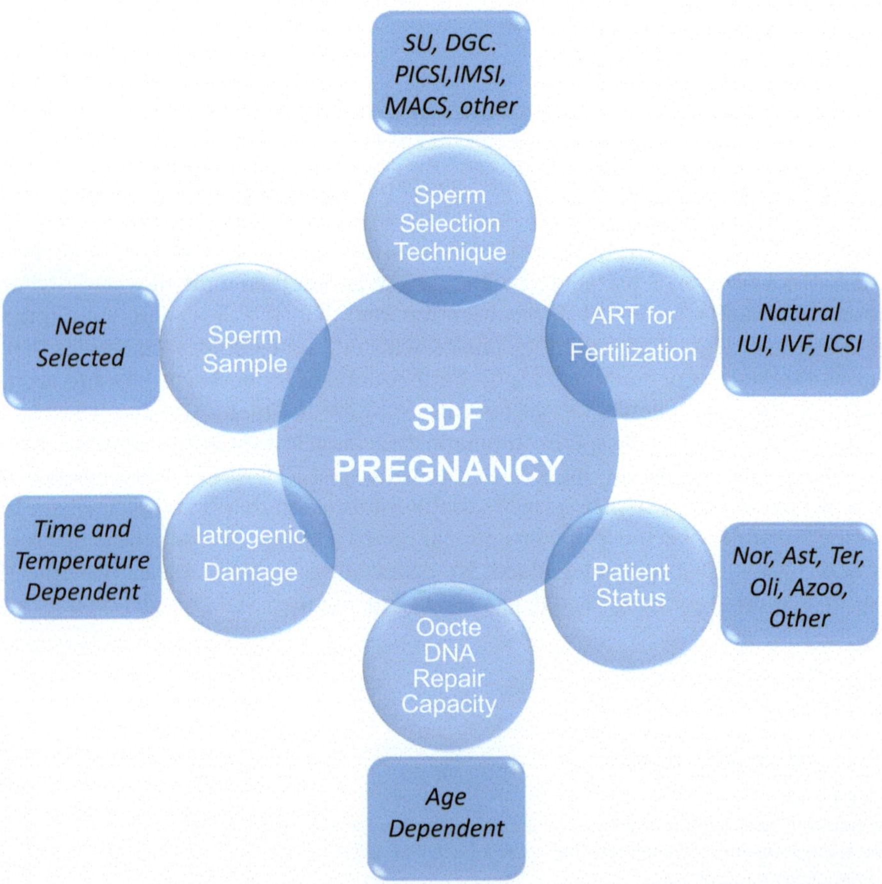

Fig. 31.1 A map of putative modulators that may influence sperm DNA fragmentation (SDF) having a negative impact on pregnancy. The complex interaction of multiple factors as depicted in the figure may help to understand why the search for a cutoff value of SDF in the neat ejaculate that is able to predict the pregnancy outcome would be challenging

important to investigate the association between other seminal characteristics and SDF values. Lastly, little is known about the effectiveness and fidelity of DNA repair at the oocyte level once fertilization has occurred. Likewise, different sperm selection techniques and various strategies used to fertilize the oocyte may also affect the fertilization rates, embryo development, and pregnancy rates.

In fact, seeking for a discrete number of SDF value that is directly associated with reproductive outcome is difficult because the whole biological process involved is rather complex with many inherent and uncontrolled patient factors as well as those related to the ART practice (Fig. 31.1). Within this scenario of uncertainties, the iterative question which reproductive medicine specialists should ask is once an abnormal level of SDF has been detected in a patient, how can we solve the problem?

In this chapter, we review the methods for assessing SDF and the strategies that can be used to diminish SDF in samples used for fertilization. Some of these strategies may produce a synergistic effect for SDF reduction, as we will see.

31.1.2 *Assessing Sperm DNA Fragmentation*

This book includes detailed information about the different available techniques to evaluate sperm DNA fragmentation. Although a correlation does exist among the different techniques used for assessing SDF, the threshold values may vary among them [9–11]. In this chapter, most of the results presented relates to the application of the sperm chromatin dispersion test (SCD) on its commercial version (Halosperm, Halotech DNA, Madrid, Spain). A comprehensive review of the sperm chromatin dispersion test is provided in Chap. 8. Using the SCD test, sperm presenting with non-fragmented DNA show a homogeneous and large halo of dispersed chromatin surrounding a compact core (Fig. 31.2a–c). Conversely, sperm with fragmented DNA show either a small halo of dispersed chromatin (Fig. 31.2d) or lacking such a halo of dispersed chromatin (Fig. 31.2e, f). All spermatozoa showing fragmented DNA according to the halo technique are arrowed in green in Fig. 31.1.

31.2 Clinical Management of Sperm DNA Fragmentation

31.2.1 *The Influence of Environment and Lifestyle*

It is known that toxicity caused by exposure to environmental pollutants or certain unhealthy lifestyle factors may induce the generation of ROS, resulting in cellular oxidative damage. Both of these effectors of cell damage have become a major health concern nowadays [12]. Obesity/overweight, pollution exposure, tobacco and/or drug abuse, excessive physical activity, UV radiation, excessive exposure to electromagnetic radiation such as the ones emitted by cell phones, and heavy metal

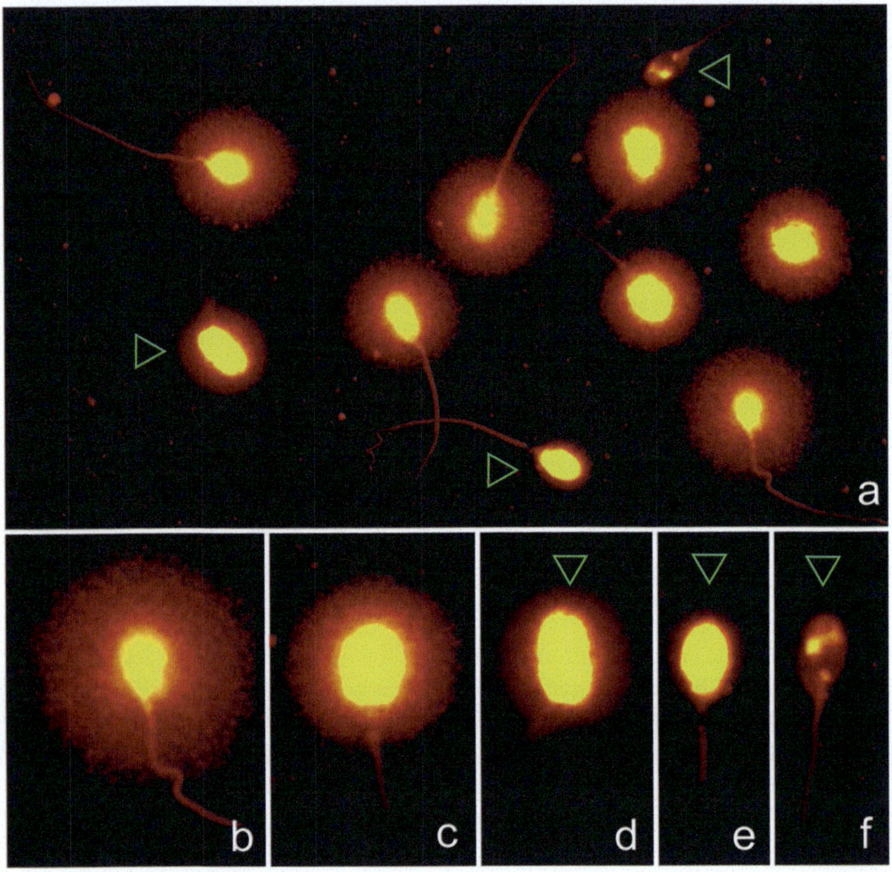

Fig. 31.2 Evaluation of sperm DNA fragmentation after Halosperm processing. (**a**) Full view of a microscope field showing sperm containing fragmented and non-fragmented DNA. Individual spermatozoon with intact (**b**, **c**) and damaged (**d**–**f**) nuclear DNA is shown. Original image captured under fluorescence microscopy and GelRed staining

exposure, among others, can produce an imbalance in the enzyme activation systems involving REDOX processes and result in cell damage at different levels [12–15]. Notwithstanding the difficulties in controlling all confounding variables when addressing the influence of each aforementioned factor on sperm SDF, fair evidence has indicated that environment and lifestyle may affect the sperm DNA molecule. For instance, an association between exposure to bisphenol A and abnormal levels of SDF has been demonstrated [16, 17]. Using boars as an experimental system, it was demonstrated that an excessive intake of zinc, a common oligoelement present in most of the antioxidant cocktails, may increase the level of SDF with only 50 ppm more than the recommended daily intake [18]. These examples illustrate that the direct negative effects of environmental conditions on SDF are difficult to be controlled or avoided. We therefore must be conscious that overexposure to these effectors can produce a severe disruption of normal sperm chromatin conformation that may result in poor reproductive outcomes. Although it has not been properly demonstrated, most of these negative effects, however, can be reversed by lifestyle modification such as having a balanced and healthy diet.

Given that oxidative stress is resulting from an imbalance between the amount of ROS and their counteracting antioxidants, a logical strategy to avoid its negative effect would be the administration of antioxidant cocktails to rebalance the REDOX system. Both the incorporation of antioxidant cocktails to the diet [19, 20] and supplementation to the sperm preparation medium have been attempted [21, 22] to prevent local ROS attack during sperm handling. However, the putative beneficial effects of such methods are not as straightforward as it has been generally assumed [23–25]. There are three important biases identified in the experimental approaches used in these studies: (i) most of the studies are underpowered and lacked a placebo-controlled arm and a double-blind design; (ii) studies were performed using different antioxidants in different combinations, dosages, and durations; (iii) most studies did not examine the effect of antioxidants on specific groups of infertile patients. Having said that, it is important to acknowledge that most of the published literature is supportive of the beneficial roles of antioxidants in improving semen quality [26]. Nevertheless, antioxidants are usually administered without any prior evaluation of ROS/antioxidant capacity. This is mainly due to the general assumption that sperm DNA damage and low sperm motility are mainly caused by an excess of ROS. However, other factors related to patients' genetic background might also affect the sperm membrane structure, the levels of protamination, and other structural sperm elements. These factors may negatively impair sperm quality regardless the level of ROS in the media. Furthermore, side effects and health risks of long-term vitamin use in unselected patients have been reported. All these factors indicate that it is inadvisable to generalize the association between oxidative stress and sperm DNA fragmentation [27].

Ideally, the antioxidant cocktails should be prescribed only following the confirmation of redox imbalance in the ejaculate of men with low sperm motility and/or low membrane quality and/or high levels of SDF.

31.2.2 *Impact of Ejaculatory Abstinence Duration*

The World Health Organization (WHO) recommends semen sample to be collected after 2–7 days' abstinence [28]. Although this practice mainly focuses at obtaining a higher volume of ejaculate, its benefit in the context of ART remains unclear because prolonged ejaculatory abstinence can be deleterious to sperm DNA integrity and male fertility capacity [29]. Moreover, in the era of ICSI where only one spermatozoon is needed to fertilize the oocyte, this practice could be easily censured. Given the potential deleterious effects of ROS during epididymis transit and the absence of active mechanism of DNA repair in maturing sperm, the practice of asking patients to abstain from ejaculation for long periods before collecting sperm for ART purposes is equivocal. In fact, sperm containing non-fragmented DNA can be affected by external and internal effectors of DNA damage (oxidative stress, DNase activity) after long storage in the epididymis. In a recent study, the effect of ejaculatory abstinence periods on routine and advanced sperm tests was assessed in a group of normozoospermic men who provided semen samples after 1, 2, 5, 7, 9, and 11 days of abstinence [30]. Although semen volume, sperm concentration, and total sperm count increased significantly with abstinence duration, sperm DNA fragmentation was also found to be increased. Both 1 and 2 days of ejaculatory abstinence had the least amount of DNA fragmentation. The authors concluded that shortening of ejaculatory abstinence time was not detrimental to sperm quality in normozoospermic men and could potentially be a strategy in reducing sperm DNA fragmentation. In another study, recurrent ejaculations, i.e., for three consecutive days, also resulted in a significant decrease in the proportion of spermatozoa containing a damaged DNA molecule [31, 32]. Moreover, the DNA quality improved further if the samples were processed using density gradient centrifugation (DGC) after repeated ejaculations (3 h of abstinence) (Table 31.1). In addition, recent studies have suggested that shorter abstinence is better for intrauterine insemination (IUI) and assisted reproductive technology (ART) than the abstinence recommended by WHO for performing a diagnostic semen analysis [40]. A possible explanation for these observations is that more immature spermatozoa enter the epididymis as a result of repeated ejaculations. Some of these immature spermatozoa may be defective because they have entered the epididymis before complete maturation in the testis. It is also possible that the repeated ejaculation prevents the complete oxidation of sperm nuclear sulfhydryl groups during epididymal transit. Combining

Table 31.1 Summary of the effect on sperm DNA fragmentation (SDF) reduction after using different strategies of sperm selection

Protocol	SDF ejaculate	SDF selected	SDF reduction	Reference
Testicular sperm	40.9	8.3	79.7	Esteves et al. [33]
Recurrent ejaculation (72 h)	26.9	19.6	27.1	Gosálvez et al. [31]
Recurrent ejaculation (3 h)	20.8	10.8	48.1	Gosálvez et al. [31]
Ejaculate fractionation	23.5	16.8	28.5	Hebles et al. [34]
SU (successful pregnancy)	25.3	16.9	33.2	Gosálvez et al. [35]
SU (no successful pregnancy)	34.9	23.7	32.1	Gosálvez et al. [35]
DGC (donors)	18.2	12.3	32.4	Gosálvez et al. [36]
DGC (patients)	27	19.6	27.4	Sánchez-Martín et al. [37]
Ejaculate fractionation (stallion)	11.1	7.3	34.2	de la Torre et al. [38]
Sex sorting (bull)	7.9	3.1	60.8	Gosálvez et al. [39]

SDF in all samples assessed with Halosperm (human) or Halomax (animals: cursive). All values are percent

SU swim-up, *DGC* density gradient centrifugation

recurrent ejaculations with sperm selection using DGC, the proportion of immature sperm increases in the ejaculated sample, but they are trapped in one of the layers of the density gradient. This is because the whole sperm surface of the immature sperm head is larger than that of normal sperm. Thus, most of these immature cells with damaged DNA will be eliminated in the sample to be used for ART. From our observations, sperm DNA damage decreases in virtually all cases after recurrent ejaculation and DGC. The magnitude of SDF decrease is up to 50% compared with the SDF values obtained in the original ejaculate (Table 31.1; 31).

In conclusion, recurrent ejaculation is a noninvasive and simple strategy that can be combined with DGC to reduce the proportion of sperm containing damaged DNA in semen specimens to be used for ART. The synergistic effects of combining recurrent ejaculations with PICSI, MACS, or other methodologies for sperm selection need to be explored further.

31.2.3 Impact of Ejaculate Fractionation

The laboratory methods of processing sperm for ART purposes do not conform to the rules designed by nature. After semen collection, the final sample represents a mixture of different ejaculated fractions. Conversely in nature, a given ejaculation consists of different semen fractions with different characteristics. In most of the mammalian species, the ejaculate comprises the pre-ejaculatory fraction, which is free of sperm and includes the fluid fraction of the Cowper's and Littre's glands, and the first and second fractions. In humans, the first fraction represents 15–45% of the ejaculate. This rich sperm fraction originates from the epididymal sperm and contains prostatic secretions, including acid phosphatase, citric acid, magnesium, and zinc, and it appears to exert a protective effect on sperm. The second fraction is the remaining 55–85% of the volume and is characterized by having a low sperm count immersed in secretions of the seminal vesicles [41, 42]. It can be therefore hypothesized that the first ejaculated fraction contains sperm with better seminal parameters. Therefore, semen fractionation could be used as an effective method for selecting sperm prior to fertilization.

Interestingly, the first ejaculate fraction has lower volume, higher sperm concentration, sperm with better motility, and lower levels of SDF (16.85 ± 7.2%) than the second fraction (30.3% ± 15.0%) [34, 38]. In asthenozoospermic and teratozoospermic males, these differences have also been observed [43]. Similar experiments performed with stallions have showed an equivalent effect (first fraction SDF = 7.3% ± 2.5%; second fraction SDF = 25.1% ± 19.3%). It seems that a certain level of interspecies concordance exists in the proportion of SDF reduction observed by semen fractionation (Table 31.1; 38).

In conclusion, ejaculate fractionation is a simple method that may generate a sperm population characterized by increased sperm motility and concentration and, most importantly for ART, lower level of damaged DNA than that observed in the whole ejaculate.

31.2.4 Use of Testicular Sperm for ICSI

Sperm obtained directly from the testicle have shown to have lower levels of DNA damage compared to ejaculated counterparts [44–47]. As a matter of fact, testicular tissue extraction has been advocated as a method with potential beneficial effects for couples undergoing ART when elevated SDF is a contributory infertility factor.

In a recent study, 147 couples with oligozoospermia and elevated SDF (SCD >30%) were offered ICSI with ejaculated or testicular sperm [33]. Among patients subjected to testicular sperm retrieval, the level of SDF level was 8.3% compared to 40.7% in their ejaculates collected at the same day after 2–3 days of ejaculatory abstinence (Table 31.1). The magnitude of SDF reduction was approximately 80%. Added to this, ICSI outcomes were significantly better in the group of patients using testicular sperm compared to the group of similar characteristics where only ejaculated sperm and ICSI were used [33]. Although the clinical pregnancy rates were not statistically different among the studied groups, the proportion of women experiencing early miscarriage was significantly lower if testicular sperm was used, resulting in higher live birth rates in this aforementioned group [33].

In conclusion, the use of testicular sperm seems to be a valid strategy to overcome infertility in couples subjected to ICSI in whom the male partner has elevated SDF.

31.2.5 Impact of Laboratory Sperm Selection Techniques

Not all spermatozoa in the ejaculate present with the optimal characteristics for fertilization even when they have normal morphological characteristics [48]. The proportion of spermatozoa that are able to reach and fertilize the oocyte, giving rise to syngamy with the female nucleus, is highly variable among individuals. This is one of the reasons why different laboratory strategies have been developed in ART in order to improve the relative proportion of sperm with full fertilization potential. Such methods are aimed to concentrate the subgroup of cells exhibiting normal motility, morphology, and normal chromatin contents, which may result in higher pregnancy rates when used for intrauterine insemination (IUI), in vitro fertilization (IVF), or intracytoplasmic sperm injection (ICSI).

Swim-up (SU) or density gradient centrifugation (DGC) can be considered as basic techniques for sperm handling in the laboratory. These methods represent the classical examples of strategies conducted to improve the relative sperm quality as compared to the original ejaculate. These methods remove the seminal plasma and select the sperm subpopulation that exhibit progressive motility. They also proved to be partially effective in eliminating spermatozoa exhibiting a damaged DNA molecule [36, 49, 50].

There are also other techniques that can be used to select spermatozoa with better physiological or morphological quality. While techniques such as the hyaluronic binding assay (HA) attempt to select mature sperm that are bound to the molecules of hyaluronic acid [51], the motile sperm organelle morphology examination

(MSOME) is aimed at visualizing sperm abnormalities that are not visible at low magnification [52–54]. Although these techniques potentially deselect spermatozoa with DNA damage [55, 56], their effectiveness for reproductive outcome remains to be confirmed.

One option to further deselect sperm with damaged DNA would be the combination of SU and DGC with MSOME, HA, or PICSI (physiological ICSI), but this strategy needs to be studied. On the contrary, the use of magnetic-activated cell sorting (MACS) represents one of the few strategies of sperm selection that specifically removes apoptotic spermatozoa. Arguably, spermatozoa negatively selected for the presence of annexin V are more likely to present with DNA free of strand breaks [57, 58].

While in theory, these techniques should be able to eliminate a large part of sperm deficiencies at different levels, it may not be so in real situation as certain parameters such as motility can be negatively affected after their applications [59, 60]. With respect to SDF, selection using SU or DGC may result, in some patients, in a higher level of DNA damage in the ejaculate [36]. In some cases, critical issues such as those concerning the length of telomeric DNA sequences at the sperm fraction, which would be used in ART, might be compromised [61].

Most of these shortcomings relate to the fact that all these techniques require labor-intensive laboratory manipulation, which may cause iatrogenic sperm damage [62, 63]. Moreover, the effectiveness of these complex techniques to deselect sperm with DNA fragmentation for ART remains equivocal [64]. Factors such as the patient profile and type of technique may affect the ability of these methods to remove sperm with damaged chromatin [65, 66]. For instance, it has been shown that DCG has low efficiency to remove apoptotic sperm [66]. Notwithstanding, using a two-tail comet assay to assess simultaneously single- and double-strand DNA breaks, it was found that SU and DGC are equally efficient in eliminating spermatozoa containing double-strand DNA damage, but DGC is more efficient than SU in selecting spermatozoa that are free from single-strand DNA damage [67]. The determination of the best technique to be used in each patient, alone or combined, is still not clear.

In conclusion, the existing laboratory sperm selection techniques may reduce the proportion of sperm with DNA damage, but at present, none of them, alone or combined, provide complete elimination of sperm with damaged chromatin.

31.2.6 Iatrogenic Sperm Damage During Sperm Handling

The use of in vitro conditions when handling sperm in the laboratory is inherently associated with potential iatrogenic damage [62, 68, 69]. In general, it is recommended to avoid long periods of sperm incubation, incubation at 37 °C, and aggressive centrifugation force. With respect to the negative impact of DNA quality, it is known that SDF increases with incubation in a time-dependent fashion, but it also depends on individual characteristics [70, 71]. This fact brings about the concept of sperm DNA longevity and the rate of SDF (rSDF): proportion of spermatozoa containing a fragmented DNA molecule increases per time unit after ejaculation [63, 70]. It is remarkable that significant differences exist between different individuals despite using the same conditions for sperm handling [36]. In some cases, sperm DNA exhibit a relatively slow degradation, resulting in a very good fit of the logarithmic curve function, while in other cases this increase is exponential [70, 71]. In Fig. 31.3, the differential dynamic behavior of SDF in two cohorts of individuals ($n = 10$ per group) after 24 h of neat sperm incubation at 37 °C is shown. While the blue line shows a logarithmic tendency of SDF increase, the orange one shows an exponential tendency confirming a long SDF longevity for these patients. This rate is variable, depending on the conditions of sperm manipulation [72]. Interestingly, the composition of the semen extenders may also affect the rates of SDF within the same individual [73]. Sperm DNA longevity is species-dependent [74] and is in part related to the protamination characteristics of the sperm chromatin [75].

It is challenging to investigate the clinical implications of iatrogenic damage. In certain experimental models, the increase of sperm DNA damage after sperm collection produces a significant decrease in embryo quality. For instance, in zebra fish, where SDF increases shortly after sperm activation, significant differences in fertilization rates are not apparent, but a higher miscarriage rate is noted [76]. A similar situation is observed in multi-ovulating species such as rabbits [77]. In humans, on the

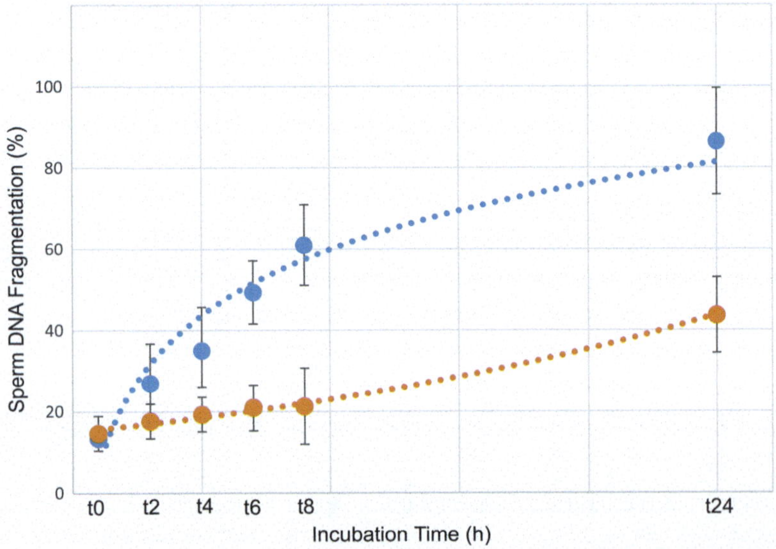

Fig. 31.3 Dynamic representation of sperm DNA fragmentation (SDF) along 24 h of incubation at 37 °C using neat sperm samples on normal seminogram ($n = 10$ per group). Criteria of inclusion (SDF lower than 50% after 24 h of incubation). Blue line shows a logarithmic tendency for SDF increase, while this tendency is exponential in the orange-line plotted group

other hand, it has been shown that a reduction in the time from the ejaculation until the sample is used for fertilization is associated with better reproductive outcome [78].

In conclusion, the obvious recommendation would be to minimize iatrogenic-induced sperm damage during their handling in the laboratory. Long periods of sperm incubation, especially at 37 °C, should be avoided. A dynamic evaluation of the rSDF in each patient would provide useful information on the stability of the sperm DNA. Subsequently, we may design customized strategies of sperm collection in order to minimize the negative impact that may be present post-ejaculation and during sperm collection and in vitro handling.

31.2.7 The Influence of Sperm Concentration

In mammalian species, it is known that changes in the membrane quality, motility characteristics, and other seminal parameters could occur in the samples prepared for cryopreservation. Notably, commercial vials of semen for insemination used in the veterinary field tend to have fewer sperm than that of the original ejaculate. In fact, the recommended number of spermatozoa per seminal dose varies among different animal species [79, 80]. Moreover, sperm concentration is critical when samples for insemination are sorted for sex separation [81]. Some studies have shown that both motility and membrane integrity improve with increased dilution of the cryopreserved specimen, although the proportion of acrosome-reacted sperm does not vary greatly. For example, in bulls, sperm dilution after incubation of the sample using relatively high and low room temperature for 24 h results in minor differences between both experimental conditions in terms of viability or susceptibility to osmotic stress. However, samples with lower sperm concentration present with a higher proportion of viable cells with reacted acrosomes [82]. The influence of sperm concentration within the same ejaculate was tested in ram; it was demonstrated that sperm DNA longevity is larger when low sperm concentrations are used in preparing the seminal doses [83]. In other words, samples prepared with low sperm concentration are less affected by iatrogenic DNA damage. Ongoing experiments using human normozoospermic patients in our laboratory also indicate that in vitro DNA longevity decreases with sperm concentrations of 100M and greater and achieves stability when reaching concentrations lower than 10M (Gosálvez et al. unpublished results). Although a conclusive explanation for these observations is lacking, it seems plausible that the level of oxidative stress occurring after the collision of moving sperm would be higher. Low sperm concentration would diminish the probability of random collisions. Moreover, the amount of cellular debris in the medium increases as sperm die, as do the levels of active enzymes from the acrosome or free topoisomerases contained in spermatozoa with defective protamination.

In the ART scenario, especially when ICSI is indicated, sperm concentration is not a limiting factor. Therefore, handling ex vivo specimens with low sperm concentration may improve DNA stability.

31.2.8 Creating a Mini-cryopreserved Sperm Bank for Personal Use

As reported above, sperm DNA damage is lower in donors and normozoospermic men than infertile men [2, 5]. Added to this, there is a variation in SDF from one ejaculate to another in the same men [3, 73]. So the question that poses to us is the following: when a man with severe male factor infertility in whom SDF is an important contributory factor subjected to ART, why should the ejaculate sample obtained on the day of fertilization be used rather than the ones obtained previously with confirmed lower levels of SDF?

Creating a mini-cryopreserved sperm bank derived from different ejaculates from the same patient where SDF levels are systematically assessed would allow selecting the specimens with lower SDF to be used for fertilization. Such autologous sperm bank could contain specimens with SDF lower than those obtained fresh at the day of fertilization. In a prospective study including five couples with repeated ART failure and severe male factor infertility presenting with high levels of SDF, two couples were able to achieve pregnancy using the sperm sample from the self mini-bank that exhibited a lower level of sperm damage than that presented on the day of fertilization.

The potential benefits of mini sperm banks for personal use seem to be an attractive option; however, its use requires further investigation.

31.2.9 Sperm Sorting

Flow cytometry sperm sorting has been used in separating X- and Y-bearing sperm based on DNA charge associated with the sex chromosomes. Sperm sorting has been successfully used to produce viable offspring in some mammalian species [84, 85]. In humans, the method has been applied successfully in some countries for sex selection [86–88]. This technique not only offered as a sex selection for family planning but also as an option to avoid sex-linked genetic diseases.

Furthermore, sperm sex sorting is used for milk production control as part of dairy farming. Using bulls as an experimental model, it has been demonstrated that sperm sorting using flow cytometry reduces the proportion of sperm containing a fragmented DNA molecule compared with the original ejaculate [39]. Sperm sorting for bulls uses a neutral food dye that is able to penetrate and dye the nuclei of those spermatozoa with permeable membranes (dead sperm). The laser beam can be arranged for targeting those specific unviable spermatozoa and separate them from the rest. Interestingly, a large part of such spermatozoa contain a damaged DNA molecule [39]. In theory, using this rationale and avoiding DNA nuclei staining could possibly separate the viable sperm from the non-viable population, and this selected subpopulation would likely contain a lower level of SDF. A protocol that applies only a neutral dye, which is unable to penetrate the live sperm presenting an orthodox cell membrane, however, is not currently available to be used for the purpose of reducing sperm DNA damage. Nonetheless, it seems plausible that such a strategy can be used for selecting sperm with intact chromatin contents.

31.3 Conclusions

Sperm DNA damage cannot be considered as neutral sperm parameter for pregnancy. Any technique or strategy that could be conducted to minimize the sperm DNA damage should be implemented to improve sperm capacity for fertilization, pregnancy rate, and embryo quality. In Table 31.1, we summarized the efficiency of different methods to deselect sperm with SDF, most of which are currently used in andrology laboratories. However, the literature is poor in studies comparing the methods tail-to-tail, as it is in comparing the synergistic effect of such strategies to reduce SDF. In order to optimize the management of patients with infertility, we recommend a first assessment of SDF when a standard seminogram is prescribed. Subsequently, if a high level of SDF is observed, the level should be controlled using some of the strategies we have outlined in this chapter.

Acknowledgments This research was supported with public funding (Spanish Ministry of Economy and Competitiveness (MINECO): BFU-2013–44290-R).

References

1. Zhao J, Zhang Q, Wang Y, Li Y. Whether sperm deoxyribonucleic acid fragmentation has an effect on pregnancy and miscarriage after in vitro fertilization/intracytoplasmic sperm injection: a systematic review and meta-analysis. Fertil Steril. 2014;102:998–1005.
2. Sakkas D. Novel technologies for selecting the best sperm for in vitro fertilization and intracytoplasmic sperm injection. Fertil Steril. 2013;99:1023–9.
3. Sergerie M, Laforest G, Boulanger K, Bissonnette F, Bleau G. Longitudinal study of sperm DNA fragmentation as measured by terminal uridine nick end-labelling assay. Hum Reprod. 2005;20:1921–7.
4. Agarwal A, Cho CL, Esteves SC. Should we evaluate and treat sperm DNA fragmentation? Curr Opin Obstet Gynecol. 2016;28:164–71.
5. Gosálvez J, López-Fernández C, Fernández JL, Esteves SC, Johnston SD. Unpacking the mysteries of spermDNA fragmentation: ten frequently asked questions. J Reprod Biotech Fertil. 2015;4:1–16.
6. Gosálvez J, García-Ochoa C, Ruíz-Jorro M, Martínez-Moya M, Sánchez-Martín P, Caballero P. ¿A qué velocidad "muere" el ADN del espermatozoide tras descongelar muestras seminales procedentes de donantes? Revista Internacional de Andrologia. 2013;11:85–93.
7. Esteves SC, Gosálvez J, López-Fernández C, Núñez-Calonge R, Caballero P, Agarwal A, Fernández JL. Diagnostic accuracy of sperm DNA degradation index (DDSi) as a potential noninvasive biomarker to identify men with varicocele-associated infertility. Int Urol Nephrol. 2015;47:1471–7.
8. The Practice Committee of the American Society for Reproductive Medicine. The clinical utility of sperm DNA integrity testing: a guideline. Fertil Steril. 2013;99:673–7.

9. Chohan KR, Griffi n JT, Lafromboise M, De Jonge CJ, Carrell DT. Comparison of chromatin assays for DNA fragmentation evaluation in human sperm. J Androl. 2006;27:53–9.
10. Feijó C, Esteves SC. Diagnostic accuracy of sperm chromatin dispersion test to evaluate sperm deoxyribonucleic acid damage in men with unexplained infertility. Fertil Steril. 2014;101:58–63.
11. Gosálvez J, Fernández JL, Yaniz J, de la Casa M, López-Fernández JSD. A comparison of sperm DNA damage in the neat ejaculate of sperm donors and males presenting for their initial seminogram. Austin J Reprod Med Infertility. 2015;2:1014.1–4.
12. Garolla A, Torino M, Sartin B, Cosci I, Patassini C, Carraro U, Foresta C. Seminal and molecular evidence that sauna exposure affects human spermatogenesis. Hum Reprod. 2013;28:877–85.
13. Sheynkin Y, Welliver R, Winer A, Hajimirzaee F, Ahn H, Lee K. Protection from scrotal hyperthermia in laptop computer users. Fertil Steril. 2011;95:647–51.
14. Zalata A, El-Samanoudy AZ, Shaalan D, El-Baiomy Y, Mostafa T. In vitro effect of cell phone radiation on motility, DNA fragmentation and clustering gene expression in human sperm. Int J Fertil Steril. 2015;9:129–36.
15. Dupont C, Faure C, Sermondade N, Boubaya M, Eustach F, Clément P, Briot P, Berthau TI, Levy V, Cedrin-Durnerin I, Benzacken B, Chavatte-Palmer P, Levy R. Obesity leads to higher risk of sperm DNA damage in infertile patient. Asian J Androl. 2013;15:622–5.
16. Wu DH, Leung YK, Thomas MA, Maxwell R, Ho SM. Bisphenol A (BPA) confers direct genotoxicity to sperm with increased sperm DNA fragmentation. Fertil Steril. 2011;96(3):S5–6.
17. Meeker JD, Ehrlich S, Toth TL, Wright DL, Calafat AM, Trisini AT, Ye X, Hauser R. Semen quality and sperm DNA damage in relation to urinary bisphenol A among men from an infertility clinic. Reprod Toxicol. 2010;304:532–9.
18. García-Contreras A, De Loera Y, García-Artiga C, Palomo A, Guevara JA, Herrera-Haro J, López-Fernández C, Johnston S, Gosálvez J. Elevated dietary intake of Zn-methionate is associated with increased sperm DNA fragmentation in the boar. Reprod Toxicol. 2011;31:570–3.
19. Agarwal A, Nallella KP, Allamaneni SS, Said TM. Role of antioxidants in treatment of male infertility: an overview of the literature. Reprod BioMed Online. 2004;6:616–27.
20. Wirleitner B, Vanderzwalmen P, Stecher A, Spitzer D, Schuff M, Schwerda D, Bach M, Schechinger B, Herbert Zech N. Dietary supplementation of antioxidants improves semen quality of IVF patients in terms of motility, sperm count, and nuclear vacuolization. Int J Vitam Nutr Res. 2012;82:391–8.
21. Michael AJ, Alexopoulos C, Pontiki EA, Hadjipavlou-Litina DJ, Saratsis P, Ververidis HN, Boscos CM. Effect of antioxidant supplementation in semen extenders on semen quality and reactive oxygen species of chilled canine spermatozoa. Anim Reprod Sci. 2009;112:119–35.
22. Sharafi M, Zhandi M, Sharif AA. Supplementation of soybean lecithin-based semen extender by antioxidants: complementary flowcytometric study on post-thawed ram spermatozoa. Cell Tissue Bank. 2015;16:261–9.
23. Ménézo YJ, Hazout A, Panteix G, Robert F, Rollet J, Cohen-Bacrie P, Chapuis F, Clément P, Benkhalifa M. Antioxidants to reduce sperm DNA fragmentation: an unexpected adverse effect. Reprod BioMed Online. 2007;14:418–21.
24. Menezo YJ, Evenson D, Cohen M, Dale B. Effect of antioxidants on sperm genetic damage. Adv Exp Med Biol. 2014;791:173–89.
25. Walczak-Jedrzejowska R, Wolsk JK, Slowikowska J. The role of oxidative stress and antioxidants in male fertility. Cent Eur J Urol. 2013;66:60–7.
26. Ross C, Morriss A, Khairy M, Khalaf Y, Braude P, Coomarasamy A, El-Toukhy T. A systematic review of the effect of oral antioxidants on male infertility. Reprod BioMed Online. 2010;20:711–23.
27. Bjelakovic G, Nikolova D, Gluud LL, Simonetti RG, Gluud C. Antioxidant supplements for prevention of mortality in healthy participants and patients with various diseases. Cochrane Database Syst Rev. 2012;14(3):CD007176.
28. World Health Organization. WHO laboratory manual for the examination and processing of human semen. Geneva: World Health Organization; 2010.

29. Levitas E, Lunenfeld E, Weiss N, Friger M, Har-Vardi I, Koifman A, Potashnik G. Relationship between the duration of sexual abstinence and semen quality: analysis of 9,489 semen samples. Fertil Steril. 2005;83:1680–6.
30. Agarwal A, Gupta S, Du Plessis S, Sharma R, Esteves SC, Cirenza C, Eliwa J, Al-Najjar W, Kumaresan D, Haroun N, Philby S, Sabanegh E. Abstinence time and its impact on basic and advanced semen parameters. Urology. 2016;94:102–10.
31. Gosálvez J, González-Martínez M, López-Fernández C, Fernández JL, Sánchez-Martín P. Shorter abstinence decreases sperm deoxyribonucleic acid fragmentation in ejaculate. Fertil Steril. 2011;96:1083–6.
32. Pons I, Cercas R, Villas C, Braña C, Fernández-Shaw S. One abstinence day decreases sperm DNA fragmentation in 90 % of selected patients. J Assist Reprod Genet. 2013;30:1211–8.
33. Esteves SC, Sanchez-Martín F, Sanchez-Martín P, Schneider DT, Gosálvez J. Comparison of reproductive outcome in oligozoospermic men with high sperm DNA fragmentation undergoing intracytoplasmic sperm injection with ejaculated and testicular sperm. Fertil Steril. 2015;104:1398–405.
34. Hebles M, Dorado M, González-Martínez M, Sánchez-Martín P. Seminal quality in the first fraction of ejaculate. Syst Biol Reprod Med. 2014;30:1–4.
35. Gosálvez J, Caballero P, López-Fernández C, Ortega L, Guijarro JA, Fernández JL, Johnston SD, Nuñez-Calonge R. Can DNA fragmentation of neat or swim-up spermatozoa be used to predict pregnancy following ICSI of fertile oocyte donors? Asian J Androl. 2013;15:812–8.
36. Gosálvez J, de la Torre J, López-Fernández C, Pérez-Gutiérrez L, Ortega L, Caballero P, Núñez R. DNA fragmentation dynamics in fresh versus frozen thawed plus gradient-isolated human spermatozoa. Syst Biol Reprod Med. 2010;56:27–36.
37. Sánchez-Martín P, Sánchez-Martín F, González-Martínez M, Gosálvez J. Increased pregnancy after reduced male abstinence. System Biol Reprod Sci. 2013;59:256–60.
38. de la Torre J, Sánchez-Martín P, Gosálvez J, Crespo F. Equivalent seminal characteristics in human and stallion at first and second ejaculated fractions. Andrologia. 2016;49:1–5.
39. Gosálvez J, Ramirez MA, López-Fernández C, Crespo F, Evans KM, Kjelland ME, Moreno JF. Sex-sorted bovine spermatozoa and DNA damage: I. Static features. Theriogenology. 2011;75:197–205.
40. Marshburn PB, Alanis MC, Matthew MLS, Hurst BS. A short period of abstinence before intrauterine insemination is associated with higher pregnancy rates. Fertil Steril. 2009;93:286–8.
41. Cohen J, Euser R, Schenck PE, Brugman FW, Zeilmaker GH. Motility and morphology of human spermatozoa in split ejaculates. Andrologia. 1981;13:491–8.
42. Mortimer D. Biochemistry of spermatozoa and seminal plasma. In: Practical laboratory Andrology. New York: Oxford University Press; 1994. p. 89–109.
43. Kumar D, Kalthur G, Mascarenhas C, Kumar P, Adiga SK. Ejaculate fractions of asthenozoospermic and teratozoospermic patients have differences in the sperm DNA integrity. Andrologia. 2011;43:416–21.
44. Bernie AM, Ramasamy R, Schlegel PN. Predictive factors of successful microdissection testicular sperm extraction. Basic Clin Androl. 2013;23:5.
45. Greco E, Scarselli F, Iacobelli M, Rienzi L, Ubaldi F, Ferrero S, Franco G, Anniballo N, Mendoza C, Tesarik J. Efficient treatment of infertility due to sperm DNA damage by ICSI with testicular spermatozoa. Hum Reprod. 2005;20:226–30.
46. Moskovtsev SI, Alladin N, Lo KC, Jarvi K, Mullen JB, Librach CL. A comparison of ejaculated and testicular spermatozoa aneuploidy rates in patients with high sperm DNA damage. Syst Biol Reprod Med. 2012;58:142–8.
47. Moskovtsev SI, Jarvi K, Mullen JB, Cadesky KI, Hannam T, Lo KC. Testicular spermatozoa have statistically significantly lower DNA damage compared with ejaculated spermatozoa in patients with unsuccessful oral antioxidant treatment. Fertil Steril. 2010;93:1142–6.
48. Avendaño C, Franchi A, Taylor S, Morshedi M, Bocca S, Oehninger S. Fragmentation of DNA in morphologically normal human spermatozoa. Fertil Steril. 2009;91:1077–84.
49. Nasr-Esfahani MH, Deemeh MR, Tavalaee M. New era in sperm selection for ICSI. Int J Andro. 2012;35:475–84.

50. Zini A, Finellia A, Phanga D, Jarvia K. Influence of semen processing technique on human sperm DNA integrity. Urology. 2000;56:1081–4.
51. Huszar G, Ozenci CC, Cayli S, Zavaczki Z, Hansch E, Vigue L. Hyaluronic acid binding by human sperm indicates cellular maturity, viability, and unreacted acrosomal status. Fertil Steril. 2003;79:1616–24.
52. Bartoov B, Berkovitz A, Eltes F, Kogosowski A, Menezo YJR, Barak Y. Real-time fine morphology of motile human sperm cells is associated with IVF-ICSI outcome. J Androl. 2002;23:1–8.
53. Cassuto NG, Hazout A, Bouret D, Bale R, Larue L, Benifla JL, Viot G. Low birth defects by deselecting abnormal spermatozoa before ICSI. Reprod BioMed Online. 2014;28:47–53.
54. Boitrelle FM, Pagnier M, Athiel Y, Swierkowski-Blanchard N, Torre A, Alter L, Muratori C, Vialard F, Albert M, Selva J. A human morphologically normal spermatozoon may have non-condensed chromatin. Andrologia. 2015;47:879–86.
55. Parmegiani L, Cognigni GE, Bernardi S, Troilo E, Ciampaglia W, Filicori M. 'Physiologic ICSI', Hyaluronic acid (HA) favors selection of spermatozoa without DNA fragmentation and with normal nucleus, resulting in improvement of embryo quality. Fertil Steril. 2010;93:598–604.
56. Gosálvez J, Migueles B, López-Fernández C, Sanchéz-Martín F, Sáchez-Martín P. Single sperm selection and DNA fragmentation analysis: the case of MSOME/IMSI. Nat Sci. 2013;5:7–14.
57. Bucar S, Gonçalves A, Rocha E, Barros A, Sousa M, Sá R. DNA fragmentation in human sperm after magnetic-activated cell sorting. J Assist Reprod Genet. 2015;32:147–54.
58. Gil M, Sar-Shalom V, Sivira YM, Checa MA. Sperm selection using magnetic activated cell sorting (MACS) in assisted reproduction: a systematic review and meta-analysis. J Assist Reprod Genet. 2013;30:479–85.
59. McCann CT, Eric Chantler E. Properties of sperm separated using Percoll and IxaPrep density gradients. A comparison made using CASA, longevity, morphology and the acrosome reaction. Inter J Androl. 2000;23:205–9.
60. Esteves SC, Agarwal A. Ensuring that reproductive laboratories provide high-quality services. In: Bento FC, Esteves SC, Agarwal A, editors. Quality management in ART clinics: a practical guide. New York: Springer; 2013. p. 129–46.
61. Santiso R, María Tamayo M, Gosálvez J, Meseguer M, Garrido N, Fernández JL. Swim-up procedure selects spermatozoa with longer telomere length. Mutat Res. 2010;688:88–90.
62. Mortimer D. Sperm preparation techniques and iatrogenic failures of in-vitro fertilization. Hum Reprod. 1991;6:173–6.
63. Gosálvez J, López-Fernández C, Fernández JL, Gouraud A, Holt WV. Relationships between the dynamics of iatrogenic DNA damage and genomic design in mammalian spermatozoa from eleven species. Mol Reprod Dev. 2011;78:951–61.
64. López-Fernández C, Johnston SD, Gosálbez A, Fernández JL, Álvarez JG, Gosálvez J. Inter-center variation in the efficiency of sperm DNA damage reduction following density gradient centrifugation. Nat Sci. 2013;5:15–20.
65. Sakkas D, Manicardi GC, Tomlinson M, Mandrioli M, Bizzaro D, Bianchi PG, Bianchi U. The use of two density gradient centrifugation techniques and the swim-up method to separate spermatozoa with chromatin and nuclear DNA anomalies. Hum Reprod. 2000;15:1112–26.
66. Stevanato J, Bertolla RP, Barradas V, Spaine DM, Cedenho AP, Ortiz V. Semen processing by density gradient centrifugation does not improve sperm apoptotic deoxyribonucleic acid fragmentation rates. Fertil Steril. 2008;90:889–90.
67. Enciso M, Iglesias M, Galán I, Sarasa J, Gosálbez A, Gosálvez J. The ability of sperm selection techniques to remove single- or double-strand DNA damage. Asian J Androl. 2011;13:764–8.
68. Donnelly ET, McClure N, Lewis SE. Glutathione and hypotaurine in vitro: effects on human sperm motility, DNA integrity and production of reactive oxygen species. Mutagenesis. 2000;15:61–8.
69. Matsuura R, Takeuchi T, Yoshida A. Preparation and incubation conditions affect the DNA integrity of ejaculated human spermatozoa. Asian J Androl. 2010;12:753–9.

70. Gosálvez J, Cortés-Gutiérrez E, Rocio Nuñez R, Fernández JL, Caballero P, López-Fernández C, Holt WV. A dynamic assessment of sperm DNA fragmentation versus sperm viability in proven fertile human donors. Fertil Steril. 2009;92:1915–9.
71. Gosálvez J, Cortés-Gutierrez E, López-Fernádez C, Fernández JL, Caballero P, Nuñez R. Sperm DNA fragmentation dynamics in fertile donors. Fertil Steril. 2009;92:170–3.
72. Gosálvez J, Núñez R, Fernández JL, López-Fernández C, Caballero P. Dynamics of sperm DNA damage in fresh versus frozen-thawed and gradient processed ejaculates in human donors. Andrologia. 2011;43:373–7.
73. Rylander L, Wetterstrand B, Haugen TB, Malm G, Malm J, Bjørsvik C, Henrichsen T, Sæther T, Giwercman A. Single semen analysis as a predictor of semen quality: clinical and epidemiological implications. Asian J Androl. 2009;11:723–30.
74. Imrat P, Mahasawangkul J, Gosálvez J, Suthanmapinanth P, Sombutputorn P, Jansittiwate S, Thongtip N, Pinyopummin A, Colenbrander L, Holt WV, Stout TAE. Effect of cooled storage on quality and DNA integrity of Asian elephant (Elephas maximus) spermatozoa. Reprod Fertil Dev. 2012;24:1105–16.
75. García-Peiró A, Martínez-Heredia J, Oliver-Bonet M, Abad C, Amengual MJ, Navarro J, Jones C, Coward K, Gosálvez J, Benet J. Protamine 1 to protamine 2 ratio correlates with dynamic aspects of DNA fragmentation in human sperm. Fertil Steril. 2011;95:105–9.
76. Gosálvez J, López-Fernández C, Hermoso A, Fernández JL, Kjelland ME. Sperm DNA fragmentation in zebrafish (Danio rerio) and its impact on fertility and embryo viability:implications for fisheries and aquaculture. Aquaculture. 2014;433:173–82.
77. Johnston SD, López-Fernández C, Arroyo F, Gosálbez A, Cortés Gutiérrez EI, Fernández JL, Gosálvez J. Reduced sperm DNA longevity is associated with an increased incidence of still born; evidence from a multi-ovulating sequential artificial insemination animal model. J Assist Reprod Genet. 2016;33:1231–8.
78. Dalzell LH, McVicar CM, McClure N, Lutton D, Lewis SE. Effects of short and long incubations on DNA fragmentation of testicular sperm. Fertil Steril. 2004;82:1443–5.
79. Maxwell WMC, Johnson LA. Physiology of spermatozoa at high dilution rates: the influence of seminal plasma. Theriogenology. 1999;52:1353–62.
80. Peña A, Linde-Forsberg C. Effects of spermatozoal concentration and post-thaw dilution ratio on survival alter thawing of dog spermatozoa. Theriogenology. 2000;54:703–18.
81. Gaviraghi A, Puglisi R, Balduzzi D, Severgnini A, Bornaghi V, Bongioni G, Frana A, Gandini LM, Lukaj A, Bonacina C, Galli A. Minimum number of spermatozoa per dose in Mediterranean Italian buffalo (Bubalus bubalis) using sexed frozen semen and conventional artificial insemination. Theriogenology. 2013;79:1171–6.
82. Prathalingam NS, Holt WV, Revell SG, Jones S, Watson PF. Dilution of spermatozoa results in improved viability following a 24 h storage period but decreased acrosome integrity following cryopreservation. Anim Reprod Sci. 2005;91:11–22.
83. López-Fernández C, Johnston SD, Fernández JL, Wilson RJ, Gosálvez J. Fragmentation dynamics of frozen-thawed ram sperm DNA is modulated by sperm concentration. Theriogenology. 2010;74:1362–70.
84. Johnson LA, Flook JP, Hawk HW. Sex preselection in rabbits: live births from X and Y sperm separated by DNA and cell sorting. Biol Reprod. 1989;41:199–203.
85. Johnson LA. Sex preselection in swine: altered sex ratios in offspring following surgical insemination of flow sorted X- and Y-bearing sperm. Reprod Domest Anim. 1991;26:309–14.
86. Cran DG, Johnson LA, Miller NGA, Cochrane D, Polge CE. Production of bovine calves following separation of X- and Y-chromosome bearing sperm and in vitro fertilization. Vet Rec. 1993;132:40–1.
87. Karabinus DS, Marazzo DP, Stern HJ, Potter DA, Opang CI, Cole ML, Johnson LA, Schulman JD. The effectiveness of flow cytometric sorting of human sperm (MicroSort®) for influencing a child's sex. Reprod Biol Endocrinol. 2014;12:106.
88. Fugger EF, Black SH, Keyvanfar K, Schulman JD. Births of normal daughters after MicroSort sperm separation and intrauterine insemination, in-vitro fertilization, or intracytoplasmic sperm injection. Hum Reprod. 1998;30:2367–70.

Chapter 32
Sperm DNA Testing: Where Do We Go from Here?

Ahmad H. Al-Malki and Armand Zini

32.1 Introduction

The assessment of male fertility potential traditionally depends on the semen analysis, and the most important parameters of this analysis are sperm concentration, motility, and morphology. Unfortunately, the clinical value of these parameters in the diagnosis of male infertility remains limited [1]. While some authors recognize the importance of semen parameters in the assessment of male fertility potential [2, 3], others question the prognostic value of this test [4–6]. Moreover, with the introduction of intracytoplasmic sperm injection (ICSI), the clinical importance of the semen analysis has declined [7].

The genomic integrity of the spermatozoon is essential for the accurate transmission of genetic information and for the proper development and maturation of the embryo [8, 9]. Animal models of sperm chromatin and DNA damage have clearly shown that sperm DNA fragmentation (e.g., experimentally induced damage) is associated with reduced male fertility potential [10–13]. These experimental studies have shown that sperm DNA damage is associated with adverse reproductive outcomes after ARTs, lower pregnancy rates, chromosomal abnormalities, pregnancy loss, reduced longevity, and birth defects [14–17]. These studies have raised concerns regarding the potential adverse outcomes associated with the use of DNA-damaged sperm in the context of human assisted reproduction.

A large number of tests have been developed to measure sperm chromatin and DNA damage in human spermatozoa [18, 19]. These tests were developed with the hope that they might further our understanding of sperm nuclear architecture, accurately measure sperm chromatin and DNA damage, and be valuable tools in clinical

A.H. Al-Malki • A. Zini (✉)
Department of Surgery, Division of Urology, McGill University, Montreal, QC, Canada
e-mail: aalmalki14@hamad.qa; ziniarmand@yahoo.com

A. Zini, A. Agarwal (eds.), *A Clinician's Guide to Sperm DNA and Chromatin Damage*, https://doi.org/10.1007/978-3-319-71815-6_32

practice. To date, the studies show that sperm DNA tests may be good markers of male fertility potential. Prospective studies of couples with unknown fertility status have shown that sperm DNA damage is associated with a lower probability of conception (odds ratio = ~7) and a prolonged time to pregnancy [20–23]. These studies also reveal that sperm DNA test results may be better predictors of pregnancy than conventional sperm parameters in this context [23].

Several systematic reviews of studies correlating sperm DNA test results and reproductive outcomes after ARTs have shown that sperm DNA damage is associated with lower intrauterine insemination (IUI) (odds ratio = ~9) and conventional in vitro fertilization (IVF) pregnancy rates (odds ratio = ~1.6–1.9) [19, 24–27]. In contrast, systematic reviews have shown that the relationship between sperm DNA damage and intracytoplasmic sperm injection (ICSI) pregnancy rates is weak (OR = ~1.3) [19, 24–27]. Several systematic reviews have also shown that sperm DNA damage is associated with an increased risk of pregnancy loss after an established natural, IVF, or ICSI pregnancy [28, 29].

The widespread clinical application of sperm DNA tests in the evaluation of infertile men and in the management of couples enrolled in IUI and IVF treatment cycles has not been firmly established despite a large number of clinical studies (40–50 relevant studies). One of the important reasons for the poor acceptance of sperm DNA tests in the evaluation of infertile men is the marked heterogeneity of the study characteristics. Studies on sperm DNA damage and reproductive outcomes differ in their design (prospective, retrospective, case-control) and in patient (e.g., female factors) and cycle characteristics (e.g., day of embryo transfer). Moreover, it is difficult to compare studies because they use one of several sperm DNA tests (e.g., SCSA (sperm chromatin structure assay), comet assay (also known as single-cell gel electrophoresis), TUNEL (terminal deoxynucleotidyl transferase-mediated dUTP nick-end labeling) assay).

Another reason sperm DNA tests have not been widely utilized in clinical practice is the limited understanding of what the individual assays actually measure [30]. All of the assays require some preparation of the sperm nucleus (variable degree of nuclear decondensation) prior to addition of an enzyme or dye that permits detection of the target sites (e.g., sites of damaged DNA). As such, it remains unclear if a test measures real damage or damage induced by the assay conditions. Ultimately, it is believed that all sperm DNA tests provide an indirect measure of DNA damage (e.g., SCSA, TUNEL) because the assay conditions alter the chromatin state [9, 31, 32]. It is the unique property of the sperm nucleus (i.e., with a tightly packaged chromatin) that limits the accessibility of assay reagents to all areas of the genome and complicates the correct interpretation of assay results [33]. The limited and variable accessibility of reagents to potentially damaged sites in the sperm DNA and chromatin is one reason that the precise nature, location, and clinical significance of sperm DNA damage remain poorly understood.

The lack of consensus on what is considered an acceptable assay and/or assay conditions has been another reason for the limited utilization of these assays in the clinic [30, 34]. Similarly, the lack of standardized protocols for these assays is another worry voiced by many clinicians. This has led to some concern regarding precision, reproducibility, and repeatability of the various assays. Another important weakness of these studies is the fact that multiple cutoffs or thresholds have been used, even for the same assay (e.g., 15% or 30% for DFI using the SCSA). The variability of DNA damage thresholds has led to some confusion and misinterpretation of test results [35]. Moreover, the thresholds for many of these tests have not been adequately validated (not adequately powered or not using appropriate control populations).

The biological variability of sperm DNA tests is also an important point to remember when interpreting sperm DNA test results and using these results in clinical decision-making. It has been shown that tests of sperm DNA damage exhibit a small to moderate degree of biologic variability (coefficient of variation (CV) in the range of 10–30%) such that one may need to repeat the assay to confirm the result [36–40]. Several studies have shown that sperm DNA test results can be influenced by sexual abstinence, with longer abstinence periods being associated with higher levels of sperm DNA damage [41, 42]. Finally, external factors (e.g., fever, infections, medications) can also affect sperm DNA integrity [43–45].

Given the important clinical and biological uncertainties of sperm DNA testing, additional work in this area is much needed. In the future, basic studies should be aimed at improving our understanding of the nature of sperm chromatin and DNA damage and what it is that the various sperm DNA tests truly measure. We should also establish standardized sperm DNA assay protocols that provide reproducible results across different laboratories. Future clinical studies evaluating the relationship between sperm DNA damage and reproductive outcomes should be designed as prospective, controlled trials with well-defined populations. These studies should help establish validated and clinically relevant sperm DNA damage thresholds. Ultimately, such studies will help establish the clinical value of sperm DNA tests as markers of male fertility potential.

32.2 Conclusions

A large number of clinical studies (over 50 relevant studies to date) have shown that sperm DNA damage is associated with reproductive outcomes. However, the widespread clinical application of sperm DNA tests in the evaluation of the infertile man has not been firmly established due to a number of limiting clinical and biological factors. The factors responsible for the limited acceptance of sperm DNA tests in the evaluation of infertile men include the marked heterogeneity of clinical studies, the incomplete understanding of sperm chromatin and DNA damage, the lack of standardized sperm DNA test protocols, and the biological variability of these assays. Future studies should be aimed at improving our understanding of the nature of sperm chromatin and DNA damage and, ultimately, help establish the clinical value of sperm DNA tests in the evaluation of infertile men.

References

1. Guzick DS, et al. Sperm morphology, motility, and concentration in fertile and infertile men. N Engl J Med. 2001;345(19):1388–93.
2. Wichmann L, Isola J, Tuohimaa P. Prognostic variables in predicting pregnancy. A prospective follow up study of 907 couples with an infertility problem. Hum Reprod. 1994;9(6):1102–8.
3. Tomlinson MJ, Kessopoulou E, Barratt CL. The diagnostic and prognostic value of traditional semen parameters. J Androl. 1999;20(5):588–93.
4. Bonde JP, et al. Relation between semen quality and fertility: a population-based study of 430 first-pregnancy planners. Lancet. 1998;352(9135):1172–7.
5. Lefievre L, et al. Counting sperm does not add up any more: time for a new equation? Reproduction. 2007;133(4):675–84.
6. Chen X, et al. Predictive value of semen parameters in in vitro fertilisation pregnancy outcome. Andrologia. 2009;41(2):111–7.
7. Lewis SE. Is sperm evaluation useful in predicting human fertility? Reproduction. 2007;134(1):31–40.
8. Gatewood JM, et al. Isolation of four core histones from human sperm chromatin representing a minor subset of somatic histones. J Biol Chem. 1990;265(33):20662–6.
9. Gawecka JE, et al. A model for the control of DNA integrity by the sperm nuclear matrix. Asian J Androl. 2015;17(4):610–5.
10. Evenson DP, Darzynkiewicz Z, Melamed MR. Comparison of human and mouse sperm chromatin structure by flow cytometry. Chromosoma. 1980;78(2):225–38.
11. Doerksen T, Trasler JM. Developmental exposure of male germ cells to 5-azacytidine results in abnormal preimplantation development in rats. Biol Reprod. 1996;55(5):1155–62.
12. Cho C, et al. Haploinsufficiency of protamine-1 or -2 causes infertility in mice. Nat Genet. 2001;28(1):82–6.
13. Delbes G, Hales BF, Robaire B. Effects of the chemotherapy cocktail used to treat testicular cancer on sperm chromatin integrity. J Androl. 2007;28(2):241–9. discussion 250–1
14. Ahmadi A, Ng SC. Fertilizing ability of DNA-damaged spermatozoa. J Exp Zool. 1999;284(6):696–704.
15. Fernandez-Gonzalez R, et al. Long-term effects of mouse intracytoplasmic sperm injection with DNA-fragmented sperm on health and behavior of adult offspring. Biol Reprod. 2008;78(4):761–72.
16. Perez-Crespo M, et al. Factors from damaged sperm affect its DNA integrity and its ability to promote embryo implantation in mice. J Androl. 2008;29(1):47–54.
17. Perez-Crespo M, Pintado B, Gutierrez-Adan A. Scrotal heat stress effects on sperm viability, sperm DNA integrity, and the offspring sex ratio in mice. Mol Reprod Dev. 2008;75(1):40–7.
18. Delbes G, Hales BF, Robaire B. Toxicants and human sperm chromatin integrity. Mol Hum Reprod. 2010;16(1):14–22.
19. Zini A. Are sperm chromatin and DNA defects relevant in the clinic? Syst Biol Reprod Med. 2011;57(1–2):78–85.
20. Evenson DP, et al. Utility of the sperm chromatin structure assay as a diagnostic and prognostic tool in the human fertility clinic. Hum Reprod. 1999;14(4):1039–49.
21. Spano M, et al. Sperm chromatin damage impairs human fertility. The Danish First Pregnancy Planner Study Team. Fertil Steril. 2000;73(1):43–50.
22. Loft S, et al. Oxidative DNA damage in human sperm influences time to pregnancy. Hum Reprod. 2003;18(6):1265–72.
23. Giwercman A, et al. Sperm chromatin structure assay as an independent predictor of fertility in vivo: a case-control study. Int J Androl. 2010;33(1):e221–7.
24. Bungum M, et al. Sperm DNA integrity assessment in prediction of assisted reproduction technology outcome. Hum Reprod. 2007;22(1):174–9.
25. Collins JA, Barnhart KT, Schlegel PN. Do sperm DNA integrity tests predict pregnancy with in vitro fertilization? Fertil Steril. 2008;89(4):823–31.

26. Practice Committee of the American Society for Reproductive, M. The clinical utility of sperm DNA integrity testing: a guideline. Fertil Steril. 2013;99(3):673–7.
27. Simon L, et al. A systematic review and meta-analysis to determine the effect of sperm DNA damage on in vitro fertilization and intracytoplasmic sperm injection outcome. Asian J Androl. 2016;19:80.
28. Zini A, et al. Sperm DNA damage is associated with an increased risk of pregnancy loss after IVF and ICSI: systematic review and meta-analysis. Hum Reprod. 2008;23(12):2663–8.
29. Robinson L, et al. The effect of sperm DNA fragmentation on miscarriage rates: a systematic review and meta-analysis. Hum Reprod. 2012;27(10):2908–17.
30. Barratt CL, et al. Sperm DNA: organization, protection and vulnerability: from basic science to clinical applications—a position report. Hum Reprod. 2010;25(4):824–38.
31. Henkel R, et al. TUNEL assay and SCSA determine different aspects of sperm DNA damage. Andrologia. 2010;42(5):305–13.
32. Evenson DP. The Sperm Chromatin Structure Assay (SCSA((R))) and other sperm DNA fragmentation tests for evaluation of sperm nuclear DNA integrity as related to fertility. Anim Reprod Sci. 2016;169:56–75.
33. Brown R, Harper J. The clinical benefit and safety of current and future assisted reproductive technology. Reprod BioMed Online. 2012;25(2):108–17.
34. Zini A, Albert O, Robaire B. Assessing sperm chromatin and DNA damage: clinical importance and development of standards. Andrology. 2014;2(3):322–5.
35. Simon L, et al. Comparative analysis of three sperm DNA damage assays and sperm nuclear protein content in couples undergoing assisted reproduction treatment. Hum Reprod. 2014;29(5):904–17.
36. Evenson DP, et al. Individuality of DNA denaturation patterns in human sperm as measured by the sperm chromatin structure assay. Reprod Toxicol. 1991;5(2):115–25.
37. Erenpreiss J, et al. Intra-individual variation in sperm chromatin structure assay parameters in men from infertile couples: clinical implications. Hum Reprod. 2006;21(8):2061–4.
38. Keel BA. Within- and between-subject variation in semen parameters in infertile men and normal semen donors. Fertil Steril. 2006;85(1):128–34.
39. Smit M, et al. Clinical correlates of the biological variation of sperm DNA fragmentation in infertile men attending an andrology outpatient clinic. Int J Androl. 2007;30(1):48–55.
40. Oleszczuk K, Giwercman A, Bungum M. Intra-individual variation of the sperm chromatin structure assay DNA fragmentation index in men from infertile couples. Hum Reprod. 2011;26(12):3244–8.
41. Gosalvez J, et al. Shorter abstinence decreases sperm deoxyribonucleic acid fragmentation in ejaculate. Fertil Steril. 2011;96(5):1083–6.
42. Pons I, et al. One abstinence day decreases sperm DNA fragmentation in 90 % of selected patients. J Assist Reprod Genet. 2013;30(9):1211–8.
43. Evenson DP, et al. Characteristics of human sperm chromatin structure following an episode of influenza and high fever: a case study. J Androl. 2000;21(5):739–46.
44. Moskovtsev SI, et al. Frequency and severity of sperm DNA damage in patients with confirmed cases of male infertility of different aetiologies. Reprod BioMed Online. 2010;20(6):759–63.
45. Tanrikut C, et al. Adverse effect of paroxetine on sperm. Fertil Steril. 2010;94(3):1021–6.

Epilogue

The study of sperm DNA and chromatin abnormalities has gained significant importance in the past several years, largely due to the major advances in assisted reproductive technologies (ARTs). Studies in this field have demonstrated that the genetic integrity of the sperm is a key aspect of the paternal contribution to the offspring, particularly, in the context of ARTs. We are now starting to better understand the unique organization of the sperm chromatin, as well as, the nature and etiology of sperm DNA damage.

In Chap. 1 of the textbook, Dr. Rod Balhorn, a pioneer in the field of sperm chromatin structure, describes the dramatic transformation of the physical and functional state of the chromatin during spermiogenesis. A more detailed description of the nuclear proteins and chromatin structure is presented by Dr. Steven Ward and Dr. Raphael Oliva's group in Chaps. 2 and 3, respectively. These chapters provide us with a better understanding of the unique organization of the sperm chromatin but also show that there are still many unanswered questions about its structure.

The laboratory evaluation of sperm DNA tests is discussed by experts in the field in Chaps. 4, 5, 6, 7, 8, and 9. The authors present us with a detailed description of the SCSA (Dr. Evenson), TUNEL assay (Drs. Muratori and Baldi), benchtop flow cytometer TUNEL assay (Dr. Agarwal et al.), comet assay (Dr. Cortes-Gutierrez et al.), sperm chromatin dispersion assay (Jaime Gosalvez et al.), and cytochemical tests (Dr. Juris Erenpreiss et al.). A broader review of these tests is presented in Chap. 10 (Dr. Tanrikut et al.), and it is concluded that no one test is deemed the optimal assay in the assessment of male infertility.

The etiology of sperm DNA damage is thought to be multifactorial, with the understanding that both primary testicular and secondary (external and post-testicular) factors are involved in its pathogenesis. The putative primary factors responsible for sperm chromatin and DNA damage (oxidative stress (Dr. Henkel et al.), abortive apoptosis (Dr. Sakkas et al.), defective DNA repair (Dr. Boissonneault et al.), and defective spermatogenesis (Drs. Sharma and Agarwal)) are presented in Chaps. 11, 12, 13, and 14. A number of the better known external factors involved in the pathogenesis of sperm DNA damage are discussed in Chaps. 15, 16, and 17

A. Zini, A. Agarwal (eds.), *A Clinician's Guide to Sperm DNA and Chromatin Damage*, https://doi.org/10.1007/978-3-319-71815-6

(lifestyle factors (Dr. Harlev et al.), cancer (Drs. Chan and Robaire), and environmental factors (Drs. Giwercman and Spano)). The role of the oocyte in the repair of sperm DNA damage is presented in Chap. 18 (Drs. Gunes and Sertyel).

The impact of sperm DNA damage on reproductive outcomes and the clinical utility of sperm DNA tests are topics of ongoing debate. In Chap. 19, Dr. Gutierrez-Adan et al. demonstrate from the results of their experimental (animal) studies that sperm DNA damage clearly has a negative impact on reproductive outcomes. In Chaps. 20, 21, and 22, the influence of sperm DNA and chromatin damage on human reproduction are presented (natural pregnancy (Drs. Spanò and Giwercman), ART pregnancy (Drs. Bungum and Oleszczuk), pregnancy loss (Dr. Samanta et al.)). In Chaps. 23 and 24, the pros (Dr. Zini et al.) and cons (Dr. Sigman et al.) of sperm DNA tests in the assessment of male infertility are discussed. These chapters illustrate the strengths and weaknesses of the available studies on sperm DNA damage and human reproduction. The factors responsible for the limited acceptance of sperm DNA tests in the evaluation of infertile men include the marked heterogeneity of clinical studies, the incomplete understanding of sperm chromatin and DNA damage, the lack of standardized sperm DNA test protocols, and the biological variability of these assays.

There are several treatment options for men with sperm DNA damage. Non-specific treatments are discussed in Chaps. 25 (antioxidant therapy, Dr. Agarwal et al.), 27 (physiological ICSI, Dr. Tavaalee et al.), 28 (advanced sperm processing techniques, Dr. Agarwal et al.), and 31 (strategies to diminish DNA damage, Dr. Esteves et al.). In Chap. 26, Dr. Esteves et al. discuss the influence of varicocele on sperm DNA damage and the beneficial effect of varicocelectomy on sperm DNA damage. The potential value of using testicular rather than ejaculated sperm for ICSI in men with sperm DNA damage is debated in Chaps. 29 (pro, Dr. Esteves et al.) and 30 (con, Dr. Chan).

We have made great advances in our understanding of the organization of the sperm chromatin, the etiology of sperm DNA damage, and the potential influence of sperm DNA damage on reproduction. However, several important clinical and biological uncertainties remain. Future studies should be aimed at improving our knowledge of what the various sperm DNA tests measure. Sperm DNA assay protocols should be standardized such that they can provide reproducible results across different laboratories. Future clinical studies evaluating the relationship between sperm DNA damage and reproductive outcomes should be designed as prospective, controlled trials with well-defined populations. These studies will help establish validated and clinically relevant sperm DNA damage thresholds. These steps will surely help address the often heard criticism of the lack of sufficient high-grade evidence in support of the routine use of sperm DNA damage testing in specific clinical scenarios. Ultimately, we hope to establish the clinical value of sperm DNA tests as markers of male fertility potential and develop sound treatment options for infertile men.

Armand Zini
Montreal, QC, Canada

Ashok Agarwal
Cleveland, OH, USA

Index

A. Zini, A. Agarwal (eds.), *A Clinician's Guide to Sperm DNA and Chromatin Damage*, https://doi.org/10.1007/978-3-319-71815-6

The manufacturer's authorised representative in the EU is Springer Nature Customer Service Centre GmbH, Europaplatz 3, 69115 Heidelberg, Germany. If you have any concerns regarding our products, please contact ProductSafety@springernature.com

Printed and bound by CPI Group (UK) Ltd, Croydon, CR0 4YY

30/09/2026

02225232-0013

The manufacturer's authorised representative in the EU is Springer Nature Customer Service Centre GmbH, Europaplatz 3, 69115 Heidelberg, Germany. If you have any concerns regarding our products, please contact ProductSafety@springernature.com

Printed and bound by CPI Group (UK) Ltd, Croydon, CR0 4YY
30/09/2026
02225232-0013